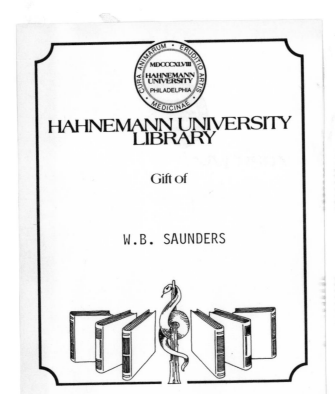

BREAST IMAGING:
Diagnosis and Morphology of Breast Diseases

ROBERT L. EGAN, M.D.

Professor of Radiology
Emory University School of Medicine
Atlanta, Georgia

1988
W.B. SAUNDERS COMPANY
Harcourt Brace Jovanovich, Inc.
Philadelphia • London • Toronto • Montreal • Sydney • Tokyo

W. B. SAUNDERS COMPANY
Harcourt Brace Jovanovich, Inc.

West Washington Square
Philadelphia, PA 19105

Library of Congress Cataloging-in-Publication Data

Egan, Robert L., 1920–

Breast imaging.

Includes index.
1. Breast—Imaging.   2. Breast—Diseases—Diagnosis.
I. Title.   [DNLM: 1. Breast—radiography.   2. Breast
Diseases—pathology.   3. Breast Neoplasms—radiography.
WP 815 E28b]

RG493.5.D52E33   1988   618.1'90757   87–27508

ISBN 0–7216–2320–4

Editor: W. B. Saunders Staff
Developmental Editor: Kathleen McCullough
Designer: Karen Giacomucci
Production Manager: Peter Faber
Manuscript Editor: Constance Burton
Illustration Coordinator: Peg Shaw
Indexer: Angela Holt

BREAST IMAGING: Diagnosis and Morphology of Breast Diseases   ISBN   0–7216–2320–4

Last digit is the print number: 9   8   7   6   5   4   3   2   1

Dedicated to

M.A.E.
K.L.E.
D.A.E.
C.L.L.
M.J.F.
P.L.H.

Foreword

In addition to numerous articles and book chapters on imaging of the breast, Bob Egan has already published 13 monographs on this subject. It is indeed an honor and a privilege for me to write the foreword to this, his latest and most comprehensive work, *Breast Imaging: Diagnosis and Morphology of Breast Diseases*.

We have been friends from almost the beginning of his career at M. D. Anderson Hospital in 1956 and have been associates at Emory University since 1963. Leborgne, Gershon-Cohen, and Egan were the pioneers of mammography; however, it was Egan who developed a technique that resulted in sufficient accuracy and reproducibility to stimulate general interest in breast imaging. In 1960 his publication "Experience with Mammography in a Tumor Institution," in the *Journal of Radiology*, was followed by a wave of enthusiasm among his colleagues that resulted in support by the Cancer Control Program of the U.S. Public Health Service for training radiologists and technologists in mammography.

Along with this, Egan developed extensive teaching materials and organized annual seminars that further promoted interest in radiographic diagnosis of breast disease among not only radiologists but also other physicians, especially pathologists and surgeons. The emphasis on the earlier diagnosis of breast cancer was a major factor in modification of the existing radical surgical management of breast cancer and development of reconstructive surgical techniques for improved cosmetic results.

He established the first breast imaging center at Emory University, where he constantly investigated the application of other imaging techniques such as magnification radiography, film-screen mammography, thermography, diaphanoscopy, uptake of various radioactive isotopes, CT, US, and, more recently, MR imaging. Egan established methods for accurate determination of radiation dosimetry to the breast and an ongoing project in gathering demographic and historical data for establishing risk factors in breast cancer. His lifetime goal has been to promote the earlier detection and improved treatment of breast cancer, and it is no exaggeration to state that he has been instrumental in the development of the modern programs dedicated to this purpose. This textbook is a testament to his undertaking.

JAMES V. ROGERS, M.D.

Preface

Embarkation upon this volume coincided with a sharply changed attitude, after more than 25 years, of widespread acceptance of mammography as the unchallenged method of detecting early, assuredly curable breast cancer. This quarter of a century is a remarkably short period in medical history. The incurable breast cancer of the nineteenth century slowly evolved by the early twentieth century into one that possibly could be controlled by radical mastectomy. But this hope was offset by a philosophy of nihilism that no medical procedure altered the predetermined course of breast cancer. Next, the concept "the smaller the lesion, the larger the treatment" led to the phase of supraradical surgery. In the premammography days, during the latter part of the first half of the twentieth century, there was no perceptible improvement in the cure of women with breast cancer. Yet in the second half of this century, dramatic 95 per cent ten-year cure rates of mammographically discovered breast cancers were recorded.

Present philosophies must encompass each of these aspects: that some breast cancers are incurable upon discovery; that limited improvement will occur in some clinically Stage I lesions that are biologically Stage II or Stage III lesions; and that some very small (labeled minimal) aggressive carcinomas require vigorous treatment. These considerations must be tempered with biologic tumor (cell) type, multicentricity, bilaterality, and host resistance. Fortunately, looming from such seemingly chaotic concepts is the most important and least controversial statistic: The size and histologic stage of breast cancer is inversely related to the length of survival.

Mammography has been hailed as the first significant contribution to the control of breast cancer since Halsted described his radical mastectomy in 1903. Prior to 1950, 16 senior authors contributed 29 articles on x-ray of the breast. From 1950 to 1955 four authors produced nine articles; from 1956 to 1959 nine authors wrote 21 articles; and from 1960 to 1967 82 authors produced five books and 147 articles. Between 1968 and the present, the literature on mammography grew explosively. From this voluminous outpouring many altered concepts of mammography and breast disease could be expected. It is indeed a tribute to the stability of mammography that no such concepts have altered its course since its development and introduction clinically in 1956 (outlined in our first volume in 1964).

The use of mammography in early detection evoked a resurgence of interest in cancer of the breast and a tremendous outpouring of basic and clinical investigation. Traditional modes of thinking were questioned and traditional attitudes re-examined. Thus, in an era of transition, the profession was being asked to espouse new concepts, develop new procedures, and fulfill unfamiliar and uncomfortable roles regarding breast cancer. The use of mammography stimulated evaluation of other methods of imaging the breast and engendered the team, or multidisciplinary, approach to detect, diagnose, and institute treatment of breast cancer. Primarily this team includes the surgeon, radiologist, and pathologist but also involves primary care physicians and gynecologists as well as all physicians treating women.

In 1956 the surgeon came to depend strongly upon the radiologist to guide his biopsy scalpel. In a specimen that was normal to inspection and palpation, the pathologist, in turn, depended on the radiologist to localize the pathology for this study. This markedly unusual information on mammography challenged the radiologist to more meaningful diagnoses, to improvement in treatment planning, and to overall understanding of breast diseases. Thus, the triumvirate was born. This necessitated communication—a phenomenal development, as the radiologist had been concerned only with what was simple interpretation of vague shadows, the surgeon had been complacent with what he could feel in the breast, and the reclusive pathologist had maintained the position of the oracle.

The intrusion of the radiologist bedfellow led to pivotal new concepts of breast cancer: Breast cancer is not a local phenomenon but a diffuse disease of the mammary epithelium; noninvasive and microinvasive stages of breast cancer exist and can be detected; mammographic breast cancer cure rates exceed 95 per cent; contralateral primary breast cancer is frequent and assumes clinical importance; the team approach to breast cancer is mandatory; specimen radiography must be available to every x-ray or pathology laboratory; and frozen-section histopathologic studies need reassessment for their specific roles in breast cancer.

As Emory University had been established as the unsurpassed training center and site of continued investigation and development of the means to combat breast cancer, our experience should be exemplary of the team approach to breast diseases. When possible, this volume will be limited to those aspects. It is not a complete treatise on the clinical approach to breast problems, not an encompassing guide to the technical aspects and interpretation of mammograms, and not a detailed compendium on the pathology of breast diseases. Rather, it stresses combined useful methods to diagnose, treat, and define prognosis of breast diseases. The practice of reporting our own experience will be paramount. A comprehensive review of the voluminous literature on breast diseases would be a monumental undertaking and would defeat our purpose.

Objections to widespread use of mammography have been cost, radiation, and lack of appeal to the general physician for clinical application in asymptomatic women. Yet today the decision to biopsy the breast is being preceded by mammography, just as a chest radiograph precedes thoracotomy. The possibility is very real that mortality from breast cancer may be reduced to the degree that such a death may become one requiring assignment of responsibility or as much an anachronism as a death from puerperal sepsis.

Personal training of over 1500 radiologists and as many of their technologists for five days or more occurred over 30 years, the larger number being trained during the earlier period. This suggests a decreasing number of strongly indoctrinated radiologists during the later years. Yet radiologists trained earlier who have seen their wives' lives saved through mammographic detection of their breast cancers provide a motivation to preserve meticulous mammography.

An increasing number of radiologists need instruction in breast diseases to prepare for the next phase of mammography—the selection of women at risk for breast cancer to be followed with uncompromised mammography. Awareness and understanding of the basic unchanging clinical, radiographic, and pathologic characteristics of breast cancer then becomes more acute. The clinician must continue to labor without the guidance of signs of early breast cancer, and the pathologist must constantly sharpen his diagnostic acumen and depend more and more on the cooperation of the radiologist. In this challenge the radiologist must become more comfortable with the long-established mammography technique and well-documented x-ray changes of the breast for consistent and dependable performance.

The restless search for improvements in mammography, or a replacement procedure, led to special receptors such as Xerox and screen-film combinations, to procedures such as thermography and ultrasound, and to hopes directed toward magnetic resonance and spectroscopy. Still, highly reproducible conventional mammography has not been challenged. Breast sonography added a complementary approach in selected women. Grids helped to restore radiographic quality lost with screen-film receptors. State-of-the-art mammography tested over a quarter of a century, which required no modification except radiation reduction through screen-film receptors, now must be championed pending substitution or complement.

Complete understanding of breast morphology and mastery of the diagnosis of breast diseases are progressive steps toward expanding the use of mammography in eradication of breast cancer. Herein lies our purpose, buttressed by contributions drawing upon unparalleled experience extending from 1956. Continued evaluation of mammography and its relationship to all aspects of breast disease dates from its inception at the Oncologic Institute of the University of Texas M.D. Anderson Hospital and Tumor Institute. There the team approach was born and nurtured so that the clinician, surgeon, radiologist, and pathologist could pursue the emerging "mammographic" early breast cancers and their precursors. Necessity was truly the mother of invention to provide ways to combat this most curable form of breast cancer. Here were sown the seeds for breast cancer screening and less mutilating surgery.

Also, endless requests for training provided the impetus for producing original and frequently updated training material and training sessions. Continued assimilation of similar materials has proved tedious; one-on-one instruction is too time-consuming and monetarily unrewarding for the development of other continuation programs. It is hoped that this volume will span some of the gaps in training materials.

Insistence upon segregation of mammography patients from the general radiographic areas used for barium enemas and for studying desperately ill patients led to the establishment of the first special breast-imaging center in 1962. In this center, prototypes of all breast imaging devices or individual components were evaluated. For five years, three full-time physicists assessed the empirical mammography technique and its modifications. Another unique concept was the mammography pathology laboratory, consisting of one full-time pathologist and two pathology technologists, devoted completely to the study of breast diseases over a period of five years. Housed within the center were two full-time biostatisticians, the necessary computer programmers, research assistants, and personnel to gather, collate, and analyze data on our mammography patients from 1963. Sufficient radiologists and radiologic technologists were available to cooperate in carrying out epidemiologically controlled clinical trials. Breast-imaging centers have now become the trend and may include many imaging procedures, although not necessarily all those listed.

A brief historical perspective will be presented as a mandatory aspect of the understanding of breast diseases. A description of the normal breast with its normal variations, embryology, and physiology also will be presented. Insight into the clinical examination, imaging, and histopathologic study of breast diseases will be necessary to understand our approach. Presentation of the basic mammography technique leads to greater appreciation of its many variations and inherent problems. Xeroradiography is included even though it is being phased out owing to increased radiation, lessened radiographic quality, and the fact that more radiologists are becoming familiar with film receptors. Most other imaging methods are not greatly contributory; only sonography is stressed, as it may be valuable in selected instances. The fate of magnetic resonance imaging must await its further development.

The importance of histopathologic studies is constantly emphasized as part of the team effort to study breast diseases. C. Whitaker Sewell, M.D., Associate Professor of Pathology at the Emory University School of Medicine, and keenly interested in breast diseases, has 15 years' association with the breast-imaging center. Pathologic studies, observations on the radiologic experience with breast diseases, and histopathologic illustrations are among his invaluable contributions to this volume. He has kindly filled the role of contributing author to this radiologist's documented experience.

Localization and biopsy with radiography of the specimen is stressed as a major role of the radiologist in the team approach. Our whole-organ breast studies, probably never to be repeated, have contributed enormously to our understanding of breast disease. A working classification of both benign and malignant breast diseases acceptable to all specialties aids in more precise communication about breast problems and diseases. The lesions will be more clearly understood when amply demonstrated by radiographic subgross studies. Presentation of noninvasive and invasive duct carcinoma will be followed by descriptions of the very special types of breast carcinomas, such as intracystic papillary carcinoma, mucinous carcinoma, and medullary carcinoma with lymphoid stroma. Our experience with the syndromes of Paget's disease, inflammatory carcinoma, multicentric carcinoma, carcinoma in younger women, intramammary lymph nodes, and bilateral carcinoma will be outlined as well. Benign and malignant radiographic changes of breast diseases are amply illustrated. Important radiologic changes, such as breast masses and skin changes, are assigned separate chapters. Subareolar carcinomas and carcinomas in the peripheral portions of the breast present special problems in diagnosis and deserve emphasis. The high degree of correlation of ductal epithelial hyperplastic radiographic and pathologic changes with carcinoma warrants special attention. Certain histologic types of carcinoma are presented separately so that our experience can be more clearly outlined. Intracystic papillary carcinoma is a lesion in the realm of the radiologist and, even though infrequent, merits emphasis.

The intriguing radiographic finding of breast calcifications, especially clustered calcifications not associated with a mass, deserves special consideration. Perhaps the most important subset of carcinoma, that in women under age 35 years or the "forgotten women," is associated with the radiologist's most difficult problems. Our experience with cancer developing under observation (after previous no-cancer clinical and x-ray examinations) is a sobering one yet provides otherwise unavailable insight into the natural history of breast cancer and a realization of our inadequacies. It supports the argument for annual mammograms. Approximately 300 of 2000 primary breast cancers developed under observation in a period of slightly over 20 years.

Postsurgical and radiotherapeutic changes present varied differential diagnoses. Indications for mammography are enumerated and, just as important, the difficulties with mammography are emphasized. Emory University breast data, including clinical, epidemiologic, radiographic, and pathologic information on women in a high socioeconomic group that yielded good follow-up for as long as 22 years, provide the backdrop for this volume. A high-risk marker has been elusive. Several approaches to establish risk are presented: a robust improved linear discriminant analysis, radiographic markers, and an entirely new approach using in vivo optical spectroscopy. With the trend toward imaging centers and screening for breast cancer reawakened, both existing and anticipated problems are reviewed.

To reduce cost and minimize space, redundant illustrations and repetitious cases (so often the landmark of an atlas) are avoided. Examples include comparative normal opposite breasts or a normal previous mammogram. Illustrating the lesion per se is often more informative than showing the whole breast x-ray. However, if present, a distant change, such as increased vascularity, is described. Some illustrations have been selected for interest rather than for quality, e.g., an unusual lesion or a change not apparent on better mammograms, or to demonstrate inherent technical problems due either to the type of breast or to the disease process. Non-screen film, with infinitely more radiographic detail, may result in illustrations esthetically inferior to those from the less detailed screen-film studies. Attempts to convey the problems in mammography are mandatory, nonetheless.

The original interpretation of the mammograms by the author, without benefit of clinical findings in each illustrative case, is presented. Such a policy allows the reader a better insight into the everyday problems encountered in mammography. This does not suggest that a radiologist in a less investigative setting should not use all clinical information available in rendering his consultative report. The final pathologic diagnosis is utilized whether with biopsy tissue, mastectomy specimen, or post-mortem examination.

In 1963–1964 it become apparent that there was a choice of staying in general radiology or committing myself entirely to mammography and breast diseases. For the latter, a center was needed to teach, evaluate, and investigate breast imaging and to demonstrate the team approach to breast disease. The Advisory Group of the Cancer Control Program of the USPH, Lewis C. Robbins, M.D., Chief, recommended funding such an endeavor and set about, through committee, to canvass the United States for a parent organization. Among the reasons I finally chose Emory University are the following: (1) Emory University School of Medicine was a well-established and highly respected medical institution; (2) it was located in a high socioeconomic residential community where preventive medicine was important, with patient cooperation being paramount; (3) an active oncologic clinic (Winship) had been in existence for nearly 30 years; (4) the institution had participated in the Reproducibility Study and had an ongoing program in mammography and breast diseases headed by James V. Rogers, M.D., radiologist, and R. Waldo Powell, M.D., surgeon; and (5) the team approach to breast diseases was highly espoused by Elliott Scarborough, M.D., oncologic surgeon and Director of the Emory University Clinic; by John Ellis, M.D., Professor and Chairman of the Department of Pathology; and by Heinz S. Weens, M.D., Professor and Chairman of the Department of Radiology. Appreciation is extended to these individuals for their great help in establishing the Section of Mammography at Emory University and the coooperation that later led to its development into the present Breast Imaging Center. The continued support of the members of the Winship Clinic, the Emory University Clinic, and the many referring physicians so helpful in cooperation of evaluation, treatment, and follow-up in our own pioneering investigation of high-risk women, thermography, xeroradiography, sonography, breast cancer screening, and its various aspects is acknowledged and greatly appreciated.

Particular acknowledgement is extended to the physicists (William Chambers, Jimmy Fenn, and Johnny Vinson), who worked diligently in the initial investigation of the field of 20 to 40 kvp and in the many imaging modalities applied to breast diseases. Thanks are owed to the following individuals. To the many radiologic technologists, especially Patricia A. Barnett, R.T., Chief Mammography Technologist for the longest time, imbued with the complete dedication so necessary in treating frightened breast cancer patients, in teaching radiologists and other technologists, and in participating in the many investigative programs of the breast center. To Sooneung Kim, M.D., Associate Professor of Pathology, who for five years laboriously carried out our whole-organ correlated breast studies with able assistance from Suzi Schwartz, Pathology Technologist and Research Assistant. To Robert Mosteller, Ph.D., and Charles Stevens, Ph.D., biostatisticians who devised and brought to fruition the regional discriminant analytic procedure to select women at high risk of breast cancer. The Emory University Computer Center; the

SEER Program, Georgia State Health Department; and the Epidemiology Section of Emory University, Raymond S. Greenberg, M.D., Director, provided indispensable aid in planning, developing, and evaluating the many protocols of the Breast Imaging Center to investigate breast diseases. Particular appreciation is extended to Kathleen L. Egan and Cheryl L. Lane, Research Assistants, for tireless accumulation, collation, and preparation of data for presentation in this volume.

Contents

Historical Perspective

In 1913 Salomon, a German surgeon, after studying approximately 3000 amputated breasts, reported the clinical, radiographic, and pathologic correlation of breast tumors, particularly the invasive characteristics and patterns of spread of cancers. He demonstrated calcification in cancer of the breast, although he did not describe it. He also recognized the potential value of radiography for demonstration of occult cancers of the breast. Many of the radiographic features of breast tumors were outlined by him and subsequently have been independently verified. Lacking the opportunity to review his original radiographs of the breast specimens, one can only conjecture, following inspection of reproductions of these radiographs and noting his concise description of breast lesions, that he had developed a radiographic technique of considerable detail. Perhaps, had his work not been interrupted by World War I, he would have progressed to early clinical application of this technique on a firm basis.

Kleinschmidt contributed an undated radiograph of an intact breast to the book on cancer by Zweifel-Payr (1927).

Stafford L. Warren was trying to standardize the technique in his new x-ray department at Rochester Memorial Hospital in Rochester, New York, for measurement and evaluation of the thoracic aorta. While fluoroscoping the breasts at various angles he found that placing the arm over the head allowed an oblique anteroposterior exposure that showed the breast and axillary fossa. As early as 1926 Warren made radiographs of the breasts in various positions. After considerable trial, stereoscopic films of each breast were decided upon. A steady position for the two stereoscopic views was obtained by placing the patient in the recumbent semioblique position on a wooden table, with sandbags under the opposite shoulder and with the patient retracting the opposite breast from the x-ray beam. Both breasts were studied.

The quite new and modern equipment in use in Warren's department in 1926 was utilized for radiography of the breast. The "new" fine-grain acetate-base Kodak film and Patterson "fine-grain" screens were used. One of the early flat-top Bucky diaphragms, with finer lead strip spacings than the current curved-top ones of the time, was used. The radiographic tube was a rather "fine" focal spot, hooded target, General Electric Coolidge tube in an open lead glass bowl; it was connected by bare copper wire to the overhead, ceiling-mounted, copper-tube, high-voltage distribution system. The transformer was mounted in a cabinet above the control cabinet, with a small Picker type mechanical rectifier and synchronous motor with semispherical collector shoes. This amount of protection for the operator and patient was just beginning to be used in the newer installations of the day; during radiography of the breast the lower body was protected by a lead-rubber apron. Vigilance was necessary to keep the elbow of the arm retracting the opposite breast from the tube terminal to avoid sparkover.

Warren's original report (1930) on the clinical application of x-ray of the breast stirred considerable interest in the procedure; numerous articles by radiologists and surgeons appeared in the early 1930s, both in the United States and in Europe. Despite the nonexistence of the procedure prior to Warren, it is safe to venture the opinion that radiography of the breast was carried out only a few days or months following Roentgen's first public announcement of his "x-ray" on January 23, 1896. Willy E. Baensch recalls radiography of the breast while he was Professor of Radiology of Leipzig in the late 1920s. Even at the time of Warren's report in 1929, Hickey remarked during discussion of the paper that a number of radiologists had done radiography of the breast in a desultory way. He referred to his own less rewarding experience while at Woman's Hospital in Detroit, with a renewed interest following his visit with Warren in Rochester in 1927.

Warren had presented a simple and detailed technique, but he had presented results indicating a high degree of accuracy in radiographic diagnosis of breast cancer. However, he also indicated the necessity for radiographs of the best possible quality, including stereoscopic views. He emphasized the definite limitations of the procedure and he clearly reported that many of his radiographs were of advanced cancers, many without histologic confirmation. Subsequent workers apparently failed to appreciate the basic principles of technically good radiography of the breast and concentrated on various gadgetry, positions, and injection techniques. Despite the deterioration with time of the new film emulsion used by Warren, his original radiographs of the breast remain better than some currently submitted for consultation, especially those with screen-film receptors.

In the 1920s, independent groups began investigating clinical radiography of the breast: in addition to Warren, there were Goynes, Gentil and Guedes, Dominguez, and members of the Leipzig Clinic. Dominguez recognized calcification in cancers; Seabold studied cyclic changes of the breast during the menstrual cycle; Vogel discussed the radiographic differentiation between chronic cystic mastitis and carcinoma; Ries learned that the practice of injection of foreign and irritating radiopaque material into the milk ducts was unsafe; and Espaillat attempted radiographic, clinical, and histopathologic correlation of breast diseases.

Despite a number of reports on radiography of the breast in the early 1930s, interest in the procedure quickly subsided. Communication with a number of these earlier workers revealed that although each thought that there was potential value in the procedure, there was disappointment with their erratic results, which were usually due to the inferior quality of their radiographs. Since that era, only an occasional proponent of this method of examination persisted. Despite almost complete lack of recognition by colleagues in his own city, Gershon-Cohen persisted in the use of radiographic examination of the breast, continued as a dedicated student of breast diseases, and wrote untiringly on the subject in an effort to convince those colleagues.

Leborgne recognized the need for techni-

cally improved radiography; he had been able to recognize calcification in 30 per cent of cancers. During that period Gros, Sigrist, and von Ronnen sustained interest in the procedure in Europe. There was almost complete lack of emphasis on teaching materials and aids, on correlation of results, and on the technical aspects of breast radiography. Gershon-Cohen made an attempt to communicate with Leborgne and correlate their efforts by sending his colleague Ingelby to Montevideo. However, upon her return to Philadelphia Ingelby reported that Leborgne and his wife were kind people but that she had failed to ask about or to learn anything about his breast radiography (1967).

In 1954 Rigler et al., as part of the Minnesota Cancer Detection Center, carried out radiographic studies of the breasts of 1500 apparently normal women. Some 25 benign tumors and one cancer were discovered. This represented a futile effort at mass screening with radiography of asymptomatic patients for cancer of the breast. Rigler described the radiographic technique as quite crude (1961).

Pendergrass (1963) in the early 1940s combined radiography of the breast with physical examination, transillumination with special water-cooled units constructed by the General Electric Company, and photography without significant contribution to the diagnosis of breast tumors. Centers in Europe continued radiography of the breast without success; the investigators stressed the difficulties of the procedure, which required meticulous attention to detail and special interpretation.

Radiography of the breast reached a low point in the estimate of physicians. Haagensen (1956) emphatically stated that radiography had no place in diagnosis of breast diseases (but in 1962 expressed enthusiasm about "Egan's improved technic"). Sporadic articles did appear, mostly contributing to the distrust of radiography of the breast, e.g., demonstration of occult carcinomas of the breast, obviously palpable, as the illustrations clearly showed a lead marker superimposed on the carcinoma on the radiographs; cases clearly demonstrating carcinomas being followed for years by radiography without the radiologist recognizing them until they were advanced; and reports of the diagnostic accuracy based on equivocal and vague radiographic interpretations of lesions being "probable" or "suspicious."

Early in 1956 during a therapy planning

clinic, Gilbert F. Fletcher, M.D., Head of the Department of Radiology at the University of Texas M. D. Anderson Hospital and Tumor Institution (Gerald D. Dodd, M. D., was then Chief of the Section of Diagnostic Radiology) said, "Egan, you are a diagnostic radiologist now—start doing radiography of the breast." Not wanting to advertise my meager knowledge of the subject (and that was not to use the expression in Philadelphia), I stopped him in the hall later and asked him what he meant by breast x-ray and how it was done. He told me it was soft tissue studies of the breast but that he had no specific knowledge of technique.

The technical quality of the radiographs of the breast was a secondary consideration in most work reported in the literature. It was apparent that diagnosis of breast lesions was directly proportional to the quality of the radiographs and that if this phase of breast radiography were perpetuated, the procedure was doomed to extinction. Historically it was evident that radiographs of good quality would be mandatory.

One could only speculate on the events leading to abandonment of radiography of the breast. In these earlier reports there was no continuity or pooling of efforts. Techniques were incompletely and vaguely outlined but always with the comment that they were most difficult; diagnostic criteria that were mentioned were said to require much experience in evaluation; small groups of patients without adequate follow-up were analyzed; and the usual conclusion was that there was potential value to radiography of the breast, although each author was discouraged by its use.

There followed trials of published techniques and one unpublished one that consisted of factors for an anteroposterior radiograph of the knee. All produced radiographs lacking in detail. To my mind, it seemed better to disregard all these reports and start completely anew.

Then followed several months of experimentation with various radiographic technical factors that included a kilovoltage range from 12 to 22 Mev; various intensifying screens, including lead screens; focal spot sizes ranging from 0.3 mm to 2 cm; anode receptor distances of 22 cm to 6 feet; exposure times of 1/20 to 20 seconds; stationary grids; approximately 75 film emulsions, even ektachrome; numerous positions, including one of the pendant breast; stereoscopy; compres-

sion; and floating the breast in liquid. A high milliamperage–low kilovoltage technique was the compromise. The milliampere–seconds was frightening, but after careful measurements on a radical mastectomy specimen, then on several patients, the physicists assured me that it was a perfectly safe procedure.

Complete dosimetry and evaluation of the x-ray beam quality seemed the first logical step toward establishing a new technique. This was done on thin slices of breast tissue from a radical mastectomy specimen kept in a deep freezer in my office. Oddly, despite the clamor over radiation to the breast during mammography that lasted for 30 years, these studies have not been repeated on breast tissue. Mammograms were then done on patients, most of whom were scheduled for surgery; an unequivocal report on each lesion was made prior to biopsy. A code number indicating the specific diagnosis was appended. Radiographic diagnoses were made without clinical findings.

After approximately two dozen examinations had been done, I was informed that a carcinoma of the breast had been found in a breast showing no abnormality on the mammogram. Obviously I was prepared for this event, as I fully anticipated an accuracy of 50 per cent at best. This did not discourage the surgeons as they pointed out that the carcinoma was in the tail of the breast, which often extended high into the axilla. They quickly said that the last 13 cases had been given the exact histopathologic diagnosis. This caught my interest and I then began to get follow-up, even going to the surgical pathology laboratory with my mammograms. An axillary view was added to include this portion of the breast and the lymph node–bearing area. Some surgeons referred patients to give the radiologist "enough rope to hang himself"; the pathologists became amused, then interested, when histopathologic diagnoses were appearing on the charts prior to biopsy, often on lesions difficult to find in biopsy specimens; other clinicians were delighted that the surgeon's opinion could be challenged; and most of the radiologists continued to refer to me in less than complimentary terms.

The mammographic technique using ridiculously low kvp and an industrial film emulsion did seem strange to my uninitiated colleagues, whose attitude was that breasts would be burned off, x-ray tubes ruined, unnecessary breast biopsies done, and a false sense of security created.

There had been no uniform choice of a term to describe the procedure. "Roentgenography of the breast" was nonspecific. "Mastography" was an unwieldly term; "mastos," a combining form, was used sparingly in reference to the breast and was easily confused with similar-sounding terms. "Mammography" had crept into Stedman's Dictionary as a radiographic procedure employing a contrast medium but did not reflect precisely the previous usage of the term. Although only a few authors had used the term, "mammography" was selected as being concise, short, and following more closely the usual system of radiographic nomenclature and the most frequently used combining form for the mammary gland. Most importantly, this little-used term separated specifically this most promising unique technology from previous unpalatable ones.

Despite my caution in allowing five years to elapse during active clinical use in a highly respected oncologic institution, initial efforts to publish the results of the technique were rejected by the M. D. Anderson Hospital, based on prior knowledge of x-ray examination of the breast. Only after firm assurance from the Department of Epidemiology, where the data were being analyzed, was the report released for publication. Then it was rejected by peer referee review of one of our leading radiologic journals, again based on past results of breast radiography. But the editor arbitrated the numerous criticisms and finally accepted the report for publication (1960).

Following the original report on our four-year study in radiology in 1960, there occurred immediate and mushrooming interest in mammography. I had already successfully trained a number of radiologists in the technique and demonstrated its usefulness combined with the team approach over the four-year period in a tumor institute. My next step was to plan a modest reproducibility study involving three institutions and a private radiology practice in Houston. As the principal investigator I sought funds from the state Public Health Service. Lewis C. Robbins, M.D., Chief, Cancer Control Program, United Public Health Service, and staff learned of this proposal, became interested, and set out to verify our study. Dr. Robbins reported:

"We soon learned to respect the scientific integrity of Dr. Egan. We discussed the development of his mammography technic with the whole team that made the breakthrough possible: the surgeons, the pathologists, the statistician, Eleanor MacDonald, who collected and analyzed the results, and with Dr. R. L. Clark, Director of the University of Texas M. D. Anderson Hospital and Tumor Institute, under whose administration this study was conducted. The mammography report was given to the surgeon before biopsy was performed. If the surgeon had not verified the results in Egan's study, he would have been quick to complain. We noted a keen competition in the teamwork at M. D. Anderson Hospital, an effort to find cases in which Egan erred. But errors (false negatives) were less than three per cent in the first 2,000 mammograms. Consequently, the surgeons in this situation learned to use mammography as a prebiopsy aid, and their confidence lent additional credence to results in the Egan report."

A number of radiologists associated with the Public Health Service and the American Cancer Society visited the hospital to observe the results at first hand. These radiologists included Drs. Thomas Carlile, Eugene Pendergrass, Wendell Scott, James Cooney, and Theodore Hilbish. Their reports were cautiously optimistic and unanimous on the point that the technique permitted a mammogram of a quality that had not been available before; they further noted the close teamwork between the surgeons, radiologists, and pathologists. Also, they found that a method of training in the technique and interpretation of the mammograms had already been developed and had been proved effective. Over 15,000 reprints of the original article had been requested during the first three years following its publication. Carlile, then President of the American Cancer Society, remarked that "this article lit a slow-burning fuse which did not flare until Robbins sensed its value and undertook to overcome the resistance and inertia of three decades of negativism."

Developments led to my being the principal investigator to test the usefulness of mammography. A unique reproducibility study was designed in collaboration with M. D. Anderson Hospital, the Cancer Control Program (USPH), the National Cancer Institute (NCI), and 24 institutions scattered throughout the United States. Fortunately this study demonstrated its aims: (1) that radiologists with five days' indoctrination could perform satisfactory mammography; and (2) that the team approach could be established in their respective institutions. This led the Surgeon General of the United

States to conclude: "Mammography shows promise of being an important diagnostic aid in control of cancer of the breast."

This originally unmatched study not only established mammography but also served as a model for subsequent clinical trials (Clark et al., 1965). It laid the foundations, enumerated the requirements, provided the protocols, and established the methods for evaluation of future clinical trials for testing and adaptation of new medical procedures. As the principal investigator I required all the available expertise possible to plan and execute this program. Simple, clear-cut aims and concise end points were required. Cooperation of 24 of the most highly competitive institutions was required. A team had to be forged in each institution consisting of diagnostic radiologists, surgeons, and pathologists who often barely spoke to each other rather than share knowledge and shortcomings. The success of the reproducibility study provided the impetus for progression into many phases of clinical applications of mammography, renewed and diversified areas of investigation of breast diseases, and even screening of well women for breast cancer. It made possible the HIP and BCDDP screening programs. Without such a study mammography would have continued to wallow in the negativism noted by Carlile.

It is most significant that many of the clinicians who were formerly very interested in mammography but lost their enthusiasm emphatically espoused the revolutionary technique. Among them were surgeons (Haagensen, Pack, and Cutler) and radiologists (Rigler, Pendergrass, and Baensch). This fact alone should persuade the student to avoid all short cuts in making mammograms and concentrate on the basic principles of radiography.

Perhaps the best insight into the development of mammography was the summation that occurred when the annual seminars on mammography and breast diseases began in 1962 as part of the evaluation of the progress of the reproducibility study. This first seminar was held in Houston and was a means of getting the participants in the study under one roof and to outline the protocol. Perhaps this was a bit of history, this mingling of specialists in radiology, surgery, and pathology with a common cause. A second seminar in 1963, also in Houston, was a means to spur the participants in the reproducibility study. The participating team of radiologists,

surgeons, and pathologists had now had one year's experience with mammography, and they contributed lively discussions of practical problems with mammography technique and interpretation and of the realization of the necessity of the team approach to the diagnosis and treatment of breast diseases. Bridging the chasms between the medical specialties was most remarkable; mammography appeared to be the necessary first thread, thin as it was.

The optimistic concept, introduced in 1961, of having the centers of the reproducibility study act as training centers for mammography was faltering. The Third Annual Seminar was held in Atlanta at Emory University in 1964 to introduce a revised plan to develop training centers in mammography around the United States. Dr. James V. Rogers, Jr., was completing a pilot training program at Emory University, with 16 southeastern radiologists serving as primary trainees. The reproducibility of mammography had again been established. The feasibility of this new approach of training centers for radiologists was already so well established that 14 training centers in mammography around the United States were in various stages of being set up.

To teach and act as consultants in mammography, about 30 radiologists strategically placed around the United States volunteered their facilities while these training centers were being established and their loads lightened. Many unique teaching aids were being developed at the designated world breast center at Emory University with support from the Cancer Control Program; then they were placed in teaching centers and made available to interested radiologists and technologists.

Numerous enthusiastic claims began to appear in the radiologic literature extolling various techniques as superior for mammography. Many radiologists, lacking the time and opportunity to take advantage of instruction, began doing mammography with their own technical modifications, not realizing that all these modifications had already been tried and found inadequate. Many mammograms submitted for consultation were inadequate, and indeed, many were worse than nothing at all. This happened despite strong and repeated admonitions that much damage would result from poor mammograms.

Historical evaluation as well as recent experience indicated that accuracy of radiographic diagnosis of breast diseases depended on mammograms of the best technical quality. An ad hoc committee was formed with Arthur Present as chairman. The First Standardization Conference on Mammography (or any other radiographic procedure) was held by the Cancer Control Program, this ad hoc committee, and the American College of Radiology in Philadelphia in February 1965. Included were radiologists and technologists with considerable experience in mammography, physicists who had done investigative work at low kilovoltage levels, many representatives of the American College of Radiology interested in breast cancer and patient dosage, representatives of the United States Public Health Service, x-ray machine manufacturers, and interested radiologists. The chairman, after long discussions, summarized the efforts, feelings, and experience of a great many people who provided us with scientific information by stating that "there are no great disagreements about skin dosage or about techniques of mammography." This group, as well as other groups, was unanimous in its opinion that properly executed mammography contributes to cancer control and has the potential of reducing the death rate from cancer of the breast.

The superb efforts of this group produced another milestone in mammography. Then after the procedure was accepted by the American College of Radiology, they accepted a singular permanent committee with Dr. Wendell Scott as chairman, reflecting our emphasis on a truly multidisciplinary team rather than an occasional representative from another specialty.

With this solid background, several events led to the next seminar. The Fourth Annual Mammography Seminar at Emory University in 1965 served to consolidate mammography, to act as testimonial to our training programs, to introduce the American College of Radiology Committee to the procedure, to welcome Dr. William Ross as new Chief of Cancer Control Program, and to pay tribute to the outgoing Chief, Dr. Lewis C. Robbins, for his tremendous contribution to mammography. The team approach was now unshakable. The Emory University team stressed their long experience with specimen radiography, a real highlight in mammography.

The Fifth Annual Mammography Seminar at Emory University in 1966 consolidated the team approach to breast diseases even more

firmly, as the various members of the team reported more widespread use of mammography, keener interest in breast diseases, and greater desire to attack breast cancer. This was particularly brought out by a panel moderated by Dr. Murray M. Copeland. Also noteworthy at this seminar was that the reevaluation of the approach to training radiologists and technologists in mammography proved to be sound.

In 1967 the Sixth Annual Seminar was held in San Juan, Puerto Rico, as an International Conference sponsored by Emory University and I. Gonzalez Martinez Oncologic Hospital, with support from the Cancer Control Program. Again the main theme of this seminar was the team approach to breast diseases with very active participation of each member of the team at this time, training of radiologists, and auxiliary approaches to the study of breast diseases. The technical aspects and radiographic factors for mammography had been so well established, standardized, and accepted by the American College of Radiology and mammographers that little attention was given to them. Biopsy specimen radiography, introduced to the group two years before, was being practiced more widely. Whole-organ breast studies were gaining more attention. Potentially cancerous and precancerous breast lesions were being more openly discussed. Dr. Lauren V. Ackerman accused me of trying to use a crystal ball in talking about precancerous breast lesions. Some of these rather sticky and controversial discussions extended into ductal epithelial hyperplasia, atypia, and noninfiltrating carcinoma. Although today such hypotheses may not be totally accepted, they do not arouse such strong reactions from discussants. Also, more attention was being focused on calcifications in the breast, lobular carcinoma in situ, and the possible importance of multiple primary carcinomas. This seminar really began the boiling of several cauldrons and was nearly 20 years ahead of its time. A system of, and teaching material for, training mammography technicians to read mammograms had been in the developmental stage since 1962 but kept under wraps. By 1965, five technologists, one medical secretary, and one nonmedical secretary had been adequately trained at Emory University. Training of mammoscreeners had already proved to be so workable that it was being spread to other centers. The team approach had been so well established by the time of this seminar that the various specialty groups not only desired to communicate with each other but also wished to share some of their frustrations with breast diseases and to seek as much help as possible.

So much had been consolidated and so much new material introduced that the proceedings of this seminar were published, edited by R. Egan. The report contains much of the background for later approaches to the study of breast diseases.

Meanwhile, from 1963 to 1966 the Health Insurance Plan (HIP) of New York conducted breast screening with physical examination and (Egan) mammography to determine whether that approach could reduce breast cancer mortality. Sixty thousand women were randomized into screening and control groups, but only 20,000 of the 30,000 women selected for screening participated. To avoid bias of a self-selected population, data collected on the screened group included the 10,000 women who chose not to participate. By the seventh year, mortality in women 50 years and older was one-third lower in the screened than in the nonscreened group. Thus, if mammography had been omitted in annual screening, the benefit would have fallen by one third.

From my viewpoint as a consultant in planning this program, as the instructor in mammography of the participants, as a provider of my chief mammography technologist for on-site instructions in the technique of mammography, and as a reviewer of 15 per cent of the mammograms, there were certain reservations about the study: (1) We had successfully completed a nationwide reproducibility study and future screening rested solely on this one effort; at least two studies should have been conducted; (2) the quality of the mammograms was inferior despite efforts to cajole the participating radiologists to update their equipment and technique; (3) only 23 of the total 35 physician groups in the insurance program agreed to participate, slightly over 50 per cent; and (4) the radiation to the skin during mammography measured by a highly respected physicist was excessive. Since none of the 23 participating stations could be replaced by more efficient ones, since long delays would result in seeking new participants, since the only stated aim of the program was to determine if routine screening for breast cancer by physical examination and mammography would detect breast cancer at an earlier and more curable stage, and since I was convinced that physical examination alone could do that, my acquiescence seemed appropriate at the time. However, the less than optimal quality of the mammograms did contribute to the failure of detection of early cancers in younger women, and the increased radiation to the skin provided fodder for the increased-risk critics of mammography in later years. The increased radiation on the skin did not necessarily reflect any increase in midline dose but rather that technical factors such as collimation were at fault.

In hindsight, had we conducted two programs as I so strongly urged (on budgets as modest as this one) later criticism of mammography as a screening procedure could have been avoided, much expense spared, and the increased use of mammography not drastically delayed. The cautiously injected step-by-step momentum of mammography would have benefited from a competitive study.

Although I had inestimable help from my colleagues in planning and presenting these annual mammography seminars, they were becoming too large for a single institution or single small group of individuals to promote properly. The American College of Radiology Committee and Breast Diseases was asked to share the planning of the following seminar, and the American Cancer Society (ACS) the seminar following that one.

Sponsored by the American College of Radiology and the Cancer Control Program, the Seventh Annual Mammography Seminar was held in May 1968, in St. Louis to honor our committee chairman. Its theme was to continue the team approach toward the "Detection of Early Breast Cancer." The results of treatment were examined as well as the epidemiology and possible identification of high-risk groups so that the cure rate for breast cancer could be improved. Experimental modalities such as thermography and xerography (12 years after mammography had been established) were considered. Unsuspected breast cancer and cancer in the opposite breast were important considerations in that these were often early lesions. Incipient cancer of the breast, whole-organ breast studies, screening of the general population, and particularly the team approach to early diagnosis of breast cancer were important issues. The x-ray technologist had been encouraged to become part of the team (after years of struggle with the College of Radiology), with a mammography technologists' seminar having been held the day before the annual seminar. The technologists then attended the annual seminar.

The Eighth Annual Seminar on Mammography and Diseases of the Breast was held in Washington, D.C., in May 1969, sponsored by the American Cancer Society, the American College of Radiology, and the Cancer Control Program. This too was preceded by a technologists' seminar. This seminar was designed to be all-inclusive in every aspect of breast disease. Twelve hundred participants were in attendance. Again the team approach to diagnosis and treatment of breast cancer was apparent. The epidemiology, causation, pathogenesis, detection and diagnosis, developments for the control of breast cancer, and management of the patient with breast cancer were subjects of investigation. This seminar was such a huge success that it led to the abandonment by both the American Cancer Society and the NCI of their own yearly breast conferences.

In the early 1960s, after we failed to develop selective filters for the mammography x-ray beam, we substituted a molybdenum target for tungsten anode, hoping that the greater k-electron effect of the molybdenum x-rays at 22 to 28 kvp energies would increase the contrast between breast tissue structures. When we found that it was more difficult to increase mas with this tube, that a three- to fourfold increase in mas was required for film darkening, and that a great deal more radiation was absorbed in the breast, the tube was returned to the shelf. In the late 1960s, others, including Gros, thought that this anode improved his mammography despite the limitations. He found also that any improved image quality was achieved at the expense of the patient's comfort by compression and that an increased surface exposure of 8 r compared with Egan technique of 2 r. In 1969 the CGR Company introduced the Senograph mammography unit in the United States. Its 0.8 mm molybdenum focal spot was no improvement over the standard 1.0 to 2.0 mm tungsten focal spots in use at the time, as the short target-receptor distance (11 to 13 inches) with the compression cone offset any geometric effect of the smaller focal spot. It was not until eight years later that the company realized that a longer target-receptor distance was necessary.

In May 1970, the Ninth Annual Mammography Seminar was held in Denver, sponsored by the American College of Radiology and the Cancer Control Program. With a theme of "Early Breast Cancer: Diagnosis and Management," it aimed toward the newer problems that had been brought about by mammography, earlier presentation of women with breast problems, and the profession's renewed interest in breast cancer. Panels on means to diagnose breast cancer earlier and to formulate treatment policies in areas nonexistent or little regarded previously were charged with obtaining a clear statement of the particular problem and its ramifications and a concisely defined course of action. This was to be my last seminar as chairman of the program committee.

The Tenth Annual Breast Seminar in Glen Cove, New York, stressed the team approach, while the eleventh seminar in Nassau in 1972 again concentrated on detection of breast cancer and its treatment. Locations of the seminars on the East Coast, West Coast, or more central areas of the United States provided a mechanism to deliver the message of mammography and early breast cancer more widely.

The Twelfth Annual Breast Seminar, held in San Diego in 1973, consisted of plenary sessions in the morning with instruction courses and works in progress during the afternoon. Bilateral and multiple cancers were stressed. Mr. John L. Hayward delivered the First Annual Wendell G. Scott Memorial Lecture, "Experience of Local Surgery in the Treatment of Early Breast Cancer."

In the early 1970s our work with the Eastman Kodak Company film engineers was directed toward faster acceptable nonscreen film emulsions and those suitable for mechanical processors. Simultaneously we were able to perfect a mechanical film processor that simulated hand processing of fine-grain nonscreen film. These efforts restimulated our interests in the limited use of screen-film receptors with single-emulsion film and a single closely contacting screen. Rare-earth intensifying screens were being investigated and were incorporated in these efforts, approaching but not equaling conventional mammography, still widely practiced without rigid receptors and with less than 1 rad midline per examination. DuPont actually marketed the Lo-Dose I System, a single-emulsion, single-screen receptor that permitted rapid automatic processing but was poorly received by experienced mammographers owing to its many disadvantages.

Two trends in the approach to breast cancer were surfacing: (1) screening well women, and (2) lack of emphasis on the team approach. Based to some extent on their experience with the Guttman (Manhattan) screening project (Phil Strax, Director), in 1971 the American Cancer Society Board of Directors decided to fund four to six community demonstration projects for two years, at which time the participants could continue the projects if their communities supported them. In the summer of 1972 Emory University was site visited and approved for the first screening center. Concomitantly the Breast Task Force of the NCI suggested a joint venture, adding $4 million to the $2 million of the ACS and increasing the number of projects to 12 to 14. This agreement was reached in October 1972; Emory University more or less became the first center approved for screening. Unlike the clear-cut ACS study, this ACS/NCI Breast Community Detection Demonstration Project (BCDDP) had no recorded aims, no protocol, no directing personnel, and no data forms or concise semblance of a clinical trial. Emory University remained poised to start screening and without direction was coerced to begin screening July 1, 1973. We used our own data forms for months, the data later being discarded. A data center in Philadelphia, periodically changing directors, provided data forms nearly one and one-half years after the project was deemed ready to start. Political and various pressures over the beginning three years eventually led to 27 projects in the United States involving 29 institutions.

Many of the project directors, internists, surgeons, and oncologists were not students of mammography, breast diseases, and the necessary team approach. "Just hire a radiologist to cover" was their attitude. Ignoring radiologic input was disastrous for the first year, as 50 per cent of subsequent cancers were not detected on the initial screening. Not only did radiologic quality suffer but wide variations and excessive amounts of radiation were delivered during mammography. Our training program continued but training on the job was preferred. The NCI then established Physics Monitoring Centers, "but we physicists," as expressed by the director, "have no experience with dosimetry below 250 kvp." Emory University had done most of the basic investigation of the mammography kilovoltage range and acted as the training center for many of these physicists.

Shortly thereafter the Bureau of Radiological Health developed the BENT program statewide that would monitor radiation during mammography and offer assistance in correcting technical errors.

After the death of Dr. Scott in 1972, the American College of Radiology sharply deemphasized the multidisciplinary aspect of its Committee on Mammography and Diseases of the Breast. Another radical change was to shun the interest and support of the Cancer Control Program, at the time part of NCI.

The purpose of the Thirteenth Annual Breast Seminar in Buena Vista in 1974 was to teach the physician how to deal with the problems of early breast cancer. The ACS and NCI paid for the attendance of 150 residents. Emphasis was on physical examination, breast lumps, nipple discharge, early breast cancer, mammography, and premalignant breast lesions. Afternoons were devoted to instruction courses. By 1975 in San Juan, screening for breast cancer appeared on the program; this year Egan delivered the Wendell G. Scott Memorial Lecture on "Team Approach to Breast Cancer." The Fifteenth Annual Breast Seminar in Las Vegas featured breakfast panels and much discussion of the BCDDP and risk/benefits of mammographic screening.

The Sixteenth Annual Breast Seminar in Houston in 1977 reverberated with the claims that screening with mammography caused more cancers than were detected. A mixed, confused undertone rumbled with discussions of the BCDDP, radiation from mammography, risk/benefits of screening, the NCI changing policy, and the ACS suggesting calmness. The NCI had already generated ample replies to the critics but failed to use them: (1) Their training centers continued to combat poor-quality mammography; (2) they had established Physics Centers to correct erratic amounts of radiation during mammography; (3) the BENT program was operational for poor quality and excessive radiation by other radiologists; and (4) already one third of the breast cancers in the BCDDP were in women under age 50 years, almost all being detected by mammography. The ACS continued to defend the BCDDP, but NCI continued its eerie silence.

In San Francisco in 1978 the Seventeenth Annual Breast Seminar continued with confusion in the message that was clearly offset by Arthur I. Holleb in his Wendell G. Scott

Memorial Lecture. His account of the enormity of the breast cancer problem and the proven inestimable value of mammography clearly overshadowed all the unproven radiation scare hypotheses of a handful of dissenters. Heavy emphasis on the treatment of breast cancer and appeasement of women with a woman's panel on breast cancer were features of the seminar.

The criticism following the imbroglio of screening detracted from these last seminars. The chairmanship of the Committee on Mammography and Breast Diseases was changed. Even the name of the committee was changed, with de-emphasis of the multidisciplinary approach. There was insufficient support for annual seminars.

The Nineteenth Annual Seminar was held in 1981 in San Diego and was entitled the Nineteenth National Conference on Breast Cancer. I had remained the only person who had attended all the previous conferences, but I was not invited to this one. A new format in the program reflected epidemiology, systemic disease, galactorrhea, amenorrhea, immunotherapy, hormones, scintigraphy, the question "are cancers found by x-ray real?," and the testing of new modalities. The Wendell G. Scott Memorial Lecture was on thermography.

The Working Group (Beahrs) evaluating the BCDDP in comparison with the HIP screening program recommended strongly a randomized clinical trial to determine if screening with mammography in women under age 50 years was of value. With Egan as Project Director, Emory University in collaboration with the Epidemiology Section of the Communicable Disease Center (NCI) in 1980 produced a collaborative proposal with 15 other institutions, Breast Cancer Randomized Controlled Screening, to answer questions about breast cancer screening in this age group. Emory University was site visited for several days. In concept and in substance the proposal was well accepted. But despite the strong urgings of their Working Group, NCI refused to become involved in such a breast program, still smarting from some of the aftermath of the ACS/NCI BCDDP. Instead they chose to await the Canadian and Swedish screening programs that were proposed or in operation.

The Falun, Sweden, screening program was begun in 1977 and involved 161,000 women over age 39 years (Tabar et al., 1984).

In the same year a screening program was begun in Malmö, Sweden, a city of 235,000 inhabitants (Anderson, 1984). The Canadian program had a slow and rocky start. Other programs were also started outside the United States.

The Twentieth National Conference on Breast Cancer was held in New Orleans in 1982. Even five years following the hypothetical radiation scare, the first day was dedicated to radiation with mammography; the next day took up the significance of "minimal" breast cancer; and then there was a day of screening and two days of treatment. The American College of Radiology felt that there was not enough interest and support for annual seminars; thus the Twenty-first Conference was held in 1984 in Hawaii and the Twenty-second in 1986 in Boston. These same conference participants doggedly repeated, annually, then every second year, their concerns over the same questions of radiation, age for screening with mammography, significance of "minimal" cancer of the breast, and superiority of screen-film vs xeroradiography.

Meanwhile, at other breast meetings during this period heated discussions centered around breast imaging centers and the many facets of spreading quality mammography. The first breast imaging center established at Emory University in 1964 was firmly in existence, with many radiologists and oncologists noting its success. There were myriad questions of how to organize, finance, accept women, handle referral, and economize as well as matters of ethical conduct, third-party payment, and modalities to use and in what order. The best ways to educate women and their physicians, particularly obstetricians, gynecologists, family practitioners, internists, and other front-line physicians, were real concerns.

The driving force was how to increase the use of mammography and how to get women to have their baseline mammogram. If only 5 to 7 per cent of eligible women were getting mammography, how could 0.06 rad midline per examination be a public health problem? Who cares about the superiority of a receptor if it is not being used? Historically a contrast was emerging: The early history of mammography followed closely the Annual Seminars on Mammography and Breast Diseases, with that outside the United States paralleling these events, but in later years the absence of concrete guidelines and strong guidance resulted in a division of courses in the United States and abroad.

Every woman's magazine in this country has published articles urging women to become familiar with breast cancer, breast self-examination (BSE), mammography, and alternatives to treatment. These followed particularly after Betty Ford and Happy Rockefeller publicized their breast cancers in 1974. This momentum has continued into the establishment of national women's organizations to establish clearing houses to disseminate knowledge on breast cancers and ways to combat it.

This general interest in mammography by women establishes a new pattern to the application of mammography, screening of well women for establishment of increased risk for breast cancer either incipient or present. The radiologist alone must direct the challenge. Although no new problems have arisen, few concrete proposals have been presented for those problems abounding for 30 years. The trend has been the breast imaging centers for small local pockets of women all lacking in motivation of the general population. The solution to providing mammography to all eligible women is the simple pre-mammography selector using optical spectroscopy outlined in our discussions in "Probability of Breast Cancer." Then all women will consider mammography the "woman's test" that will be boldly demanded by all those eligible women.

The strong and persistent rejection by radiologists of this proven, highly acceptable risk marker for mammography can only lead to abandonment of women's dependence on radiologists and to their seeking alternative guidance.

REFERENCES

Anderson I (1984): Breast cancer screening in Malmo. *In* Brunner S, Langfeldt B, Andersen PE (eds): Recent Results in Cancer Research. Berlin, Springer-Verlag, p 114.

Baensch WE (1962): Professor of Radiology, Georgetown University, Washington, DC: Personal communication.

Clark RL, Copeland MM, Egan RL, et al (1965): Reproducibility of the technic of mammography (Egan) for cancer of the breast. Am J Surg *109*:127.

Dominguez CM (1930): Estudio radiologico de los descalcificadores. Bol Soc Anat Pathol *1*:175.

Egan RL (1960): Experience with mammography in a tumor institution. Evaluation of 1,000 studies. Radiology *74*:894.

Espaillat A (1933): Contribution a l'Etude Radiographique du Sein Normal et Pathologique. Thèse Paris, No. 417, Librairie Paris.

Gershon-Cohen J (1967): Personal communication.

Gershon-Cohen J (1967): Mammography, thermography and xerography. Cancer J Clin *17*:108.

Goynes J, Gentil DF, Guedes B (1931): Sobre la Radiografia de la Glandula Mamaria y su Valor Diagnostico. Arch Espan Oncol *2*:111.

Gros CM (1963): Diseases of the Breast. Paris, Masson et Cie.

Haagensen CD (1956): Diseases of the Breast. Philadelphia, WB Saunders.

Haagensen CD (1962, 1963): College of Physicians and Surgeons of Columbia University, New York, NY: Personal communications.

Kleinschmidt O (1927): *In* Zweifel-Payr: Klinic der bosartigen Geschwulste, Bd. IV. Hirzel, Leipzig.

Lame EL, Pendergrass, EP (1947): An addition to the technic of simple breast roentgenography. Radiology *48*:266.

Leborgne R (1951): Diagnosis of tumors of breast by simple roentgenography: calcifications in carcinoma. Am J Roentgenol *65*:1.

Pendergrass EP (1963): Personal communication.

Ries E (1930): Diagnostic lipoidal injection into milk ducts followed by abcess formation. Am J Obstet Gynecol *20*:414.

Rigler LG (1961): Visiting Professor of Radiology, University of California, Los Angeles School of Medicine, Los Angeles, CA: Personal communication.

Robbins LC (1962): Purposes of the mammography reproducibility study. Cancer Bull *6*:102.

Salomon A (1913): Beitrage zur Pathologie und Klinik des Mammakarzinoms. Arch Klin Chir *101*:573.

Seabold PS (1931): Roentgenographic diagnosis of diseases of the breast. Surg Gynecol Obstet *53*:461.

Tabar L, Akerlund E, Gad A (1984): Five-year experience with single-view mammography randomized controlled screening in Sweden. *In* Brunner S, Langfeldt B, Andersen PE (eds): Recent Results in Cancer Research, Berlin, Springer-Verlag, p 105.

Vogel W (1932): Die Roentgendarstellung der Mammatumoren. Arch Klin Chir *171*:618.

Von Ronnen JR (1956): Plain Roentgenography of the Breast. Amsterdam, Academic Press, p 229.

Warren SL (1950): A roentgenologic study of the breast. Am J Roentgenol *24*:113.

Breast Self-Examination

2

BACKGROUND

The woman who conscientiously practices breast self-examination (BSE) improves her chances of detecting early breast cancer through several avenues: (1) Subtle differences can best be appreciated by her as the earliest physical changes of breast cancer; (2) consultation with her physician results more frequently; (3) informative discussion of the changes may prepare her for better future examinations; (4) a differential diagnosis may be established; and (5) further investigation may lead to a second opinion from an oncologic breast surgeon, a mammogram, or a tissue examination.

Embarrassment, fear of discovering a lump, or the feeling of inadequacy in evaluating the many lumps and bumps in the breasts is soon overcome as the routine of BSE becomes commonplace and as the woman becomes more familiar with her breast texture and contents. She then becomes the epitome of defense against lethal breast cancer as minute changes are elicited. Discussion of these findings with her physician establishes a range of normality, reducing timidity or overconcern. Physicians are becoming more aware, and receptive, of women referring themselves for help in evaluation of their breasts. This sequence provides an alternative to a limited number of physicians attempting periodic and frequent breast examination of all their women patients in the age group at risk for development of cancer. The awareness of this increasing demand by some physicians' organizations, e.g., the American Society of

Obstetrics and Gynecology, has created a necessity for setting standards for BSE, routine breast examinations, and referrals for mammography. Other physicians not trained in breast oncology may feel inadequate and seek a second opinion or refer the woman for mammography—all a plus for the woman with a breast problem. Also, routine mammography for all the women in the relevant age group is limited by time, personnel, and expense. These steps initiated by BSE tend to establish a higher risk patient, reduce the number of mammograms required, and convince the woman that the time and expense (and radiation exposure) of mammography is worthwhile.

Oncologic breast surgeons and physicians with a high percentage of women patients could provide in their waiting rooms audiovisual means of demonstrating breast self-examination and then teach, or have their nurses teach, BSE during some portion of the breast examination. Breast imaging centers are ideal for indoctrinating women in BSE. The women can then be approached at the height of concern and interest in breast problems and be more receptive to instruction. Audiovisual teaching of BSE is not only acceptable but appropriate in the mammography area.

Until the ideal "risk marker" for breast cancer is established, all means to get women to mammography must be pursued. Further reduction in radiation will offer no enticement; time and expense of meticulous mammography cannot be reduced drastically enough to make it appeal to all women. Erudite discriminant analysis for risk or a simple test has not been established. The radiologist is hampered by limited time. This reverts to more emphasis on BSE.

The radiologist must emphasize to the mammography technologist that his or her role is becoming increasingly important in disseminating information about BSE and persuading women to practice it religiously. In the early 1950s the importance of convincing women that BSE may well be a lifesaving measure was well known to the medical profession, but even with a great push from the American Cancer Society the practice was picked up by only a few women and then often reluctantly (Haagensen, 1952.)

In a Gallup poll conducted for the American Cancer Society in late 1973, it was found that the physician plays a key role in convincing women to practice BSE on a regular basis. With routine methods of dissemination of information regarding BSE, only a small percentage of women practiced the procedure. Of the other women who had received personal instruction from a physician about BSE, 92 per cent continued to practice it regularly. It is well known among breast surgeons that a woman who becomes familiar with the texture of her breast and practices BSE regularly in many instances finds a small tumor before the oncologic surgeon can feel it.

Although no clinical trials with BSE have been conducted, many retrospective studies have shown varying degrees of value, e.g., reduced metastatic disease (Greenwald et al., 1978) or no significant benefits (Smith et al., 1980). Many of the pros and cons of BSE need further evaluation, and, just as importantly, so do the behavioral patterns of both the woman and her physician. Under certain circumstances BSE can be taught with an amazing efficiency (when compared with the oncologic surgeon's examination). This portends real contributions from BSE when the primary care physicians are not nearly so skilled examiners. Yet by the same token BSE should not be oversold as a substitute for or to the exclusion of established screening procedures of meticulous physical examination and mammography. In the BCDDP over 50 per cent of the invasive cancers less than 1 cm in size were found by mammography, while 8 per cent were found by physical examination alone. In those cancers over 1 cm in size, one third were found by mammography alone with no increase in the number found by clinical examination only.

BSE is aimed at finding cancers of the breast, an infrequent routine whose reward is a negative finding. It can be contrasted with the positive effects on a diabetic woman who takes insulin to control her blood sugar level. Although almost 100 per cent of the women presenting themselves to their physicians can pinpoint an area of concern in their breast, and the physician too may be concerned, the rate of false positive findings

by BSE is high. Even after repeated assurance by the physician that self-referral is the expected practice, it becomes monotonous and costly and some degree of discouragement on the part of the patient is inevitable.

The small mass of carcinoma must have a different growth pattern and host tissue response to become palpable, suggesting the advanced and aggressive nature of the process. To be assuredly curable this carcinoma must be asymptomatic. There are exceptions, but in general symptomatic women don't have highly curable cancers. We must not forget the lessons of the BCDDP where, especially at Emory University, we concentrated on well women and found cancers that averaged 4 mm in size with a maximum of 1 positive low axillary lymph node. Yet the incidence of breast cancer was over five times that expected in the general population.

That lesson suggests that women have an inherent sense of selection into a high-risk group, a self-selected bias that should be encouraged by freely admitting women to mammography without physician-imposed restraints, community discouragement, and prohibitive costs. Reducing fear as a barrier to consultation without reducing it as a stimulus is mandatory; no false sense of security should be generated; and women should be imbued with a selfish desire to remain healthy and cancer free. It is in this milieu that women will eventually develop the conviction that mammography is their examination, and theirs alone—the sole momentum for universal implementation of this lifesaving tool.

THE EXAMINATION

Breast self-examination is a simple, painless procedure that takes just a few minutes. Many women need to be persuaded that they can evaluate the variations in the consistency and irregularities in their breasts without developing anxieties. If the woman is convinced that the breast is not a homogeneous mass but contains various structures producing nodularity, thickenings, or small lumps, she can realize that her breasts are normal despite such irregularities. All women's breasts vary in texture throughout their life and menstrual cycles, but once the intelligent woman's fingers are adapted to BSE she can be the first to distinguish and point out any small irregularity. In other words, she becomes the most expert person in examining her breasts. However, she is not encouraged to make diagnoses but only to report any unusual change to her physician.

One of the most important parts of BSE is establishing a regular time in which to conduct it, e.g., once a month just after the menstrual period or, if the patient is postmenopausal, on some day of the month that is easy to remember.

The examination should be started during a shower (Fig. 2–1) or bath, when the skin is wet and soapy. The fingertips then slide easily over the skin of the breast, requiring only light pressure. The patient's body as well as the hands should be relaxed. The palmar surfaces of the fingers are used in a gentle touch. With the fingers flat, every part of the breast is touched and felt gently for a lump or thickening that is clearly distinct from the rest of the tissue.

After the shower, the breasts are observed while the woman is standing or sitting in front of a mirror (with her arms relaxed at her sides) and in a well-lighted area (Fig. 2–2). She looks for any variation in the size or shape of the breast and changes in the skin of both breasts, e.g., puckering, dimpling, flattening, retraction, or changes in color or texture. The nipple is inspected for discharge, recent retraction or change in previous retraction, scaling, weeping, or size. The next step is to raise both arms over the head and repeat the skin and nipple inspection. She then places both hands on her hips, presses vigorously downward (which flexes her pectoral muscles, thereby retracting the breasts upward), and repeats the inspection, particularly for uneven retraction of the skin, nipple, or any part of the breast.

The next step is to lie supine (Figs. 2–3 to 2–11). The arm on the side being examined is raised above the head. A small, rather firm pillow or a folded bath towel is placed under the shoulder on the side being examined. This makes the base of the breast parallel with the chest wall so that it is balanced, flattened out, and as thin as possible on the chest wall. This also prevents the tendency of the breast to fall laterally and fold upon itself toward the axilla.

In this position the inner half of the breast is gently palpated with the flat of the fingers of the opposite hand. Some women may prefer a little talcum powder on the fingers of the examining hand for, as with the soapy water, the fingers glide more easily over the skin with less pressure, maintaining tactile sensitivity. The fingers proceed in transverse direction beginning just below the clavicle on a line with the nipple. Palpation extends all the way to the sternal border, and in transverse lines it is continued until the lower part of the breast, the inframmammary fold, is reached. This fold is an area of compressed breast tissue called the inframmammary ridge and is a normal finding.

The arm on the side of the breast being examined is next placed at the side and the axilla is palpated as high under the arm as possible. The outer half of the breast is then examined in transverse lines beginning far laterally to the nipple line and all the way from the level of the axilla down to the

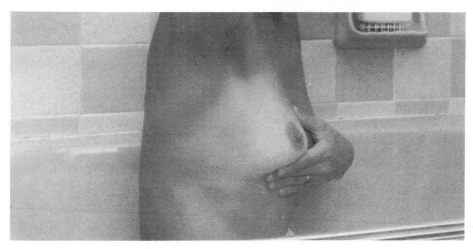

Figure 2–1. Breast self-examination (BSE) is started while in the shower or bath. (From Egan RL: Breast Imaging, 3rd ed. Rockville, MD, Aspen Publishers, Inc., 1984. Used by permission.)

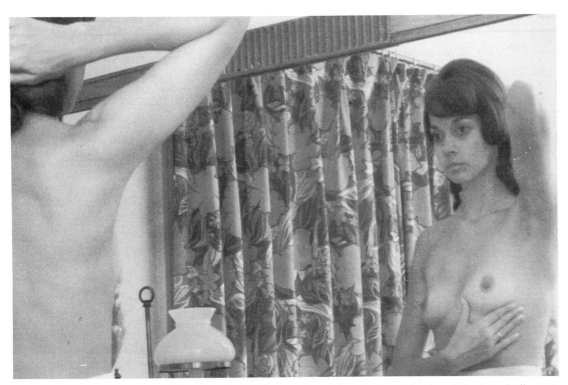

Figure 2–2. Inspection in front of a mirror is the next step. (From Egan RL: Breast Imaging, 3rd ed. Rockville, MD, Aspen Publishers, Inc., 1984. Used by permission.)

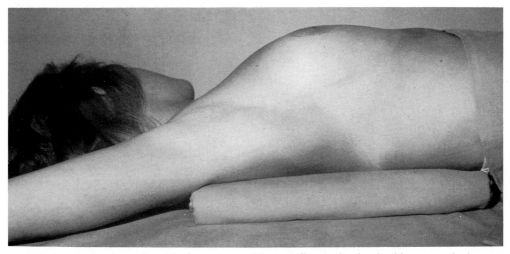

Figure 2–3. Examination is continued in the supine position. A pillow under the shoulder causes the breast to flow evenly over the chest wall. The arm is raised for examination of the medial half of the breast. (From Egan RL: Breast Imaging, 3rd ed. Rockville, MD, Aspen Publishers, Inc., 1984. Used by permission.)

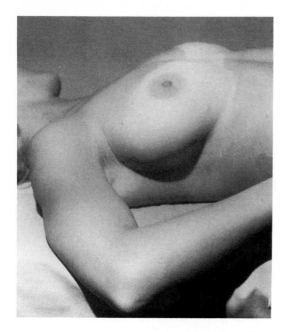

Figure 2–4. The breast improperly balanced on the chest wall for BSE, with the shoulder flat on the table, causes the breast to fall laterally. (From Egan RL: Breast Imaging, 3rd ed. Rockville, MD, Aspen Publishers, Inc., 1984. Used by permission.)

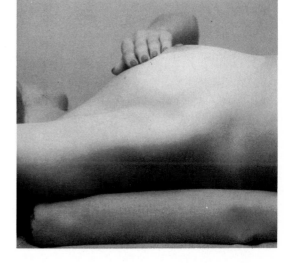

Figure 2–5. The inner half of the breast is palpated with the opposite hand. (From Egan RL: Breast Imaging, 3rd ed. Rockville, MD, Aspen Publishers, Inc., 1984. Used by permission.)

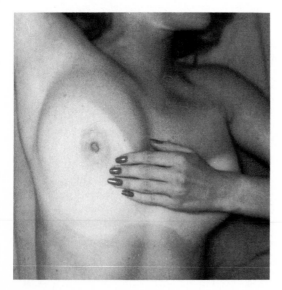

Figure 2–6. The medial half of the breast is examined by a series of transverse lines extending from the nipple line to the sternum, or breast bone. (From Egan RL: Breast Imaging, 3rd ed. Rockville, MD, Aspen Publishers, Inc., 1984. Used by permission.)

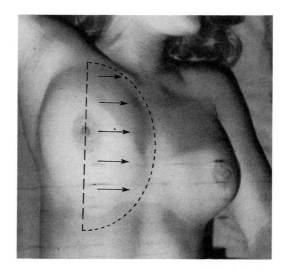

Figure 2–7. The transverse palpation extends from the clavicle to include the inframammary crease. (From Egan RL: Breast Imaging, 3rd ed. Rockville, MD, Aspen Publishers, Inc., 1984. Used by permission.)

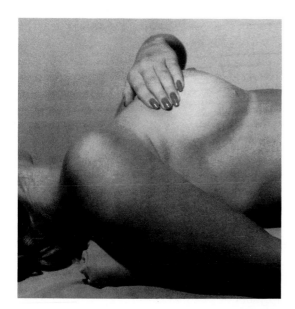

Figure 2–8. For palpation of the lateral half of the breast, the same supine position is maintained but with the arm at the side. (From Egan RL: Breast Imaging, 3rd ed. Rockville, MD, Aspen Publishers, Inc., 1984. Used by permission.)

Figure 2–9. The series of transverse lines of palpation extends from the axilla to the inframammary crease and from the breast far laterally to the nipple line. (From Egan RL: Breast Imaging, 3rd ed. Rockville, MD, Aspen Publishers, Inc., 1984. Used by permission.)

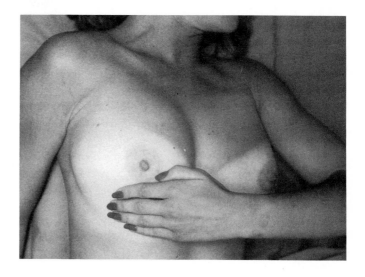

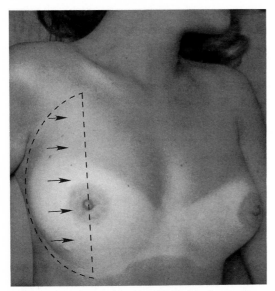

Figure 2–10. Extent of the lateral half of the breast. (From Egan RL: Breast Imaging, 3rd ed. Rockville, MD, Aspen Publishers, Inc., 1984. Used by permission.)

inframammary crease. Particular attention is given to the upper part of this half of the breast because it contains more breast tissue and more nodular arrangements of tissue; most tumors occur in this area. The central breast, or areolar area, is palpated. The other breast is examined in the same way, with reversal of the pad under the shoulder and the examining fingers.

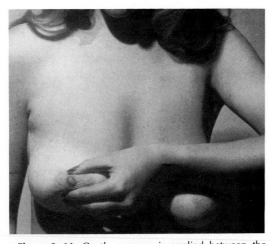

Figure 2–11. Gentle pressure is applied between the thumb and fingers over the areola surrounding the nipple, with a slight stripping motion toward the nipple to determine the presence of a nipple discharge. (From Egan RL: Breast Imaging, 3rd ed. Rockville, MD, Aspen Publishers, Inc., 1984. Used by permission.)

Many physicians do not routinely recommend palpation in the sitting position as the breast will frequently become more pendulous and confusing to evaluate. However, if anything is felt in the recumbent position it may be rechecked in the sitting position. In a sitting position the nipple may be milked very gently between the thumb and forefinger for evidence of any secretions. The American Cancer Society suggests a rotary type motion around the nipple in examining the breasts. However, many women do not like this motion because the nipple can be more readily stimulated to erection, producing anxieties.

If this instruction is given by the mammography technologist in a professional manner, it can readily become part of the examination of mammography and prove lifesaving to the patient. Our technologists have been teaching BSE for a number of years without any real problems. However, at times a woman may be adamant about not learning the technique, in which case the technician should be content to suggest that the patient discuss the procedure with her family doctor.

OBSERVATIONS

BSE has failed to become the panacea for breast cancer as was once hoped. Yet it has become one of the most productive means for women to participate in the prevention of a nearly unique female disease, breast cancer. The unprejudiced and unrestricted practice of BSE by increasingly larger numbers of women can only focus attention on this long-shrouded disease and alert the medical profession that a clamor for metamorphosis in diagnosis and treatment of breast cancer will be heard loudly and clearly.

REFERENCES

Greenwald P, Nasca PC, Lawrence CE, et al (1978): Estimated effect of breast self-examination and routine physical examination on breast-cancer mortality. N Engl J Med 299:271.

Haagensen CD (1952): Self-examination of the breasts. JAMA 149:356.

Lewison EF (1954): Breast self-examination; education and clinical effectiveness of the film. Md Med J 3:123.

Smith EM, Francis AM, Polissar L (1980): The effect of self-exam practices and physical examinations on extent of disease at diagnosis. Prev Med 9(3):409.

Clinical Examination of the Breast

BACKGROUND

Until mammography becomes an integral part of the medical evaluation of every woman, history and physical examination remain the key elements in providing care for breast problems. The clinician is the pathway to decision making. The challenge of this pivotal role evokes responses from clinicians that are based on individual philosophies ranging from "there is nothing in the breast that I can't feel" to "routine mammography for all women above certain ages." When a woman consults her physician she likes to be assured that she has no malignancy of the breast or, short of that, to be properly directed to assure that conclusion (e.g., mammography or surgical consultation). Many women end up in the consulting room of an oncologic breast surgeon as an extension of a breast examination by a less experienced primary care physician or for a second opinion of their breast problem. This surgeon must then rely heavily upon his own physical examination for sound conclusions as to return visits, aspirations, biopsy, or supplementary imaging modalities.

Surgeons have always assumed the responsibility for breast cancer detection, but it is becoming the role of the mammographer, sonographer, and others to supply the information needed for accurate detection of cancer before the patient is sent for definitive treatment. Surgeons not using the excellent tools available in the search for cancer are not offering women the best in detection of early and potentially curable breast cancer. They will miss those cancers that cannot be felt, will remove many areas of normal tissue, and may cause days of needless anxiety when a tentative preoperative diagnosis has not been established. The woman going to surgery knowing that her breast lesion is almost certainly malignant (or benign) has a great psychologic advantage over the one who has not been forewarned.

The clinician today, unlike his revered tutors, must not only be an accomplished breast examiner but also be aware of his shortcomings and be intimately knowledgeable of diagnostic aids that are available to optimize his skills. Wariness of and overexpectations of these aids are equally deplored. The first appointment should include instructing the patient in her own care and furthering her understanding of the ancillary studies breast cancer detection.

There are two distinct backdrops against which women undergo clinical examination of their breasts. The most frequent, the most unfathomable, and the most challenging situation is that of the examining physician equipped with only his tactile and visual senses examining the trusting patient, then walking with her from the examination chamber with her diagnosis clearly and unhesitatingly established. As many as 50 per cent (as established by the BCDDP) of early breast cancers lurk in clinically normal breasts. Very few of these women will have further studies as part of the initial clinical evaluation. The other situation is the clinical examination, in a breast imaging center, of women already scheduled to have mammography and whatever ancillary studies are indicated as an extension of physical examination and/or mammography. Two distinctly different types of clinical examinations of the breast are not available, so that these two groups of women have an equal chance of detection of their clinically occult carcinomas.

THE EXAMINATION

Physical examination of the breast includes inspection and palpation conducted with the patient in both the erect and the recumbent positions. The entire breast, including the nipple and areola, and the regional lymph node areas, axillary and supraclavicular, must be included in the examination.

Despite its usefulness, mammography is not infallible, and the radiologist is at times chagrined to learn that a carcinoma proved by biopsy was not apparent on the film. Mammography is not a substitute for physical examination; the two are complementary. Nor is either a substitute for biopsy. For this reason, whether elicited by palpation alone, by mammography alone, or by both, every suggestive nodule in the breast should be removed for histologic examination before mastectomy is performed. This policy will lead to a larger number of biopsies; however, it should also lead to the discovery of a large number of cancers during the early course of their development.

The clinician, radiologist, pathologist, and surgeon should share the care of the patient with carcinoma of the breast.

Inspection of the breasts must be conducted with a good strong light and with an assistant to move the light about to bring out variations in skin color, texture, early retractive signs, and slight changes in contour. The skin over the breast is examined for dilatation of subcutaneous veins, redness, and edema. Changes in the nipple are noted. Palpation of the breasts is carried out using appropriate positions and maneuvers on an examining table with access from both sides. Palpation should be an orderly, precise, and gentle procedure.

Only a few of the many changes that occur in the breast will be mentioned. Figures 3–1 to 3–24 demonstrate the complete and methodical examination as performed by Ralph Waldo Powell, M.D., Associate Professor of Surgery at Emory University School of Medicine, as he explained during a symposium for Patient Care.*

ABNORMALITIES

Mass

At Emory University the most frequent clinical finding was a mass in 86 per cent of palpable cancers: 44 per cent of these masses were classified as well defined and 56 per cent as poorly defined; 90 per cent of the masses were firm or hard, only 10 per cent being soft or cystic. Pain, tenderness, and thickening each occurred in 12 per cent of the cancers, and nipple discharge was present in 2 per cent. The most common location of cancer was in the upper outer quadrant, where there is a greater amount of breast tissue: 50 per cent of the cancers were in the upper outer quadrant; 18 per cent were in the upper inner quadrant; 10 per cent were in each of the lower inner and lower outer quadrants; 7 per cent were central; and 5 per cent were diffuse.

Text continued on page 28

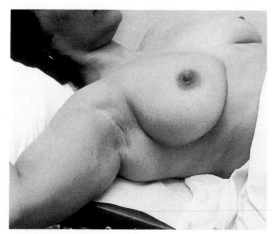

Figure 3–1. Have the patient lie with her arm abducted to 75 degrees (you may want to put a folded sheet or towel under her shoulder, but it isn't necessary) and inspect the breasts for symmetry and for subtle changes in color or texture of the skin.

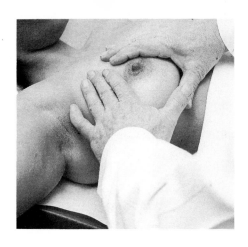

Figure 3–2. Stand on the patient's right side to examine the right breast. Using four fingers of each hand, begin palpation in the upper central portion and proceed clockwise from the superior to the medial quadrants. Palpate gently initially; with too firm presssure you may miss a soft mass. Repeat this step, palpating much more firmly.

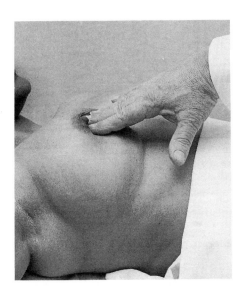

Figure 3–3. The last maneuver in the supine position with the arm abducted is the examination of the central portion of the breast. Very gently palpate the nipple and tissue underneath for evidence of small masses or duct thickening.

Figure 3–4. Gently strip the nipple to check for discharge.

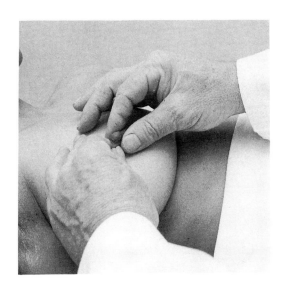

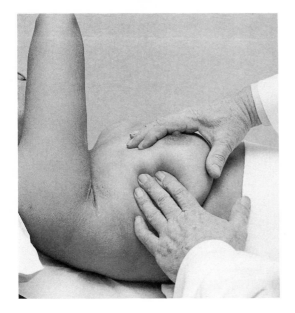

Figure 3–5. Complete the examination of the right breast with the patient in the supine position by having the patient rotate her arm across the chest wall.

Figure 3–6. This position tends to bring the breast farther across the chest wall and affords a more accurate examination of the tail of the breast.

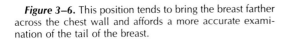

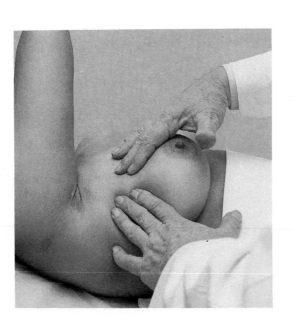

Figure 3–7. In this position, a small deep-lying lesion that might otherwise be missed can be brought out from the inner spaces, trapped over a rib, and palpated readily. Move to the other side of the table and examine the left breast.

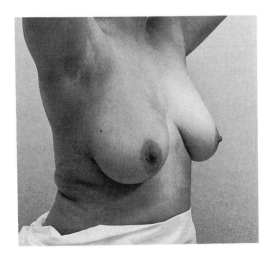

Figure 3–8. Have the patient sit on the end of the table with her feet dangling, so you can get close enough to have freedom of motion in examining both breasts. It's sufficient for the patient to place her hands above her head, but if she rests them on her head the position is much less tiring.

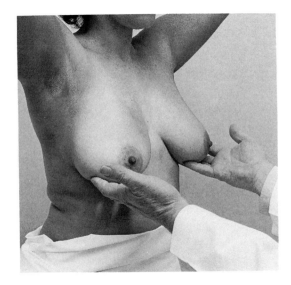

Figure 3–9. Place both your hands under the breasts for front inspection. Compare the breasts for size and nipple parallelism and check for differences in the veins of the subcutaneous tissue, skin changes, and nipple irregularities.

Figure 3–10. Palpate the breast tissue very gently, beginning in the upper central portion; proceed clockwise about the circumference of the breast.

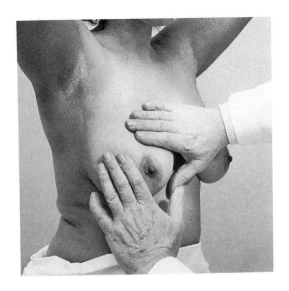

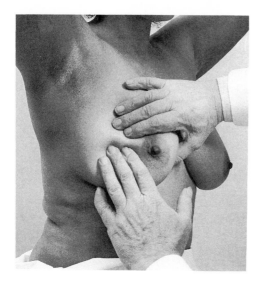

Figure 3–11. Repeat the circumferential palpation of the breast, using firmer pressure to detect possible deep-lying lesions.

Figure 3–12. Gently palpate the nipple for small, centrally located lumps or duct thickening. Check for nipple discharge by stripping the nipple softly.

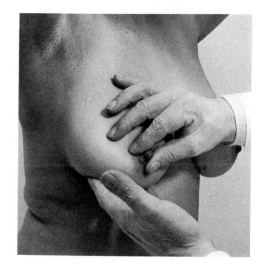

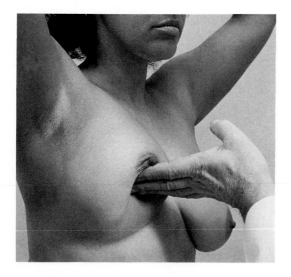

Figure 3–13. Lift the breast with your fingertips and inspect the lower and lateral portions for subtle change in the color or texture of the skin.

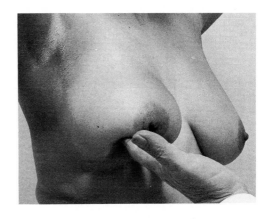

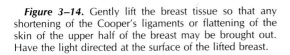
Figure 3–14. Gently lift the breast tissue so that any shortening of the Cooper's ligaments or flattening of the skin of the upper half of the breast may be brought out. Have the light directed at the surface of the lifted breast.

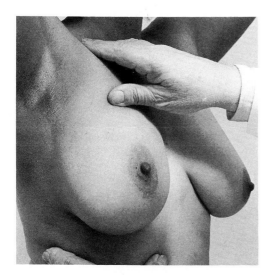

Figure 3–15. Pull upward on the breast tissues. This gentle elevation may demonstrate nipple and skin changes such as foreshortening of the nipple or flattening of the skin.

Figure 3–16. To conclude the examination of the right breast with the patient in the first sitting position, gently and then firmly (shown above) palpate the tail of the breast as it enters the lower portion of the axilla.

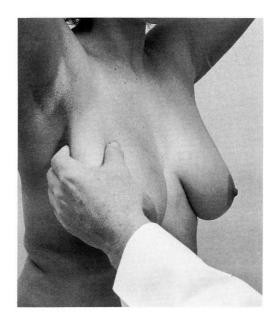

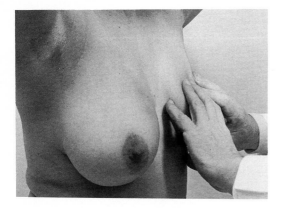

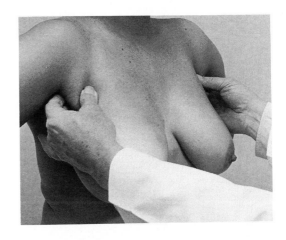

Figure 3–17. With both the patient and you maintaining the same position, repeat the previous maneuvers for the opposite (left) breast, making certain that the assistant has redirected the light.

Figure 3–18. Stand directly in front of the patient; to ensure flexing, check as shown here. Carry out frontal inspection, looking for nipple or skin abnormalities and for asymmetry. Carry out all maneuvers that were done with the patient in the second position; repeat for left breast.

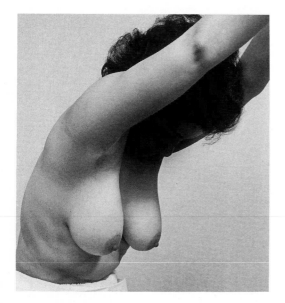

Figure 3–19. Use one hand to support the patient's hands above her head as she leans forward. The weight of the breasts will project them from the chest wall; subtle skin changes that might otherwise be missed can be demonstrated in this position.

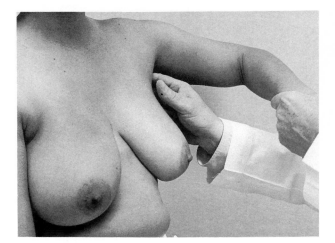

Figure 3–20. With the patient relaxed, support her relaxed arm loosely to facilitate manipulation; palpate the axilla gently with a kneading motion. Repeat with the other hand for the other axilla.

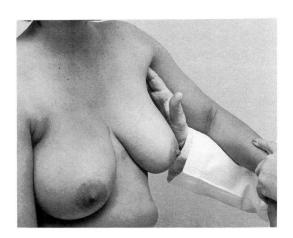

Figure 3–21. To examine the upper portion of the axilla, use vigorous palpation even if it makes the patient uncomfortable. Push your hand firmly upward and milk the axillary contents downward.

Figure 3–22. Repeat with the other hand for the other axilla.

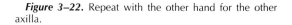

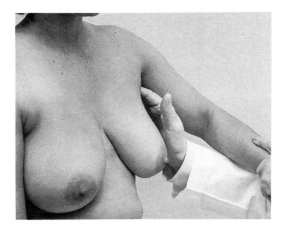

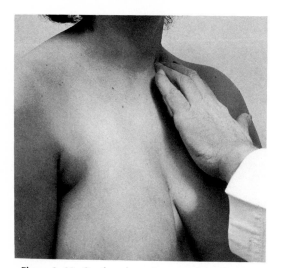

Figure 3–23. Gently palpate the supraclavicular portion of the neck; repeat with the other hand on opposite side.

First the examiner must decide whether a definite mass is present as opposed to thickening, caking, granularity, or nodularity. A dominant nodule is a significant finding, and its size, consistency, border or shape, and movability are noted; 28 per cent of Emory University breast patients had a clinically dominant mass, either solitary or multiple.

Suspicious Mass

The most suspicious mass was single, hard, fixed, or nonmovable. Of our palpable cancers 83 per cent had a single dominant mass that was palpable, whereas 3 per cent of cancers were associated with multiple masses.

Benign Mass

This is usually softer, firmer, spongier, more movable, or more discrete than a suspicious mass. The two most common benign breast masses are fibroadenomata and cysts. The fibroadenoma is a firm, often lobulated or notched, freely movable, nontender mass that varies greatly in size and number and usually occurs in younger women. It is composed of dense encapsulated components of normal breast tissue. A cyst is a localized dilatation of a duct by fluid. It may be soft and nontender or tense and quite tender, with the latter findings often fluctuating with the menstrual cycle. Cysts are usually smooth and movable but may be indistinct, being embedded in surrounding fibrocystic tissue.

Vague Mass

This is usually a part of fibrocystic disease without a dominant mass and is considered a normal variant unless one area predominates when compared with other parts of the same breast or the opposite breast; any such findings should be noted.

Nipple Changes

Retraction or Inversion

The important aspect of this finding is reliable documentation, if possible, of how long it has been present. Congenital nipple changes are not significant, but recent changes may be extremely important. Many times, particularly in older women, nipple retraction may be due to benign changes in the major subareolar ducts, but it may well be due to an underlying neoplastic disease that must be carefully searched for.

Nipple Discharge

In our series cancer was associated only with bloody or serosanguineous nipple discharge from a single duct; however, cancer can produce any type of discharge from the major ducts. Only eight of our patients presenting with bloody discharge proved to have breast cancer.

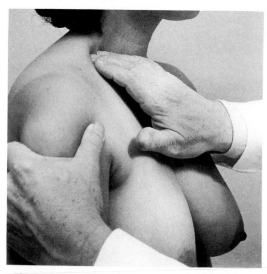

Figure 3–24. Grasp the arm near the shoulder and palpate the supraclavicular area firmly. Repeat with the other hand for the opposite side. This completes the examination of the breast. When no abnormality is found, you can assure the patient that she has completely normal breasts by physical examination.

Nipple Erosion

Erosion, scaling, or oozing of the skin of the nipple that may extend onto the areola may signal the presence of an underlying breast cancer.

Axillary Lymph Nodes

Normal

Small, firm, flat, oval (elongated), and movable nodes usually are normal. Enlarged nodes that are tender usually are associated with an inflammatory process.

Abnormal

Large, hard, rounded, or irregular and nonmovable nodes are more often associated with carcinoma of the breast or some generalized cancer.

Secondary Changes

Retraction

Demonstration of the retractive phenomenon of breast cancer is the most positive approach to the diagnosis of breast cancer clinically. It does represent relatively advanced cancer. Any skin of the breast, the nipple, the areola, a quadrant, or the whole breast may be retracted; the breast may become smaller.

Skin Thickening

The skin may become thickened to the point of "peau d'orange," like an orange peel. The skin over the carcinoma may become ulcerated. Scattered nodules of cancer (satellite nodules) may appear in the skin.

Inflammatory Carcinoma

The skin may be thickened, raised, reddened, and hot, with the breast heavy, hard, and painful. Inflammatory changes are advanced manifestations of breast cancer and indicate a very poor prognosis.

The Physical Examination

Some radiologists prefer to perform physical examinations of the breast on all their mammography patients. This has not been the author's policy owing to absence from the breast imaging center or because of the desire to assess clearly the mammographic contribution to diagnosis of breast diseases. At the patient's or technologist's request, however, it has always been done. We adamantly required the referring physician to be responsible for the clinical examination of the breast. Yet the physical examination is very helpful in that it supplies additional information about the patient's breasts so that the entire mammographic examination can be better performed with special attention to particular areas of interest. It may lead to the use of supplementary views that make a difference between the correct and a missed diagnosis. In our center the technologist is given a complete understanding of the clinical problems and the manifestation of breast cancer and supplies the necessary information to the radiologist. Clinical examination provides an invaluable means of obtaining data for identifying the high-risk breast cancer patients.

Breast Embryology, Anatomy, and Physiology

The constantly changing breast of an individual throughout her life in relation to the cyclic changes of menses, the altered physiology and anatomy during pregnancy and lactation, and the progressive factor of aging make very difficult the task of describing the normal anatomy and physiology of the breast. This is compounded by the lack of definition of the normal, the variant of normal, and borderlines of neoplasia such as fibrocystic disease.

There are wide variations in the clinical appearance and texture as well as the imaged appearance of the normal breasts of different individuals at different times. Varying appearances may occur in one breast of a patient as compared with the other and in different areas of the same breast, emphasizing the functional nature of the organ. Specific changes may be associated with puberty, the menstrual cycle, pregnancy, lactation, and postlactation involution. The regular hormone influences, especially during menopause, malnutrition, or debilitating disease, may lead to unpredictable alterations of the breast.

A clear tridimensional concept of the normal structures of the breast is necessary to categorize any variations into the subtle common variations, discrete benign changes, and the wide-scale evolution of some of these benign changes through the gamut of hyperplasia, in situ carcinoma, and the various manifestations of malignancy.

The challenge of understanding breast appearances is compounded by differing characteristics of the whole breast as imaged by x-ray or ultrasound and the structures as depicted in preparations of varying thicknesses of breast tissue for gross, subgross, or microscopic study. Thus, many types of images and breast tissue studies are needed to enhance the clinical, radiographic/sonographic, and pathologic features of the breast.

EMBRYOLOGY

The "milk line" is seen in the six-week embryo as an invaginating bandlike ectodermal thickening extending from each axilla to the inguinal region (Fig. 4–1). By the tenth week there is further invagination. By the fourth month an outpouching is seen. The epithelium of the pectoral portion, which is deep in the connective tissue, remains, whereas other areas of this band of tissue normally undergo regression, unless it persits to produce supermammary breasts. By the sixth month ducts are forming, and by

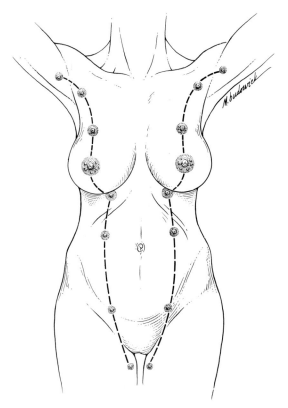

Figure 4–1. Bilateral milk lines. Breast tissue with a nipple, a nipple only, or breast tissue only can occur at any point along this line.

the tenth month the rudimentary ducts are fully developed. These ducts extend into the fat pad and sit on the pectoralis major muscle. At birth, owing to the effect of maternal hormones, these vestigial ducts may be prominent and produce drops of "witch's milk" for several days. In the male the ducts regress, leaving only the nipple and areola apparent, often as a depression. In the female, there are varying periods of relative inactivity, but the epithelial shafts slowly elongate and branch (Fig. 4–2). The process is speeded up prior to puberty and at puberty is greatly accelerated. Much of the shaping of the breasts at this stage is caused by the accumulation of fat. Even at puberty acini have not yet developed. During the adolescent period, usually between the ninth and thirteenth years of age, breast growth is accelerated and continues until sexual maturity. During adolescence one breast may grow faster than the other but by menarche they usually are the same size.

Budlike glandular structures, the acini, grow from the end of ducts during pregnancy in preparation for secretion of milk during delivery. When lactation ceases, the acini disappear and the glandular elements again consist only of the branching ducts. Following the menopause the glandular tissue grad-

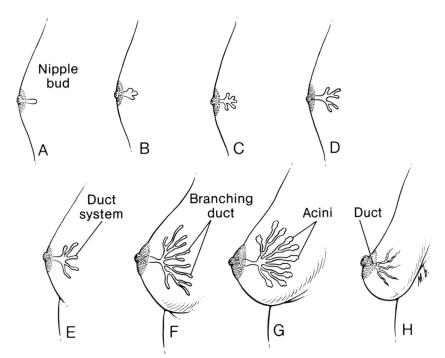

Figure 4–2. Infolding ectoderm. *A,* At 6 weeks is the beginning of the breast, a skin appendage tumor similar to a sweat gland. *B,* 12 weeks. *C,* Late fetus. *D,* At birth. *E,* Prepubertal. *F,* Mature breast. *G,* Lactating breast. *H,* Postmenopausal atrophic breast.

ually atrophies and becomes less prominent. The maintenance of the shape of the breast is due largely to the accumulation of varying amounts of fat as the glandular tissue atrophies.

ANATOMY AND HISTOLOGY

The breasts (mammae, mammary glands) are two large, hemispheric eminences lying within the superficial fascia and situated on the front and sides of the chest. Each extends from the second rib (level of the clavicle) above to the sixth rib below, and from the side of the sternum to near the midaxillary line (Fig. 4–3). Their weight and dimensions vary at different periods of life and in different individuals. They are small prior to puberty, enlarge with generative organ development, increase in size during pregnancy and especially after delivery, and become atrophic in old age. The left breast is generally larger than the right. The deep surface of each is nearly circular, flattened, or slightly

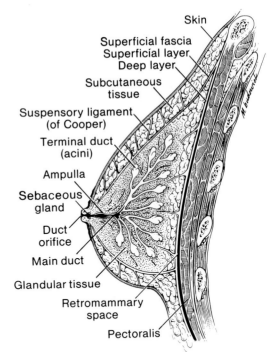

Figure 4–4. Glandular and supporting framework of the breast. The drawing is of 1 cm breast tissue sections, fixed in methylsalicylate and studied by transillumination.

concave, and each has its long axis directed toward the axilla.

The junction of the inferior portion of the breast with the chest wall is referred to as the inframammary crease; that portion extending outward and upward toward the axilla is the tail or axillary prolongation of the breast. In some patients, the breast tissue may extend laterally beyond the midaxillary line or be contiguous with its mate over the sternum.

The mammary gland forms a cone with its base at the chest wall and its apex at the nipple. During mammography the breast may flow or be flattened into a hemisphere, but during sonography in the prone water path technique it maintains this conical shape. It is located between the superfical and deep layers of the superficial fascia. In location, structure, and development it resembles a sweat gland. The superficial layer of fascia, separated from the skin by 0.5 to 2.5 cm of subcutaneous fat and areolar tissue, forms an irregular boundary for the anterior surface of the glandular tissue (Fig. 4–4). In a three-dimensional fashion, tentacle-like prolongations of fibrous tissue extend from this fascia to the skin to surround lobules of subcutaneous fat in forming the suspensory

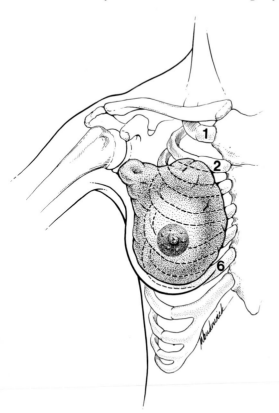

Figure 4–3. On the chest wall the breast extends from the second to sixth ribs and from the lateral border of the sternum to the midaxillary line. The long axis is toward the axilla, the tail of Spence.

ligaments of the breast (Cooper's ligaments). Thin linear strands, the retinaculae cutis, extend from these prolongations of the superficial fascia to become anchored in the skin. No distinct layer of subcutaneous fat is seen beneath the nipple. In the subareolar area, the superficial layer of the superficial fascia is intimately associated with the skin. Posteriorly, the breast is bounded by the deep layer of superficial fascia, separated from the superficial layer of deep fascia by the retromammary space, which contains fat and loose areolar tissue. The anatomic structures usually identified on the mammogram are shown in Figure 4–4. This would correspond to a longitudinal breast sonography scan through the nipple or to a mediolateral mammogram.

Major Ducts

In the adult mammary gland there are 15 to 20 irregular lobes, converging to the nipple, separated by thin fibrous septa that are irregular and poorly defined. Each lobe is drained by its own lactiferous duct (Fig. 4–5). On cross sections of the nipple each major duct can be seen, 2 to 4.5 mm in diameter, lined by stratified squamous epithelium. The ducts end in a local dilatation beneath the areola, the sinus lactiferus. Each duct is constricted as it passes to the summit of the nipple and ends as an independent opening, 0.4 to 0.7 mm in diameter; or several ducts may join below the summit of the nipple and drain through a common orifice. Thus, the excretory ducts may be as few as six to eight.

Distention of the subareolar ducts with inspissated secretions and epithelial debris is considered a normal anatomic variant (Figs. 4–6 to 4–9).

Some dilatation of the major subareolar ducts can be seen on most breast sonograms. This may be diffuse or localized thickening. A tubular dilated duct may extend into a cystic dilatation. Debris may produce internal echoes.

Nipple and Areola

Breast nipples may be erect, flat, or retracted. Slight indentations in the summit of the nipple are produced by the orifices of the lactiferous ducts. The sides of the nipple are irregular because of crevices in the epithelium into which ducts of sebaceous glands enter (Fig. 4–10). The nipple is located in the center of the areola, if in profile, where the normal skin thickness of 0.5 to 1.5 mm may appear on the mammogram to increase, either abruptly or gradually, to 1 to 5 mm (Fig. 4–11). Since the areola is saucer-shaped, variations of projection produce this apparent variation of the skin thickness on the x-ray, although histologically the skin of the areola is no thicker than the remaining skin of the breast. The apparent variability of the areolar skin thickness on mammograms is symmetric about the nipple. The areola is not recognized on sonography. The glands of Montgomery produce tiny excrescences on the areola. Several hair shafts may be present about the areola.

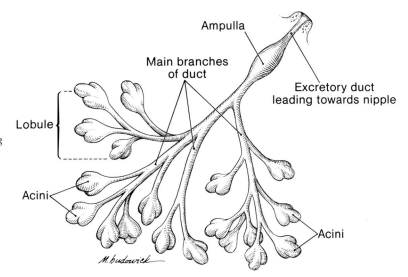

Figure 4–5. Schematic drawing of a complete lobe of the breast.

Ampulla

Main branches of duct

Excretory duct leading towards nipple

Lobule

Acini

Acini

M. budowick

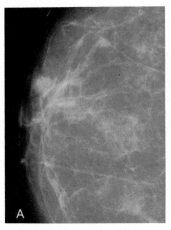

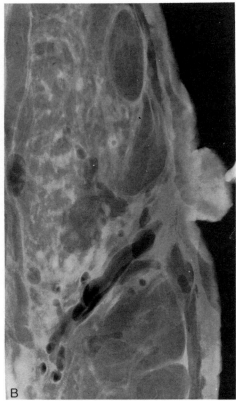

Figure 4–6. *A*, Local dilatation of a major subareolar duct in a 68-year-old woman studied for large fatty breasts. *B*, Dilatation of major ducts, one of which is cut longitudinally. The superficial layer of superficial fascia is well shown in the lower half of the illustration, and two large deposits of fat are entrapped in the upper half.

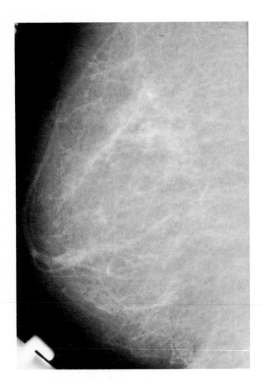

Figure 4–7. Elongated, dilated duct. Baseline study of a 63-year-old woman. (A vein is superimposed.)

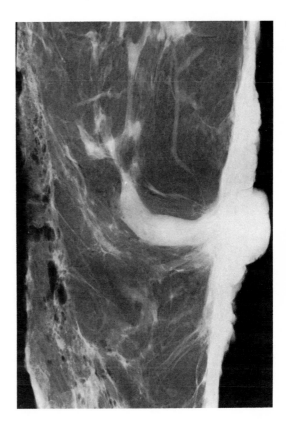

Figure 4–8. Blunt dilatation of major subareolar ducts in a 75-year-old woman with carcinoma. Whole-organ slicer radiograph: wide dilatation for a short distance, tapered end, then local dilatation. The ducts produce the only density in this area.

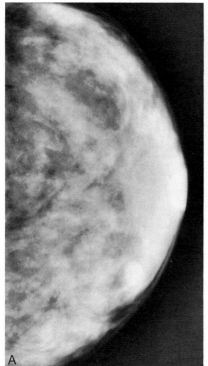

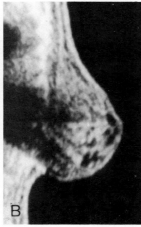

Figure 4–9. Duct ectasia. A 48-year-old woman followed for benign biopsy 17 years previously. *A*, Mammography: dense fibroglandular tissue, paucity of subcutaneous fat, near-homogeneous density of subareolar area. *B*, Sonography: The subareolar density is made up of a collection of ducts with ectasia.

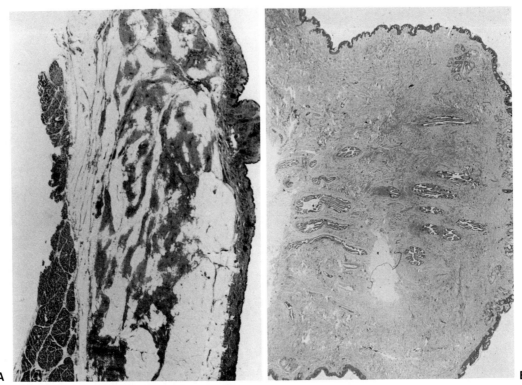

Figure 4–10. A, Radiograph of a 5 mm slicer section of the breast at nipple level. Major ducts are surrounded by compact fibromuscular tissues of the nipple. This density lessens sharply as the ducts fan out from the base of the nipple. B, Longitudinal section of the nipple showing major ducts, ampullae, and surrounding compact dense tissue. Note abrupt change of density at the base of the nipple.

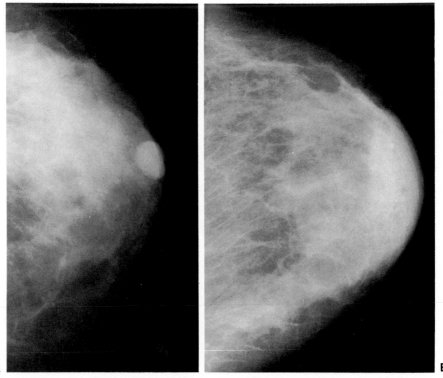

Figure 4–11. Craniocaudad mammogram with nipple off profile (A) and in profile (B).

Skin

Variations in thickness of the breast skin between large and small breasts may be especially apparent on the mammograms. The small breasts usually are firmer and do not lie as flat on the film holder. More skin in the smaller arc traversed by the tangential x-ray beam shows a denser band of skin on the radiograph. The large breast lies flatter, and, in effect, at the periphery the x-ray beam traverses a more parallel plane through the skin. Sonographic scans of the breast normally do not show any skin thickening.

With age the skin atrophies and may contribute to the apparent variation in thickness on the mammograms. On sonography, atrophic skin may readily wrinkle and interfere with good imaging. Near the inframammary crease, there is actual skin thickening because the pendant breast compresses this portion of the skin for 1 to 1.5 cm from the chest wall.

Fibroglandular Tissue

The essential parts of the mammary gland are the functional elements, or the parenchyma, and the supporting structures, or the stroma (Fig. 4–12). The walls of the secretory portions, the alveolar ducts and alveoli, consist of a row of low columnar cells. Myoepithelial cells are arranged near their bases. These myoepithelial cells, which associate the breast morphologically with sweat glands, have the capacity to become a functional part of the breast or to assume the role of fibrous supporting tissue. Connective tissue surrounds the ducts.

Many of the internal echoes of the breast on the sonogram are from the fibrous sheaths that produce compartments, imperfectly separate the lobes, and have prolongations that interdigitate with both the superficial and the deep layers of the superficial fascia. This interlobular connective tissue is dense and produces the interface with fat and other less dense tissues. The fibrous sheaths, along with the ducts, are the supporting framework and in the dependent portion of the breast are well developed. Since the sheaths form conical structures with irregular compartments of diminishing volume toward the nipple, they will never in their entire course be tangential to the x-ray beam. As a result, they project as incomplete lines.

The intralobular connective tissue immediately surrounds the ducts and is referred to as pericanalicular or periacinous. It consists of many cells and contains few collagenous fibers and little fat. Because this layer of loose connective tissue functions as a distensible medium for hypertrophy of the epithelial portions of the gland during pregnancy and lactation, it is considered a portion of the parenchyma despite its fibrous nature. The anatomic division between stroma and parenchyma is the basement membrane of the ducts. The intralobular connective tissue is beyond this basement membrane, but because it responds to hormonal influences and participates in cyclic changes usually associated with the parenchyma, it is considered parenchymal. The stroma consists of the dense, collagenous, interlobular connective tissue, containing the large blood vessels, nerves, lymphatics, and varying amounts of adipose tissue. This connective tissue produces the poorly defined septa between the lobules and lobes of the gland.

Thus, the three main tissues of the breast are fatty, fibrous, and ductal elements. On mammography fat is more radiolucent,

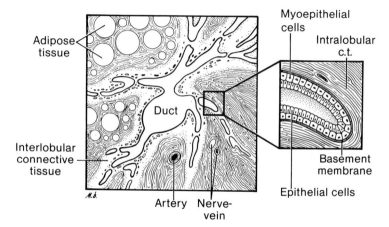

Figure 4–12. Microscopic appearance of the essential histologic elements of the mammary gland. The intralobular connective tissue is in the lighter area surrounding the ducts. The myoepithelial cells are schematically depicted. (After Maximow and Bloom.)

Adipose tissue

Interlobular connective tissue

Duct

Artery Nerve-vein

Myoepithelial cells

Intralobular c.t.

Basement membrane

Epithelial cells

whereas glandular and fibrous tissues have the same density. A corresponding sonographic density is present.

The trabeculae or striae, which converge toward the nipple, consist of both parenchymal elements of ducts and stromal elements of interlobular connective tissue. As the duct components and connective tissue components of these shadows are inseparable, "trabeculae" is a convenient descriptive term.

Veins

The veins of the breast vary considerably in arrangement and size in different individuals but are usually symmetric in the same individual. The superficial veins are seen clearly on photographs taken with infrared light (Figs. 4–13 and 4–14). On the mammogram, they are even more clearly outlined because of surrounding fat. They are not seen on sonography. The superficial veins follow one of two general patterns. In the longitudinal arrangement the veins converge near the sternal border and join the perforating veins, which empty into the internal mammary chain. In the transverse arrangement the veins converge near the suprasternal notch and drain into the lower neck veins, which empty into the anterior jugular veins. The infrared photographs also reveal that

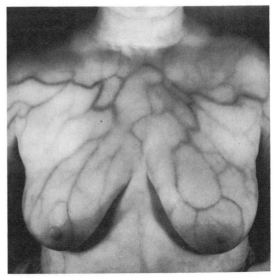

Figure 4–14. Transverse pattern shows converging veins near the sternal borders. (Used by permission of Massoput and Gardner.)

veins of one breast may anastomose with those of the other at the midline over the sternum. The course of the veins within the breast is readily followed on mammograms. The caliber of the veins at the point of anastomosis under the areola is several millimeters in diameter, which may explain the ease of spread of carcinoma in the directions of drainage of these anastomotic veins.

The deep veins of the breast are divided into three main groups (Haagensen, 1971): (1) those that empty into the internal mammary vein and are the largest veins of the breast; (2) those that empty into the axillary vein and are more variable in their size and arrangement; and (3) those that empty into the intercostal veins (Fig. 4–15). Direct communication with systemic veins is established through the azygos veins. There is also direct anastomosis with the vertebral system of veins by the azygous route.

Arteries

The main arterial blood supply to the mammary gland is from the perforating branches of the internal mammary artery. Additional blood supply is from the thoracic branches of the axillary artery and from the intercostal arteries (Fig. 4–16).

Lymphatics

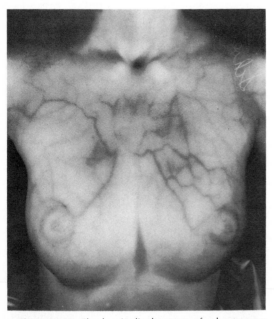

Figure 4–13. The longitudinal pattern of subcutaneous veins of the breast, shown converging near the suprasternal notch and outlined by infrared photography. (Used by permission of Massoput and Gardner.)

The lymphatics in the breast are located as three systems: (1) immediately periductal and

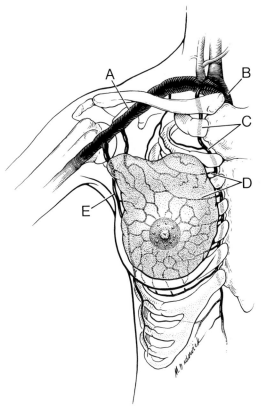

Figure 4–15. Deep veins of the breast. *A,* Axillary vein. *B,* Innominate vein. *C,* Internal mammary vein. *D,* Perforating branches of the internal mammary. *E,* Thoracodorsal vein.

outer and upper quadrants. They may or may not be associated with breast cancer and may or may not contain metastatic cancer cells. With the axilla proximal, metastasis to these nodes may be distal, that is, in a direction away from the axilla. In whole-organ studies, such nodes occur in approximately one fourth of the breasts studied for carcinoma and are positive in three fourths of the cases. The intramammary node may be positive and the axillary lymph nodes positive or negative, with the reverse holding for positive axillary lymph nodes. These nodes are readily differentiated from a focus of cancer by identification of residual lymphoid tissue in the node.

With the three-dimensional study of the breast by mammography, many confusing shadows had to be clarified in the gross and microscopic pathology laboratories. Intramammary lymph nodes were an example. In the mid-1950s, physicians and anatomists who were queried had never heard of such anatomic structures.

extending deep into the breast; (2) on the surface of the glands beneath the subcutaneous adipose tissue; and (3) immediately subcutaneous (Fig. 4–17). As far as the whole-organ studies demonstrate, the three systems probably intercommunicate only in the subareolar area, and there quite freely. Also on the whole-organ studies, intramammary lymph nodes were demonstrated in 25 percent of the breasts. To be truly intramammary and not just low axillary nodes the lymph nodes had to have glandular tissue surrounding their entirety.

Occasionally, intramammary lymph nodes are visualized on the mammograms as smoothly outlined rounded nodules with the sinus producing a notch. These are not the deep or pectoral lymph nodes referred to by surgeons but are truly intraglandular; there appears to be no systematic relation to the usually described axillary lymphatic chains of lymph nodes. They may be located in any section of the breast but usually are in the

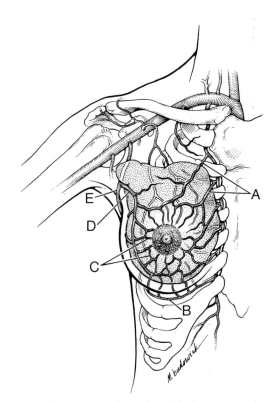

Figure 4–16. Arterial supply of the breast. *A* and *B,* Anterior perforating branches of the internal mammary artery. *C,* Areolar arterial anastomosis. *D,* Branch of lateral thoracic artery. *E,* Lateral thoracic artery.

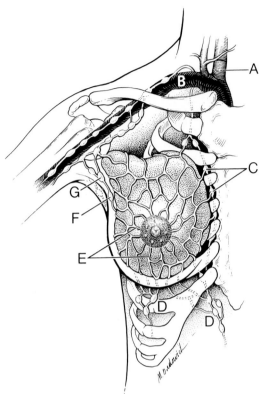

Figure 4–17. Lymphatic drainage of the breast. *A*, Jugular vein. *B*, Subclavian vein. *C*, Internal mammary lymphatics. *D*, Abdominal lymphatics. *E*, Circumareolar lymphatics (plexus of Sappey). *F*, Low axillary node. *G*, Central or midaxillary lymph nodes.

RADIOGRAPHIC APPEARANCE

The mammary gland projects as a triangle on the mammograms. Within this triangle and separated from the skin by varying amounts of the more radiolucent adipose tissue is a dense triangular pattern, with the base toward the chest, composed of glandular tissue and lactiferous ducts with their connective tissue sheaths extending to the nipple. A very similar pattern is projected onto the sonograms.

There are three major types of breast tissue seen on breast imaging: fibrous, glandular, and adipose. Since the fibrous and glandular tissue have nearly the same Z number (approximately 7), they cannot be separated adequately on the mammogram or the sonogram, and, as they are anatomically intimately associated, the term "fibroglandular tissue" best describes these structures. Adipose tissue, with a Z number of approximately 6, is more radiolucent then fibroglandular tissue and provides the necessary contrast on the mammograms, while producing a disrupted echo pattern on the sonograms.

The relative amounts of fat and fibroglandular tissue characterize primarily the breast types and influence the diagnostic accuracy of mammography. During the reproductive years, there is usually a predominance of fibroglandular tissue, with perhaps equal amounts of adipose and fibroglandular tissue at menopause; after menopause, the fibroglandular tissue is steadily replaced by adipose tissue. Generally, the more fat in the breast, the lesser the contribution of sonography to breast imaging.

The subcutaneous layer of adipose tissue between the superficial layer of superficial fascia and the skin in some breasts is extremely small, particularly in the young pubertal or virginal breast and in the breast containing marked fibroplasia. Whole-organ studies have established a definite cleavage plane (see Chapter 11) at the level of this upper layer of superficial fascia, beyond which the main body of glandular tissue does not extend. Small segments of glandular tissue may extend for a short distance in a sawtooth fashion between prolongation of the suspensory ligaments toward the skin. These extensions could be of importance in an attempted thorough subcuticular mastectomy, as one could leave islands of tissue behind with a thick flap of skin. Usually by the time a woman approaches the premenopausal stage, when serious breast problems are more common, there is at least an average of 1 cm thickness of gland-free subcutaneous adipose tissue.

On the craniocaudad view the dense inner triangle composed of glandular tissue (Fig. 4–18) produces varying degrees of diffuse opacity; the contrast is dependent upon the amount of fat present. A reticular appearance is caused by the stroma or connective tissue framework, which may be nearly homogeneous in the very dense virginal breast. In the less dense breast, intermediate degrees of fatty deposition, ducts, and trabeculae are clearly outlined. The fatty atrophic gland may have a nearly homogeneous ground-glass appearance, with few ducts and trabeculae obvious, or it may have a prominent trabecular pattern superimposed on the fatty background.

The craniocaudad mammogram corresponds to the transverse sonogram of the breast. One must visualize numerous tomographic sonographic scans (usually taken at

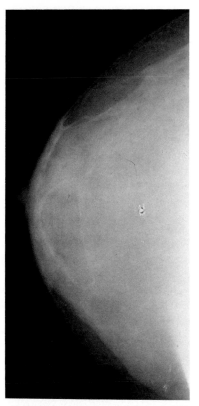

Figure 4–18. Normal craniocaudad view of 33-year-old woman studied for cancerophobia. Shown are the skin, the nipple, the subcutaneous adipose tissues, the areola projecting symmetrically about the nipple, and the triangular pattern of glandular tissue.

with a lobulated appearance. The upper border of the glandular tissue is less distinctly outlined against the subcutaneous fat. A sawtooth pattern is often produced if the glandular tissue is supported at unequal levels by the suspensory ligaments. The suspensory ligaments may not be well developed and may end as thin prolongations in the skin. With progressive fatty deposition, the appearance of the upper portion of the breast is similar to that of the craniocaudad view, with the inferior trabeculae prominent in their convex pattern. A ground-glass appearance results from almost complete fatty replacement when accompanied by atrophy of the interlobular connective tissue. This is not constant, however, as women in their nineties may have prominent trabeculae. Glandular tissue near the inframammary crease usually has smooth margins. The upper posterior glandular tissue may contain irregular fatty infiltration, which causes a thin prolongation of tissue toward the axilla, apparently separate from the main portion of breast

an average of 2 mm apart) superimposed to produce the craniocaudad mammogram. As the scans proceed through the superior aspect of the breast to the inframammary crease, varying amounts of subcutaneous fat, intramammary fat, and fibroglandular tissue will be demonstrated. Some structures, such as the veins seen on mammography, will not be identified on sonography. Yet the sonograms closely correspond anatomically with the mammograms and gross sections of the breast.

The reticular pattern is almost entirely replaced on the mediolateral or oblique mammogram by gross striation composed of the ducts, their associated connective tissues, and the trabeculae (Fig. 4–19). These supporting structures course fairly straight toward the nipple in the upper portion of the breast but are concave in the lower portion of the breast. In this projection, the lower border of the glandular tissue has a smooth convex outline, caused by the weight of the gland on the supporting strands, perhaps

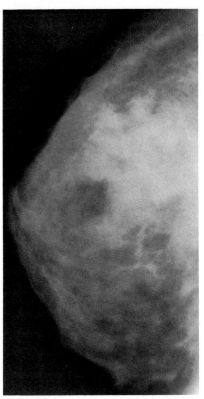

Figure 4–19. Normal mediolateral view of 19-year-old woman student studied for possible breast lump. Note the more gross striations and the sawtooth pattern in the upper breast produced by the glandular tissue being supported at unequal levels by the suspensory ligaments.

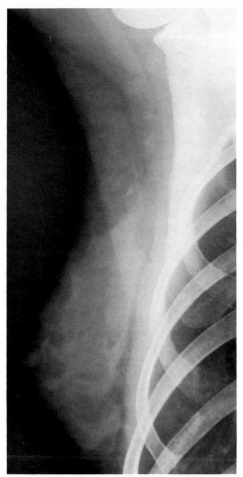

Figure 4–20. Axillary view. On the axillary view, the axilla and axillary prolongation of the breast are seen. Small normal axillary nodes may be seen on occasion as well as muscle planes outlined by fat in the axilla.

CHRONOLOGIC AND PHYSIOLOGIC BREAST CHANGES

On mammography there is a wide variation in the appearance of the breasts in different women or in the same woman at different stages of her life. At present there is a less distinct classification of parenchymal breast tissue patterns by sonography than by mammography, but comparisons can still be useful. Although there is a relationship between the age of the patient and the x-ray appearance of the breast, it is inconsistent. The breasts of a young adult, especially after several pregnancies, may have the same appearance as the breasts of a premenopausal woman. The breasts of a nulliparous menopausal patient may contain the same type of dense glandular tissue that so often is associated with the young adult. It is convenient to use categories that imply chronologic and physiologic development of the mammary gland. There is, of course, wide variation and subtle overlapping of these categories: (1)

tissue and completely surrounded by fat. This tissue prolongation may appear to be an irregular mass and thus suggest carcinoma, but close scrunity will show a pattern of involuting glandular tissue with faint trabecular connections to the remaining gland.

Glandular tissue that extends into the axilla is easily identified on the axillary view. This glandular tissue is important in differentiation of primary breast carcinoma from enlarged axillary nodes (Fig. 4–20). Axillary nodes varying in size from 0.5 to 1.0 cm, of no apparent clinical significance, may be outlined by the fat in the axilla.

The longitudinal breast sonogram corresponds to the mediolateral or oblique mammogram in the same way as the craniocaudad mammogram is related to the transverse sonogram.

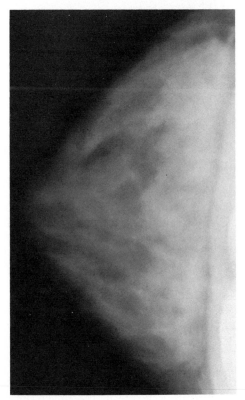

Figure 4–21. Pubertal breast. This 13-year-old girl presented with one breast slightly larger than the other. Near-homogeneous glandular tissue with a paucity of fat and a thin layer of adipose tissue separate this glandular tissue from the skin.

pubertal, (2) virginal, (3) young adult, (4) premenopausal, (5) menopausal, (6) post-menopausal, (7) atrophic, (8) pregnant, and (9) lactating and postpartum (Figs. 4–21 to 4–27).

It is during the first pregnancy that there is the earliest and most marked progressive increase in size and density of the breasts, with the greatest changes occurring during the third trimester (Figs. 4–28 to 4–30). Glandular tissue fills all of the central portion of the breast. Most of the radiolucent adipose tissue disappears, and there is a reduction in the amount of subcutaneous fat. Just prior to delivery, the glandular tissue appears extremely dense, with blurred outlines and increased opacity. Scattered radiolucent areas may be seen, and the trabeculae are indistinct and wider than usual. During lactation, more radiolucent areas appear, and the overall appearance of the gland is cloudy, especially just before nursing (Fig. 4–31). These changes are less noticeable and begin later in

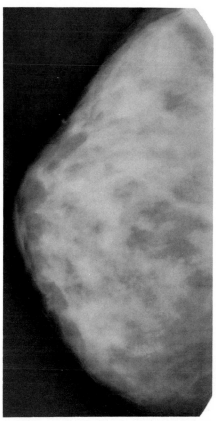

Figure 4–23. Young adult breast. This has a wide range of appearance that could represent a teenage mother or nulliparous premenopausal female. Usually there is an increase in adipose tissue as in this 23-year-old nulliparous patient without complaint in this breast.

pregnancy in grand multiparae than in women who have had fewer pregnancies. After lactation the breast begins to return to a more normal appearance (Fig. 4–32).

During the menstrual cycle there is not only subjective evidence of change in breast size but also actual change in volume by measurement, with the maximum increase occurring just prior to the onset of menstruation. On the mammogram there is no significant change in appearance or density; this increase in fullness of the breast is related to the overall retention of water by the body at this time. Since there is no change in ratio of adipose to fibroglandular tissue in the breast and each of these tissues retains proportionate amounts of fluid, the mammographic appearance is unaltered.

Slight variations in the appearance of the normal breast often produce distinctive patterns as prominent trabeculae (Figs. 4–33 and 4–34). A lobulated pattern may be produced by the weight of the glandular tissues on the

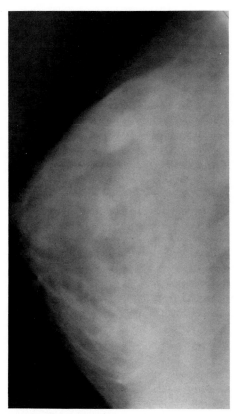

Figure 4–22. Virginal breast. Increase in size is usually the result of increased glandular tissue but very little increase in adipose tissue. This 17-year-old girl had no complaint in this breast; the skin of such small dense breasts is poorly seen on the mediolateral view.

Text continued on page 50

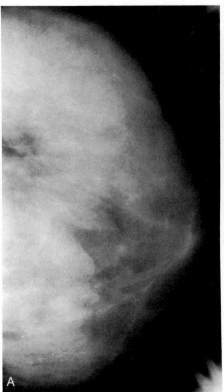

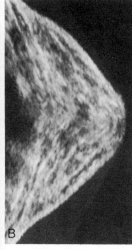

Figure 4–24. Premenopausal breast. This also has a wide range of appearance but usually shows increased fatty deposition. A 45-year-old patient, gravida 2, para 2, routine checkup without complaints. *A*, Mammography. *B*, Sonography.

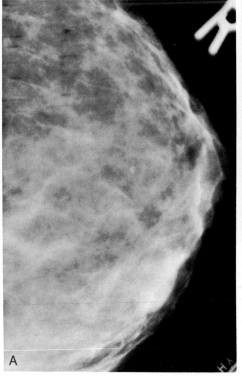

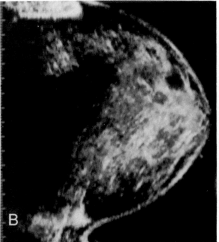

Figure 4–25. Menopausal breast. There is considerable overlap in this age group, but generally there is progressive replacement of fibroglandular tissue with adipose tissue both by increase in amount of subcutaneous fat and by fatty infiltration of the glandular tissue. A 47-year-old woman, gravida 3, para 3, normal menstrual history until recent irregular menses. *A*, Mammography. *B*, Sonography.

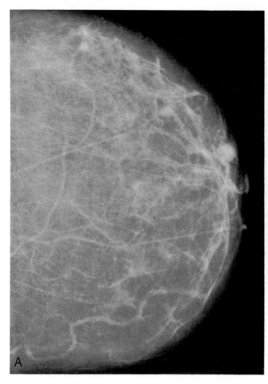

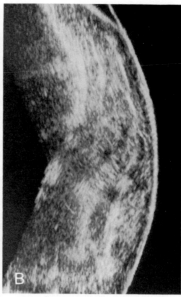

Figure 4–26. Postmenopausal breast. There is wide variation in this group, but usually replacement of all the fibroglandular tissue has occurred. The fat then clearly outlines the major ducts, trabeculae, and veins. A 69-year-old woman seen for routine mammogram. A, and B, Sonography.

Figure 4–27. Atrophic breast. The trabeculae as well as other structures may be sharply outlined, as above, or there may be nearby homogeneous ground-glass appearance indicating almost complete replacement of all structures by fatty tissue. A 77-year-old woman with a questionable lump in the opposite breast.

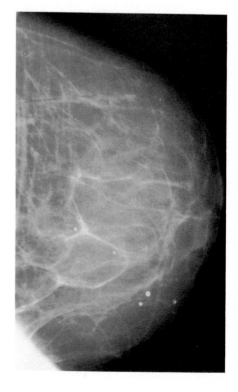

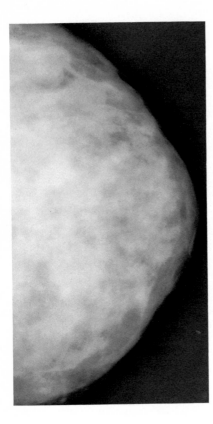

Figure 4–28. Breast at two and one-half months of pregnancy. Much variation exists with relation to the length of pregnancy and the number of previous pregnancies. As the changes of pregnancy progress, the glandular tissue becomes prominent, ill defined, and increasingly opaque. There is also loss of subcutaneous tissue. This patient was 23 years old, gravida 3, para 2.

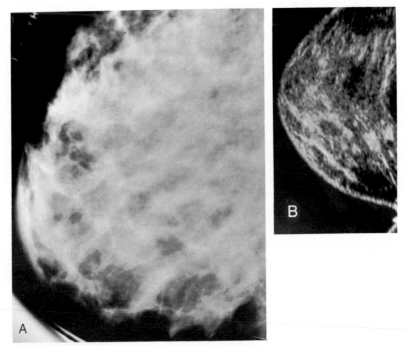

Figure 4–29. Four months of pregnancy. A 37-year-old patient studied for a vague nodule. *A,* Mammography. *B,* Sonography.

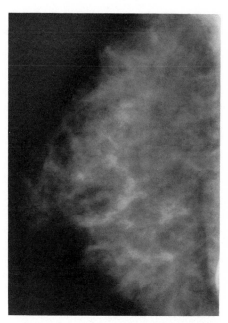

Figure 4–30. Pregnant breast. As pregnancy advances the glandular tissue becomes more prominent, fluffy, or ill defined with loss of clear edges, and there is an overall increase in breast density as the fat is replaced. Lactation preserves most of these changes. A 23-year-old seven-months-pregnant woman with vague nodule of the opposite breast.

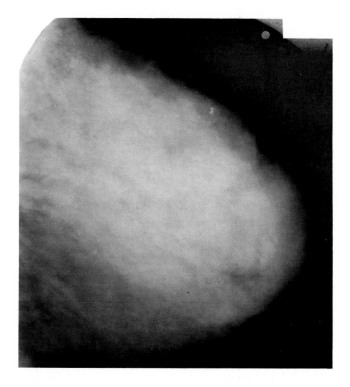

Figure 4–31. Lactating breast. This type has more glandular tissue, increased vascularity, and fluffy densities with interposed radiolucent areas. The density of the glandular tissue is more noticeable just prior to nursing. A 36-year-old black female, gravida 8, para 6, lactating for one year; questionable nodule in the other breast.

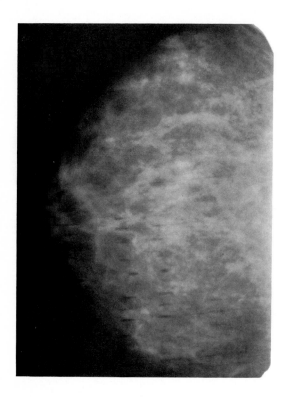

Figure 4–32. Postpartum breast. A 34-year-old white female, gravida 4, para 4, two weeks following normal delivery; no attempt to nurse; questionable nodule in the opposite breast.

Figure 4–33. Prominent trabeculae in a postmenopausal breast. This 69-year-old woman had mammography to study her large breasts. As opposed to the ground-glass appearance of the fatty senile breast, the trabecular pattern remains marked against a fatty involution.

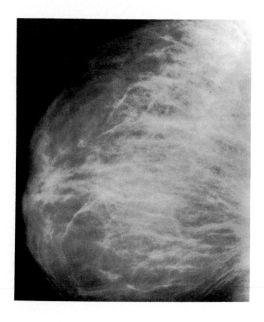

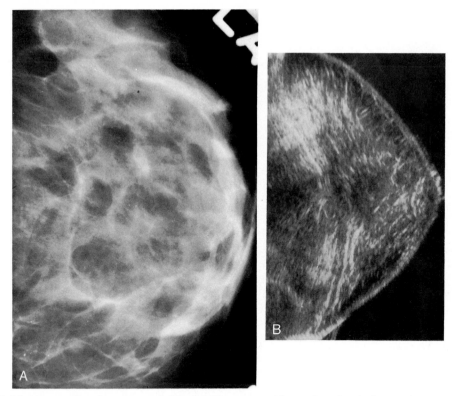

Figure 4–34. Heavy trabecular pattern. A 34-year-old woman with a subareolar thickening for two months. *A*, Mammography: mild subareolar fibrosis with dense trabeculae. *B*, Sonography: high-level distorted echoes from the fat surrounded by heavy trabeculae.

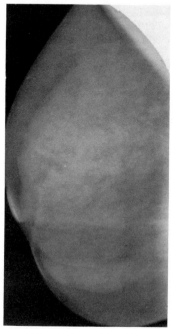

Figure 4–35. Lobulated breast tissue. A 65-year-old white female with normal pregnancies, menses, and menopause; questionable mass in the opposite breast.

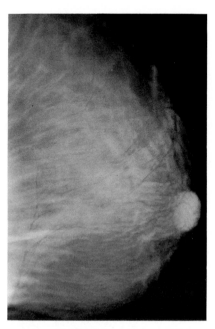

Figure 4–36. Wrinkled skin. A 67-year-old black female with recent 25 lb weight loss to 104 lb, admitted with carcinoma of the esophagus and vague nodularities in the breast.

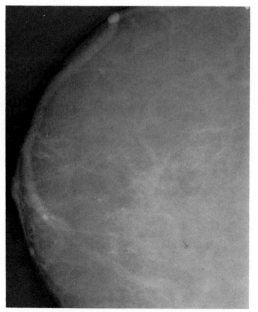

Figure 4–37. Large, but normal, veins. A 63-year-old white female with vague complaints. Large veins in both breasts; followed for five years without evidence of breast disease.

suspensory ligaments (Fig. 4–35). Wrinkled skin may interfere with good studies (Fig. 4–36). Large veins are no problem if symmetric (Fig. 4–37). Normal fibroglandular tissues may appear masslike or even cystic (Fig. 4–38). Often one breast is larger, or placed higher or lower on the chest wall, than its mate. Fibroplasia also makes good studies

difficult (Fig. 4–39). Entrapped fat is more confusing clinically and sonographically than radiographically (Fig. 4–40). Occasionally a protruding rib may be confusing clinically (Fig. 4–41). Calcified axillary lymph nodes are hard with an unexplained etiology clinically (Fig. 4–42).

CONTRACEPTIVE PILL EFFECT

To many women oral contraceptives have become a way of life; breasts of such women must then be considered normal or a variant of normal. The estrogen and progesterone component hormones affect individual women to an unpredictable degree—pain may be marked with one preparation, whereas another is readily tolerated; some patients may note no unusual changes; and some patients may not tolerate any preparations. Since these hormones are used over long periods of time, they may well influence the mammographic appearance of the breasts.

Once large numbers of mammograms of various age groups prior to the widespread use of these oral contraceptives had been viewed, it was necessary to establish a moderately reliable and objective baseline as to the usual mammographic appearance of the breast at various ages. Thus, a reliable protocol was established to assess the effects of the contraceptive pills on the mammographic

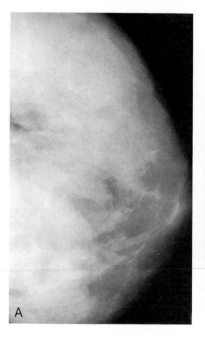

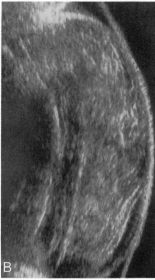

Figure 4–38. A and B, Dense nodular glandular tissues. A 27-year-old woman with the right breast larger than the left.

A

B

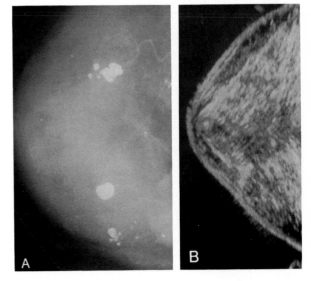

Figure 4–39. A and B, Homogeneous fibroplasia pattern. A 42-year-old woman with painful breast. Dense fibroplasia and calcifying fibroadenomata that did not shadow on sonography.

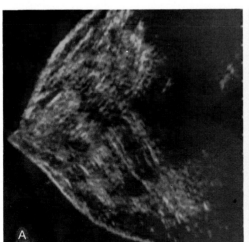

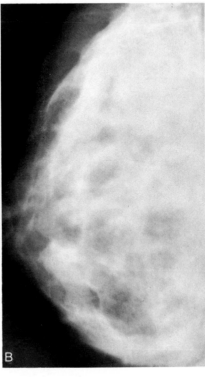

Figure 4–40. Entrapped fat. A 17-year-old with a soft movable lump UIQ of the breast. Sonography (A) revealed a poorly outlined anechoic area that was fat on mammography (B) and upon biopsy.

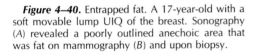

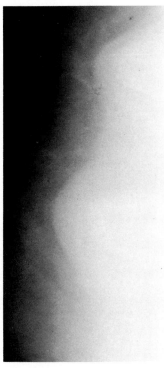

Figure 4–41. Prominent rib producing a breast "lump." A 42-year-old woman presented with a lump in her right breast. Clinically a hard area was palpated in the area of the protruding rib. Chest deformities do cause problems in clinical evaluation of the breasts and technical problems in radiography.

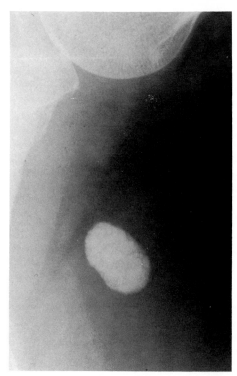

Figure 4–42. Calcified axillary lymph node. The node was palpable; the breasts were normal. The etiology of the calcified node was not apparent and the history was noncontributory. The solid calcification suggests some diffuse process within the node.

appearance of the breast. One hundred consecutive menstruating women of two categories were compared: (1) women who had not used oral contraceptives; and (2) women who had used oral contraceptives for six months or longer prior to mammography. Patients who had a previous breast cancer, who were pregnant or had lactated during the past six months, who had discontinued use of the pill, who were under age 21 years, or who were postmenopausal were excluded.

The only clinical information accompanying the mammograms was the age of the patient. After review of the mammograms a "yes" (noting use of the pill) or "no" (indicating its not being used) was simply noted (Table 4–1). Use of the contraceptive pill was correctly predicted on the mammograms in 12 of 36 women and was not predicted in 24. Of 64 women not using the pill, 31 were predicted and 33 not predicted from the mammograms.

The conclusion was reached that the use or nonuse of the contraceptive pill cannot be predicted from the mammogram by attempt-

ing to judge the increased or decreased amount of fibroglandular tissue expected for the particular age of the woman. This is similar to the inability to predict the state of the menstrual cycle by mammography. The relative amounts of fibroglandular tissue are not affected in either instance even though the retention or nonretention of fluid may be. Since such fluid would be equally distributed in the fat and fibroglandular tissues, the relative amounts of these tissues would not be disturbed.

ADOLESCENT BREAST

The adolescent development of the breasts usually lasts from two to four years and

TABLE 4–1. Mammographic Evaluation of 100 Consecutive Menstruating Women Who Had or Had Not Routinely Used Oral Contraceptive Pills

| Use of Pill | Mammographic Prediction | |
	Yes	No
Did use pill	12	24
Did not use pill	33	31

normally occurs between the ninth and thirteenth years of age. At this time there is an accelerated growth in the breasts of the female that continues until sexual maturity. One breast may enlarge more rapidly than the other, normally beginning at approximately the ninth year, but eventually there will be nearly equal accelerated growth in both breasts. Usually by menarche the growth has become approximately equal.

The female breast, nipple, and areola enlarge gradually during adolescence, with the fibroglandular tissue enlarging in a like fashion, while the proportion of surrounding fatty tissue gradually is reduced. The fibroglandular tissue takes on a somewhat homogeneous, dome-shaped, smooth contour that gradually expands until there is a rather thin line of radiolucent adipose tissue between the surface of the glandular tissue and the skin. Posteriorly, some lengthening and branching of the ducts may be apparent where there is less smooth contour to the surface of the gland. As fat is deposited within the fibroglandular tissue, the trabeculae become more clearly outlined. The entire process is a gradual one, not specifically related to any certain alteration in physiology, and continues as a deposition of fat until the mature type gland is formed.

Unilateral Early Ripening

Sometimes, between the sixth and eighth years of age, one breast of the female may gradually appear to have grown to 1 cm or slightly larger, with the other breast remaining clinically unchanged (Figs. 4–43 and 4–44). The parent or grandparent usually discovers this unilateral nodule, which may be tender and is usually freely movable. This marked difference in size and palpatory findings usually persists until the ninth year, when the second breast begins its normal physiologic increase in size. With this growth, both breasts become equal in size, contour, and consistency. The term "unilateral early ripening" was coined to describe this syndrome and to specify that this is a normal variation consisting of development of one breast in advance of the other. The breast should not be biopsied, as all the breast tissue would be removed, with consequent lack of development of the breast on this side. This lack of development of the breast following biopsy frequently goes unnoticed by the physician, and it is not recognized until two to four years later, as the patient frequently transfers from a pediatrician to another physician. In such cases mammography may serve to prevent the loss of a breast.

Figure 4–43. Unequal enlargement of breast. Patient was a 12-year-old girl seen prior to onset of menstruation or appearance of secondary signs of puberty. Two years later, both breasts were much enlarged but of equal size.

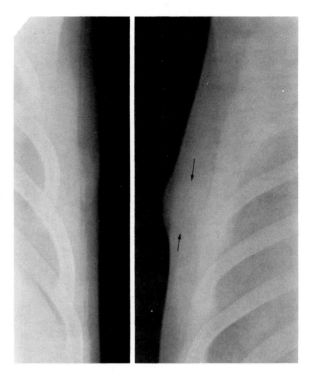

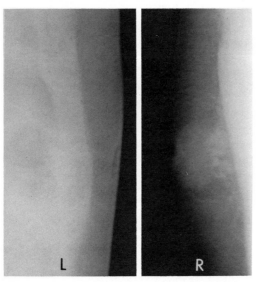

Figure 4–44. Unilateral early ripening of right breast. This eight-year-old white girl was seen for pain in the right nipple of two days' duration. Physical examination was normal, but five months later there was marked unilateral enlargement (above). As puberty was approached, both breasts became enlarged symmetrically.

ANOMALIES OF DEVELOPMENT

The postnatal engorgement of the breast and the clear or cloudy discharge subsides spontaneously unless there are repeated attempts to express the fluid. Such an ill-advised practice may lead to infection. Sporadic epidemics of neonatal breast abscess, usually caused by *Staphylococcus aureus*, occur in hospital nurseries and are extremely difficult to eradicate. Persistent hypertrophy is uncommon and may need endocrine investigation.

Amastia, absence of breast tissue, rarely occurs. Athelia, absence of nipple, is also rare and invariably accompanies amastia. Nipple inversion, or flattening, may be congenital (Figs. 4–45 and 4–46). Hypoplasia of one or both breasts may occur, also uncommonly. Breast atrophy in adolescents is usually the result of a protein-deficient diet leading to loss of fat and glandular tissue to produce the wrinkled, sagging breast of senility. Hypertrophy, often congenital, can be so extreme that surgical correction is necessary (Fig. 4–47). Extension of the breast into the axilla, as a prolongation of the tail of the breast, is common.

Supernumerary breasts occur (Fig. 4–48), or supernumerary nipples (Fig. 4–49). The nipple may be prominent (Fig. 4–50).

MALE BREAST

The infant male and female breasts are similarly slightly enlarged for several weeks, as they are under the influence of the mother's hormones at birth; witch's milk may be present. Following this hormonal influence, the male breast normally regresses to a small button of homogeneous fibroglandular tissue immediately under the nipple, surrounded by varying amounts of fat. The glandular tissue consists of vestigial main ducts surrounded by minimal fibrous tissue. During adolescence there is mild stimulation to the growth of the fibroglandular tissue, lasting no more than one to two years. During periods of increase of body fat, and especially after middle age following redeposition of

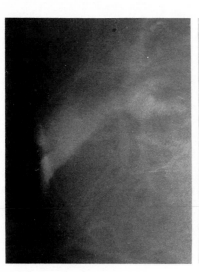

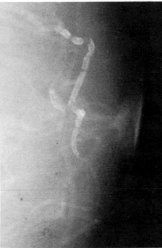

Figure 4–45. Congenital retraction of the nipple. A 67-year-old woman studied for a questionable lump in the left breast. Only arteriosclerosis was seen in this fatty breast, but nipple retraction and an enlarged duct were noted in the right breast. This nipple had been retracted "all her life."

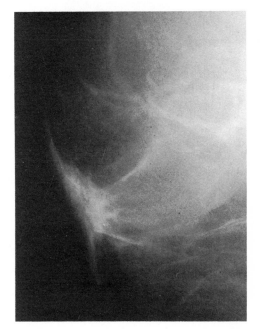

Figure 4–46. Congenital retraction of the nipple in a 62-year-old woman. This checkup study showed no abnormality in either breast. Very few subareolar changes were noted except for shortened ducts.

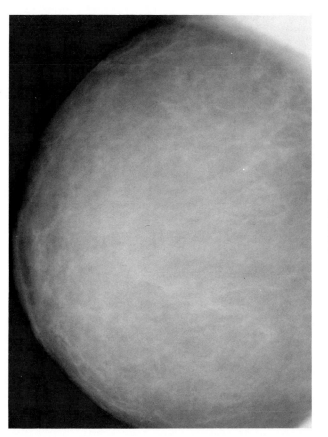

Figure 4–47. Adult hypertrophy. A 46-year-old black female without specific complaints. Clinically: massive breasts, too large to examine. Mammography: normal large breasts. The patient's mother and sisters had even larger breasts. The breast above covered the 8 × 10 inch film.

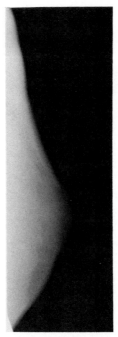

Figure 4–48. Supernumerary breast. A 57-year-old white female who was being followed after a right radical mastectomy for carcinoma. The supernumerary breast was inferior to the normally located right breast and was without evidence of disease.

the body fat, the male breast may become more prominent, with the increase in size being due to adipose tissue.

With prolonged intake of certain drugs, such as digitalis for cardiac disease or stilbestrol for prostatic cancer, and with systemic imbalance of the normal male hormones, as with cirrhosis, both the fibroglandular and the fatty tissues tend to increase and at times radiographically simulate the female breast.

Gynecomastia

Gynecomastia is a frequent occurrence in the young adult male. The mammographic appearance of the enlarged male breast most frequently is a rather smoothly rounded, fairly homogeneous density of fibroglandular tissue under the nipple and areola, surrounded by a larger area of adipose tissue. At times, however, linear extensions of branching ducts fan out in this adipose tissue and, with small areas of adipose tissue interspersed in the fibroglandular tissue, may produce an appearance similar to that of the female breast. Several aspects of fibrocystic disease may be noted on the mammograms

of such breasts; other common benign breast diseases of the female may also occur.

At times it is difficult to evaluate skin thickening in the male. In the smaller male breast, the tangential x-ray beam traverses the skin to produce apparent skin thickening, or the skin may actually be thicker in the male.

Cancer in the male accounts for 1 to 2 per cent of all breast cancers. It produces all the signs of malignancy as seen in the female, including calcification.

PHYSIOLOGY

The physiology with its resultant altered anatomy of the breast must be viewed as a continuous dynamic process from the intra-uterine development of the breast until cessation of life. During this full cycle there are many individualized specific changes related to the menstrual cycle in preparation for pregnancy and peaks of activity during pregnancy and preparation for lactation.

Cyclic Changes

The pituitary gland influences many of the hormonal changes in the breast during its

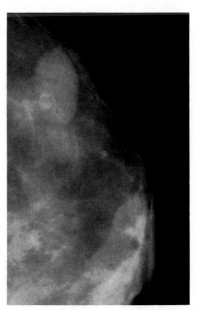

Figure 4–49. Full-sized extra nipple medial to the main nipple. The nipple was erectile but only scanty thin milky secretions were present during normal nursing periods. Very little associated ductal tissue is noted.

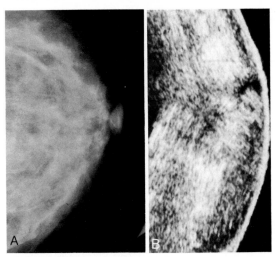

Figure 4–50. A, Prominent nipple producing an air pocket on sonography. This 51-year-old woman had lumpy breasts with prominent nipples. B, Sonography: Even with compression an air pocket persisted about the nipple. This, and the air over a retracted nipple, may be corrected with application of petroleum jelly.

cycles (Fig. 4–51). By the end of the first trimester, estrogen (testosterone in the male) has made sex differentiation apparent. Except for a few postnatal days, when withdrawal of the maternal hormones may allow prolactin to stimulate the mammary tissues to secrete "witch's milk," a latent phase of hormonal activity continues until puberty. Gonadotropin hormones then stimulate production of pituitary follicle-stimulating hormone (FSH) and luteinizing hormone (LH). The follicular maturation ensues with production of estradiol-17-β. Just prior to establishment of the balance between the hypothalamus, pituitary, and ovary that regulates the menstrual cycle, the breasts are stimulated at first largely by estrogen. During these anovulatory cycles, the duct system elongates and branches, fat deposition occurs, and the intralobular connective tissue increases. With the onset of ovulation the acinar structures are influenced by progesterone from the corpus luteum.

Fullness and tenderness of the breasts is usual during the premenstrual phase of the normal menstrual cycle. The breast volume is enlarged by increased blood flow and water retention in the tissues. This is enhanced by estrogen stimulating parenchymal proliferation preparatory to acinar formation, progesterone inducing ductal engorgement with epithelial cells that extend into acinar

cells if pregnancy occurs; prolactin causes fat droplets to appear in these cells.

Toward the end of the menstrual cycle these changes regress, to recur during the next cycle. These repeated episodes of proliferations, and with never complete regressions, result in physiologic changes that produce the essentially normal syndrome of fibrocystic disease. The concept of multiple tissue response in the breast is pertinent to the understanding of fibrocystic disease, in which at least five fairly distinct changes occur at different rates and in only approximate sequence. These are ductal dilatation and cyst formation, lobular hyperplasia, stromal fibrosis, lymphocytic infiltration, and ductal epithelial hyperplasia or metaplasia.

Pregnancy and Lactation

There is a massive increase in maternal and placental steroids during pregnancy.

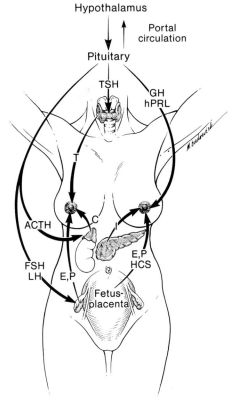

Figure 4–51. Hormonal influences on the breast: T, thyroxin; I, insulin; C, cortisol; P, progesterone; E, estrogen; HCS, human chorionic somatomammotropin; FSH, follicle-stimulating hormone; LH, luteinizing hormone; ACTH, adrenal corticotrophic hormone; TSH, thyroid-stimulating hormone; GH, growth hormone; hPRL, human prolactin.

Prolactin increases to inhibit steroid effect on the hypothalamus. Human chorionic somatomammotropin appears at the fifth gestational week as a lactogen. Estrogens suppress lactation. Free cortisol and insulin are increased. Marked ductal, lobular, and acinar changes precede delivery and lactation.

After parturition there again is a marked change in the milieu, with the sudden withdrawal of placental hormones that had suppressed galactopoiesis. Previously elevated levels of prolactin decline but are transiently elevated by the neurosensory effect of suckling on the hypothalamus and pituitary. While prolactin is necessary for the synthesis and secretion of milk, a prerequisite for lactation is the presence of cortisol, thyroxine, insulin, and parathormone. Ejection of milk is caused by oxytocin from the posterior pituitary, also stimulated by suckling.

With cessation of suckling there is cessation of lactation. This may be speeded up by fluid restriction and binding of the breast without emptying the gland and by administration of estrogens, progestins, and androgens.

Involution

Involution of the breast occurs with the decline and termination of ovarian functions. During the premenopausal phase, at age 35 to 45 years, there is a gradual decrease in glandular epithelium and acinar and lobular tissues. In the menopausal-postmenopausal phase, age 45 to 75 years, there is marked loss of lobular and acinar structures with an increase in fat deposition and predominance of connective tissue. In the advanced senile part of this phase only small islands of duct epithelium surrounded by hard fibrous connective tissue remain.

For convenience, involution of the various structures of the breast can be considered as lobular, ductal, and stromal.

Involution of the noncystic lobular elements involves the ducts and intralobular connective tissue. The basement membrane thickens, the two layers of epithelial cells shrink to one flattened layer, and the duct lumina narrow and become nearly obliterated with cessation of secretions. The intralobular connective tissue becomes dense hyalinized collagen and blends into the ordinary interlobular connective tissue. A variant of this type of involution is the cystic form. Acini join to form microcysts with rounded outlines. The intralobular connective tissue remains as the specialized type. These two forms of involution may be found together in the same breast in varying proportions. With ductal involution the ductules and small ducts disappear, with an increase in connective tissue.

The supporting connective tissue disappears in part and is replaced with adipose tissue in stromal involution. The adipose metaplasia may proceed by expansion of the layer of subcutaneous fat or by deposition of areas of fat throughout the gland. Both usually occur at the same time but at different degees.

Estrogen Receptor

Tumor estrogen receptor (ER) predicts with considerable accuracy those women who are likely to respond to endocrine therapy and those who are not. Those patients with endocrine-dependent tumors (ER-positive) will respond to endocrine therapy 80 per cent of the time, whereas those with receptor-negative tumors (ER-negative) will fail to respond to endocrine therapy 90 per cent of the time. If the tumor contains a large amount of both estrogen and progesterone receptors, favorable response to treatment will approach 90 per cent. This information makes treatment planning for women with breast cancer more realistic and more simplified.

REFERENCES

Haagensen CD (1971): Diseases of the Breast, 2nd ed. Philadelphia, WB Saunders, p 21.

Massopust LC Jr, Gardner WD (1950): Infrared photographic studies of superficial thoracic veins in the female. Surg Gynecol Obstet 91:717.

Maximow AA, Bloom WA (1945): A Textbook of Histology. Philadelphia, WB Saunders, p 594.

Mammography Techniques

BACKGROUND

Interest in radiography of the breast was strongly revitalized after publication of the results of a new and vastly different technique that was simple, safe, and readily reproducible (Egan, 1960). This technique had been in routine use at a tumor institution for four years. In February 1965, a Standardization Conference on Mammography of The American College of Radiology, representing widely diversified interests in breast cancer (see Chapter 1), concluded that "there was no great disagreement about radiation to the breast and this improved technique of mammography." Thus, mammography introduced as an investigative procedure quickly became an indispensable adjunct for detection of curable breast cancer, with rapidly increasing use throughout the world.

However, the NCI Working Group on the Risks Associated with Mammography in Mass Screening (Breslow et al., 1977), reported an excess of cancer in three groups of women having radiation to the breasts: (1) those having chest fluoroscopies during treatment for pulmonary tuberculosis; (2) those treated with radiation for postpartum mastitis; and (3) Japanese women following atomic bomb irradiation. Unfortunately, so many women, even highly symptomatic ones, and their physicians became so frightened of breast radiation that the use of mammography was sharply curtailed or completely eliminated. This despite the NCI report that 1 rad to the midbreast produced an increase of less than 1 per cent over a lifetime to the natural risk of 7 per cent (7 per cent to 7.07 per cent) and that little or no risk was observed when such irradiation occurred after age 30 years, at which time breast cancer becomes the greatest problem.

Fortunately, we had already worked with the Eastman Kodak and Du Pont Companies to develop screen-film receptors with reduced dosage. Although these receptors produced an image of inferior quality compared with the then widely used nonscreen-film mammography, there was a reduction from

0.4 rad midline per exposure on properly executed nonscreen mammography to 0.06 rad per exposure on screen-film mammography.

The use of screen-film receptors introduced new problems, especially: (1) the need for severe compression of the breast, best accomplished by adding special, more expensive mammography x-ray units; and (2) the conflict between lowered radiation and image quality. Compromises in techniques are required, but there are suitable combinations of mammographic equipment (Egan, 1984). Routine views may be craniocaudad and mediolateral or a single oblique view, with supplemental views as needed. A general purpose x-ray unit, a simplified special mammography unit, or a more complex unit incorporating grid and magnification may be available and adapted for use. In all cases the principles previously outlined (Egan, 1960) for nonscreen-film mammography must be incorporated, as each mammographic system depends upon the physical combinations of the components. Broadly, these are: sharpness of the image—geometry, focal spot size, motion, receptor, and processing; and contrast—physical properties of the breast tissues, thickness of the part, scatter, detector, processing, and x-ray spectrum.

There are two basic reasons why soft tissue radiography of the breast cannot be successfully performed with the radiographic techniques and film emulsions employed in general medical x-ray procedures: (1) Low kilovoltage and minimal filtration of the x-ray beam must be utilized to emphasize the small differences in absorption of the soft tissues of the breast so that sufficient contrast can be produced for meaningful mammograms; and (2) radiographic detail (definition of fine objects) on the mammograms is more critical because it is necessary to resolve objects of 0.05 mm or less as opposed to 0.5 to 2 mm objects in general radiography.

The factors for the basic low-kilovoltage–high-milliamperage technique must be maintained. This mammographic technique, with the only variable being a change in the target-film distance, was applicable to breasts of all sizes in patients of all ages and states of nutrition. The paramount aim was maximum radiographic detail. The procedure could be carried out with equipment found in the average radiology department and required no alteration of the technical conditions used more than 30 years ago. The technique has

remained safe, simple, nontraumatic, inexpensive, reproducible, and acceptable to the patient. Its long history indicates a unique stability. As noted by five physicists in a review of present mammographic techniques in the *Radiologists' Guide to Detection of Early Breast Cancer by Mammography, Thermography and Xeroradiography,* "there is no question that nonscreen industrial film allows the maximum detail to be recorded." Our skin dose of approximately 2 rads (0.4 rad midline) per exposure remained constant in several institutions and was measured often by countless physicists.

Variations will occur with different receptors, e.g., nonscreen-film, screen-film, and xeroradiography. But knowledge of the basic technique will enable its easy adaptation to specimen radiography requiring low kvp, minimal filtration, and collimation; to xeroradiography with balloon compression and altered positioning of the mediolateral views; to grid or magnification radiography; and to screen-film mammography, where the most drastic changes are necessary owing to the required severe breast compression. These changes for the screen-film receptor are necessary because (1) the kvp range is so restricted by the type system, usually 25 to 27 or 28 kvp; (2) vigorous compression must be applied to the breast so that the thickness at the base approaches the thickness in the subareolar area in order to produce better and more even transmission of the x-ray beam, to reduce scattered radiation, and to reduce the object-film distance; (3) strong pulling of the breast from the chest wall is necessary to position the glandular tissues over the receptor; and (4) drastic, almost acrobatic positioning of the breast in the oblique (modified mediolateral) position is required. Application of many of these established principles of mammography is required for views of the breast at right angles for localization purposes, for a special projection such as the lateromedial, for special coned-downed spot views, and for recumbent mammography.

Completely covering the period of transition from the simple, well-established, proven nonscreen film mammography technique into the endless modifications required to encompass all these variations is not a simple task. Once one variable is introduced, the floodgate is opened. Even today some of the x-ray units used for screen-film mammography are general purpose units. Even special units may vary, e.g., target anode material, and different combinations of anode material and filtration are used in xeroradiography of the breast.

Limiting the description to the best use of screen-film mammography and breast xeroradiography would simplify the task. Ideally, screen-film mammography would all be done on a special unit with the ultimate in positioning and compression, molybdenum filtration, and the best of all technical factors for mammography. In xeroradiography there would be assured quality control, use of a tungsten anode, aluminum filtration, no artifacts, and again the best of all technical factors. These ideals are not possible owing to space requirements, costs, a limited number of special units, poorly trained technologists, lack of experience in referring physicians with resultant occasional referrals, absence of standardized procedures, limited physicists' input, and the different preferences of radiologists.

It is well to keep in mind while discussing the technical aspects of mammography that it was mandatory in the beginning to follow certain unwavering routes, foreign to most mammographers today. Only one radiologic parameter, the grid, had not been investigated in the tedious development of a compromised combination of technical factors to produce convincing mammograms. Some investigated parameters follow: 12 kvp to 22 meV; 60 to 75 film emulsions; 0.1 to 20 sec exposures; very slow to fast intensifying screens, including lead screens; focal spot sizes from 0.3 to 25 mm; short to long target-film distances; varied object-film distances (magnification); milliamperage settings of 50 to 300 ma; flaring to extended cylinder collimators; multiple positions, including the three-point pendant breast (on both knees, one hand for support and one holding the breast not being studied, cross-table radiography) and the oblique or Cleopatra position; and compression.

All students of breast cancer knew that breast x-ray had been tried and was worthless. So the first consideration was to make absolutely sure that there was no confusion about what was being done and to be adamant as to how it would be done. Although I had the only solid experience in the world with this technique, the slightest suggestion of wavering would have been destructive. The next approach was to combat the radiologists' thinking that they must buy some

expensive equipment to be used, perhaps, a very few times before it was discarded. The counterapproach was to adapt the simplest technique to existing x-ray units with minimal alterations. The third consideration was the radiologists' need for patients, making it necessary to forge a route into the surgical societies. This required incomparable mammography so that for the first time the surgeon's all-sensing fingers would be challenged by detected and proven nonpalpable cancers. The pathologist then had to be drawn into the act and be willing to spend some extra effort to find and diagnose these unheard-of cancers. The unique team approach was necessary to demonstrate these tiny cancers that were later to be proved curable. The selling required meticulous and authoritative dosimetry under Warren K. Sinclair, Ph.D., at M.D. Anderson Hospital. We did the only known actual breast tissue dosimetry in the 20 to 40 kvp range to this date.

Only after years of education of physicians, instruction of radiologists and technologists, clinical trials, a nationwide reproducibility study, and successful screening programs could the pursuit of these original routes be relaxed. It was fortunate indeed that this quarter of a century of investigation of mammographic factors (at one time, five years alone with three full-time physicists studying why certain aspects worked and how to improve them) served to provide screen-film receptors as our alternative to nonscreen-film mammography, when criticism of breast radiation threatened the demise of this valuable medical tool.

Breast imaging is discussed in much greater detail in the author's *Breast Imaging*, Third Edition (1984).

COMPONENTS OF BREAST RADIOGRAPHY

Physical Properties of Breast Tissue

Glandular and fibrous tissues of the breast absorb the x-ray beam equally, whereas fat is more radiolucent and provides the necessary subject contrast. The interaction of the x-ray photons with these tissues at the low kilovoltage is photoelective effect at the lower range of energy and Comptom scattering at the higher range. Barnes and Brezovitch (1979) observed that scattered radiation in mammography was considerable and severely limited the visibility of small structures. They concluded that scattered radiation varied from 35 to 100 per cent of the primary beam intensity and that with its suppression a moderate increase in kilovoltage could be tolerated.

X-Ray Spectra

In the mammography energy range of 20 to 50 kvp, the shape of the x-ray spectrum may be varied by changing anode material, type and amount of added filtration, and kvp.

Anode materials for mammography generally are tungsten, molybdenum, or alloys of these two metals. With a tungsten anode a continuous bremsstrahlung spectrum is obtained by filtering any characteristic L x-rays and remaining below 50 keV to avoid characteristic K x-rays. The glass window provides sufficient filtration, approximately 1 mm Al equivalent, in the usual x-ray tube. Aluminum filters must be added to beryllium window tubes, at least 0.5 mm for mammography and generally 1.0 to 3.0 mm for xeroradiography.

With the molybdenum anode in addition to the continuous bremsstrahlung spectrum there are peaks of 17.4 and 19.6 keV from the characteristic K x-rays. This beam produces higher contrast at the lower mammography kvp range, in practice below 30 kvp. The window is usually beryllium; filters of Al or Mo may be used. The Mo filters absorb more intensely energies above 20 keV, thus permitting a higher concentration of the characteristic K x-ray peaks. The Mo filter is usually 0.03 mm thick. On the other hand, the Al filter increases the overall concentration of higher energy photons by removal of relatively more lower energy photons. A thickness of 0.5 mm Al is mandatory; an Al filter of more than 1 mm tends to reduce the relative amount of characteristic K x-rays. This is contrary to the aim of severe breast compression, which is to reduce the thickness of the part with less absorption in the tissues of the characteristic K x-rays.

The tungsten/molybdenum alloy anodes will be intermediate between the two pure component anodes. The relative amounts of each metal will contribute to the properties of the emergent x-ray beam.

In radiography of actual breast tissue phantom comparisons can be made between images from tungsten and molybdenum anodes. In general, the Mo anode with smaller thicknesses (1 to 5 cm) produces greater contrast, while in greater thickness, over 6 cm, the contrast is reduced but is equal with both types of anode. As thickness of the phantom increases, the mas required to darken the film becomes greater with the Mo anode. At an 8 cm thickness it is 3.5 to 4 times greater with the Mo anode. Practically all the characteristic K x-rays are absorbed and there is an increase in the absorbed dose without darkening the film. In clinical mammography the absorbed radiation is two to three times greater with the Mo anode than with the W anode.

Geometry

Geometric unsharpness, blurring of the x-ray image, is related to the size of the focal spot and object-receptor distance. The size of the usual mammographic focal spot is no larger than 1 mm, preferably smaller if not limited by the necessary tube output. The object-film distance can be reduced somewhat by vigorous compression, or its relative distance reduced by changing the anode-receptor distance. The stationary anode fad was short-lived owing to uncontrolled geometric unsharpness and marked heel effect with an anode-receptor distance of 11 to 13 inches.

The ranges of technical factors for various types and sizes of breast are listed in Table 5–1. These factors are merely a rough guide, as there will be wide variations with different x-ray units, anode type, filtration, and so forth.

Motion

Motion is the greatest single problem in the production of radiographic detail. At 1-sec exposures, rhythmic or gross motion is just as disadvantageous as at 6-sec exposures. It is only when the exposure time is reduced to 1/20 sec or less that the time factor becomes of real importance.

In no aspect of breast radiography is the technologist so challenged to avoid motion. Rapport is most necessary with tense, frightened, embarassed women who are normally well composed. A few moments of friendly reassurance and explanation will make the difference between a useless and an excellent study.

Patient relaxation and proper support with stabilization of the breast during radiography are far more important considerations than concern over a 1-sec vs a 6-sec exposure.

TABLE 5–1. Range of Technical Factors Used in Mammography

Age, Group, Breast Type	Nonscreen Factors*	Screen-Film Factors†	Screen-Film Grid†
Menopausal, average consistency			
Small			
Craniocaudad	300 ma, 22 kvp, 30 in, 6 sec	200 ma, 25 kvp, 30 in, 1.5 sec	200 ma, 27 kvp, 30 in, 1.5 sec
Mediolateral	300 ma, 24 kvp, 30 in, 6 sec	200 ma, 25 kvp, 30 in, 2 sec	200 ma, 29 kvp, 30 in, 1.5 sec
Medium			
Craniocaudad	300 ma, 26 kvp, 36 in, 6 sec	200 ma, 26 kvp, 30 in, 2.5 sec	200 ma, 27 kvp, 30 in, 2 sec
Mediolateral	300 ma, 28 kvp, 36 in, 6 sec	200 ma, 27 kvp, 30 in, 3 sec	200 ma, 29 kvp, 30 in, 2 sec
Large			
Craniocaudad	300 ma, 26 kvp, 40 in, 6 sec	200 ma, 27 kvp, 30 in, 3 sec	200 ma, 27 kvp, 30 in, 2.5 sec
Mediolateral	300 ma, 28 kvp, 40 in, 6 sec	200 ma, 29 kvp, 30 in, 3 sec	200 ma, 29 kvp, 30 in, 2.5 sec
Postmenopausal	Average 2–4 kvp less; if flabby and flat, 5 sec	Similar to small	Similar to small
Premenopausal	If soft, same as menopausal; if firm, add 2–4 kvp	Similar to menopausal; 2–3 kvp added if firm breasts	Similar to menopausal; may require up to 33 kvp
Virginal	Similar to premenopausal; if small, 26–30 in; may require 32–34 kvp	Similar to premenopausal; may require 30 kvp, 5 sec	Similar to premenopausal; if large and dense, possibly 5 sec
Dense area	Distance reduced to 22 in	As virginal	As virginal

*With conventional x-ray units.
†With special mammography units.

Sandbags placed on that half of the film holder not being used add greatly to the stability. The breast should be completely supported as though unattached to the chest wall. It has been demonstrated repeatedly that more motion is noted with 2-sec than with 6-sec exposure. Faced with the longer time, the technician positions the breast and patient more meticulously and impresses on the patient the need for complete cooperation.

Although with a screen-film receptor exposure time is considerably shorter, all the tricks to minimizing motion are as important as with nonscreen mammography. The use of rather severe compression helps, but if the breasts are painful the woman cannot be relaxed, thus contributing to motion.

The same considerations for nonscreen-film mammography hold for screen-film mammography except that exposure time is reduced. To check for motion on the mammograms, seek out calcifications, prominent trabeculae, veins, or the rib cage. With proper positioning of the patient for mammography, it has been the author's experience that causes other than motion account for most blurring on the mammograms.

Collimation

Proper collimation of the x-ray beam is mandatory for adequate radiographic detail and reduction of skin dose. It is estimated that as much as 85 per cent of film darkening in mammography is from scattered radiation. Target-film distances of less than 20 inches on the average x-ray unit frequently utilize only the aperture of the tube housing for collimation when the average breast is included in the x-ray beam. The use of cones flaring at the same angles as the divergence of the x-ray beam accomplishes no useful collimation of that beam. To encompass the breast in the x-ray beam, the aperture in the tube housing for emission of the x-ray must be as large as 2.5 cm. This allows off-focus irradiation and large quantities of scattered radiation to be in the area covered by the primary x-ray beam. Also, the heel effect is most apparent. This greater radiation increases the skin dose markedly. Target-film distances of less than 22 inches do not allow either good collimation of the x-ray beam or ease in patient and tube positioning.

With nonscreen-film mammography the use of a cylinder cone and change of target-skin distance to include only the breast in the x-ray beam allow "built-in" compensation for the wide variations in breast size and shape encountered in practice.

Figures 5–1 through 5–4 illustrate the use of collimation.

Central Beam

The central beam is directed toward the base of the breast in the craniocaudad and

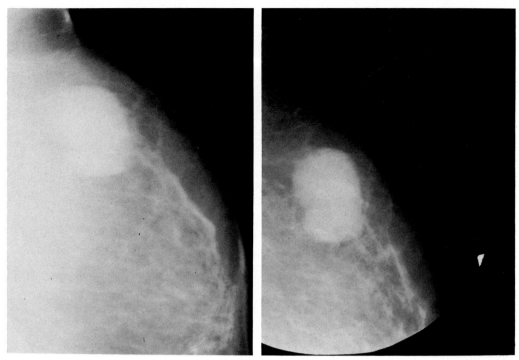

Figure 5–1. Full mediolateral view of the breast showing a lesion. A coned spot over this area was made by reducing the target-film distance and extending a telescoping cylinder cone.

mediolateral views. This beam is the most energetic and is directed toward the thickest part. Because the breast slopes gradually toward its periphery and there is a compensatory fall-off of the beam energy with this reduction in the thickness of the part, there is a near-equal density of the skin and base of the breast on the mammograms (Fig. 5–5).

Proper centering of the central beam is more critical with the screen-film receptor. Even with the vigorous compression used, the latitude in exposure factors is limited.

Receptors

Nonscreen-Film

A few remarks may be appropriate for the comprehension of the sacrifices in radiographic detail or definition (ability to see small structures on a radiograph) as one progresses from very fine-grain film emulsions to faster, coarser grained emulsions. Today the slower fine-grain emulsions may not be used in clinical mammography but are invaluable in specimen radiography and even flower radiography. Such thin motionless objects may be beautifully recorded at 12 kvp, beryllium window tube, no added filter, and long exposures.

The film emulsion must be selected with a particulate grain size in accordance with the aim of the x-ray examination. Sufficient experience has been gained in mammography to know that not only must trabecular structures the size of a spider's web be identified, but their distortion must be recognized; fine, stippled calcifications may not exceed 0.05 mm and will go undetected when masked by graininess of the film emulsion. Thus, it becomes desirable that the grain of the film emulsion not be visible under the hand lens. With larger grain emulsions the hand lens serves only to magnify the grain pattern. The display of numerous unexplained shadows cast by breast structures should be accomplished to provide a stimulus for further investigation of mammography as well as of breast diseases.

Radiographic detail in mammography depends on radiographic contrast and acutal definition of the part. Contrast and definition are so intimately associated that one cannot be considered without the other. Their relative effects on detail depend on several factors. Radiographic contrast is related to subject contrast (affected by variations in actual x-ray density of the parts, quality of the x-ray beams, thickness of the part as a scatter-

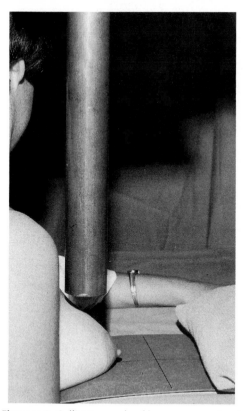

Figure 5–2. Collimator made of heavy copper pipe, 1.5 inch inside diameter and 14 inches long, is meticulously aligned for extremely close collimation and elimination of off-focus radiation.

ing medium, and control of the scattered beam by collimation) and film contrast (dependent on the type of film emulsion and base and on the factors that go into processing this emulsion). Definition, in turn, is related to geometric sharpness (relative focal spot size, target-film distance, and object-film distance), and graininess and mottle (affected by film emulsion type and speed, film processing, and quantum scintillation).

It is readily seen that the recording of the x-ray image is greatly dependent on the film type. To record the edge of fine trabeculae, a very fine-grain industrial emulsion must have sufficient film contrast to record the natural subject contrast. The fine grain and reduced speed prevent undesirable effects on quantum scintillation (statistical fluctuation of the total x-ray beam energy per unit area of film) because more photons are required per unit area for darkening the film, resulting in a more even exposure. The wide latitude of such an emulsion allows near-equal density of the skin and base of the breast; a fine-grain emulsion used with a change of target-

film distance allows all breasts to be studied under the same technical conditions and can be viewed under bright illumination.

Less contrast is required in the film emulsion as finer structures are studied in mammography. The retinal appreciation of a difference in the density of structures is more definite the nearer the two are to each other; two 0.05 mm apposed densities would be quite close.

The speed of the emulsion is directly related to graininess; the faster the film, the more noticeable are the individual grains that contribute to an absence of radiographic detail. This becomes important when cancer clearly seen on fine-grain industrial film cannot be seen on a coarser grain industrial film that is only three times the speed of the fine-grain emulsion. Artifacts due to static, light leaks, or high-temperature processing are more evident on grainier films, but processing errors (e.g., streaking or uneven development) are generally more common on the less grainy film.

The film may be used in the cardboard holder or in a previously prepared disposable paper pack. Most technologists prefer the slightly stiffer carboard holder for ease in positioning and for exclusion of skin wrinkles or air pockets. The paper pack should be placed over lead rubber in the craniocaudad projection because the beam is directed to-

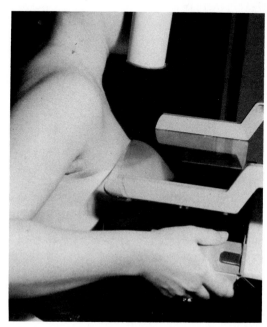

Figure 5–3. Small cone with fixed target-film distance used with special compression device.

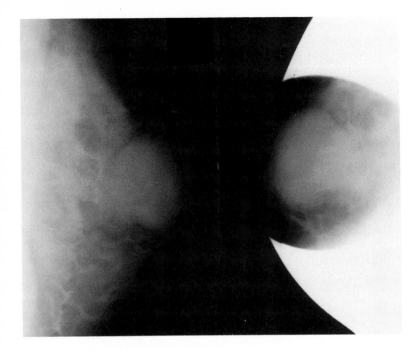

Figure 5–4. Mediolateral view showing a lesion: coned view with copper pipe and compression at the end of the cone for better detail. Note the silhouette of the breast (at left) for localization purposes. Similar results may be obtained with cone in Figure 5–3.

ward the gonads. For use with cardboard holders, it is necessary to remove the interleaving protective papers supplied with the film to reduce extraneous shadows.

Double-loading techniques for variable densities are unnecessary if a single film with with an emulsion of wide latitude is selected; it is well to remember that one good mammogram is far superior to two inadequate ones. Furthermore, the technique is compromised if the technologist thinks that "if one film is not good, the other will be," with the result that in all probability neither is properly exposed. Mammograms should be inspected by the technologist for quality and the need, if any, for additional views before the patient's release. Double or triple loading with some types of film emulsion for duplication of studies is readily accomplished without changing the technical conditions.

Screen-Film

The combination of the film emulsion and screen receptor is faster than nonscreen-film emulsion. It is grainier, with less definition of small structures. Yet as a compromise, with less radiation required it is acceptable for mammography. Most of the darkening of the emulsion is due to fluorescent light photons from the intensifying screen with a resultant increase in the contrast at 25 to 30 kvp.

The photons of light spread out in all directions as they travel from screen to film emulsion proportional to the distance from the source to be captured by the emulsion. The distance can be reduced by (1) good screen-film contact; (2) use of a single film emulsion; (3) placement of the film emulsion side in contact with the screen; (4) placement of the film behind the screen as more x-rays interact with the front side of the screen; and (5) proper spread and thickness of the fluorescent layer. This film can be developed in a mechanical processor.

Latitude of the screen-film receptor and range of milliamperage and kilovoltage is markedly limited compared with that of the fine-grain nonscreen-film. Contrast may be excessive at 25 kvp or lower, and graying is quite evident at 29 kvP or higher. Phototiming may be of benefit with this receptor.

There has been sufficient improvement in screen-film combinations that they can be used in mammography. Screens introduce screen mottle and artifacts and require rigid casettes. Rather vigorous compression is needed to reduce the thickness of the breast in position. Even women with no tenderness in their breasts do not appreciate such compression. The compression device makes positioning of the patient and breast more difficult; may push the breast tissues up along the chest wall, especially at the base; and may prevent radiography of the base of the breast. Compression devices are usually

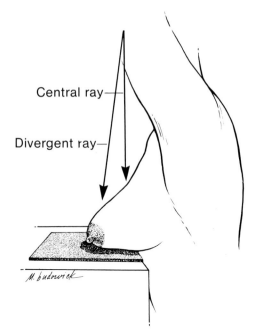

Figure 5–5. The central ray is directed to the midpoint of the base of the breast and parallel to the chest wall. The more energetic central beam traverses the thickest portion of the breast, with fall-off of the beam toward the periphery of the breast.

part of an x-ray unit designed for mammography. The amount of radiation required is reduced compared with nonscreen-film.

Special rare-earth intensifying screens have been developed for mammography. Much effort was required to develop film emulsions for satisfactory combinations. Today there are so many screens and acceptable film emulsions that almost endless pairing of the screens and film can result in satisfactory images.

The screen-film receptors are generally used in one of two ways: (1) in a light-tight, plastic, somewhat flexible holder, or a polyethylene bag, that requires a vacuum to ensure good screen-film contact; or (2) in a rigid cassette with the screen mounted on foam plastic to produce screen-film contact. Both are rigid, even the flexible one, after the vacuum is applied. Care must be taken to place the single-screen intensifying surface against the emulsion side of the single-emulsion film. The rigid cassette is preferred over the holder or polyethylene bags. The bags may be reused no more than six to eight times and the plastic holders only a few months. The cassettes produce just as good screen-film contact and last indefinitely.

Cleanliness is extremely important with both types of screen-film holders. The screens should be cleaned daily with a commercial screen-cleaning solution and air sprayed with each new loading. Dust on the screen prevents the light from the screen from reaching the film emulsion, easily mimicking tiny calcifications. Fastidious darkroom care is one of the prices for use of the intensifying screen in mammography.

Screen-film mammography uses primarily light to expose the silver halide crystals, whereas the nonscreen-film technique relies entirely on the x-ray photons to interact with the film emulsion. Obviously, the potential radiographic quality of nonscreen techniques can never be approached with the screen-film receptors.

Rather severe compression of the breast is required with the screen-film receptor in order to get an acceptable study without the anterior breast appearing black and the base of the breast white. The proper balance is difficult to achieve; overly exposed areas cannot be retrieved by a bright light as with nonscreen fine-grain emulsions.

Another large difference in the two receptors is the relatively enormous increased effort in positioning the breasts for mammography. The mammographer must be widely inventive, acrobatically agile, endowed with endless patience, and hypnotic while compressing the tender breasts at almost all times during the study.

There is not only the theoretical advantage with screen-film receptors of increasing the object-receptor distance but also perceptible improvement in image quality in tissues that are farthest from the film. Even with a 1 mm focal spot, the object size is magnified while the screen mottle remains the same, thus increasing the ratio of part size to mottle. This contributes to the clarity of image.

Special Mammography Units

Several dozen x-ray units designed especially for mammography have been marketed over the past 20 years. Generally, they had fixed target-film distances and poor collimation, making positioning difficult. These features often led to the preference for conventional x-ray units with their versatility.

With the great concern over radiation to the breast, intensifying screens were used to reduce radiation exposure. This necessitated compression of the breast, and vigorous compression was required. This was best obtained on special mammography units, so that some radiologists insist that mammography can be done only on a special mammography unit.

The possible combinations in assembling a mammography x-ray unit makes even the experienced mammographer confused in trying to select the proper unit. Despite a continued demand for these x-ray units (more breast clinics cropping up and more radiologists changing from xeroradiography to screen-film) most American manufacturers stopped making a unit. Fortunately, for a while there were a limited number of models both from the United States and foreign manufacturers. In the last few years units have again proliferated. The units now have target-film distances of 50 cm or more, can use either tungsten or molybdenum anode targets, can be used for magnification, have compression devices, and usually have a grid or a provision for adapting a grid. Poor collimation and lack of versatility are drawbacks of most models. The grid is the only innovation. Compression has always been mandatory in using tubes with limited x-ray output. Our experience now includes experimentation with focal spot sizes as small as 10 μ for mammography. Their precise application has not been determined.

Compression Devices

Compression of the breast may provide better radiographic detail by decreasing the thickness of the breast tissue and producing a shorter object-film distance. Better immobilization of the breast may also be obtained if no anxiety or nervousness is created. Some lesions near the chest wall may never be demonstrated with various compression techniques. Failure to include the chest wall can be a serious and common problem with routine compression mammography. Compression of the breast that has been pulled as far from the chest wall as possible immobilizes it and retains more of the deeper glandular tissues over the receptor.

Radiation of the patient can also be reduced if compression is done by using the cylinder collimator and the compression device. Elimination of the scattered radiation improves radiographic detail. However, with compression of the breast obtained by the end of the collimator, there will be a marked and unpredictable increase in flux of the radiation, causing increased skin dosage. Because breasts differ greatly in size, contour,

and density, equal pressure is not always obtained. The pressure should not be severely painful.

Compression may be accomplished with two types of special device. One type is attached to the base of the cone, and the target-film distance is varied only by the thickness of the breast (Fig. 5–6). The other type of device is mounted independently of the x-ray tube and provides versatility in angling the tube, which changes the central x-ray beam in relation to the breast and varies the target-film distance (Fig. 5–7). Some of these special mammography units with independent compression devices have fixed object-film distances (Fig. 5–8). Both devices may be used similarly.

A compression device mounted independently of the tube is preferable by far. This arrangement provides more versatility and can be adjusted more easily by the technologist. A lock is necessary to hold the plate in position, and a safety device is preferred so that too much pressure cannot be applied inadvertently and bruise the breast; also it should be easily removed to increase the versatility of the x-ray unit. The plate should be flat, made of some inflexible material such as Lexan, at least 1 mm thick, and reinforced with metal on the sides and the one edge nearer the x-ray unit away from the patient.

At the chest wall the curvature of the edge of the compression plate is crucial. A gently upward-curving edge defeats attempts to compress the breast properly. As downward

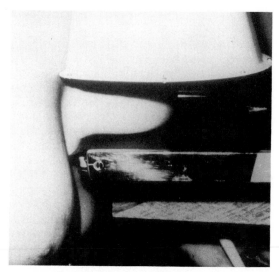

Figure 5–6. Special mammography compression arrangement with the compression device attached to the base of the collimator.

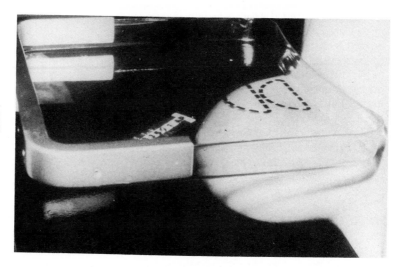

Figure 5–7. Special mammography compression device mounted independently of the x-ray tube and collimator.

pressure on the breast is applied by the plate a great deal of breast tissue at the base of the breast is pushed toward and upward onto the anterior chest wall beyond the posterior edge of the receptor and cannot be imaged. The base of the breast projected onto the receptor will be underpenetrated and the subareolar area overpenetrated. This design is more humane but cannot be effective. Neither a straight uncurved nor a gently curving posterior plate edge can be used for similar reasons.

The chest wall edge is made by bending the flat plastic compression plate straight up to a right angle, then an additional 10 to 15 degrees toward the x-ray unit (away from the chest wall). This bent part should be at least 2 to 3 cm long. Such an arrangement

adds strength to the edge over the base of the breast, where most pressure is required and where most plates crack. The angle away from the chest wall prevents any portion of the plate from contacting the chest wall other than at the one point on the curving chest wall (near the midpoint of the base of the breast). The upper portion of the plate may even prevent bulging of the tissues along the chest wall anteriorly and laterally and hanging over the receptor. Less tissue is pushed up and off the receptor. The posterior edge of the plate is aligned over the back border of the receptor. The plate is kept parallel to the upper surface of the receptor.

For all types of compressions of the breasts, the device is brought gently but firmly into place. Every attempt must be made to ensure that compression is produced in the craniocaudad view from directly above and downward rather than from the front and toward the chest wall. The same applies

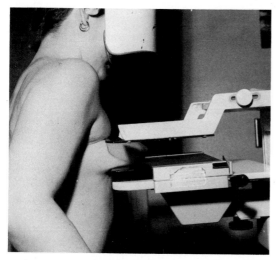

Figure 5–8. Fixed target-film distance, with the compression varied independently of the tube.

TABLE 5–2. Screen-Film Receptors and Compression in Breast Imaging

Advantages	Disadvantages
Reduced milliamperage	Artifacts
Possibly less motion effect	Screen mottle (noise)
Magnification better tolerated; with added grid higher kvp can be used	Rigid screen-film holder
	Reduced latitude
	Less resolution (scattered light)
Less scattered radiation	May be painful
More uniform density of image	Can push breast tissue beyond receptor
Less geometric unsharpness	
May demonstrate more glandular tissue on the craniocaudad view	

for the mediolateral view, achieved by pressing laterally on the breast, not angling the device toward the patient. This is necessary to prevent pressing too much breast tissue back and upward along the chest wall. At times a mass near the chest wall may be forced outward by slight angulation of the compression device.

The usual ranges of technical factors used in mammography are included in Table 5–1. Advantages and some of the disadvantages of screen-film receptors are listed in Table 5–2.

POSITIONING

A description of positions for mammography is not so readily accomplished when one considers the number of modified mammography units available and the use of various compression devices. The basic mammography positions will serve as a springboard to illustrate numerous physical problems introduced by these special units. The established mammography positions will be shown to acquaint the technologist with the general procedure. These will be followed by the necessary steps to adapt the positioning to screen-film mammography.

Two views at right angles of each breast are routinely obtained, the craniocaudad and mediolateral (or modified mediolateral, the oblique), and, if indicated, one of the axilla. These views make possible good delineation of the quadrants of the breasts, ease in positioning, patient comfort and cooperation, and coverage of the axillary prolongation of the breast and the area of axillary lymph nodes.

Such objects as adhesive tape, bandage, gown, or medications (including deodorants and powders) must be removed, as they can produce distracting or confusing shadows at this low kilovoltage.

Nonscreen Receptor

Craniocaudad Position

The patient is seated at one end or at one side of the x-ray table or at the x-ray unit (Fig. 5–9). If an adjustable stool is used, the height is adjusted to permit the breast to rest firmly on the film holder. At a level suitable for breast-film contact, the patient will appear to be seated uncomfortably low. A table with adjustable height, such as the hospital

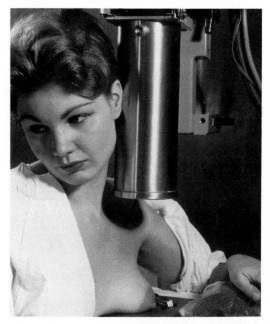

Figure 5–9. Craniocaudad view. For the craniocaudad mammogram, the patient is seated at the end of the table. The breast is firmly supported and is positioned with the nipple in profile.

overbed table, which is available and versatile, is also convenient.

Elevation of the breast to a height of near-discomfort will allow the breast to be completely supported by the film holder. This is mandatory to prevent transmission of any gross chest motion to the breast and to provide firm breast-film contact.

Mediolateral Position

The mediolateral position provides the second projection of the breast, is the single most important view in mammography, and is the most difficult for the mammographer to master. If properly executed, almost all the breast tissue is projected onto the film; also, near-equal density of the skin and the base of the breast on the mammogram will be obtained (Fig. 5–10).

On the mediolateral view, all the technical factors remain the same except for an increase of 2 kvp over the craniocaudad view. There will be slightly greater variation in overall density than with the craniocaudad view, so that the skin may require a bright light for study.

Axillary Position

The third basic view to complete a mammographic study is the axillary view, designed for study of the axillary contents, the

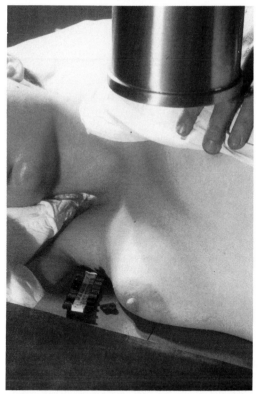

Figure 5–10. Mediolateral view. For the mediolateral view, the patient lies comfortably on her side. The breast is supported by a 3-inch thick wooden block. The position of the markers placed toward the axilla allows identification of the quadrants of the breast.

tail of the breast, and portions of the upper quadrant of the breast (Figs. 5–11 and 5–12).

Screen-Film Receptor

Craniocaudad Position

With screen-film receptors the craniocaudad view will be identical to that described except for the addition of routine compression. Most of the x-ray units for mammography have the compression device separate from the collimator. After the breast has been positioned on the platform of the x-ray unit, the compression paddle is adjusted while the breast is carefully maintained in firm contact with the film holder and the chest wall is firmly held against the edge of the platform and film holder. This view may be done with the patient standing, but we prefer the sitting position, which results in better cooperation (Fig. 5–13).

Mediolateral Position

In the mediolateral view compression may be obtained with the patient in the routine recumbent position and the compression device brought into position and locked. The upright mediolateral compression is obtained from the vertical with the film holder lateral to the breast being examined (Fig. 5–14). The patient is positioned against the film with the breast as far forward as possible so that the maximum amount of breast is included on the film. The patient is rotated toward the film holder to bring the nipple into profile. The compression device is then brought into position against the breast. At the same time, the sagging breast is supported by one hand until the pressure of the compression paddle maintains the breast in position. The patient may be required to retract an opposite pendulous breast while the compression device is secured into position. The larger, more sagging breast may require considerable manipulation to ensure more complete coverage and, in particular, more detail of the breast. Consequently, such compression devices have been facetiously labeled "convenience units," whereas they tax the ingenuity of the technologist, especially when trying to capture the glandular tissue near the chest wall.

Oblique Position

This view, with as many variations as there are mammographers, is the second view of conventional mammography or may be used only as a supplemental view. In the routine mediolateral view the x-ray beam is directed across the chest wall and obliquely through the breast in a transverse manner in a medial to lateral direction. This projects more breast from the chest wall onto the receptor. In the view we designate as the oblique, the x-ray beam is from a superomedial to inferolateral direction with the obliquity of the breast position in the mediolateral maintained (Figs. 5–15 and 5–16). In addition, there is an attempt to project some additional tissues in the tail of the breast (Fig. 5–17).

This variation of the standard mediolateral view we developed (Egan, 1960) as the Cleopatra view (the fetching position in the bow of her Nile River boat) to act as single-view mammography replacing the craniocaudad and mediolateral views, particularly in screening programs. Later it was sporadically revised and popularized to use with special mammography units, as the chest wall could not be included on the mammograms.

We consider the oblique a routine view. We do not practice single-view mammography. Getting the patient to mammography, properly logged in, identified, and prepared

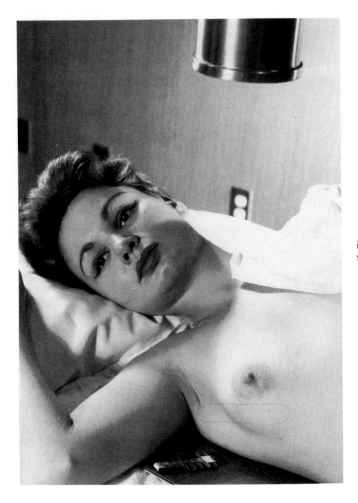

Figure 5–11. Axillary view. The axillary view is obtained with the patient in a recumbent but slightly oblique position.

for the study represents most of the work and expense. A few moments for a second view of the breast is neither expensive nor time consuming. Avoiding calling the patient back, reducing concern over a vague change, knowing the precise localization of a change, and adding confidence make the second view worthwhile. Also, additional views at right angles to each other are required for precise localization of an area of the breast.

Despite the compromises in technique, radiographic detail, and added patient discomfort with use of screen-film receptors, there may be an advantage at times with special mammography units (Fig. 5–18).

XERORADIOGRAPHY OF THE BREAST

Background

In planning our breast imaging center at Emory University in 1964, one modality that was to be studied was xeroradiography of

the breast. Arrangements had been made with the General Electric Company for the use of their unit, reportedly one they had obtained from those being stockpiled for general radiography in the event that atomic bombing during World War II destroyed all x-ray film emulsion. The particular unit would be released by Ruzicka et al (1965) when they had completed a study of the breast. At the RSNA in 1965 the General Electric Company representative asked me when the unit should be shipped to Emory University. My center was deeply involved in breast radiography, thermography, sonography, isotope studies, and much else. Discussion with the contract officer of my grant revealed that John Wolfe was interested. We all met and agreed that Wolfe should do the study with whatever help was necessary from me. Almost weekly visits to Hutzel Hospital in Detroit followed, with my becoming a consultant to Xerox Corporation, and many efforts were made to get Xerox Corporation to upgrade the unit for clinical ap-

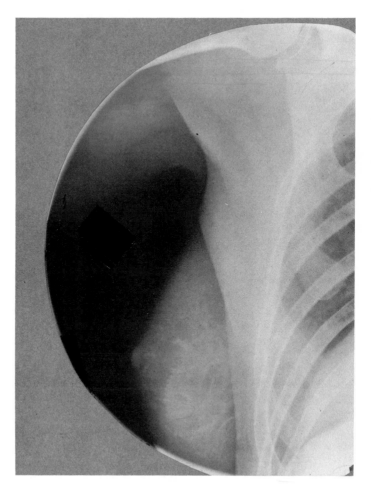

Figure 5–12. Axillary view. Note the obliquity to demonstrate maximally the muscular and fascial planes outlined by fat in the axilla.

plication. This was a time-consuming process, but over the years units were produced and placed in breast centers.

The xerographic reproduction process was patented in 1942. In 1947 Haloid Company, later to be the Xerox Corporation, began commercial development. Application in medicine began in 1952 and application to the breast in 1956. Our involvement began in 1965.

As a photoelectric process xeroradiography is similar to xerography. It is used with conventional or special mammographic equipment. The major differences between conventional radiography and xeroradiography are as follows: (1) The latent image is formed by photoconduction on a selenium surface plate and developed by a dry process; (2) a permanent image is recorded on opaque paper; (3) positive or negative images can be produced; and (4) edge enhancement is often greater.

The latitude in radiographic exposure factors in xeroradiography of the breast is nar-

row. Two characteristics are inherent in xeroradiography: accentuation of margins (edge enhancement) and broad recording latitude at the expense of large-area contrast.

Structures within the breast and axilla, as well as bones of the thorax and air in the lungs, vary in radiopacity but are recorded and recognized with a single exposure, reflecting wide recording latitude.

The latent image on the selenium plate is developed by an aerosol of charged fine particles of blue powder that are attracted to the charge distributed on the plate produced by the x-ray beam. The powder pattern is built up to correspond to the strength of the charge on the plate. The pattern shows low contrast between large areas as the whole plate is subjected to the burst of particles. But where there is a sharp change in density of the charge there is a marked increase in contrast. Edge enhancement occurs with an abrupt difference in the tissue densities of adjacent structures. The edges of the denser area are usually more pronounced than in

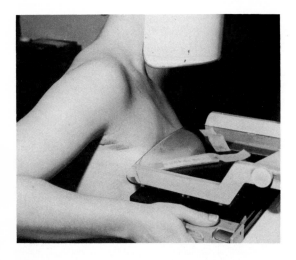

Figure 5–13. Craniocaudad position with compression. The breast is severely compressed in an attempt to pull the base as far as possible from the chest wall.

fine-grain film mammography. This is partic-ularly marked around coarse calcifications or where the bone or muscle is apposed to the tissue of the breast. The marked edge en-hancement (toner robbing) can be reduced by negative xeroradiography. Yet sometimes on a film the edge enhancement, or halo, about a cyst or fibroadenoma is much greater than on xeroradiography.

Positive and Negative Modes

In the positive mode the toner particles are given a negative charge. These particles col-lect on the positively charged plate denser under dense areas of the breast that have absorbed more incident radiation required to neutralize these positive charges, and be-come dark blue against the lighter back-ground of less dense tissues (Fig. 5–19A). This is the reversal of the film image. For years this was the usual method of recording xeroradiographic images until methods to reduce radiation to the breast were sought.

In the negative mode the development process is reversed (Fig. 5–19B). The toner particles are positively charged and produce an image reversed from the positive mode. The dense structures, such as calcifications, appear lighter against the less dense breast tissues. There is an approximately 20 per cent decrease in radiation compared with the positive mode. Some radiologists claim that there is also improved contrast and better definition of small objects. Other radiologists have found no improvement in image qual-

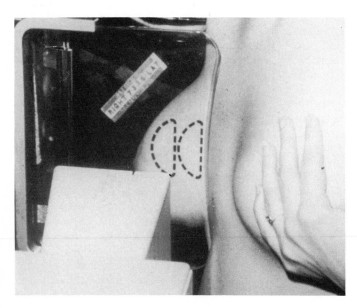

Figure 5–14. Compression mediolateral view. The patient is standing, slightly oblique to the apparatus. The film platform and compression device are positioned as far pos-teriorly as possible and snugly against the chest wall. The breast is held in position with one hand and compression applied with the other.

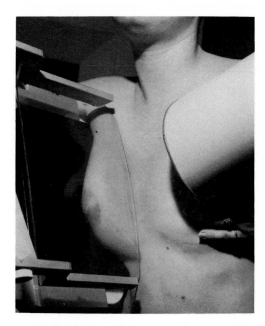

Figure 5–15. Erect oblique view. With the breast compressed and the opposite breast retracted, the tube is angled 30 degrees (possibly 60 degrees but usually 30 degrees suffices) to conform to the woman's anatomy.

ity. Having grown up with the positive mode, I believe there is scant, if any, convincing advantage to the negative mode.

Radiographic Techniques

Technical conditions that produce an optimum image of the breast with a conventional overhead tungsten target x-ray tube are (1) 300 to 450 ma; (2) 0.7 to 2.0 mm focal spot size; (3) 35 to 45 kvp; (4) 30- to 36-inch source image receptor distance (SID); and (5) total filtration of 0.5 to 2.0 mm of aluminum (Al) or equivalent (with 1.0 mm considered optimum for quality and 2.0 mm for dose reduction).

The x-ray unit should be calibrated for outputs of 35 to 45 kvp set in increments of

1 to 2 kvp. The output with the small and large focal spots should be compared for significant differences at the same milliamperage settings. Identical settings are not the same on all x-ray units. Calibration is usually necessary. Suggested technical factors are listed in Table 5–3.

There are several reasons for the wide milliamperage range of 300 to 450 ma.

1. The outputs of x-ray units vary because of factors such as age and the condition of the tube.

2. Outputs of multiphasic and constant potential equipment vary.

3. The total filtration, e.g., 0.5 mm Al at 300 ma, 1.0 mm Al at 350 ma, 1.5 mm Al at 400 ma.

4. Permits conversion from positive to negative modes.

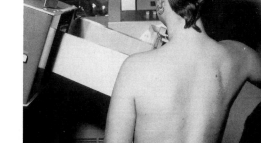

Figure 5–16. Erect oblique view. The tube angle is better appreciated from this view.

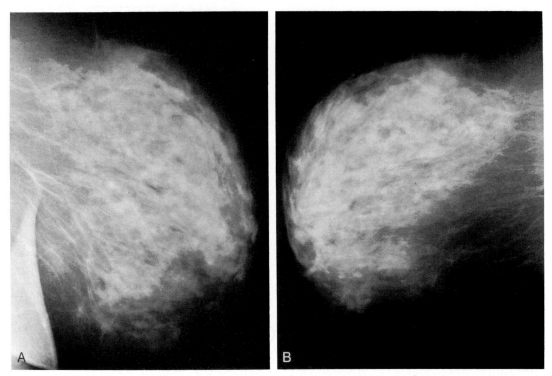

Figure 5–17. *A,* Erect mediolateral compression study poorly done as the breast has sagged against the chest and abdominal wall. *B,* Breast properly pulled out while compression was applied.

TABLE 5–3. Suggested Xerographic Technical Conditions for Three Different Types of Breast for 1.0 mm Infiltration

	Density	ma	kvp	Charge	Mode
Craniocaudad projection	Minimal	350	35–36	D	Positive
	Average	350	38	D	Positive
	Excessive	175	44	D	Positive
	Alternative technique for excessive density				
		175	42–45	C	Positive
		230	46	D	Positive
Mediolateral projection (chest wall)	Minimal	350	37–38	D	Positive
	Average	350	41	D	Positive
	Excessive	350	45–47	D	Positive
	Alternative technique for excessive density				
		425	45	D	Positive
Mediolateral projection (contact)	Same technique as for the craniocaudad projection				

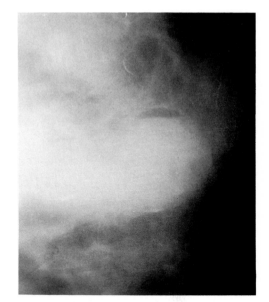

Figure 5–18. Layering of a galactocele in the erect position. This would not have been apparent in the craniocaudad or recumbent mediolateral position.

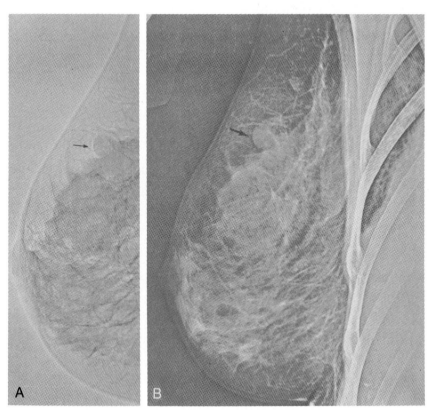

Figure 5–19. *A,* A positive mode contact (lateral view) with a breast mass. *B,* A negative (mediolateral view) of the same breast.

A kilovoltage of 35 to 45 kvp is used because a higher setting does not demonstrate soft tissues of the breast as well; calibration prevents error. A kilovoltage meter with one-step increments is an advantage. More than 45 kvp may be required for large dense breasts, dense cancer, and skin thickening.

Kilovotage is the most specific factor in xeroradiography of the breast, as a change of 1 to 2 kvp can affect the diagnostic quality of the procedure. Not nearly so specific changes can be produced by manipulation of the milliamperage. The effect of the change of 1 to 2 kvp is much greater at lower kilovoltage of breast radiography than it is for other anatomic parts using 120 kvp.

Compression of the breast is mandatory. An inflated balloon on the end of a long cone is used. Compression reduces thickness of the base of the breast and immobilizes the breast; the balloon prevents superimposition of the contralateral breast. Care should be taken not to overcompress the periphery of a fatty breast because it produces overexposure and defeats the purpose of compression. The balloon should be shaped with Scotch tape to present a bulge at the back of the cone for more compression on the base of the breast.

Establishing Techniques

After the kilovoltage is calibrated and the milliamperage factor determined, a patient whose breasts are apparently of average density is selected. The conditions determined for the craniocaudad projection comprise the baseline for other projections and for breasts of different density. The plate is charged at the "D" setting, and 37 or 38 kvp is selected. An exposure of the breast in the craniocaudad projection is made. The xeroradiograph is examined for the following (Fig. 5–20).

1. The varying densities of blue powder within the breast allow differentiation of tissues such as fat and fibroglandular tissue. If the blue tones are flat and the overall appearance is dark blue, underexposure of 2 kvp or more is suspected. A breast lacking fat could cause this type of image. With a pale blue study without distinct trabeculae, overexposure is probably responsible.

2. The halo surrounding the skin of the breast should be no greater than 2.0 mm in width. If wider, the kilovoltage is low; and if

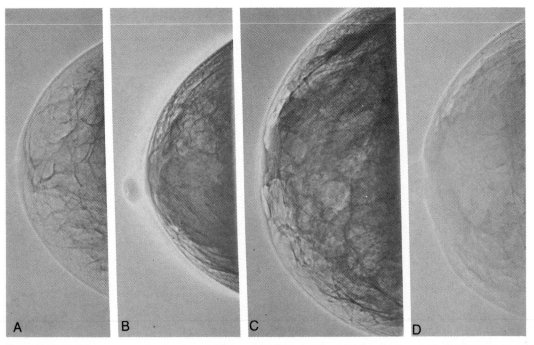

Figure 5–20. A, Proper exposure, showing equal amounts of fat and fibroglandular tissue. B, Underexposed. Note the white halo around the skin and the density. C, Correct exposure of a dense breast. D, Overexposure of a fatty breast. It is washed out and light blue.

the skin and subcutaneous tissues are nearly the same density with the skin line (halo is washed out), the kilovoltage is too high.

3. Trabecular structures should be examined with a magnifying lens to see if they are sharply defined.

Suggested technical conditions for three types of breast for 1.0 mm total infiltration are shown in Table 5–3.

A thick fatty breast requires the same conditions in the craniocaudad projection as an average density breast that contains fat and fibroglandular tissues. For the thickest parts of this type of breast in the mediolateral position, an increase of 4 to 5 kvp or an increase in time by one step and 2 kvp is required to penetrate tissues near the chest wall and in the axilla. The axillary projections may require a 50 per cent increase in the milliamperage and 4 to 6 kvp over the craniocaudad projection. If in an obese patient a positive-mode study fails because of the kilovoltage and tube limitations, a negative mode may be used. The negative technique recommended requires lowering the milliamperage by one third and increasing the kilovoltage by 1 or 2 kvp. The plate should be charged on contrast "D" and developed on density "B" or "C," with the mode control on "N."

Molybdenum Anode Tube

In xeroradiographs of the breast with a molybdenum anode x-ray tube, the kilovoltage and filtration differ from those in film mammography. The characteristic radiation from this anode is between 27 and 30 kvp (17 to 20 keV). The desired range is 35 to 45 kvp; the characteristic x-rays from this tube are of lower kilovoltage, which increases contrast and decreases latitude. The setting is between 40 and 50 kvp as compensation. A 0.5 mm Al filter is added, replacing the usual 30 μm molybdenum filter, or the two are used in combination.

Positioning

Craniocaudad and mediolateral projections are routine (Fig. 5–21). In addition to the mediolateral projection that includes the chest wall and axilla, a mediolateral view with the breast and cassette in contact is usually obtained. The marker is placed at least 2 inches from the skin and next to the outer (axillary) quadrant.

Positioning follows closely that of routine mammography, and variations of these positions may also be used with xeroradiography (Egan, 1984). A radiographic table, special plastic-top tunnel, or load-bearing cassette is used.

Imaging Problems

The selection of the proper kilovoltage is the greatest inherent difficulty in xeroradiography of the breast. Underexposure of only 2 kv may produce a nondiagnostic study. Overexposure may not be as detrimental as underexposure. It is recognized by a pale blue tone.

Poor contact between the breast and cassette causes the loss of radiographic detail, i.e., fine trabecular structures and minute calcifications. Excessive skin folds and wrinkles can cause adjacent tissues to be omitted or deleted from the image by white streaks, which are referred to as toner robbing. Whenever increased thickness or density is present on the surface anatomy of the breast, in contrast to increased density within the breast, toner is strongly attracted away from adjacent tissue. A pronounced area of white encircles the nipple when it is off profile and superimposed on breast tissue, simulating a dense mass with typical edge enhancement.

Table 5–4 compares the advantages and disadvantages of xeroradiography with those of film mammography.

TABLE 5–4. Xeroradiography of the Breast

Advantages	Disadvantages
Dry process	More radiation by a large
Viewed by reflected	factor
light—two or more	Messy
people view	More expensive
simultaneously	Less resolution, less
One sheet covers large	information
breast	Poor wide-field contrast
Edge enhancement	Very fine calcifications not
Wide exposure latitude	seen
	Numerous artifacts
	Filing problems with large
	sheets
	Use of minifying lens
	Increased object-film
	distance
	Added views routinely
	Higher kilovoltage, more
	scatter to body
	Increased down time
	Difficult to use Mo anode

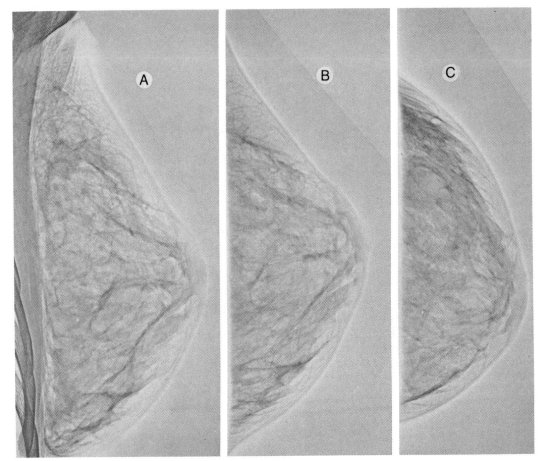

Figure 5–21. Correctly exposed and positioned complete xeroradiographic study. *A*, Mediolateral view. *B*, Contact lateral view. *C*, Craniocaudad view.

EVALUATING MAMMOGRAPHIC TECHNIQUES

Background

The most desirable mammographic technique is simply the one that is clinically applicable and provides the best image possible. Mammographic image quality is measured by the ability of the human retina to perceive small structures on the mammograms. Other terms for image quality include radiographic quality, definition, sharpness, and clarity. Interpretation of mammograms does depend to a great degree on the image quality—the perception of structures—but does not indicate the quality of the study. A cancer may be easily diagnosed on a poor mammogram, whereas tiny calcifications can be seen only on a high-quality study without their etiology being apparent.

Mammographic technique is 90 to 95 per cent of the procedure and interpretation only 5 to 10 per cent. We all make the same errors for the same reasons. Generally, if three criteria are fulfilled good mammograms are being produced: (1) The outline of the skin is sharp as well as the thin dark line just beneath the skin; (2) when viewed through the hand lens there are structures seen throughout the breast, including adipose tissue, without homogeneous areas being visible; and (3) in many areas sweat glands are clearly seen. Another set of criteria indicates the quality of the mammograms: (1) Ninety per cent of cancers are diagnosed; (2) 10 per cent of cancers are clinically unsuspected; and (3) 10 per cent of benign lesions are false positive (benign lesions interpreted as cancer).

Some element of contrast is necessary to make a structure visible against surrounding tissues. This is radiographic contrast, and it is influenced by subject contrast and receptor contrast. Subject contrast (intensity of transmitted x-rays through various tissues) of the breast is narrow, requiring efforts to delineate fine structures of the breast that are of near-equal density. All the technical factors used for mammography individually and collectively influence the quality of the mammogram. Some factors, such as kilovoltage, can be controlled and used at an optimal condition, whereas others, such as the density of adipose tissue, cannot be altered. In the final mammogram, as already noted, the technique is a compromise of many factors. We shall outline some of the factors and then illustrate how we analyze the final manipulations.

Subject contrast is affected by absorption differences (thickness, density such as closely packed fibrous scar tissue against normal fibroglandular tissue, and Z number); radiation quality (anode material, kvp, filtration); and scattered radiation (collimation, grid, compression). Properties and handling of receptors affect radiographic contrast, e.g., film, screen-film, edge effect, the processing (temperature, time, agitation, chemicals), and fog level (x-ray and light leaks, time of storage, softlight). Radiographic blurring is reflected by motion, geometry, and receptor type. Noise depends on radiographic mottle (receptor grain size, quantum, and tissue mottle) and artifacts.

The several component factors producing a radiograph can be evaluated individually in the laboratory, but the complexity of the interrelationship is such that the relative importance of each factor in the production of the final radiograph cannot be easily measured. The usual techniques for measuring radiographic image quality—e.g., visual inspection of wire mesh, various-sized holes in objects of various densities, and embedding various-sized objects in wax or suspending them in some liquid such as oil—have resulted in significantly different results, as reported by Rossman (1966). Additional com-

plications to evaluating the basic parameters of the imaging system and type of image are the retinal response, the subjectivity, and the psychic response of the observer of the final radiograph.

Need for Phantoms

Contrasting results were being obtained in the 20 to 30 kvp range of mammography by use of many simulated breast phantoms. Having had considerable experience with such phantoms, we became aware that our results were inadequate and misleading for application to our well-established mammography technique, which had been derived from tedious trial-and-error radiography of mastectomy specimens and the intact breast. It became necessary to devise a suitable phantom utilizing breast tissue in order to evaluate the individual technical conditions that produce mammograms and to assess adequate radiographic detail. Data obtained at the conventional kilovoltage range and with screen techniques were not applicable to mammography with objects 20 to 40 times smaller than those seen with conventional radiography. Frequency modulation transfer systems were not helpful in the evaluation of low subject-contrast range between adipose and fibroglandular tissue, as opposed to the wide range of contrast of air and bone in general screen-film radiography.

Mammographic Phantoms

Two thicknesses of breast tissue were embedded in plastic for precise control of the many variations in the technical factors usually encountered in mammography (Egan and Fenn, 1968). In Figure 5–22 the thinner slice of breast tissue is 2 cm thick and is

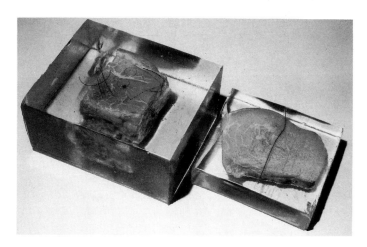

Figure 5–22. Two phantoms consisting of test objects within breast tissue mounted in plastic. In the thicker, the test objects are mounted at two levels; in the thinner, at one level. (From Egan RL, Fenn JO: AJR 102:936, 1968. Used by permission.)

embedded in a 3 cm thick plastic mount. The thicker slice (6 cm), representing the average maximal thickness of breast in mammographic positions, is embedded in an 8 cm thick plastic block, 13 × 15 cm in size. The larger phantom contains a 0.5 mm diameter copper wire, 0.25 and 0.30 mm diameter steel wires, particles of crushed chalk, a lead shot, crushed marble, and fine aluminum oxide particles embedded at fixed but different depths in the phantom.

The thinner phantom contains a 0.50 mm wire, a 0.8 cm circle fashioned out of a 0.25 mm steel wire, and Al_2O_3 particles in irregular thicknesses and sizes up to 0.25 mm in diameter. Al_2O_3 was chosen for its Z number of approximately 11, compared with a Z number of 7 for soft tissues and of 14 for calcifications in the breast. Also, the irregularity of the fragmented particles of Al_2O_3 serves to represent variable edges for radiography. With the test objects placed closer to the film, the object-film distance is 0.5 cm; with the objects on the upper surface or farther from the film, the object-film distance is 2.5 cm.

A phantom in radiography is an invaluable aid for establishing x-ray techniques without the constant problem of patient variation. The more nearly the same as the part being studied, the more valuable is a phantom. Any technical condition for radiography may be varied independently and evaluated, as illustrated in the comparison of film emulsions in Figures 5–23 to 5–25. Only the milliamperage was varied through trial and error by changing the time of exposure to produce radiographs of phantoms of comparable density.

Actual radiographic films of the area of the wire circle were cut to fit a 35 mm slide mount and, when projected onto our screen, were magnified 60 times. To maintain objectivity when evaluating the data, several disinterested people counted and recorded the total number of flecks of Al_2O_3 in the wire circle as well as the number of flecks seen in the small crescent near the center of the wire circle (Fig. 5–23). Average data obtained by eight observers comparing four film emulsions are listed in Table 5–5, demonstrating the use of this method.

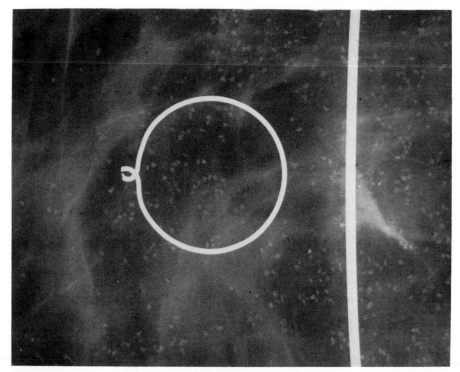

Figure 5–23. Reproduction of a portion of the radiograph of a breast phantom. The wires are 0.25 and 0.5 mm in diameter. The Al_2O_3 particles are readily seen, displaying various densities and edge formation. Kodak industrial x-ray film, type M (Estar base) was used. See also Figures 5–24 and 5–25. (From Egan RL, Fenn JO: AJR 102:936, 1968. Used by permission.)

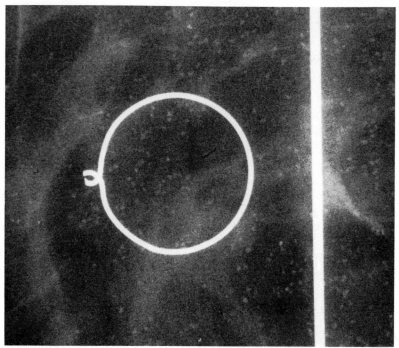

Figure 5–24. Reproduction of a radiograph similar to Figures 5–23 and 5–25, with all conditions of radiography and photography the same (density adjusted) except that Kodak industrial x-ray film, type AA (Estar base) was used. (From Egan RL, Fenn JO: AJR 102:936, 1968. Used by permission.)

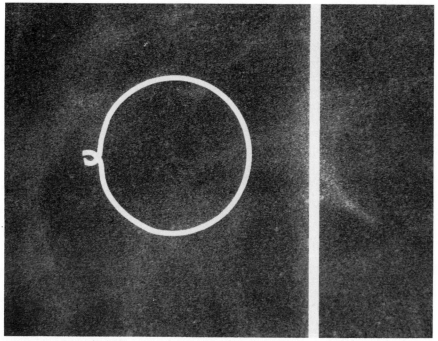

Figure 5–25. Reproduction of a radiograph similar to Figures 5–23 and 5–24, with all conditions of radiography and photography the same (density adjusted) except that nonscreen medical x-ray film was used. The radiographic detail here is similar to new screen-film techniques without added artifacts from screens. (From Egan RL, Fenn JO: AJR 102:936, 1968. Used by permission.)

TABLE 5–5. Comparison of Various Factors Using X-Ray Film Emulsions at 60 × Magnification

Film Type	Projected Size of Al_2O_3 Particles (mm)	Actual Size of Particles (mm)	Milliamperage Required for Comparable Density (ma)	No. of Particles in Ring Counted	No. of Particles in Crescent Counted
Kodak M	3	0.05	900	143	15
Kodak E*	± 4	0.07	900	114	12
Kodak AA	± 5	0.08	300	113	12
Medical NS	± 10	0.16	170	64	8

*Medical x-ray film for mammography designed for a mechanical processor.

Even more dramatic than using the numbers of particles counted for comparison is the clarity of the particles, as noted in the illustrations. For instance, only the Al_2O_3 particles on Kodak type M film projected with sharp enough edges for measurement.

To evaluate the technical factors for radiographic detail, the observer needs only the ability to see and count. Using these phantoms, observers have obtained comparable results; the results are readily reproduced from day to day, and subjectivity is reduced to a minimum. The method is reliable, objective, reproducible, adaptable, and precise. It is of particular value when two or more variables are introduced, as the relative importance of each variable cannot be assessed objectively. Thus we have evaluated all the individual technical conditions (from subject contrast through geometry) that influence the quality of the mammograms as well as a number of combinations of conditions. There is no need to speculate on possible effects of altering the technique; one simply makes the required measurements.

The increasing use of xeroradiography of the breast has required development of a phantom that allows objective comparison of xeroradiography and conventional film mammography. Most phantoms useful in evaluating conventional mammography tend to degrade xeroradiography by toner robbing; line-pair phantoms placed in close contact with the xeroradiographic plate are not comparable to studies of the breast tissues.

A phantom patterned after the thin one in Figure 5–22 was developed with Al_2O_3 particles within a metallic ring and a plastic ring simultaneously exposed on xeroradiographic paper and film for objective comparisons

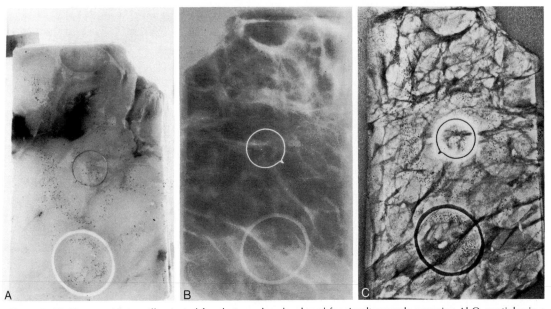

Figure 5–26. Phantom (*A*) transilluminated for photography; developed for simultaneously exposing Al_2O_3 particles in a plastic ring and metallic ring on type M film (*B*); and on xeroradiographic paper (*C*—mirror image of *B*). Many finer flecks of *B* did not reproduce.

(Fig. 5–26). This readily demonstrated the superiority of M-film compared with xeroradiography and the screen-film technique.

Some Results from Phantoms

Phantoms can illustrate several of the difficulties encountered with techniques that utilize a short target-film distance. The target-film distance utilized in some mammographic techniques is so short that collimation of the beam is done only by the aperture in the tube housing if the average-sized breast is included in the beam. This lack of collimation of the x-ray beam not only detracts from the radiographic detail but also causes a considerable increase in patient dose. A technique utilizing a 16 inch target-film distance and nonscreen film (six times as fast as fine-grain industrial film) produces a volume dose to the patient nine times as great as the conventional technique with equal density on the mammograms. This is an indication of the importance of off-focus radiation in radiography, the role of collimation, the control of scattered radiation, and the use of geometry associated with longer target-film distances.

A once widely used, gadget-oriented convenience mammography unit confined to an 11- to 13-inch target-film distance produced 10 to 15 times the radiation to the skin as did conventional mammography with great sacrifice in detail.

Collimation is of value in eliminating the heel effect. With relatively longer target-film distances, better collimation can be utilized, with the breast still included in the x-ray beam. In this manner a greater portion of the x-ray beam is made up of the central beam; with shorter distances the x-ray beam emanating from a wider area of the target must be utilized, resulting in a marked heel effect. Beneficial use of the heel effect (anode side of the tube toward the thinner part) necessitates an elaborate mechanical arrangement for rotating the tube so that the anode side of the tube is always over the nipple. Because this is not done, the anode is over the base of the breast half of the time, compounding the difficulties with short target-film distances.

One of the most important factors contributing to radiographic detail is a short object-film distance. With the breast lying directly on the film holder in any specific position, the detail can be improved by increasing the target-film distance. The penumbra and increased scattered radiation beyond the area of primary interest with the shorter target-film distance can be improved with a larger target-film distance and proper collimation.

The difficulties encountered with speculation about radiographic factors at the mammographic kilovoltage range are illustrated in Figure 5–27. One of our mammographic x-ray units had been so redesigned and rebuilt that meticulous monitoring and control of milliamperage and kilovoltage were possible. Empirically it was evident that small changes in kilovoltage in the mammography range caused marked changes in milliamperage, but this could be proved in the laboratory only after construction of such an x-ray unit. Radiography of the phantom with equal

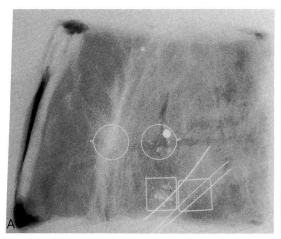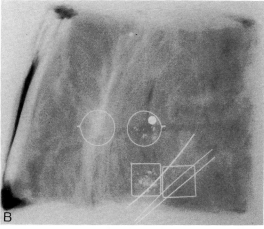

Figure 5–27. Radiographs of the large phantoms in Figure 5–22 with 23.8 and 31 kvp but with monitored and equal milliamperage, all other conditions being identical. No observer was able to detect any significant differences even on the radiographs. (Without milliamperage control, 2 kvp produces approximately 1.5 times the milliamperage effect.)

milliamperage and 19 to 34 kvp produced similar or equal film density and an absence of the expected grayness of increased kilovoltage. In another experiment the kilovoltage was kept constant and the milliamperage was varied. The radiograph with increased milliamperage was judged darker and grayer and appeared to have been produced with higher kilovoltage.

Table 5–3 lists some of the advantages and disadvantages with screen-film receptors.

Dance and Davis (1983), after review of reported evaluations of direct exposure and screen-film combinations, noted, "Radiation for film/screen systems is 5 to 20 times less than that for direct exposure systems. This advantage is partly offset by superior resolution and noise properties of direct exposure films."

REFERENCES

Barnes GT, Brezovitch IA (1977): Contrast: effect of scattered radiation. *In* Logan WW (ed): Breast Carcinoma: The Radiologist's Expanded Role. New York, John Wiley & Sons, pp 113–116.

Breslow L, Thomas LB, Upton AC (1977): Final report of the NCI Ad-Hoc Working Group on the risk associated with mammography in mass screening for detection of breast cancer. J Natl Cancer Inst *59*:467.

Dance DR, Davis R (1983): *In* Parsons CA (ed): Physics of Mammography in Diagnosis of Breast Diseases. Baltimore, University Park Press, p 95.

Egan RL (1984): Breast Imaging, 3rd ed. Baltimore, University Park Press, pp 31–58; 108–109.

Egan RL (1964): Mammography. Springfield, IL, Charles C Thomas.

Egan RL (1960): Experience with mammography in a tumor institution. Radiology *74*:894.

Egan RL, Fenn JO (1968): Phantoms for evaluating mammographic techniques and roentgenographic detail. AJR *102*:936.

Egan RL, Wright GM, Timms D (1973): Automatic processor for Eastman Kodak industrial x-ray film, type M (Estar base). Radiology *109*:734.

Ewton JR, Shalek RJ, Egan RL (1962): Estimated radiation dosage during mammography. Cancer Bull *14*:116.

Haus AG (1983). Physical principles and radiation dose in mammography. *In* Feig SA, McLelland R (eds): Breast Carcinoma: Current Diagnosis and Treatment. New York, Masson Publishing.

Kirka C (1961): X-ray tube considerations for mammography. Macklett Cathode Press *18*:2.

Rossman K (1966): Comparison of several methods of evaluating image quality of radiographic screen-film systems. AJR *97*:772.

Ruzicka EF, Kaufman L, Shapiro G, Perez V, Grossi CE (1965): Xeromammography and film mammography; a comparative study. Radiology *85*:260.

Ancillary Radiographic Techniques

GRIDS IN MAMMOGRAPHY

Background

Grids have been adapted to mammography to improve contrast and visibility of small structures by reducing scattered radiation (Freidrick and Weskamp, 1978; Jost, 1979; Lammers and Kuhn, 1979; Stanton and Logan, 1979). Depending on the field size and tissue thickness, the intensity of the scattered radiation during mammography varies from 40 to 85 per cent of the primary beam intensity (Barnes and Brezovisk, 1979).

General-purpose grids are not useful in mammography because of attenuation of the relatively low energy x-ray beam by dense spacer material. The recent introduction of a fiber-interspaced, carbon-covered grid makes grid-augmented mammography possible.

With use of grids in earlier experimentation to devise a technique for mammography (Egan 1960), problems were posed in conventional mammography: (1) increased dose to the breast; (2) need for rigid receptors; (3) greater difficulty in visualizing chest wall; (4) attenuation of the x-ray beam (with older type grids); and (5) increased object-film distance.

In investigating the use of a grid in mammography, several questions arose: Is it adaptable to mammography; does it improve visibility of small calcifications in dense, thick breasts; is the resultant image quality worth the increased radiation; and, if necessary, can the dose be reduced without sacrifice of quality?

Use of Grids

We adapted a 5:1 mammography grid with lead lamellae, fiber interspaces, carbon fiber covers, and 80 lines per inch to an x-ray unit designed for mammography. The grid allowed an increase in kilovoltage sufficient to penetrate the base of the breast without severe compression; it retained diagnostic contrast and visibility, and it maintained an acceptable level of radiation to the breast (Egan et al., 1983). A single-phase Picker Mammorex, used with a molybdenum anode target, a 30 μ molybdenum filter, and a 0.6 mm focal spot size, was modified to use a grid.

A breast tissue phantom (Egan and Fenn, 1968) was used to determine the visibility of irregularly shaped and sized Al_2O_3 particles under varying conditions of kvp, grid, non-grid, and magnification. This phantom was composed of breast tissue that was embedded in 6 cm thick plastic, and it was 8 $\times$ 10 cm in size. The relationship of contrast to a range of 25 to 35 kvp was determined using different thicknesses of a second plastic breast phantom that contained a lead shot, a similar-sized aluminum disk, and fine to coarse chalk particles. The second phantom was 9 × 14 cm in size and could be built to a 6 cm thickness in increments of 0.5 cm. The screen-film combination used for this section of the study was a Kodak Min-R system in a vacuum bag cassette.

In clinical application of grids in mammography it was found that magnification could be increased to 1.1 times without loss of spatial resolution. If a thicker cassette-type screen-film holder rather than a vacuum cassette were used, it would produce no added magnification since the film is in the top part of the cassette. Use of the grid improved visibility of the small objects in the breast phantom and permitted use of higher kvp as compared with the nongrid technique (Fig.

6–1). Also, the grid preserved comparatively more contrast with an increase in both kvp and the thickness of the phantom (Figs. 6–2 and 6–3).

Entrance surface exposure was increased when using the grid. The mas required at 27 kvp with and without the grid are plotted in Figure 6–4 vs phantom thickness, and the increase was 1.5 to 1.7 times as great at the same thickness. A 3 cm breast (compression) required 125 mas, while a 5 cm breast (no compression) required 350 mas. Also, at 33 kvp the entrance surface exposure was one-third that at 27 kvp with the grid. Figure 6–5 shows images that were obtained with a faster film; these can be compared with images that were obtained under similar conditions (Fig. 6–1 B and D). Faster film reduced the entrance surface exposure by a

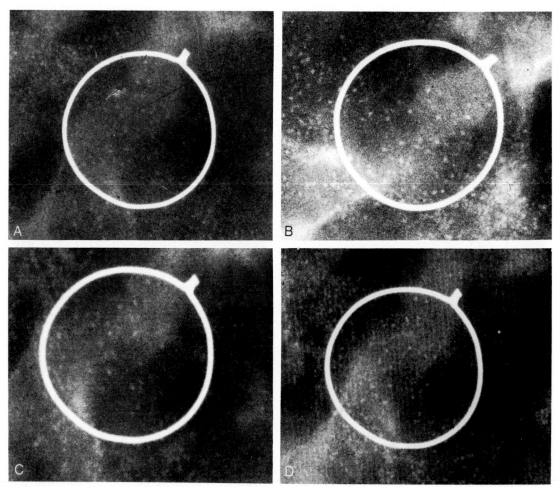

Figure 6–1. The 8 × 10 breast phantom, 6 cm thick. A, Nongrid contact at 27 kvp. B, Grid, 1.03 × magnification (the minimum possible with the grid at 27 kvp). C, Grid, 1.1 × magnification at 27 kvp. D, Grid, 1.03 × magnification at 33 kvp. More detail is visible in D than in A despite the grid lines. The prototype moving grid mechanism was not sufficiently refined to prevent occasional grid lines, i.e., the movement was not always totally synchronous with the x-ray pulses.

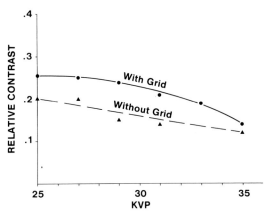

Figure 6–2. Contrast as affected by increasing the kilovoltage from 25 to 35. Relative improvement with the grid is diminished above 33 kvp.

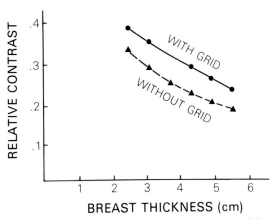

Figure 6–3. Contrast as affected by the thickness of the object. The grid improved contrast at all thicknesses studied.

factor of 2 but produced grainier radiographs with more contrast. In a clinical setting, the mammogram that was obtained with a two times faster film (Kodak Ortho-M with Min-R screen), at an increased kvp (33 kvp), and with the grid compared favorably with the Kodak Min-R screen-film system mammogram that was obtained at 27 kvp without the grid (Fig. 6–6).

With a grid there is a definite increase in the quality of the mammograms throughout the kvp range under investigation. There is also a definite increase in the amount of radiation, which is more pronounced at the lower kvp; this still remains, in our opinion, within acceptable limits. It should also be noted that the amount of radiation that is now administered during screen-film mammography can be reduced by a factor of 2 with the faster film or by a factor of 3 with higher kvp.

During screen-film mammography, the critical thickness of breasts is 3 to 5 cm, depending on the density of the fibroglandular tissue. Because many breasts cannot be compressed to less than 5 to 6 cm, scattered radiation becomes an important factor. With vigorous compression, more breast tissue is pushed out of the x-ray field and less base of the breast is included. Compression becomes of less importance, with a reduction of scattered radiation by the grid to improve contrast, use of higher kilovoltage for penetration of thicker breasts, and a reduction of the effects of geometric unsharpness by decreasing the receptor blur. Lighter compression, as with a balloon, could then be carried out in the recumbent mediolateral position with easier coverage of the chest wall and

base of the breast. Our real interest in grids in breast imaging has been the potential that severe compression of the breast could be lessened and more relaxed positioning could be adapted to screen-film use.

Scattered radiation through poorly penetrated areas, e.g., at the base of the breast, results in radiation-darkened areas on the radiograph. A grid removes much of this scattered radiation and results in significant improvement in contrast (Sorenson et al., 1980). In this situation, elevated kilovoltage combined with grid-improved images will result in the increased visibility of diagnostically important detail, more uniform penetration of the breast, and reduction in scatter.

Since the National Institutes of Health/National Cancer Institute (NIH/NCI) Consensus Development Meeting on Breast Screening in 1977, radiologists either abandoned

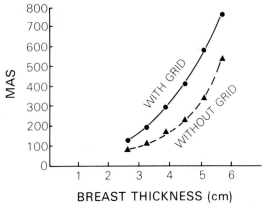

Figure 6–4. The ratio of radiation to the skin (air dose) with the grid vs no grid at 27 kvp. The maximum increase in radiation with the grid was a 4.5 to 5.0 cm thickness.

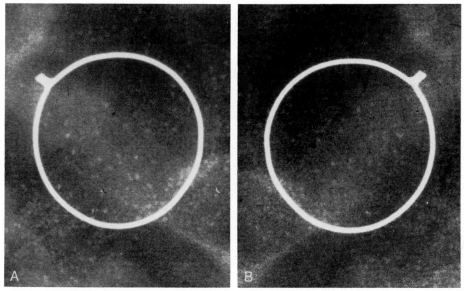

Figure 6–5. Kodak Ortho M film with a grid at 27 kvp (*A*) and 33 kvp (*B*).

mammography or accepted screen-film receptors. The first alternative was often dictated by the scarcity of patients that was caused by confused primary-care physicians and frightened women of all ages, asymptomatic as well as symptomatic. Screen-film mammography was usually done on special mammography units with molybdenum anode tubes. This approach required vigorous compression of the breast to retain sufficient radiographic contrast in the 25 to 29 kvp range and to reduce geometric unsharpness. Many women complained bitterly about this painful compression of their breast.

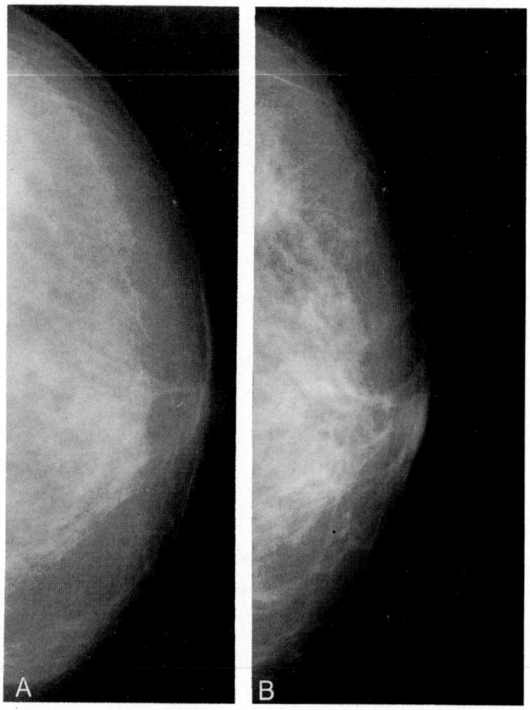

With the opportunity to increase the kilovoltage to 33 kvp, much less compression is required to penetrate the dense base of the breast. Even the base of the large, very glandular breast in a young woman on the mediolateral view is comparably imaged to that on the craniocaudad view. Balloon type compression could be used to show ribs to assure radiography of the base of the breast.

Observations

The introduction of a grid suitable for mammography has been the only recent real contribution to the technique of clinical mammography. Grids may be adapted to mammography, and they offer the advantage of improved small-detail perception, particularly in the dense, thick breast. In our opinion, the improved image quality seems worth the increase in radiation.

We have also demonstrated that the skin exposure of the breast can be reduced by using faster film and particularly by increased kvp. This increased kvp then permits (1) better penetration of the base of the breast with a more even density to the mammo-

Figure 6–6. *A,* Kodak Min-R screen-film system at 27 kvp without grid. *B,* Kodak Ortho-M film with Min-R screen at 33 kvp with grid.

TABLE 6–1. Grids in Breast Imaging

Advantages	Disadvantages
Reduces scattered radiation	Increases radiation to breast
Permits use of higher kilovoltage	Increases object-film distance
Allows resolution of smaller structures	Requires rigid box
Increased object-receptor distance improves resolution with screen-film receptor	Spacers and covers must be radiolucent
Allows simple imaging of the base of the breast	May produce artifacts (grid lines) if poorly synchronized
	Can increase exposure time

gram; (2) inclusion of the entire base of the breast; (3) less compression, such as the balloon type, for better patient comfort and cooperation; and (4) more adaptable recumbent mediolateral positioning.

Some advantages and disadvantages of the use of grids in mammography are presented in Table 6–1.

SCREEN-FILM MAGNIFICATION MAMMOGRAPHY

Background

To overcome the marked degradation of the quality of the screen-film mammograms caused by the faster film and screens (even though they are rare earth), magnification with a fine focal spot theoretically should improve the radiograph. This procedure depends on (1) focal spot size, (2) screen-film system, (3) quality of the x-ray beam, and (4) air gap between object and receptor.

Doi (1977) has presented the following technical advantages of magnification versus contact screen-film mammography (usually 1.5 to 2 ×):

1. *Sharpness effect.* The resolution is increased with magnification. The explanation is that the effective unsharpness of the screen-film system is reduced when the x-ray pattern is enlarged. The resolution increases by a factor equal to the degree of magnification.

2. *Noise effect.* Noise is greatly reduced (by a factor equal to the degree of magnification squared). The x-ray pattern is enlarged, but the noise of the screen-film system remains unchanged. This means that the "effective noise" is reduced relative to the original object size. This leads to improved visibility of the x-ray pattern.

3. *Air-gap effect.* By using an air gap, the scattered radiation is reduced, which directly leads to increased contrast of the x-ray pattern. The size of air gap should exceed 15 cm.

4. *Visual effect.* Perception (visual recognition) and analysis of small details on the radiographs (small calcifications and the like) improve considerably when the image is enlarged, the contrast is increased, and the effective noise is reduced.

With direct film mammography, especially with slow industrial film, an x-ray tube anode with a relatively high heat capacity is required, e.g., a focal spot size of 1 or 2 mm. To reduce the focal spot size as a source of image blur, an increased focal spot–receptor distance is necessary even with the breast and receptor in contact. Thus the size of the x-ray tube focal spot must be selected for compromise between heat capacity and image blur.

With the introduction of intensifying screens, there are added sources of image blur: the receptor itself and an increased object-film distance. Increased speed of the screen-film receptor permits use of smaller focal spots, compensating to a degree for the added image blur; however, short target-film distances are still sought. Receptor blur decreases as the object-film distance increases because the magnification produced increases the image size and not the amount of screen blur. Therefore, the actual amount of blur relative to the size of the object is decreased, and the image quality is improved.

Laboratory Investigation

Using phantoms (Egan and Fenn, 1968) we compared the resolution during magnification with Kodak M film, a tungsten target, and 2 mm focal spot size on a Continental mammography unit with that of a Min-R screen-film system and Radiological Sciences, Inc. (RSI) 180 μ focal spot size on the same mammography unit. If fine-grain industrial film with a short object-film distance and a 2 mm focal spot size gave maximal, or 100 per cent, detail, then a short object-film distance combined with screen-film with a 180 μ focal spot size produced ±20 per cent radiographic detail.

On M film, resolution rapidly deteriorated with magnification and became 0 per cent at 2 × magnification (Fig. 6–7). On the Min-R

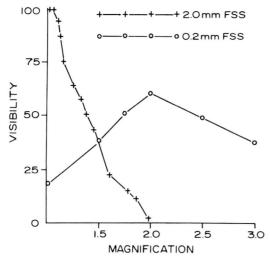

Figure 6–7. The maximum quality of the screen-film radiograph at 60 per cent of type M film quality is at 2 × magnification. Type M film quality is degraded to this level at 1.25 × magnification. FSS, focal spot size.

system, resolution was 20 per cent on contact (M film on contact was 100 per cent); it rose to 60 per cent at 2 × and then dropped to 35 per cent at 3 × magnification. At 1.25 × magnification, M film equaled the best resolution of Min-R (2 × magnification).

With conventional mammography, for M film resolution to equal that of Min-R an object-film distance of 9 inches is required at a 36 inch target-film distance. No such geo-

metric arrangement is used in conventional mammography; even with breast xeroradiography, the maximum object-film distance is no more than 3 to 4 inches.

Radiography of the dried phalangeal bones of a human hand was carried out, varying the focal spot size and object-film distance. These small bones have a fine trabecular pattern and require a relatively low kvp and ma for radiography. The Al_2O_3 flecks are blurred too rapidly for use in gross experiments. With the bones close to the film, lying on the cardboard holder, the 0.3 mm and 2 mm focal spot produced radiographs of equal quality (Figs. 6–8 to 6–11). As the bones were moved to increase the object-film distance while maintaining a fixed target-film distance, blurring readily became apparent, although it was less marked with the 0.3 mm focal spot. By this method, at magnification of 1.5 times, the radiographs had practically no detail. This clearly shows the futility of attempting such magnification while trying to maintain radiographic detail. Largeness of the recorded object is not necessarily related to sharpness of its edges. It is far easier and sounder physically to obtain an image with a short object-film distance and then to enlarge it with the use of light, which can be more readily controlled than x-rays. The image obtained with a 2 mm focal spot, blown up 20 times by use of light, has infinitely

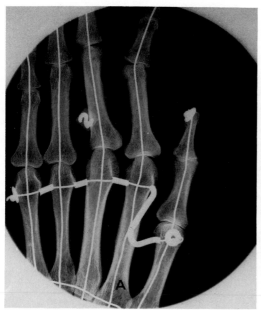
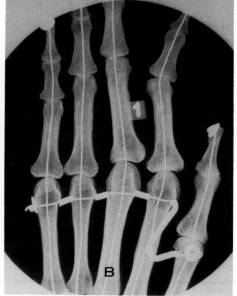

Figure 6–8. Radiographs of dried phalangeal bones of the hand. The bones rest on the cardboard film holder, and the target-film distance is 36 inches. All factors are the same except for 2 mm focal spot size in *A* and 0.3 mm focal spot size in *B*. Actual size. *A* was the slightly darker radiograph.

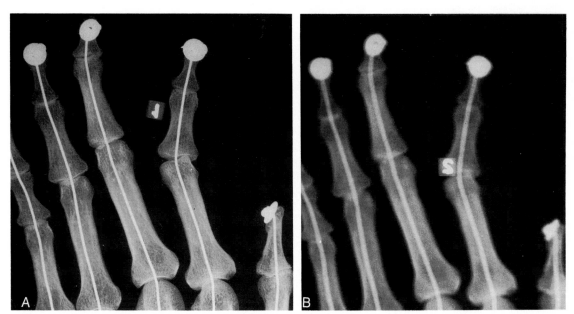

Figure 6–9. Radiographs of the same dried phalangeal bones as in Figure 6–8. The only change in technique was the 15 inch to object-film distance for each; 0.3 mm focal spot (*A*) and 2 mm focal spot size (*B*). Even with 1.5 × magnification there is unacceptable blurring (absence of radiographic detail) in both, more marked with the larger focal spot size. (Radiograph reduced in size for reproduction.)

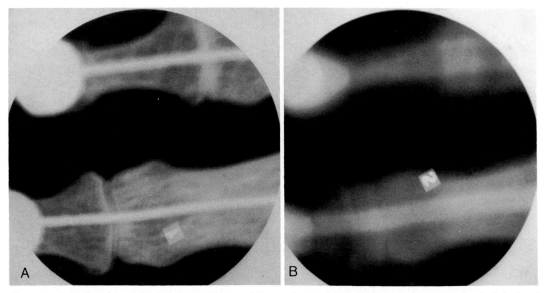

Figure 6–10. Radiograph of dried phalangeal bones of Figures 6–8 and 6–9. Technique change consisted of placing the object near the tube housing for maximum magnification, approximately 6 to 1. Note severe blurring with both focal spot sizes; *A* is 0.3 mm and *B* is 2 mm focal post size. (Radiograph reduced in size for reproduction.)

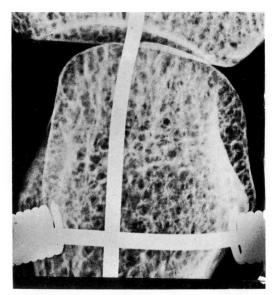

Figure 6–11. Radiograph (A) of Figure 6–8 made with the 2 mm focal spot enlarged. Size was increased 20 × by photographic enlargement (use of light) without loss of any detail; see Figures 6–9 and 6–10. (Radiograph reduced in size for reproduction.)

more detail than the one magnified only two times with a 0.3 mm focal spot using x-rays. The advantages in mammography of good positioning and compression of lateromedial projections when indicated become obvious.

Clinical Application

X-ray tubes with a focal spot size as small as 180 μ are commercially available and can be used for mammography with a target-receptor distance of 50 cm. During 2 × magnification with a 6 cm breast, the radiation at the upper surface of the breast would be increased 5.4 times because of the inverse square law ($44^2 \div 19^2$). The interposition of an air gap between the breast and the receptor tends to reduce scattered radiation.

Magnification mammography may be carried out on specially designed units or on modified conventional mammography units. In the former is a platform on which the breast rests, and the height above the receptor is varied to change the degree of magnification. A sturdy box with a cutout covered with a sheet of plastic on which the breast is placed may be readily constructed. Any height may be used. We selected a height of 6 inches to provide 1.3 × magnification at a 20 inch target-film distance. That magnification can be varied by changing the target-film distance.

When compared with screen-film receptors with less radiographic detail than that which can be produced on Kodak M film, in some cases magnification mammography improved diagnostic interpretation. This is understandable when Figure 6–7 is examined, where it can be seen that visibility improved sharply on the film-screen receptor as the object-film distance increased to produce 2 × magnification. An object near the film could be blurred at a reduced object-film distance. Several techniques may be combined (Fig. 6–12).

The dose at the skin with the 180 μ tube at 2 × magnification is two times the dose for 100 per cent quality with the 2 mm tube. The sacrifice is very great when, to use the screen-film system under our present best conditions, doubling of the dose is required to approach the image quality of conventional mammography done with an unreal object-film distance of 9 inches.

There are a limited number of proponents of magnification mammography, however, who claim that magnification of flecks of calcifications allows ready differentiation into benign and malignant types. We reviewed 500 biopsy specimens obtained for borderline calcifications not associated with a mass. These were sliced into 2 or 3 mm thickness, arranged on a cleared x-ray film and placed on a cardboard holder, and radiographed at 12 kvp with a small focal spot and 30 inch target-film distance on fine-grain industrial film. The radiographs were blow up 60 times. The two types of calcifications had so many overlapping features that they could not be confidently differentiated. Our conclusion was that a cluster of five or more borderline calcifications must be studied (see Chapter 27).

Table 6–2 outlines the advantages and disadvantages of magnification radiography of the breast compared with those of conventional mammography.

COMPUTER-ASSISTED TOMOGRAPHIC MAMMOGRAPHY (CT/M)

Computer tomography (CT) of the body has become a major diagnostic modality with the potential to resolve differences in tissue densities better than conventional radiography. When applied to the study of the breast, the cross-sectional image produced by the narrow x-ray beam rotating about the breasts

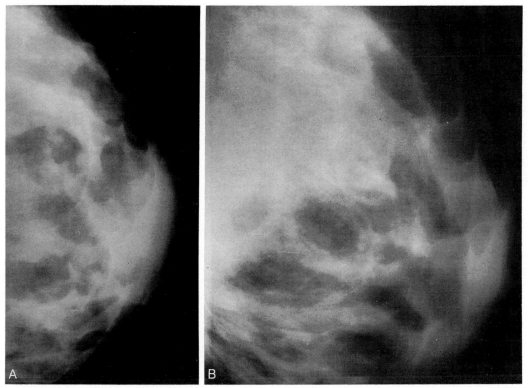

Figure 6–12. A 22-year-old nulliparous woman with large, firm, tender breasts. *A,* Routine craniocaudad view. *B,* Mediolateral view; grid, 35 kvp and magnification.

is digitized and manipulated by the computer. Very slight differences in tissue densities then can be amplified into an enhanced image. Hypothetically the malignant breast mass should produce denser shadows than a benign lesion.

Prototype CT/M breast units have been tested in two institutions. At the Mayo Clinic the results in difference in densities of benign and malignant masses were not very encouraging (Gisvold et al., 1977). At the University of Kansas (Chang et al., 1979), however, the breasts were first scanned, then intravenous

TABLE 6–2. Magnification Mammography

Advantages	Disadvantages
Utilizes an air gap	Requires very small anode
Improves resolution up to 1.5 × or 2 × with screen-film receptors	Increased radiation to breast
	Only a small area of breast projected with each exposure
	Requires short target-film distances (output of tube limits)
	Degrades nonscreen radiography
	Limited to 2 × magnification

contrast material (iodide) was administered, and the breasts were rescanned. From 5 to 10 per cent increase in density occurred in malignant masses, with much less enhancement of benign masses. Gisvold later used this enhancement technique but could not establish clear-cut differences between benign and malignant lesions (1979).

The University of Kansas group reported results of scans of 44 carcinomas ranging in size from 2 mm to 9 cm. The carcinomas increased the iodide content more than 50 Hounsfield Units (HU) enhancement on post-contrast scans (Fig. 6–13). The carcinomas were correctly identified as follows: CT/M, 93 per cent; mammography, 80 per cent; physical examination, 64 per cent; and CT/M plus mammography, 100 per cent. The CT/M was particularly useful in mammographically dense breasts.

Of 70 benign biopsy-proven lesions, 84 per cent had less than 40 HU enhancement on postcontrast scans (Fig. 6–14). In only 50 per cent of these lesions could malignancy be excluded by mammography.

At present one must assume that there is not enough evidence to envision widespread use of this approach to breast imaging, con-

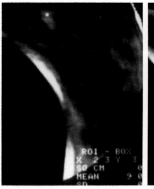
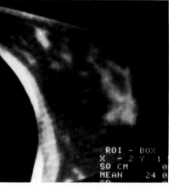

Figure 6–13. CT/M of a carcinoma. A 56-year-old woman with a breast mass, mammographically suspicious. Pre- (left) and postcontrast (right) scans showing the maximum contrast enhancement of 28 CT number (56 HU) in the mass (cursor). (Courtesy of C. H. Joseph Chang, M.D., University of Kansas Medical Center, Kansas City, KS.)

sidering that CT/M adds the risk of iodide injection to a time-comsuming and very expensive procedure without conclusively reproducible results.

GALACTOGRAPHY

Background

Galactography (ductography) is radiography of the opacified lactiferous ducts after injection of a contrast agent. Ries (1930) first demonstrated this procedure and warned of complications of infection and abscess formation following use of harsh contrast agents.

Galactography may be useful as an extension of routine mammography in the study of nipple discharge. Spontaneous nipple discharge is usually from an enlarged duct orifice, more amenable to cannulation. It is most productive with a single-duct bloody discharge not explained on the mammogram, but it may be used for any nipple discharge considered pathologic, unless the discharge is associated with pregnancy or lactation.

Technique

A smear of the nipple discharge precedes the examination. Under sterile conditions, with good light and a magnifying loop the orifice of the discharging duct is identified and a lymphangiography cannula inserted approximately 1 cm. With a hand-held syringe 0.25 to 1.5 ml of air-free contrast material is injected while the nipple is compressed about the cannula to ensure a good seal. The amount of injection depends on the pressure during injection and the sensation of fullness experienced by the patient.

Craniocaudad and mediolateral views are immediately obtained. To prevent leakage of the contrast agent, the woman compresses the nipple. We prefer to conduct the examination with the patient in the supine position, almost in the radiographic mediolateral position. This assures that a satisfactory study will be obtained in at least this position before the patient is moved into the craniocaudad position.

Extravasation of the contrast medium may occur, and the patient may experience a burning sensation. With present-day contrast

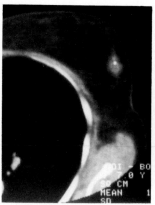
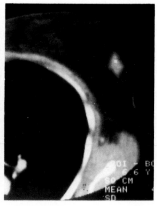

Figure 6–14. CT/M of localized fibrocystic disease. A 51-year-old woman with nodularity of the breasts, mammographically inconclusive. Pre-(left) and postcontrast (right) studies showing the maximum postcontrast enhancement of 15 CT (30 HU) in the mass (cursor). (Courtesy of C. H. Joseph Chang, M.D., University of Kansas Medical Center, Kansas City, KS.)

agents this lasts only a short time and the material is quickly absorbed. Markedly ectatic ducts may not fill easily, as they are already packed, even with increased pressure during injection. A radiograph will demonstrate this situation.

Observations

The normal galactogram clearly outlines the major ducts and the repetitive arborization of the ducts as they become smaller and extend deeper into the substance of the breast (Fig. 6–15). Although there may be 15 to 20 independent duct systems in each breast, some of these join in the subareolar area and only six to eight duct orifices may be found on the summit of the nipple.

In fibrocystic disease, varying degrees of duct ectasia will be demonstrated. Occasion-

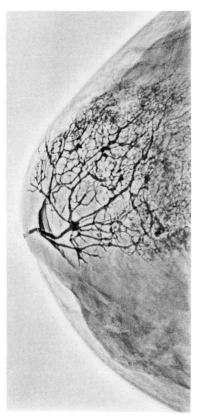

Figure 6–15. Galactogram of the normal duct system. A 26-year-old woman with a greenish nipple discharge for three weeks in clinically normal breasts. Mammography: dense breasts. Galactography: Injection of the discharging left nipple duct shows a normal duct system filling the lower outer quadrant on this craniocaudad view. (Courtesy of David D. Paulus, Jr., M.D., M. D. Anderson Hospital and Tumor Institute, Houston, TX.)

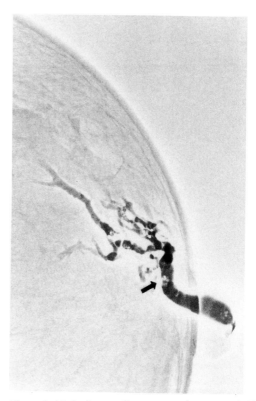

Figure 6–16. Benign papilloma on a galactogram. A 62-year-old woman with a bloody nipple discharge for three months. Clinically: bloody discharge only. Mammography: no significant abnormality. Galactography: duct ectasia and a smooth filling defect, papilloma, of the injected bleeding duct. Pathology: cytology negative; surgeon elected to follow without biopsy. (Courtesy of David D. Paulus, Jr., M.D., M. D. Anderson Hospital and Tumor Institute, Houston, TX.)

ally a communicating cyst may be opacified. The ectatic duct may be only smoothly dilated (Fig. 6–16) or markedly tortuous as demonstrated elsewhere.

The single most common cause of a bloody discharge from the nipple is papilloma. Almost all of these are in the major subareolar ducts and are benign (Fig. 6–16), presenting as a smooth-margined filling defect. Occasionally one may show atypia or be judged a papillomatous carcinoma. These would be more apt to produce ill-defined margins. However, galactography cannot differentiate the benign and malignant varieties, and surgery may be required.

On the galactogram the carcinoma distorts, displaces, or even obliterates the normal ductal pattern (Fig. 6–17). Calcifications may be obscured, but there is always the routine mammogram for reference. Some papillary and intraductal carcinomas that grow along the ducts to spread while confined to the

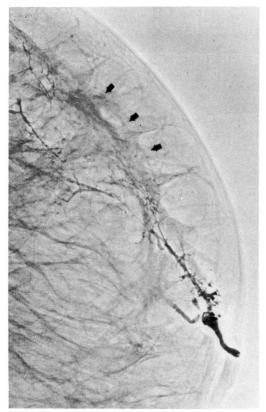

Figure 6–17. Galactography in malignancy. A 41-year-old woman with bleeding right nipple. Clinically: breasts normal except for bloody discharge. Mammography: broad band of asymmetric tissue extending from subareolar area into UOQ. Galactography: area of nonfilling ducts (arrows) after injection of contrast medium. Surgeon was directed to this area. Pathology: multiple foci of noninvasive and minimally invasive duct carcinoma in area of nonfilling. (Courtesy of David D. Paulus, Jr., M.D., M. D. Anderson Hospital and Tumor Institute, Houston, TX.)

At times this differentiation may be difficult by mammography, especially with smoothly marginated breast masses, and particularly when a portion of the periphery is obscured by overlying fibroglandular tissues. A mass may be palpable but not seen on mammography; being palpable, an air-contrast study may be done for delineation on x-ray. Simple cyst aspiration or breast sonography easily makes the differentiation.

Technique

The procedure is carried out as any cyst aspiration is done, with the addition of injection of a volume of air slightly less than that of the fluid aspirated. A meticulous sterile technique should be observed, local anesthesia may be used, and epinephrine may be added to the anesthetic preparation to reduce bleeding. Two radiographs at right angles are usually obtained, with at least one in the upright position to check for an air-fluid level.

Observations

In our practice, pneumocystography is not routinely done. The cyst aspiration is usually done to establish the presence of blood, e.g.,

ducts may produce no recognizable mammographic change if not calcified, and the galactogram may be the only source of detection.

Occasionally extravasation of contrast material into the rich plexus of lymphatics under the areola may outline the lymphatic channels leading to the axilla (Fig. 6–18).

PNEUMOCYSTOGRAPHY

Background

Air-contrast study of the lining of a cyst wall is readily accomplished by needle aspiration of the cyst fluid and injection of air to fill the cyst, followed by radiography.

Pneumocystography may be used to differentiate a solid from a cystic breast lesion.

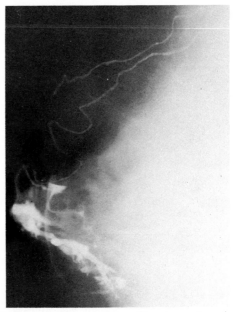

Figure 6–18. Galactography with extravasation of contrast medium. A 44-year-old woman studied for a nipple discharge from mammographically dense breasts. Galactography: partial filling of one duct system; extraductal contrast material and two lymphatic channels filled in their course toward the axilla. No sequelae.

in an intracystic papillary lesion. Sonography readily identifies the solid vs cystic breast mass. All dominant solid masses whose histologic nature is not apparent from our studies are removed for complete histopathologic studies.

HEAVY-ION MAMMOGRAPHY

Experimental studies indicate a potential for heavy-ion imaging (beam of carbon, oxygen, or neon nuclei) of density resolution superior to that of CT or film mammography. Cancers attenuate the beam to a greater extent than normal tissues or benign processes of the breast. Since an on-site cyclotron is required and the technique is expensive, a very limited number of breasts have been studied. There is a marked decrease in radiation to the breast.

REFERENCES

Barnes GT, Brezovisk IA (1979): Characteristics of scatter. *In* Logan WW, Muntz EP (eds): Reduced Dose Mammography. New York, Masson, p 223.

Chang CHJ, Sibala JL, Fritz SL, Dwyer SJ III, Templeton AW (1979): Specific value of computed tomographic breast scanner (CT/M) in diagnosis of breast diseases. Radiology *132*:647.

Doi K (1977): Advantages of magnification radiography. *In* Logan WW (ed): Breast Carcinoma. New York, John Wiley & Sons, p 83.

Egan RL (1960): Experience with mammography in a tumor institute. Evaluation of 1,000 studies. Radiology *74*:894.

Egan RL, Fenn JO (1968): Phantoms for evaluating mammography techniques and mammographic detail. AJR *102*:936.

Egan RL, McSweeney MB, Sprawls P (1983): Grids in mammography. Radiology *146*:359.

Freidrick M, Weskamp P (1978): New modalities in mammographic imaging: comparison of grid and air gap magnification techniques. Medicamundi 23:1.

Gisvold JJ, Karsell PR, Reese DF (1977): Computerized tomographic mammography. *In* Logan WW (ed): Breast Carcinoma, The Radiologist's Expanded Role. New York, John Wiley & Sons, p 219.

Jost G (1979): Evaluation of grid technique in mammography. *In* Logan WW, Muntz EP (eds): Reduced Dose Mammography. New York, Masson, p 253.

Lammers W, Kuhn H (1979): Improved image quality in mammography by means of scattered radiation grids. Electromedia 47:2.

Logan WW (1979): Overview of the radiologist's role in breast cancer detection. *In* Logan WW (ed): Breast Carcinoma: The Radiologist's Expanded Role. New York, John Wiley & Sons, p 343.

Ries E (1930): Diagnostic lipoidal injection into milk ducts followed by infection. Am J Obstet Gynecol *20*:414.

Sorenson JA, Nelson JA, Niklason LT, Jacobsen SC (1980): Rotating disc device for slit radiography of the chest. Radiology *134*:227.

Stanton L, Logan WW (1979): Mammography with magnification and grids: detail visibility and dose measurements. *In* Logan WW, Muntz EP (eds): Reduced Dose Mammography. New York, Masson, p 259.

Breast Sonography

7

BACKGROUND

Our interest and involvement in ultrasound of the breast has waxed and waned since 1963. That interest mostly waned after 1967, when frustrations in attempts to display the simplest breast lesions became overwhelming. Interest was rekindled more than a decade later only when Johnson and Johnson Company extended an invitation to make an attempt to upgrade the technique after their efforts to improve the equipment for breast sonography.

Workers in the area were reporting contradictory results with ultrasound of the breast carried out on different types of units. These early investigators were not students of breast diseases but mostly designers, engineers, or computer-oriented individuals. No one had more than a meager handful of cases. There was no training material.

Ultrasound of the breast was being done in several places, primarily with three-breast units but also with several additional prototype units. But unlike mammography, which required many years for worldwide adoption even though solid clinical studies and a unique reproducibility had been carried out in a highly successful manner, breast sonography re-entered on a lofty optimistic plane even as a screening tool. Thus mammography, backed by greatly organized and proven data in a clinical setting, paved the way for this too-enthusiastic espousement of breast sonography before units were completely designed, constructed, or tried. This placed breast sonography as a mere extension of pelvic and abdominal ultrasound as a clinically acceptable modality. This was hardly appropriate for an unproven and poorly tried procedure that rarely detected a breast cancer less than 2 cm in size. One company entering the marketplace at the level of screening for breast cancer went bankrupt.

In our experience, despite its many limitations, breast sonography should be included in breast-imaging centers for its contributions in improvement in diagnostic accuracy and for continued evaluation of technological improvements.

HISTORICAL ASPECTS

In 1956 x-ray examination of the breast was so improved that it was to become a routine complement to physical examination of the breast. Although these two procedures have been the standards for breast cancer detection, each has its limitations. During the past three decades additional methods for detecting breast cancer have been sought. These have included attempts to improve the radiographic technique, thermography, infrared scanning and light transmission, radioisotope scanning, galactography, pneumocystography, utilization of Doppler, computer tomography scanning, heavy-particle imaging, and magnetic resonance imaging.

With the development of ultrasound, the breast was one of the first organs studied. Wild and Neal (1951) and Wild and Reid (1952) were pioneers in using a pulse echo A-mode display to study benign and malignant breast diseases. During the same period Howry and Bliss (1952) and Howry et al. (1954) used a 2 mHz compound scanning technique to study the breast. Kelly-Fry et al. (1969) introduced a computer-based visualization system. Kiluchi et al. (1957) were among the earlier workers in Japan using a B-mode and 5 to 10 mHz system, while in Europe Laustela et al. (1966) reported on their A-mode 2 mHz system of studying the breast. Jellins et al. (1975) from Australia reported B-mode gray-scale presentation studies of breast diseases. However, clinical application of breast sonography did not follow owing to limitations of the available ultrasound equipment and expertise. Kobayashi (1975) presented an excellent review of these earlier developments in breast sonography.

These earlier breast studies were performed on the supine patient, with variations in coupling the transducer and skin: paraffin block casts of the breast, liquids, gels, water baths inside thin plastic bags placed over the breast, or open-ended containers sealed to the anterior chest wall and filled with water. According to the sonographer historian Holmes (1981), in 1963 Egan, with support from Magnaflux Corporation of Chicago, designed the first technique with the woman prone, the breast suspended in a water bath, and the transducers placed beneath the breasts. Comparative transverse scans of the breasts at the same anatomic level were then recorded side by side on 35 mm black and white film. This approach reflected the radiologist's desire to have comparative organ studies that could be reproduced readily

without uneven pressure, rather than the ease of penetration of the sound beam through a flat surface that was sought by his engineering-oriented contemporaries. Only quite gross lesions, huge cysts, and massive carcinomas could be demonstrated, so that little contribution to mammography was envisioned from these techniques. There were so many technical problems with scanning the pendant cone-shaped breast that the undertaking was abandoned in 1967.

Improvements in ultrasound equipment and imaging techniques led to the clinical application of ultrasound studies in the pelvis and abdomen. Ultrasound scanning of the breast with standard contact equipment was investigated as a method for evaluation of palpable breast diseases. In particular, cysts could be identified and differentiated from solid tumors.

The Australian Ultrasonics Institute with George Kossoff, Ph.D., Director, commenced construction of an ecroscope to undertake breast examination in 1963. The first breast echograms were obtained at the Royal North Shore Hospital in 1966 under the direction of Jack Jellins. These studies were done on the U. I. Octoson, a large, bulky, eight-transducer body scanner. This group has continual cooperation with the Ausonics Corporation of Australia to improve breast sonography equipment. Since the Octoson was applied to the breast with some success, a smaller version with four transducers (two on each side of the breast, with variable angles and a changeable Z axis) overcame many of the technical problems of imaging the cone-shaped breast.

Much of the emphasis on breast ultrasound followed the NIH/NCI Consensus Development Meeting on Breast Cancer Screening, September 14–16, 1977. This meeting had been prompted by reports in the literature that the radiation from mammography might itself produce breast cancer (Bailar, 1976). Although these claims were hypothetical and never proved that mammography contributed to causation of breast cancer, the news media propagated the scare so widely that the United States Federal Government felt obligated to encourage the investigation of breast sonography. Additional funds were channeled to select investigators.

The impetus was so strong that shortly after this meeting Life Instruments Company proceeded to build and sell breast sonography units for screening even though the modality was unproved clinically. Their unit operated three transducers, one centrally and one on each side of the breast, with focusing at different levels. Other dedicated water-path breast units were designed for Johnson and Johnson, Kelly-Fry, and Baum and Toshiba, in addition to hand-held small-parts scanners.

The technical problems had commanded so much of the effort toward developing breast sonography that little attention had been directed either toward developing criteria to establish the presence of breast abnormalities and their specific changes or to the efficacy of clinical application. Johnson and Johnson had planned a clinical trial but quickly aborted that effort to join in the competition to screen for breast cancer. Unsubstantiated claims abounded that ultrasound was the superior imaging technique in young women, in dense breasts, in follow-up examinations, in pregnant women, and in women fearful of radiation.

Viewing the great number of images recorded on tape, disk, or photographic emulsions posed problems. One approach was to reduce many images to a small size and record these on a film disk to be viewed in sequence at varying speeds. Video tapes could be replayed in diverse ways. Another approach was to record on video tapes, dump the images onto a disk, and view from the disk. Dual viewing was provided. The image was digitalized and fed into a computer with reconstruction and other postprocessing advantages. Image quality is degraded with transfer to a photographic disk or dual-review disk, although there is improved viewing ease. Yet, during the later period of development of these breast sonographic units there were individual efforts to establish the characteristics of breast structures and disease.

Schneck and Lehman (1982) studied the sonographic anatomy of the breast by correlation of sonographic images with gross and microscopic breast materials. Croll et al. (1982) had carried out correlated x-ray, clinical, ultrasonic, and, when available, pathologic studies of breasts of 7500 women. Cole-Beuglet (1982, 1983), Harper et al. (1983), Maturo et al. (1980), and others were doing combined studies to image the breast. However, no controlled clinical protocol to compare sonographic and x-ray studies of the breast had been done.

SONOGRAPHIC EXAMINATION

Equipment and Personnel

Rapid changes in breast sonographic equipment make only generalizations appropriate. The unit chosen should be especially designed for sonography of the breast and designed to incorporate any future developments in technique. Since most units are rather expensive, all available types should be investigated prior to purchase. The sonographer is the key to the whole procedure. We prefer a radiologic technologist with special training in ultrasound and additionally extensive training in mammography and breast diseases.

The Examination

The patient usually has already had mammography and is undressed from the waist up except for a short gown. She is seated on the side of the ultrasound table, the gown removed, and detergent applied to the breasts and anterior chest wall to prevent air bubbles on the skin. She is then placed prone with one or both breasts pendant in the water bath (depending on the unit) (Fig. 7–1). The usual identification is entered and the Z axis is adjusted.

Each radiologist or group of radiologists will develop an individual routine for breast sonography eventually and will devise numerous variations on that routine. A basic routine consists of both transverse and longitudinal scans of each breast at 2 mm intervals. Variations in use of transducers, including single-sector and compound scans, can

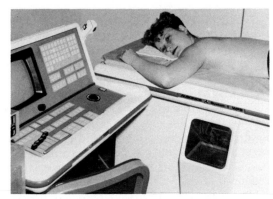

Figure 7–1. Console, water path, and patient in prone position for breast sonography. The procedure is readily accepted by women. Each breast is scanned individually. The studies then may be viewed side by side.

be part of the routine or can be supplementary studies. Formatting of the images on hard copy can be done as desired. Trial scans with various transducers may be needed to determine the optimum combinations. Generally, the more perpendicular the sound beam to the breast skin, the more efficient the scan.

Changing the position of the patient, such as moving her downward in relation to the transducers, allows inclusion of the axillary area. Rotation of the patient to change the relationship of the breast to the transducers may provide a more efficient scan.

Compression

Scans of the breast hanging loosely in the water bath provide a most realistic evaluation of the breast contour, the nipple, and the skin. The direction in which the nipple points or the shape of the breasts varies from patient to patient but normally should be symmetric. Indentations in the skin are usually smoothly concave and also are usually symmetric. A certain degree of skin wrinkling, particularly in atrophic breasts, may occur with the breast in the water.

Compression of the breast, even lightly, prevents these observations and should be avoided as much as possible. Often it is better to display the uncompressed breast first—then, when necessary, the compressed studies. Normally 35 decibels should not be exceeded, yet a trial of 40 to 45 decibels may be a better study than compression. With large breasts the routine technique will not demonstrate the retromammary space, particularly centrally. In some breasts, even with good compression this area may not be demonstrated well.

Thin plastic sheets have been used for compression but produce a problem with air bubbles. The best compression device to date is the thin plastic screen mesh obtained in hardware stores. A band of mesh slightly narrower than the width of the water bath hole is stretched across the table over the water bath. The patient's body usually will stabilize the band, and adjustment of the amount of compression is made by stretching the band.

In the scans of the compressed breast, the nipple is not recognized as a landmark, an occasional air bubble may be present, wrinkles in the skin are frequent, and the breast tissue is compressed unevenly. This technique is merely one further attempt to dem-onstrate breast pathology and is accepted with mixed feeling of concern: Are we improving the study or are we making it worse?

EMORY UNIVERSITY COMPARATIVE STUDY

An investigation of independent interpretation of breast sonography, compared with physical examination and mammography, was necessary in order to (1) establish relative accuracy for detection of breast cancer; (2) determine any complementary value to physical examination and mammography; (3) select types of breasts in which it would be potentially useful; and (4) evaluate acceptance by women and referring physicians.

Subjects and Methods

From January through June 1982, breast sonography was carried out on 786 women having physical examination and mammography. When possible, ultrasound studies were done on consecutive women who had been referred for mammography for a breast problem, as a routine follow-up study, as a baseline examination, or as part of a clinical work-up.

With the patient in the prone position, sonographic studies were performed on both breasts suspended in the water path of the Ausonic System 100. This system with four transducers, used singly or in various combinations, operated at 4.2 mHz and produced transverse and longitudinal scans at 2 mm intervals. Split-screen and full-screen single-sector or compound scans were produced routinely. Occasionally rotational scans were made. Compression was occasionally used but only after routine scanning. Mammography was carried out on a special unit using screen-film receptors, 25 to 27 kvp, 0.6 mm Mo anode, 30 μm Mo filter, and 30 inch target-receptor distance.

Results of clinical examination of the breasts had been recorded by the referring oncologic surgeon prior to referral for mammography. Each month one radiologist interpreted the mammograms without other information and recorded the findings on an appropriate form. Another radiologist did the same with breast sonograms. At the end of each month the roles of these two radiologists were reversed. Long-established criteria for x-ray diagnoses were followed by the two

TABLE 7–1. Age, Clinical Abnormality, Prior Surgery, Usefulness of Breast Sonography on 786 Patients in a Comparative Study to Detect Breast Carcinoma

	Age in Years						
	≤30	31–40	41–50	51–60	61–70	70+	Total
No. Patients	42	161	194	208	126	55	786
Clinical Abnormality							
None	8	81	109	140	92	35	445
Noncancerous	34	80	85	68	34	20	321
Carcinoma	0	1	3	3	7	6	20
Prior Surgery							
Noncancerous	9	25	54	94	40	19	241
Carcinoma	0	0	1	1	2	2	6
Biopsies							
Number	8	14	11	14	20	10	77
Malignant	0	2	5	4	13	7	31
Cancer Diagnosis							
Clinical	0	1(2)*	3(6)	3(7)	7(15)	6(7)	20(37)
X-ray	0	1(1)	2(2)	3(4)	12(6)	6(2)	24(15)
Ultrasound	0	0(1)	4†	3(2)	11	3	21(3)
Usefulness of US							
No. of patients							
None	2	68	87	106	84	27	362
Slight	34	74	91	89	28	18	346
Great	6	19	16	13	14	10	78
No. cysts found	2	11	22	5	1	0	41

*Number of false positive diagnoses in parentheses.
†US was sole indicator in one case.

radiologists; sonographic criteria had been developed together, so that there was no disagreement in reviewing the original coded reports. Final comparative evaluations of each series of studies were jointly made by the two radiologists with all information, including pathology, when available.

Breast size, relative density on x-ray, and mammographic and sonographic characteristics of all lesions were recorded. Each sonogram was then rated retrospectively for its relative clinical benefits: (1) no benefit if mammographic findings were definitive as in a clear-cut carcinoma; (2) slight benefit if it could help to clarify indeterminate mammographic findings, such as a cystic vs solid mass or poorly penetrated area on the mammogram; or (3) great benefit if it enabled the

proper diagnosis or helped prevent delay in treatment.

Results

From the 786 patients studied there were 77 excisional biopsies with 31 proven carcinomas. The age of the patient, clinical abnormality, and previous surgery are noted in Table 7–1. Clinical abnormality noted on physical examination included thickening, mass, discharge, or other changes.

On breast sonography 21 of the 31 (68 per cent) carcinomas (Table 7–2) were demonstrated, with three false positive findings (benign lesions labeled malignant). This compared with physical examination, which detected 20 (65 per cent) of the cancers with 37

TABLE 7–2. Cancer Diagnosis of 77 Biopsies

	Clinical	Mammography	Sonography
True positive rate (sensitivity)	20/20 + 11 (65%)	24/24 + 7 (77%)	21/21 + 10 (68%)
False positive rate	37/37 + 20 (65%)	15/15 + 24 (38%)	3/3 − 21 (13%)
True negative rate (specificity)	9/9 + 37 (20%)	31/31 + 15 (67%)	43/43 + 3 (13%)
False negative rate	11/11 + 9 (55%)	7/7 + 31 (18%)	10/10 + 43 (19%)
Total diagnosis	77	77	77
Accuracy	20 + 9/77 (38%)	24 + 31/77 (71%)	21 + 43/77 (83%)
Positive predictive value	20/20 + 37 (35%)	24/24 + 15 (62%)	21/21 + 3 (88%)
Negative predictive value	9/9 + 11 (45%)	31/31 + 7 (82%)	43/43 + 10 (81%)

false positive results, and with mammography, which detected 24 (77 per cent) of the cancers with 15 false positive results. Sonography had greater sensitivity than mammography for carcinoma detection in the 41 to 50 year group and equal sensitivity in the 51 to 60 and 61 to 70 year groups, with fewer false positive diagnoses. It was least useful in the elderly (> 70 years). In the 31 to 40 year group, the two carcinomas with calcifications only were not detected by sonography. In 54 per cent of the examinations breast sonography was considered helpful, and in one patient with a cancer in a dense breast it was the sole reason for biopsy (Fig. 7–2).

Sonography was readily accepted by the patients. It caused no fear of radiation and was not physically objectionable. The referring physicians later learned to appreciate both the added information about the breast and the increased confidence in the radiologist's interpretation.

From this experience it was concluded that breast sonography was a complementary procedure to mammography and physical examination of the breast, and had specific applications after the mammograms had been viewed. These applications were in mammographically dense breasts or in study of dense, poorly demonstrated areas on the mammograms (Fig. 7–3); in differentiation of masses into cystic or solid (Fig. 7–4); and in breasts with augmentation mammoplasties (Fig. 7–2). Breast sonography demonstrated

no added benefits in mammographically normal fatty breasts.

Breast cysts were correctly identified by sonography in 22 of 23 cyst aspirations (96 per cent), and cysts were demonstrated in an additional 41 women. Breast sonography was especially useful when (1) cysts were nonpalpable and etiology was uncertain on the mammogram; (2) cysts were palpable, aspiration attempts were unsuccessful and mammograms uninformative (Fig. 7–3); or (3) cysts were aspirated to determine if the cyst had been completely evacuated.

Sonography as the sole imaging modality in teenaged women may have potential in assessing the urgency to biopsy (Fig. 7–4) but would require close cooperation with the surgeon. Breast sonography was helpful in evaluation of the breast following augmentation prosthesis, as the scans at 2 mm intervals provided study of the entire breast, unlike mammography, which is dependent upon the proper tangential view to image tissues behind the dense prosthesis.

Breast sonography is a time-consuming and expensive procedure compared with mammography. In our breast-imaging center one technologist can handle only one-half the number of patients as the mammographer. There are technological limitations that prevent consistent diagnosis of small carcinomas, i.e., carcinomas with only stippled calcifications or small areas of altered architecture. Breast sonography does not use ion-

Figure 7–2. A and B, Sonography with augmentation mammoplasty. A 39-year-old woman for baseline mammogram of four-year-old mammoplasties. Mammography: dense nodular fibroglandular tissue overlying subpectoral prostheses. Ultrasound: 2 cm hypoechoic solid mass, slightly irregular margins, bright central echoes, no attenuation, anterior to subpectoral prosthesis, highly suspicious. Modified radical mastectomy. Pathology: infiltrating duct carcinoma, no axillary lymph node metastasis. In retrospect, after the mass was noted on sonography the lesion was palpable. There is no known causal relationship of carcinoma and a prosthesis.

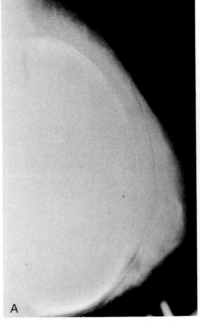

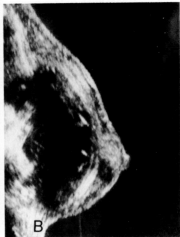

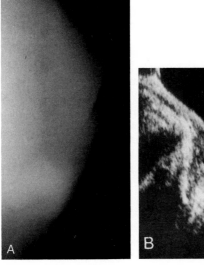
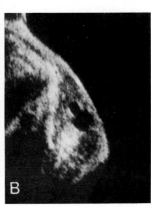

Figure 7–3. *A* and *B,* Study of dense breasts. A 38-year-old woman with a breast mass. Clinically: dominant mass cystic in nature. Aspiration attempted, no fluid obtained. Mammography: almost homogeneously dense breasts of fibroplasia. A 2 × 2.5 cm rounded mass with indistinct borders, etiology uncertain. Sonography: smooth-bordered, rounded, well-demarcated multiloculated mass with increased through-transmission, a simple cyst. Upon reaspiration, clear fluid was obtained and the mass disappeared.

izing radiation, can differentiate cysts and solid lesions, and can demonstrate cysts, solid lesions, and occasional carcinomas not found by x-ray or physical examination. In our experience (Table 7–3), with another commercially available breast sonography unit using 3.5 mHz, all of nine cancers went undetected. We concluded that the breast sonography unit must be selected and operated with great care.

In 50 per cent of the cases, even when mammography appeared to be sufficient, sonography contributed to the evaluation of the breast. It enhanced confidence that a mass was cystic or solid, that a dense area did not harbor an added density with sound attenuation, or that a prosthesis was not obscuring a carcinoma. A high specificity rate coupled with a fairly high sensitivity rate is useful in establishing priorities for breast biopsies (Table 7–2). Identifying cysts aids greatly in patient care. When sensitivity and specificity are combined, i.e., accuracy, sonography is the most accurate of the three methods. Further investigation is certainly indicated to assess the complementary role of sonography to x-ray and clinical examination of the breast.

Following mammography an additional 2530 patients were selected for sonography based on our established criteria. Of these cases, there were 107 biopsy-proved cancers, 69 discrete benign lesions, and 121 biopsies of poorly defined lesions, usually some form

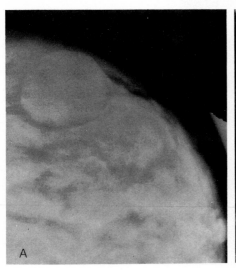
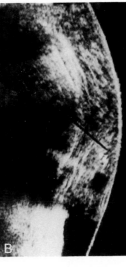

Figure 7–4. *A* and *B,* Differentiation of solid vs. cystic mass. A 19-year-old woman with breast lump increasing in size. Mammography: smooth, homogeneous, slightly lobulated mass; suspected fibroadenoma rather than a cyst. Sonography: well-demarcated, smooth-bordered, lobulated mass with rather homogeneous internal echoes, a solid lesion characteristic of fibroadenoma. Pathology: intracanalicular fibroadenoma. Note the enhanced posterior border, slightly increased through-transmission, no attenuation of the beam, suggestion of bulging of the skin despite compression, no altered architecture.

TABLE 7–3. Carcinoma Detection

		31 CA		Ultrasound	
	Clin.	Mammo.	US	4.2 mHz	3.5 mHz
Positive	63%	75%	47%	68%	0%
False positive	4.7	1.9	0.4	0.6	0
False negative	37	25	53	32	100

of fibrocystic disease without a discrete mass. The age, clinical abnormality, family history, prior surgery, biopsy, and results of this one-year study are shown in Table 7–4. Both the positive and the negative predictive values of breast sonography remained high, 88 and 86 per cent, respectively (Table 7–5) (see p. 111). Of six cases of carcinoma not demonstrated by mammography, all in dense breasts, three were detected solely by sonography, and in three others a palpable abnormality was noted in that breast.

On the basis of this comparatively extended experience, we concluded that sonography deserves a specific role in breast imaging as a complement to mammography and physical examination for improved diagnostic accuracy and heightened confidence in diagnosis. Even greater usefulness is envisioned with continued improvement in technology and equipment, especially with hand-held devices for pinpoint studies.

SONOGRAPHIC DIAGNOSIS: GENERAL CONSIDERATIONS

The tridimensional mammographic features of breast imaging are well known and should be freely compared with breast sonographic diagnostic criteria. Distinctive features of echo patterns must be sought and applied. As usual, the greatest challenge is the differentiation of normal breast, or variants of normal, from pathologic states within the breast. Certain criteria are associated with both diffuse and localized processes.

Sonography presents a new parameter in breast imaging that requires a different concept of the gross and microscopic changes of breast diseases. Simply labeling a breast lesion as cystic or solid and benign or malignant fails to supply a basis for establishing interpretation for breast sonography. Yet breast sonograms may depict specific patterns of normal breast tissues, variations of the normal breast, localized benign and malignant lesions, or poorly localized and diffuse areas of pathologic changes.

Normally there is a wide variation in the relative amounts and location of fat and fibroglandular tissues within the breast. The pattern may extend from a very thin subcutaneous layer of fat with dense fibroglandular tissues into an intermediate pattern of fat in a wider subcutaneous layer with equal distribution of fat throughout the fibroglandular tissue to almost 100 per cent of fat in the

TABLE 7–4. Age, Clinical Abnormality, Family History, Prior Surgery, Biopsy, and Results in the Total 2530 Patients Having 107 Cancers (CA) in a One-Year Clinical Study

Age (yrs)	≤30	31–40	41–50	51–60	61–70	>70	Total
No. Patients	177	691	940	429	213	80	2530
Clinical Abnormality*							
none	89	340	473	210	102	42	1256
non-CA	145	351	431	146	98	28	1199
CA	0	5	15	26	18	15	75
Family History*							
non-CA	22	141	148	182	62	10	565
CA	0	2	3	4	6	4	19
Prior Surgery*							
non-CA	20	138	190	235	132	62	777
CA	0	2	5	5	10	6	28
No. of Biopsies	26	49	50	60	85	27	297
No. of Malignancies	0	8	27	35	20	17	107
Diagnosed							
Clinical	0(4)†	3(10)	14(21)	24(22)	18(55)	15(9)	74(121)
X-ray	0	7(2)	23(13)	29(14)	19(8)	16(4)	94(41)
US	0(1)	5(2)	18(3)	28(4)	12(1)	14	77(11)

*One patient may have multiple entries.
†Number of false positive diagnoses in parentheses.

TABLE 7–5. Cancer Diagnosis of 297 Biopsies

	Clinical	Mammography	Sonography
True positive rate (sensitivity)	74/74+33 (69%)	94/94+13 (88%)	77/77+30 (72%)
False positive rate	121/121+74 (62%)	41/41+94 (30%)	11/11+77 (13%)
True negative rate (sensitivity)	69/69+121 (36%)	149/149+41 (78%)	179/179+11 (94%)
False negative rate	33/33+69 (32%)	13/13+149 (8%)	30/30+179 (14%)
Total diagnoses	297	297	297
Accuracy	74+69/297 (48%)	94+149/297 (82%)	77+179/297 (86%)
Positive predictive value	74/74+121 (38%)	94/94+41 (70%)	77/77+11 (88%)
Negative predictive value	69/69+33 (68%)	149/149+13 (92%)	179/179+30 (86%)

breast. A preponderance of any of the five normally present components of fibrocystic disease (duct dilatation and cyst formation, fibrosis, lymphocytic infiltration, ductal epithelial hyperplasia, and adenosis) contributes to variations in the normal breast pattern.

Areas in the breast may be anechoic, hypoechoic, hyperechoic, or a mixture of these. The architecture of the breast may be orderly (normal tissue), moderately disorganized (fatty tissue), or markedly disorganized (adjacent to a scirrhous duct carcinoma).

Alterations in the breast parenchyma may modify the amplitude, form or texture, and location or distribution of the echoes. For example, the low-level disorganized echo pattern of fatty breasts may have even lower echoes or more disorganized or increased amplitude of echoes, while the high-level heterogeneous echo pattern of dense glandular breasts may show similar alterations with increased attenuation of the beam.

The amplitude of the echoes may be considered high, medium, or low level and the texture either homogeneous or heterogeneous. The form of the echoes may be fine, medium, or coarse and may be in either an organized or a disorganized pattern. Localization of the area of altered echoes to the skin, the subcutaneous area, or the parenchyma is often helpful.

Diffuse Breast Changes

Most of these changes are benign and usually are extended manifestations of fibrocystic disease such as ductal hyperplasia, adenosis, or fibrosis, singly or in combination, with or without widespread areas of entrapped fatty tissue. Ductal hyperplasia may be recognized by its uniformly fine nodular pattern; patchy fibrosis by high-level echoes coupled with attenuation; and the density of adenosis by its somewhat similar pattern but one that is more localized to the upper outer quadrant of the breasts. Usually these changes are symmetric bilaterally. Other diffuse changes are related to specific breast lesions.

TABLE 7–6. Incidence of Benign and Malignant Breast Lesions Related to Breast Size and Density with Diagnoses by Modality in 2530 Women

Diagnosis	No.	Breast Size Small	Medium	Large	Breast Fatty Content >75%	26–74%	<25%	Also DH	False Positives Clin.	X-Ray	US
Benign											
Fibroadenoma	37	6	15	16	13	17	7	8	5	2	2
Variant—FA	15	0	6	9	5	4	6	4	7	2	2
F.C.D.	60	13	6	41	21	24	15	11	103	35	4
Miscellaneous	21	0	11	10	6	8	7	2	6	2	3
Total	133	19	38	76	45	53	35	25	121	41	11
Malignant									False Negatives		
ID CA	4	0	4	0	0	2	2	2	4	0	2
Duct CA	44	2	25	17	5	19	20	12	12	7	10
Comedo CA	13	0	6	7	5	6	2	4	6	0	10
Scirrhous CA	23	0	13	10	3	12	8	10	3	2	4
Medullary CA	10	1	6	3	3	4	3	3	1	0	0
Miscellaneous	13	2	6	5	1	4	8	6	7	4	4
Total	107	5	60	42	17	47	43	35	33	13	30

F.C.D. = fibrocystic disease; ID = intraductal carcinoma; DH = ductal epithelial hyperplasia.

Localized Breast Lesions

Localized lesions vary in the following characteristics on breast sonography:

A. Shape—lobulated, elongated, oval, round, poorly defined
B. Margins—demarcated
   1. irregular: mildly, moderately, markedly complex
   2. enhanced borders: anterior, posterior, poorly defined
C. Lateral refractive sign—none, mild, marked
D. Through-transmission
   1. attenuated: mildly, moderately, markedly
   2. increased: mildly, moderately, markedly
   3. no change
E. Internal echoes
   1. type: homogeneous, nonhomogeneous, mixed
   2. distribution: peripheral, central, diffuse, nonuniform
   3. density: anechoic, hypoechoic, hyperechoic
F. Surrounding tissue—altered architecture, compressed, not altered
G. Skin changes—bulging, flattening, retraction, thickening
H. Cooper's ligaments—thickened, straightened, retracted

Echo Density

To be recognized, the local breast process must be set off from the surrounding tissues by an area of either hypo-, hyper-, or anechoic density. Variation in the decibel level in scanning is often required to evaluate this echo pattern.

Echo Shape

The lesion may be well demarcated, such as a cyst, or poorly demarcated, such as a dense area of fibrosis or carcinoma. Most benign lesions are homogeneous, smooth bordered, round, oval, lobulated or bosselated and expand by pushing tissue aside. Malignant masses, on the other hand, are irregular, are denser at the center, and expand by invading the surrounding tissues.

Breast lesions that usually are considered as well demarcated or as having irregular borders include the following:

Well Demarcated	Irregular Borders
Fibroadenoma	Duct carcinoma
Adenolipoma	Medullary carcinoma
Cystosarcoma phylloides	Fat necrosis
Cyst	Cystosarcoma phylloides, invasive
Galactocele	Intracystic papillary carcinoma, invasive
Intracystic papillary lesions	Most carcinomas
Lipoma	Abscess
Sebaceous cyst	
Hematoma	
Papilloma	

Echo Location

Most breast lesions occur in the parenchyma and may bulge into the subcutaneous fat layer (usually benign), or they may extend into this layer or the retromammary area by invasion (malignant). The location of the lesion is often a strong clue as to its etiology; e.g., a benign lesion attached to the undersurface of the skin is most likely a sebaceous cyst.

Surrounding Tissues

The benign lesion usually causes no response from the surrounding tissues but may expand sufficiently to compress these surrounding tissues, increasing the amplitude of the echoes and altering the texture of those echoes. Malignant masses vary greatly in the excitation of the surrounding tissues. Well-circumscribed carcinomas may cause no more reaction than a benign lesion. However, some carcinomas cause varying degrees of disruptive echoes owing to the localized invasion. The more invasive carcinomas produce varying degrees of reactive fibrosis and retraction with collapse of the surrounding tissues to produce a high-level disorganized echo pattern.

Internal Echoes

The contents of a mass lesion determine the nature of the internal echoes. Liquid-filled lesions remain anechoic even at relatively high decibel settings unless they contain debris of solid matter. Many benign lesions and circumscribed carcinomas, such as medullary carcinoma with lymphoid stroma, have homogeneous low-level echoes. The more invasive carcinomas usually have internal echoes differing both in magnitude and in texture, while the highly invasive carcinomas, such as scirrhous, may completely attenuate the beam in shadowing.

Specific breast lesions that may cause

change in the echo density include the following:

Anechoic	Hypoechoic
Simple cyst	Fibroadenoma
Sebaceous cyst	Cystosarcoma phylloides
Intracystic	Hematoma
papillary	Papilloma
lesion	Galactocele
Hematoma	Adenolipoma
Papilloma	Lipoma
Infected cyst	Fat necrosis
	Sebaceous cyst
	Duct carcinoma
	Medullary carcinoma
	Intracystic papillary
	carcinoma
	Most solid, or mixed
	carcinomas
	Abscess or infected cyst

Attenuation of the Beam

The echoes posterior to a lesion may be the same as surrounding tissues or may be reduced or increased. Enhancement of the beam is usually associated with benign lesions, particularly cysts; reduction or shadowing with malignancy; and no change with lesions similar in tissue density to that of the normal parenchyma. In certain well-demarcated masses the velocity of the beam through the lesion exceeds that of surrounding tissues to produce the lateral refractive edge shadowing. This is more often noted with single-sector scans.

Boundary Echoes

With smooth boundaries usually associated with benign lesions, only the anterior and posterior boundaries may be well demonstrated. The lateral borders may be poorly displayed owing to the angle of the sound beam. Compound scans may be needed. Echoes from the boundaries of malignant masses have a more characteristic jagged border.

Common lesions having altered boundaries include the following:

Enhanced Posterior Borders	Enhanced Anterior Border
Fibroadenoma	Fibroadenoma
Medullary	Medullary carcinoma
carcinoma	
Cystosarcoma	*Refractive Lateral Edge Sign*
phylloides	
Cyst	Cyst
Galactocele	Galactocele

Enhanced Posterior Borders	Refractive Lateral Edge Sign
Intracystic papillary lesion	Sebaceous cyst
Lipoma	Intracystic papillary lesion
Sebaceous cyst	Hematoma
Hematoma	Papilloma
Papilloma	
Infected cyst	

Common lesions causing changes in the sound beam include the following:

Increased Through-Transmission	Shadowing
Simple cyst	Air bubble, e.g., at
Sebaceous cyst	nipple
Galactocele	Skin scar
Dilated duct	Nipple
Papilloma	Carcinoma, usually
Lipoma	duct
Hematoma	Fat necrosis
Intracystic papillary lesion	Lobular hyperplasia
	Fibrosis
Infected cyst	Calcification, large
Medullary	Biopsy scar within
carcinoma	breast
	Nevus
	Lobular carcinoma
	Abscess

Skin Changes

Reflections of skin changes are more evident in the water-suspended breast. Apparently the slightest tension is readily transmitted on the ultrasound scan. This is often the red flag that alerts one to the presence of an underlying carcinoma. A smooth bulge may be displayed with an expanding benign lesion or an expanding circumscribed carcinoma. Wrinkling in the elderly may be so severe that a satisfactory scan is impossible. These changes are poorly assessed with compression.

Skin retraction on sonography is a nonspecific change and is considered diagnostic to the same degree as increased vascularity on the mammograms.

Lesions usually associated with skin changes include the following:

Retraction	Thickening
Biopsy	Biopsy—keloid
Fat necrosis	Scleroderma morphea
Fibrosis	Nevus
Abscess	Inflammatory
Subareolar	carcinoma
fibrosis	Diffuse carcinoma

Retraction
All carcinomas,
    but mostly duct
Mondor's disease

Bulging
Fibroadenoma
Cystosarcoma
Cyst
Galactocele
Prosthesis
Sebaceous cyst

Thickening
Metastatic breast
    carcinoma
Recent marked weight
    loss
Edema of the skin
    from any cause
Hypothyroidism
Abscess
Idiopathic

Most of these alterations are summarized in Table 7–7.

CLASSIFICATION OF BREAST DISEASES

Benign

Sonographic benign diseases will be considered as discrete or diffuse breast sonographic changes; intraglandular, extraglandular, or subareolar in location; and cystic or noncystic in nature. They will be classified with the full knowledge that at present many of the lesions cannot be differentiated by sonography. A rather encompassing classification will provide comparison of diagnostic criteria as they are seen on mammography.

General consideration of the individual lesions will be discussed in other chapters, especially Chapter 12. Also, on many occasions sonographic demonstrations will be included with other imaging modalities.

Malignant

Sonographic malignant breast lesions, as in the general classification of breast diseases, can be considered as noninfiltrating, infiltrating duct carcinoma, special histologic types of carcinoma, clinical syndromes, sarcomas, and metastatic malignancies.

SPECIFIC FEATURES

Our comparative study with breast sonography led to the addition of the procedure to our breast-imaging armamentarium: (1) to determine further its usefulness in demonstrating cancers and its complementary value to physical examination and mammography, and (2) to evaluate potential characteristics that differentiate benign and malignant solid lesions.

Following inspection of the mammograms, approximately 50 per cent of the women were selected for breast sonography in the presence of (1) dense breasts, (2) areas of breast poorly penetrated, (3) masses with indeterminate etiology, (4) cysts not definitely demonstrated and failure in attempted cyst aspiration, or (5) augmentation mammoplasties. One sonography technologist was limited to doing only one half of the daily 20 to 25 breast-imaging workload of one mammography technologist.

During the one-year study the 2530 selected women with breast sonography following mammography and physical examination were representative of our total patient population (Table 7–4). Breast size and fat content had little bearing on sonographic diagnosis, although sonography was used sparingly in the fatty breasts (Table 7–6).

Cystic Masses

Simple cysts of fibrocystic disease of the breast had similar sonographic appearances as cysts elsewhere in the body (Fig. 7–3). To be diagnostic, they required the following: (1) anechoic A-mode scans at several levels in the lesion; (2) increased through-transmission except when resting on the pectoral muscles; and (3) echoes filling in from the periphery at the higher decibel settings. Approximately 96 per cent of 127 aspiration-proven cysts had these typical sonographic characteristics.

In dense breasts, sonography did detect many cysts that were not apparent clinically or on mammography and did differentiate solid and cystic masses (Fig. 7–4). Nonpalpable cysts usually were of little clinical interest. Needle aspiration did establish their presence if fluid was obtained. Sonographic evaluation of cysts was especially useful when they were (1) nonpalpable and etiology was uncertain on the mammogram, or (2) palpable with unsuccessful aspiration attempt (Fig. 7–5) or not seen on mammography.

Solid Masses
Benign

The characteristics of the biopsied benign discrete solid lesions not categorized as a poorly defined form of fibrocystic disease (Table 7–8) showed dissimilarities from can-

TABLE 7–7. The Shape, Boundary, Alteration of Sound Beam, Type of Internal Echoes, and Skin Changes of Lesions on Breast Sonography

Shape		Enhanced Boundary			Transmission of Sound Beam		Echo Density		Skin Changes		
Demarcated	Irregular	Anterior	Posterior	Lateral Refractive Edge	Increased	Decreased	Anechoic	Hypoechoic	Retraction	Bulging	Thickening
Fibroadenoma	Duct carcinoma	Fibroadenoma	Fibroadenoma	Cyst	Simple cyst	Air bubble	Simple cyst	Fibroadenoma	Biopsy	Fibroadenoma	Biopsy—keloid
Adenolipoma	Medullary carcinoma	Medullary carcinoma	Medullary carcinoma	Galactocele	Sebaceous cyst	Skin scar	Sebaceous cyst	Cystosarcoma phylloides	Fat necrosis	Cystosarcoma	Scleroderma
Cystosarcoma phylloides	Fat necrosis		Cystosarcoma phylloides	Sebaceous cyst	Galactocele	Nipple	Intracystic papillary lesion	Hematoma	Fibrosis	Cyst	Nevus
Cyst	Cystosarcoma phylloides		Cyst	Intracystic papillary lesion	Dilated duct	Carcinoma duct	Hematoma	Papilloma	Abscess	Galactocele	Inflammatory carcinoma
Galactocele	Intracystic papillary invasive		Galactocele	Hematoma	Papilloma	Fat necrosis	Papilloma	Galactocele	Subareolar fibrosis	Prosthesis	Diffuse carcinoma
Intracystic papillary	Most carcinomas		Intracystic papillary	Papilloma	Lipoma	Lobular hyperplasia	Infected cyst	Adenolipoma	All carcinomas, most duct	Sebaceous cyst	Metastatic carcinoma
Lipoma	Abscess		Lipoma		Hematoma	Fibrosis		Lipoma	Mondor's disease		Weight loss
Sebaceous cyst			Sebaceous cyst		Intracystic papillary	Calcifications		Fat necrosis			Edema of skin
Hematoma			Hematoma		Infected cyst	Biopsy scar		Sebaceous cyst			Hypothyroidism
Papilloma			Papilloma			Nevus		Duct carcinoma			Abscess
Medullary carcinoma			Infected cyst			Lobular carcinoma		Medullary carcinoma			Idiopathic
						Abscess		Intracystic papillary			
								Solid, mixed carcinoma (hyalinized FA)			
								Abscess or infected			

TABLE 7–8. Mammographic and Sonographic Features of Commoner Benign Lesions

	Radiographic										Sonographic									
	No.			SIZE				Margins			Attenuation	Transmission	Increased	Internal Echoes		Altered Architecture	Bulging Skin	Borders Potentiated		LRE
LESION		Multiple	Single	0	≤1	1.1–2	>2	Demarcated (+)	Irregular (++)	Complex (+++)				Homogeneous	Nonhomogeneous			Anterior	Posterior	
Fibroadenoma	37	13	24	2	11	4	20	37			4	2	2	35	2				9	7
Juvenile FA	2		2				2	2							2			1	1	
Lactating FA	2		2				2	2							2		1		1	
Calcifying FA	4		4			2	2	4			4				4					
Adenolipoma	5		5				5	5			1				5		2			
Cystosarcoma	2		2				2	2							2		2	1		
Lipoma	2		2				2	2			2			2						
Adenosis	6		6			2	4	4		2	2			2	4	2			2	
Hematoma	2		2			1	1	1		1	2			1	1	1		1		
Fat necrosis	2		2				2		1	1	1	1		2		2				
Fibrosis (scar)	2		2				2		2		2	2		1	1	2				
Nevus	3		3		2	1		3			1	2		3						

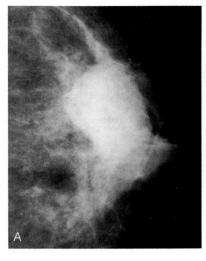

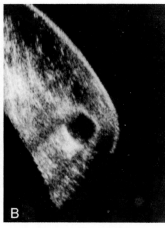

Figure 7–5. A and B, Aid in managing a simple cyst. A 51-year-old woman on estrogen therapy. Mass aspirated one week ago reappeared. Baseline mammography: 3 cm homogeneous mass with indistinct borders, which could represent a circumscribed carcinoma or, by history, a refilled cyst surrounded by hematoma and edema. Sonography: characteristic features of a simple cyst. A-mode, anechoic at 35 decibels, thick walls, surrounding increased echoes; shown, at 44 decibels may be debris from trauma contributing to apparent peripheral internal echoes. History most helpful. Pathology: simple cyst on aspiration.

cer such as larger size, better demarcation, less attenuation, greater homogeneity of internal echoes, less altered architecture, more potentiation of the anterior and posterior borders, and more frequent lateral refractive edge effect (Figs. 7–4 and 7–5).

Fibroadenomata and variants made up 83 per cent of the benign solid lesions and had typical benign sonographic characteristics: well demarcated, smooth lobulated margins, homogeneous internal echoes, 20 per cent lateral refractive edge, 25 per cent enhanced posterior border, no altered architecture, fre-quently multiple, and occasional bulging of the skin (Fig. 7–4). There was no attenuation of the beam except for four hyalinizing (Fig. 7–6) and four heavily calcified ones. Of the other benign solid lesions (except nevi), ten had attenuation of the beam, seven of these producing adjacent altered architecture (Fig. 7–7); seven were irregular; and six had non-homogeneous internal echoes.

At times an area of dense adenosis, a hematoma, or, more frequently, fat necrosis or dense fibrosis produced sonographic features that were suspicious for malignancy

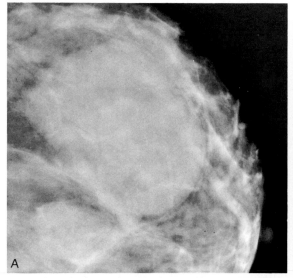

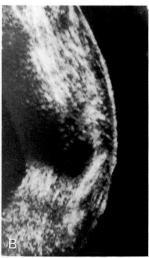

Figure 7–6. A and B, Shadowing by a hyalinized fibroadenoma. A 43-year-old woman with a breast mass for two months. Clinically: movable dominant nodule. Mammography: large, lobulated, homogeneous benign mass, most likely fibroadenoma with similar nearby smaller mass. Sonography: well-demarcated mass, homogeneous internal echoes with marked attenuation. Smaller separate mass was a cystic lesion. Pathology: hyalinizing fibroadenoma and a simple cyst.

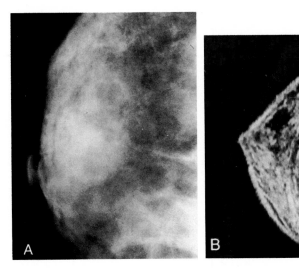

Figure 7–7. A and B, Adenosis mimicking carcinoma. A 40-year-old woman with nodular breasts. Mammography: nodular breasts with fibrocystic disease and subareolar fibrosis. Sonography: hypoechoic, fairly well-demarcated (some of the periphery irregular) solid mass, nonhomogeneous internal echoes; highly suspicious.

(Fig. 7–7). The benign or malignant character of cystosarcoma phylloides could not be distinguished sonographically.

Malignant

The sonographic characteristics of the various malignant breast lesions encountered are compiled in Table 7–9. Histopathologic diagnoses were used, to which was added a judgment by the pathologist of the relative amount of desmoplasia or reactive fibrosis (scirrhous element). "Invasiveness" indicates the degree of scirrhous element judged radiographically.

The sonographic changes of breast cancers were diverse and lacked useful consistency when lumped together. However, when the cancers were clearly divided into the "pure" duct carcinomas (ductal, comedo, scirrhous), "nonduct" carcinomas (medullary, lobular; Table 7–9), and sarcomas, consistent patterns did emerge (Table 7–10). The "pure" duct carcinomas then were further divided: (1) comedo with its more indolent growth pattern, widespread origin in the breast, and often clinically occult, producing highly variegated calcifications more associated with intraductal detritus; and (2) "solid" duct with its more aggressive growth pattern, more localized in the breast, more rapidly producing secondary signs, and with fine, punctate calcifications produced by secretion of the cells. With both types of pure duct carcinomas, irregularity, attenuation, nonhomogeneity of internal echoes, and altered architecture were more consistently related to radiographic changes of invasiveness rather

than to histopathologic degree of desmoplasia or fibrosis. Size, if 0.5 cm or larger, had only slight influence on the features of pure duct carcinomas. The highly invasive scirrhous carcinomas appeared much larger on sonography than on mammography or histopathologic study.

One fifth of all intraductal carcinomas have fairly marked changes on sonography (Fig. 7–8), probably owing to surrounding tissue reaction despite lack of invasion, whereas the remaining ductal and comedocarcinomas without radiographic mass (mainly with calcifications but often with altered architecture) produce no sonographic changes.

Infiltrating comedo and duct carcinomas, making up 75 per cent of the cancers, have consistent characteristics varying only in degree of changes related to the amount of reactive fibrosis (Figs. 7–9 to 7–13) and could be classified as typical (diagnostic) (Table 7–3). Simultaneous bilateral carcinomas detected by sonography are both characteristically primary carcinomas.

With comedo- and duct carcinomas that produced a mass associated with a scirrhous component, size was unrelated to the degree of attenuation of the beam or altered architecture, e.g., a 0.5 cm such lesion produced the same degree of change as a similar 1.5 cm carcinoma (Figs. 7–13 and 7–14). Regardless of the size of the less aggressive cancers, only 86 per cent attenuated the beam and 76 per cent caused altered architecture.

The lobular carcinoma is intermediate in type and can produce vague or profound changes. Circumscribed cancers have some

TABLE 7–9. Mammographic and Sonographic Features of Malignant Lesions

	Radiographic								Sonographic																	
	Invasiveness				Size				Margins							Attenuation			Transmission (Increased)			Internal Echoes		Altered Architecture	Skin	
									Demarcated	Irregular			Complex									Homogeneous	Nonhomogeneous		Retraction	Bulging
Carcinoma	0	+	++	+++	0	1	1.1–2	2		+	++	+++	+	++	+++	+	++	+++	+	++	+++					
Intraductal	4				4						2						1	1				1	1	2		
Ductal	4	17	16	7	4	11	16	13		10	24	6				21	9	9				6	33	34	3	3
Comedo	5	2	6		5	2	3	3			8					5	3						8	8		
Duct-Scirr.		1	3	10		5	5	4		1	7	6				3	4	7				1	13	11	3	
Comedo-Scirr.		2	5	2	1	2	1	5		2	3	3	1			3	2	4				4	5	5	1	
Medullary			5	5			2	8		8	2								3	5		2	8	2		
Lobular			1	1		1	1			1	1												2	1		
Mucinous			1					1					1							1			1			
Intracystic			2	1			1	3	2				1						3				3			
Metaplasia			1										1				1						1	1		
Papillary			2			2				1	1					2						2				
Adeno			1					1			1					1										
Apocrine								1		1							1									
Cystosarcoma			2					2	2											1		2 mixed				5

Mild, +; Moderate, ++; Marked, +++; Scirr. = scirrhous.

TABLE 7–10. Grouping of Lesions from Table 7–5 Based on an Estimate of Reliability of Sonographic Criteria of 107 Breast Cancers and Relative Frequency of Each Group

Typical Criteria (75%)	Borderline Criteria (12%)	Atypical Criteria (13%)
Comedo	Medullary	Intraductal
Duct	Intracystic	Mucinous
Scirrhous-comedo	papillary carcinoma	Cystosarcoma phylloides
Scirrhous-duct		Miscellaneous

suggestive characteristics of solid benign lesions, yet are still suspicious for malignancy. Figure 7–15 illustrates this group generally. Other types are demonstrated in their respective chapters. The medullary carcinoma with lymphoid stroma and mucinous carcinomas produce a rather consistent pattern of fairly large lesions, minimal irregularity of the borders, increased through-transmission and nonhomogeneity.

These sonographic characteristics result from the monotonous (almost sarcomatous) cellular pattern of the medullary carcinoma with lymphoid stroma without sonar reflecting interfaces unless there has been hemorrhage, fibrosis, and scarring. In the mucinous carcinoma most of the tumor is a large pool of mucin in which small clumps of cells are floating, producing a nearly fluid-filled structure. Sarcomas also have a uniform cellularity without significant reflecting surfaces but with various-sized internal echoes and limited secondary changes. The intracystic papillary carcinoma has similar characteristics but is well demarcated unless invasive by x-ray. The cystosarcomas phylloides are large, rather well-demarcated masses that can have increased through-transmission. Thus the nonduct carcinomas, even though larger than the pure duct type, have inconsistent distinguishing features, with some being demarcated, not altering the breast architecture, and having increased through-transmission.

Yet most of these circumscribed cancer lesions can be identified as malignant; i.e., the medullary carcinoma with lymphoid stroma can be differentiated rather reliably from fibroadenoma. Fibroadenoma and its variants have fairly consistent characteristics, although at times the unusual one does attenuate the sonar beam or has increased through-transmission. The medullary carcinoma with lymphoid stroma contains more nonhomogeneous internal echoes, has a more irregular border, tends not to be bosselated, and has more increased through-transmission.

CLINICAL APPLICATION OF BREAST SONOGRAPHY

In selected women following mammography and with the invaluable help of the

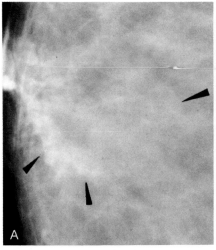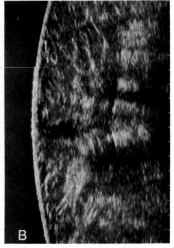

Figure 7–8. A and *B,* Changes of intraductal carcinoma. A 63-year-old woman with a vague mass above the level of the nipple medially. Mammography: very faint, almost imperceptible, fine calcifications in areas of arrows associated with pseudomasses. Sonography: hypoechoic, irregular area, surrounding architectural alteration, some shadowing indicative of infiltrating carcinoma. Pathology: entirely intraductal carcinoma, in several areas: solid, comedo, papillary, and micropapillary. The parenchymal changes are apparently a response to the presence of noninvasive carcinoma rather than actual invasion.

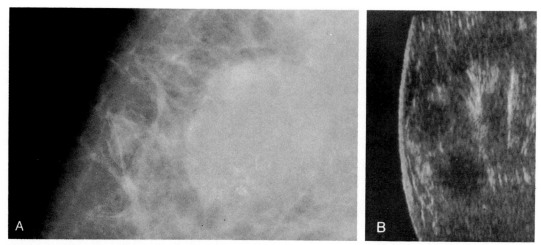

Figure 7–9. *A* and *B,* Localized mass of comedo carcinoma. A 50-year-old woman with a lump and swelling for three weeks. Mammography: 5 cm, slightly lobulated, circumscribed carcinoma containing coarse and fine calcifications of comedo type. Sonography: irregular hypoechoic mass containing nonhomogeneous internal echoes with potentiation of the posterior border and increased through-transmission. These changes suggest a circumscribed carcinoma such as medullary type. Pathology: infiltrating, poorly differentiated duct carcinoma, predominantly comedo carcinoma. Sonographically this is the least aggressive form of infiltrating duct carcinoma.

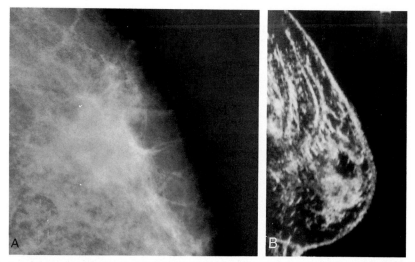

Figure 7–10. *A* and *B,* Moderately invasive duct carcinoma. A 38-year-old woman with a breast mass for four months. Mammography: irregular, coarsely spiculated 2.5 cm carcinoma with skin retraction and increased vascularity. Sonography: irregular, hypoechoic, slightly lobulated solid lesion with nonhomogeneous internal echoes, no shadowing. These findings correspond well with the less aggressive tumor on x-ray. Pathology: infiltrating duct carcinoma, no significant desmoplasia; axillary lymph nodes free of metastasis.

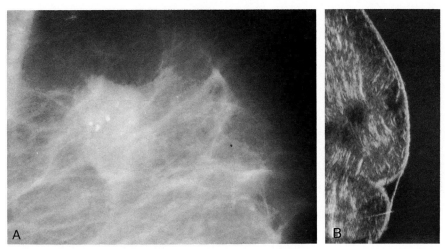

Figure 7–11. *A* and *B*, Slightly more aggressive duct carcinoma. A 58-year-old woman with a mass for one month. Clinically: 4 cm suspicious mass. Mammography: coarsely spiculated 2 × 3 cm moderately invasive carcinoma containing coarse and fine stippled calcifications. Sonography: irregular hypoechoic mass with nonhomogeneous internal echoes, minimal attenuation of the sound beam. Pathology: infiltrating duct carcinoma.

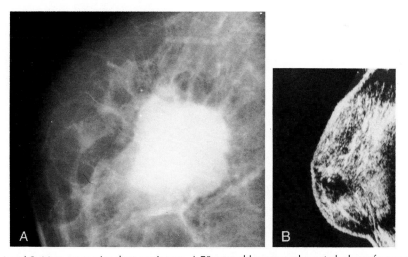

Figure 7–12. *A* and *B*, More aggressive duct carcinoma. A 70-year-old woman who noted a lump four months previously. Mammography: 3.5 cm lobulated mass with fine and coarse spiculations, fine stippled calcifications, overlying skin retraction, and marked increased vascularity. Sonography: discrete, irregular, lobulated mass with nonhomogeneous internal echoes, flattening of the skin, and surrounding disrupted architecture. Shadowing is present. Pathology: comedo carcinoma with a considerable scirrhous element.

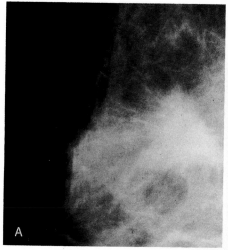

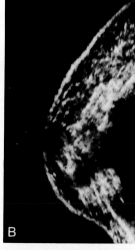

Figure 7–13. A and B, Highly invasive carcinoma. An 80-year-old woman with breast lump and inverted nipple. Mammography: 1.5 cm non-homogeneous finely spiculated mass, with retraction of the nipple and tissues toward the mass and straightening of Cooper's ligaments all the way to the skin. Sonography: jagged, hypoechoic mass, internal echoes, distortion of the surrounding tissues, skin flattening, and marked shadowing. Pathology: infiltrating duct carcinoma with marked desmoplasia.

Figure 7–14. A and B, Five mm duct carcinoma with shadowing. A 65-year-old woman who had a breast biopsy four years previously. Mammography: dense breast, altered architecture with spicules running out from the area: biopsy changes vs highly infiltrative carcinoma. Sonography: irregular bordered mass, disrupted architecture with skin retraction, shadowing. Pathology: 5 mm infiltrating duct carcinoma with productive fibrosis. Such lesions appear much larger on sonography.

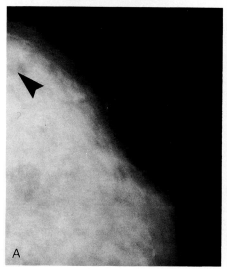

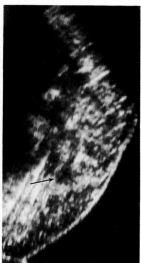

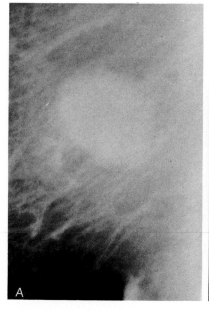

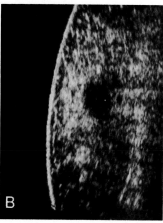

Figure 7–15. A and B, Medullary carcinoma with lymphoid stroma. A 49-year-old woman with a breast mass for three months. Mammography: rather well-circumscribed carcinoma with increased vascularity (in this age group, suggests medullary type). Sonography: demarcated, slightly irregularly walled hypoechoic mass with markedly nonhomogeneous internal echoes, potentiated posterior border, and suggestion of a lateral reflective edge. Pathology: 2.5 × 3.0 cm medullary carcinoma with lymphoid stroma.

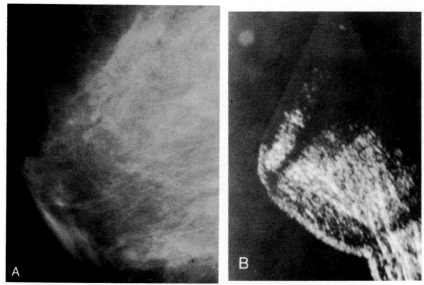

Figure 7–16. A and B, False positive sonography. A 72-year-old woman seen for baseline mammography had previous biopsy for benign disease bilaterally. Clinically: normal breasts, biopsies. Mammography: comedo carcinoma type calcification without an associated mass but with increased density, above and medial to the nipple, overlying local skin thickening in the biopsy site. Sonography: distortion of skin medial to nipple with marked shadowing extending deep into the breast. Pathology: Stage 0 comedo carcinoma, modified radical mastectomy, nodes negative; patient alive three years later. The shadowing extends through the area of the carcinoma, but this indolent carcinoma would not produce retrograde shadowing to the skin and deep into the breast.

sonography technologist, clinical rewards are to be reaped from breast sonography. Re-emphasis on false positive studies (Fig. 7–16) as well as false negative ones, must be kept in perspective. Some studies will be less than optimal (Fig. 7–17). Patterns may not always be specific for a cellular diagnosis (Fig. 7–18).

In certain cases breast sonography will lead to proper patient care. Vague mammographic changes may take on real importance in the presence of definite sonographic changes or with less definite changes of malignancy (Fig. 7–19). Sonographic changes may add the right amount of confidence at the proper time (Fig. 7–20).

Diagnosis and treatment of a fibroadenoma are real clinical problems, compounded in the young woman in whom cancer is a more difficult lesion to diagnose. Sonography does add some confidence to the detection, diagnosis, and treatment planning for these lesions (Figs. 7–21 and 7–22).

Figure 7–17. A and B, Wrinkled skin on sonography. An 84-year-old woman with a clinically palpable breast carcinoma. Mammography: moderately invasive subareolar carcinoma with thickening of the skin of the areola. Sonography: a large irregular hypoechoic area with attenuation; marked distortion of the overlying skin partially due to secondary changes of the carcinoma but primarily due to the skin wrinkling in the flabby atrophic breast. Pathology: comedo and duct carcinoma without axillary lymph node metastasis. Patient still alive at age 86 years.

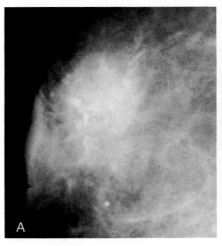
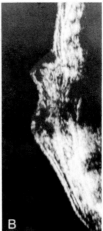

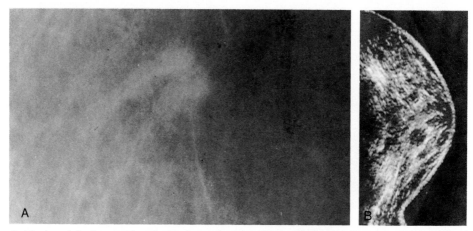

Figure 7–18. A and B, Sonography of mixed-type duct carcinoma. A 69-year-old woman seen for baseline study. Mammography: 8 × 11 mm moderately invasive carcinoma. Sonography: demarcated mass with irregular borders, nonhomogeneous internal echoes, slight peripheral architectural enhancement, no attenuation; a circumscribed low-grade carcinoma. Pathology: 1 cm moderately invasive duct carcinoma with foci of productive fibrosis, glandular formation, and mucin production. Modified radical mastectomy. All 18 axillary lymph nodes free of tumor; patient alive and well three years later.

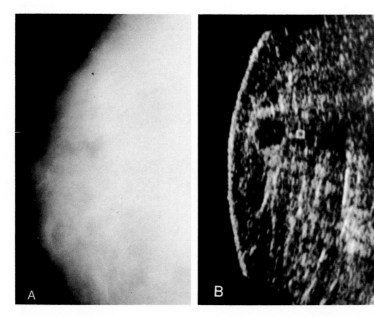

Figure 7–19. A and B, Usefulness of sonography in management. A 41-year-old woman with a palpable nodule in very nodular breasts. Area of thickening below nipple of this breast centrally biopsied one year ago, benign. Mammography: dense nodular breast with scattered calcifications. Sonography: hypoechoic area with some decreased through-transmission, fibroadenoma vs carcinoma. Pathology: solid form (no papillary or cribriform pattern) of mostly intraductal carcinoma with areas of invasion. Modified radical mastectomy; 1 of 18 axillary lymph nodes with tumor; patient alive and well three years later. Although sonography favored a benign mass, it added enough information to proceed with biopsy.

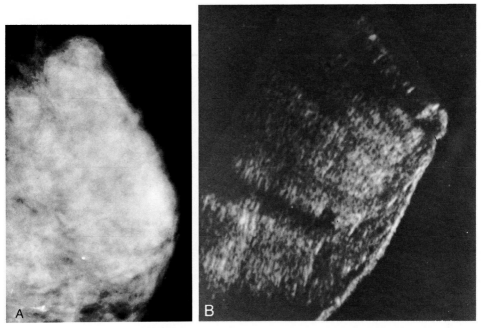

Figure 7–20. A and B, Intraductal comedo carcinoma with possible sonographic changes. A 68-year-old woman for checkup of clinically lumpy breasts. Mammography: marked nodularity on a background of dense ductal hyperplasia; three separate areas of comedo carcinoma type calcifications, one best seen is inferiorly near the chest wall. Sonography: a dilated major duct; many areas of transient shadowing but one area more marked and consistent that corresponded to one area of calcification. Pathology: at least five separate sites of intraductal comedo carcinoma, marked hyperplastic changes. Modified radical mastectomy, 0 of 15 axillary lymph nodes positive; patient alive and well two years later. Comment: One would have to question an intraductal comedo carcinoma producing shadowing of this degree. A more plausible explanation would be a nodule similar to the ones superiorly, with much fibrosis or dense adenosis producing the shadowing.

CASE HISTORY

Breast cancer and sonography in the young.

A 28-year-old woman with a breast lump for 20 months; clinically fibrocystic disease; mammograms normal (Fig. 7–23). Pathology: infiltrating comedo-carcinoma. Modified radical mastectomy; all 19 axillary lymph nodes free of disease. The patient was alive and well four years later. This type of come-docarcinoma usually produces poorly defined changes in the breast.

This case illustrates a potential aid, sonography, for the neglected young woman harboring breast cancer.

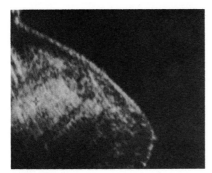

Figure 7–21. Sonography as aid in fibroadenoma in the young. A 19-year-old woman with a firm breast nodule. Sonography: a lobulated demarcated mass with nonhomogeneous internal echoes, a dominant nodule, sonographically benign. Pathology: intracanalicular fibroadenoma. Mammography not done.

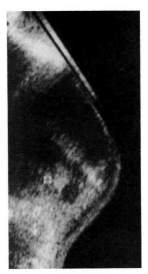

Figure 7–22. Another fibroadenoma in a 19-year-old woman. Mammography not done.

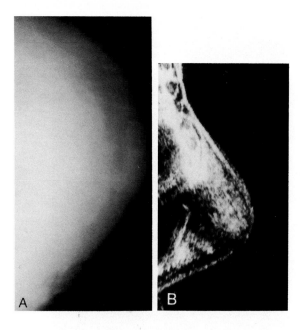

Figure 7–23. A and B, Mammography: homogeneously dense breasts with scattered calcifications. Sonography: disrupted architecture, hypoechoic upper outer half of the breast and irregular mass effect with shadowing suggestive of carcinoma.

OBSERVATIONS

Overlapping sonographic features of benign and malignant solid masses include: 30 per cent of benign masses attenuate the beam compared with 87 per cent of malignant ones; 10 per cent of the benign masses show altered architecture compared with 75 per cent of the malignant; internal echoes are nonhomogeneous in 20 per cent of the benign lesions and homogeneous in 19 per cent of the cancers; increased through-transmission is present in 10 per cent of the benign and 10 per cent of the malignant masses; and bulging of the skin can be noted with both benign and malignant masses.

Yet there are typical criteria in 75 per cent of the cancers (mostly duct); less typical criteria in 12 per cent, but still suggestive of malignancy and often reflecting the true histologic diagnosis; and atypical in 13 per cent (Table 7–10). Similarly, in the benign solid masses diagnostic criteria are typical in 75 per cent of the lesions, borderline in 12 per cent, and atypical in only 13 per cent. Thus, a fairly reliable differentiation by sonography alone of benign and malignant solid masses is possible in 87 per cent of the cancers and 83 per cent of the benign lesions (Table 7–11). This occurs while demonstrating by sonography the 6 per cent of cancers that mammography does not detect.

The observation that attenuation of the ultrasound beam becomes greater as it traverses normal breast tissue, new fibroadenomata, breast carcinomas without desmoplasia (such as duct, medullary with lymphoid stroma, and mucinous carcinoma), old and hardened fibroadenomata (with varying degrees of hyalinization), carcinomas with increased fibrotic response, and finally dense fibrosis explains the overlapping diagnostic characteristics of benign and malignant lesions. However, the astute sonographer will not impose any delay in clinical management but will, in fact, ensure less delay. The mass that may be confused with a young fibroadenoma will still be depicted as solid and suspicious, even if it is medullary carcinoma with lymphoid stroma (most likely in a woman well beyond 30 years of age and not in a teenager, who usually develops the young fibroadenoma). At the other extreme, the very dense fibrotic area of trauma, hemorrhage, organization, and dense fibrosis or

TABLE 7–11. Grouping of Benign Lesions from Table 7–8 Based on an Estimate of Reliability of Sonographic Criteria for Benign Lesions and Relative Frequency of Each Group

Typical Benign (83%)	Differential Diagnosis with Carcinoma
Fibroadenoma	Adenosis (dense and
Variants of fibroadenoma	localized)
Cystosarcoma phylloides	Hematoma
Lipoma	Fat necrosis
	Fibrosis

an area of fat necrosis should be considered malignant by the mammographer. Such lesions are infrequent but do require biopsy.

REFERENCES

Bailar JC (1976): Mammography—a contrary view. Ann Intern Med *84*:77.

Cole-Beuglet C (1982): Sonographic manifestation of malignant breast disease. Semin Ultrasound *3*:51.

Cole-Beuglet C, Soriano RZ, Kurtz AB, Goldberg BB (1983): Ultrasound analysis of 104 primary breast carcinomas classified according to histopathologic type. Radiology *147*:191.

Croll J, Kotwich J, Tabrett M (1982): The diagnosis of benign disease and the exclusion of malignancy in patients with breast symptoms. Semin Ultrasound *3*:38.

Egan RL (1960): Experience with mammography in a tumor institute. Evaluation of 1,000 studies. Radiology *74*:894.

Egan RL (1963–67): Automated water path whole breast sonography. Unpublished data.

Egan RL, Egan KL (1984): Detection of breast carcinoma: Comparison of automated water-path whole-breast sonography, mammography, and physical examination. AJR *143*:493.

Egan RL, Egan KL (1984): Automated water-path full-breast sonography: correlation with histology of 176 solid lesions. AJR *143*:499.

Egan RL, McSweeney MB, Murphy FB (1984): Breast sonography and the detection of cancer. *In* Brunner S, Langfelt B, Andersen PE (eds): Early Detection of Breast Cancer. Berlin, Springer-Verlag, p 90.

Harper AP, Kelly-Fry E, Noe JS, Bier JR, Jackson VP (1983): Ultrasound in the evaluation of solid breast masses. Radiology *146*:731.

Holmes JH (1981): Personal communication.

Howry DH, Bliss WR (1952): Visualization of the soft tissue structures of the body. J Lab Clin Med *40*:579.

Howry DH, Scott DA, Bliss WR (1954): The ultrasonic visualization of carcinoma of the breast and other soft tissue structures. Cancer *7*:354.

Jellins J, Kossoff G, Buddee FW, Reeves TS (1971): Ultrasonic visualization of the breast. Med J Aust *1*:305.

Jellins J, Kossoff G, Reeve TS, Barraclough BH (1975): Ultrasonic grey scale visualization of breast disease. Ultrasound Med Biol *1*:393.

Kelly-Fry E, Harper P (1979): Examination of the female breast by means of mammography automated B-mode and rapid real-time ultrasound scanning. Proceeding of the Annual AIUM Meeting, p 89.

Kelly-Fry E, Gibbons LV, Kossoff G (1969): Characterization of breast tissue by ultrasonic visualization methods. Proc Acoust Soc Am, San Diego, November.

Kelly-Fry E, Harper P (1983): Factors critical to highly accurate diagnoses of malignant breast pathologies by ultrasound imaging. *In* Lerski RA, Morley P (eds): Ultrasound '82. Oxford, Pergamon Press, p 415.

Kiluchi Y, Uchida R, Tonaka K, Wagai T (1957): Early diagnosis through ultrasonics. J Acoust Soc Am *29*:824.

Kobayashi T (1975): Review: Ultrasonic diagnosis of breast cancer. Ultrasound Med Biol *1*:383.

Laustela E, Kermine T, Lieto J, Tala P (1966): Studies of the ultrasonic diagnosis of breast tumors. Ann Clin Gyn Fenn *55*:173.

Maturo VG, Zusmer NR, Gilson AH, et al (1980): Ultrasound of the whole breast utilizing a dedicated automated breast scanner. Radiology *137*:457.

Schneck CD, Lehman DA (1982): Sonographic anatomy of the breast. Semin Ultrasound *3*:13.

Wild JJ, Neal D (1951): The use of high frequency ultrasonic waves for detecting changes of texture in living tissue. Lancet *1*:655.

Wild JJ, Reid JM (1952): Further pilot echographic studies on the histologic structure of the living intact breast. Am J Pathol *28*:839.

Wild JJ, Reid JM (1954): Echographic visualization of lesions of the living intact human breast. Cancer Rev *14*:277.

Nonradiographic Imaging

8

The lack of perfection of mammography has spurred attempts to improve upon it or replace it, particularly with a less expensive procedure. Almost all these efforts have been greatly disappointing. Many of the proposed procedures have proved noncontributory, such as radioisotope scanning; some show potential, as with the increased risk factor with thermography; some have special application, such as galactography; some may have routine applications, such as sonography; some are economically not feasible, such as CAT/M; some have not been thoroughly investigated, such as heavy-particle imaging; and some have particular value as laboratory procedures, such as magnetic resonance imaging.

The promising search continues, with the discovery of new information about breast diseases. A few of these procedures will be briefly considered, particularly those commanding more than the usual attention.

BREAST THERMOGRAPHY

Background

A breast thermogram is a pictorial representation of the infrared radiation of the skin over the breast. Breast cancers can produce a local or diffuse elevation in the skin temperature of one breast as compared with the opposite breast. The temperature gradient between tumor and host tissue can be increased by cooling the skin of the breast. By cooling the skin and erasing the superficial venous heat pattern, the deeper vessels, mainly arteries, contribute more to the thermographic pattern.

The radiant heat may be detected at a distance from the breast, telethermography, or with a receptor against the skin, contact thermography. In telethermography an infrared detector, the thermistor, captures the radiant energy and is electronically displayed on a television tube for viewing or photography. The contact method depends on temperature sensitivity of various cholesterol crystals encapsulated on a thin Mylar plate. With the plate against the breasts a color image is formed, each color being representative of a specific temperature. This too may be photographed for a permanent record. The images may be computerized from disks or tapes.

The resultant heat patterns may aid as an indicator of increased risk for breast cancer or in estimating prognosis of a breast malignancy.

In 1957 Lawson, a Canadian surgeon, recognizing an increase in heat from a cancerous breast, was stimulated to investigate this association. About that time the U.S. Armed Forces declassified information on their "Operation Sidewinder," a system of guiding missiles into the hot exhausts of airplanes. Lawson prompted the Barnes Engineering Corporation to produce a device to record the heat from the breast, a thermography unit. In 1965 the third such unit was placed in the Emory University Section of Mammography for clinical evaluation.

Clinical Application

By 1967 we had tabulated the results of breast thermography in 184 women coming to biopsy (Table 8–1). The recognition of only

TABLE 8–1. Thermography Compared With Mammography and Clinical Examination in 184 Women

	Number	+ Thermography	+ Mammography	+ Clinical Examination
Cancer	22	11	19	19
Noncancer	162	21	8	9
Total	184	32	27	28

50 per cent of the cancers and 13 per cent overcall of the noncancers by thermography led us to discard the procedure as being nonspecific and adding very little to the management of breast cancer patients.

This was the first form of medical thermography and became rather widely used in the United States with high expectations that it could be applied as a mass screening tool. Izard et al. (1972) reviewed 10,000 thermographic studies of the breast over a four-year period, with 85 per cent of 306 cancers in symptomatic women demonstrated by mammography and 61 per cent by thermography. Four lesions were found by blind biopsy on the opposite breast. The overcall rate (benign lesions incorrectly called malignant) was 40 per cent by thermography.

Breast thermography was subjected to a harsh evaluation in the 280,000 women in the NCI/American Cancer Society (ACS) Breast Cancer Demonstration Detection Project (BCDDP). Thermography was positive in 43 per cent of breast cancers detected during the first two screenings. If thermography and physical examination only had been used, 37 per cent of the minimal cancers would have been missed on the first screening and 44 per cent on the second. Accordingly, with these degrees of sensitivity and specificity the procedure was abandoned.

A variation of this type is "stress thermography." In this procedure the patient's hand is plunged into icy water to see if hot spots remain (theoretically showing cancer) or disappear (benign lesions). Another variation is computerized thermography, using the same data but subjecting it to computer analysis.

Contact Thermography

Certain cholesterol crystals produce patterns of color when subjected to various temperatures. The liquid crystals at one time were painted on the skin of the breasts and the color changes recorded, usually on Polaroid film. A more acceptable approach was to suspend the crystals in a liquid thinly coating a plastic sheet so that the crystals adhered in a uniform fashion when dried. With the plastic sheet mounted in a holder, it could be placed in contact with the skin of the breast. Variations in skin temperature caused the plastic sheet to glow in various colors, which could be recorded on colored Polaroid film. To remove the heat from the superficial vessels (mostly veins), the breast could be cooled with a hair blower, thus enabling a better study of deep vessels (mostly arteries). Contact breast thermography has been used more widely in Europe to add information on the prognosis of breast cancer. Gauterie and Gross (1980) reviewed 58,000 thermographic studies and found 1245 TgIII thermographic studies in women whose clinical examination, mammography, breast sonography, and fine needle biopsy had been normal. Within five years over one third had confirmed breast carcinomas. Our earlier experience (1965 to 1967) and recent BCDDP experience with telethermography revealed no pattern with significant risk prediction on similar thermographic studies.

Arguments that favor the use of breast thermography (Table 8–2) are: (1) No ionizing radiation is used; (2) the examination can be repeated as often as desired; (3) it requires very little time; (4) it causes little or no discomfort to the patient; (5) it is relatively inexpensive; and (6) when used with physical examination and mammography it should increase the overall efficiency of breast cancer detection. However, because of its lack of sensitivity and specificity, its use as the sole method of detection is not recommended. A thorough discussion on thermography can be found in the *Technologist's Guide to Detec-*

Table 8–2. Thermography of the Breast

Advantages	Disadvantages
No ionizing radiation	Low specificity
Relatively inexpensive	Low sensitivity
Requires little time	Relatively inefficient even
May be repeated often	when combined with other
No significant	procedures
discomfort	Cannot be sole method of
Requires little space	imaging the breast
Can be computerized	Patients dislike disrobing in
	cold room
	Requires carefully controlled
	environment
	Complex electronics sensitive
	to trauma
	Technologist training is
	considerable

TABLE 8–3. Thermographic Patterns

Normal
Avascular breast
    No recognizable vessels
    Cooler than chest, shoulders, neck
    Nipples faintly seen, areolae cool
Vascular breast
    Minimally vascular
    Moderately vascular
    Hypervascular
    Mottled
Abnormal
Single changes
    Unilateral exaggeration of veins
    Localized "hot spot"
    Increased heat emission at the areola
    Edge sign
Diffuse changes
    Combination of single-site changes
    Generalized increase in temperature in several
      areas
    Generalized increase in temperature in whole
      breast
    Intense heat over mastectomy scar

tion of Early Breast Cancer by Mammography, Thermography and Xeroradiography (Egan RL [ed], Chicago, American College of Radiology, 1972).

The various patterns seen with thermography of the breast are outlined in Table 8–3.

Observations

The complicated biologic thermal signals to date are poorly understood and thus judged too optimistically for safe clinical application.

When combined with physical examination, one half of all subclinical cancers still will not be detected (Fig. 8–1).

Thermography as an adjunct to mammography adds little diagnostic information yet some may bolster confidence in interpretation (Fig. 8–2).

The potential prognostic value of thermography may be of major importance.

As a high-risk marker for breast cancer, thermography may realize its greatest potential.

MAGNETIC RESONANCE

The inclusion of this short segment is merely an alert that there is a real potential in magnetic resonance (MR) imaging of the breast. Whole-body units have been used to study the breast, but smaller surface coils are more appropriate for this organ. Considera-

ble investigation of numerous magnetic field strengths and imaging properties is required to establish the optimum system for imaging the breast by MR.

In contrast to x-ray CT imaging, which utilizes x-ray absorption and transmission of cross sections of the body, the parameters of MR include hydrogen density, the state of motion of the hydrogen, and tissue relaxation times of T_1 and T_2. MR images of the breast are based on the magnetic properties of protons that have spin and act as magnetic dipoles. In a quite strong magnetic field they align themselves parallel to the direction of that magnetic field and produce a net magnetic vector (moment). Once this alignment is accomplished, a radio frequency pulse (RF) is applied. This then displaces the magnetic moment to a degree that is determined by both the strength and the length of time of the RF application. As the RF used is proportional to the strength of the magnetic field, it is known as the resonant frequency. After cessation of the RF pulse, the protons reorient themselves and an RF signal is emitted—the source of the potential image. The variation of the RF strength and the frequency at which it is repeated provides variable image potentials.

Our work at Emory University with mag-

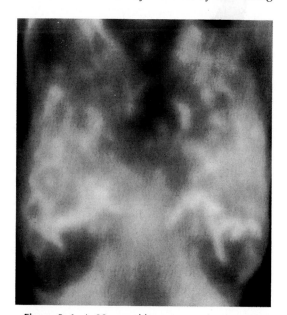

Figure 8–1. A 38-year-old asymptomatic woman was seen for routine mammography and thermography. The breasts were clinically normal, but mammograms showed suspicious calcifications without a mass, prompting localization, biopsy, and specimen radiography. The thermograms showed a normal venous pattern (white on black). Pathology: intraductal comedocarcinoma.

With MR of the breast, both benign and malignant conditions can be visualized. It discriminates between them, not on the basis of T_1 relaxation values but on a morphologic basis. In vivo T_1 measurements made in both normal and abnormal breasts indicate a large overlap between normal and abnormal tissue. T_1 values of normal or fatty breast tissue vary between 0 and 300 msec. With breast carcinomas the T_1 values vary between 100 and 300 msec. Frequently encountered benign mammary changes, which include fibrosis, fibrocystic disease, and adenosis, may also cause varied T_1 relaxation times.

Cystic breast masses can be visualized by magnetic resonance because of their long T_1 values. The small punctate clusters of calcification that often herald the presence of malignancy on mammography are not visualized on MR scans, since calcium gives no signal.

The morphologic appearance of breast lesions has been found to be more helpful in characterization than the intensity of the signal obtained with different radio frequency pulse sequences. The advantage of MR over conventional mammography appears to be its ability to produce images in axial and other planes, which give better morphologic information.

Observations

The potential for characterization of pathophysiologic conditions in the breast in biochemical and physiologic terms in association with the traditional morphologic changes should improve our ability to diagnose and evaluate breast disease processes.

Magnetic resonance imaging involving spectroscopy and elements other than hydrogen may well add to our ability to characterize tissues in the breast.

TRANSILLUMINATION

Background

Visualization of the transilluminated female breast employing a high-intensity light beam was reported over 50 years ago (Cutler, 1931). It failed to gain acceptance as a significant diagnostic test in the differentiation of benign from malignant lesions. In the late 1970s a Swedish instrument was described that recorded transilluminated images on 35 mm film. One light source was used for

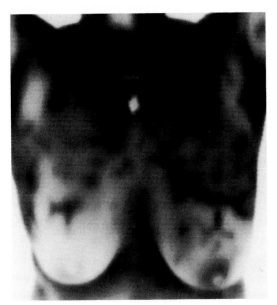

Figure 8–2. A 56-year-old asymptomatic woman was seen in a breast screening program with a clinically normal right breast. There was an area of highly suspicious altered architecture in the upper outer quadrant of the left breast. On thermography there was increased heat in the left breast. Note the larger and denser veins (black on white background), rendering this a suspicious thermogram. Pathology: infiltrating 8 mm carcinoma in the upper outer quadrant of the left breast with 20 axillary lymph nodes free of tumor.

netic resonance imaging of the breast began in the late 1970s in collaboration with the well-equipped department of chemistry for tissue spectroscopy. Initial efforts were directed to the optimal methods of handling and studying breast tissue samples, followed by comparative (with x-ray) imaging of fatty, fibrous, and glandular tissues, then hundreds of fresh breast biopsy specimens, both benign and malignant. Although there was some overlapping of relaxation times with benign and malignant tissues, we were able to differentiate disease processes in a high percentage of cases.

Most of our effort to study the intact breast awaited the construction of a surface coil—rather than attempt imaging of the breast with the body coil. Imaging with the surface coil still presents problems but many discrete diagnostic images are possible (Figs. 8–3 and 8–4).

The promise of MR in breast cancer is in imaging dense breasts and indicating biologic and physiologic alterations. Because there is currently no known biologic hazard associated with MR, its application in the diagnosis of breast disease is particularly attractive.

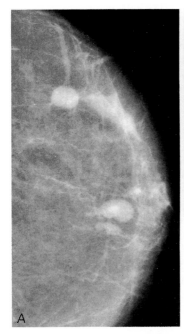

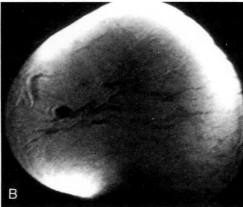

Figure 8–3. Magnetic resonant (MR) image of a benign breast mass. A 60-year-old woman with a cancer of the opposite breast. Clinically this breast was normal. *A,* Mammography: smooth bordered mass, notched with calcifications. *B,* MR image: spin echo, low-intensity signals at all levels, dense smooth bordered mass. Pathology: fibroadenoma. (Courtesy M. B. McSweeney, M.D., Emory University, Atlanta, GA.)

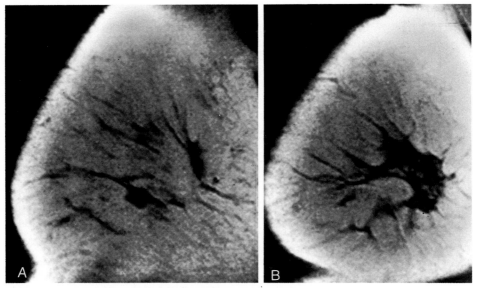

Figure 8–4. Malignant mass by magnetic resonance. A 67-year-old woman with a clinically suspicious mass. Mammography revealed a moderately invasive carcinoma. MR image: *A,* T_1 weighted image, spin echo 30/300, low signal intensity. *B,* T_2 weighted image, spin echo 30/1500, increased signal intensity. Pathology: intraductal and infiltrative duct carcinoma. (Courtesy M. B. McSweeney, M.D., Emory University, Atlanta, GA.)

visualizing the transilluminated breast by eye, and another high-intensity flash unit was coupled to the camera for imaging recording. Preferential transmission of infrared wavelengths is a characteristic of human tissue and can be recorded on infrared-sensitive color film. The examination (diaphanography) is conducted in a darkened room with the light firmly applied to the undersurface of the breast. Films are exposed by the flash tube. Infrared-sensitive color film requires special processing, so that there may be a delay in reviewing the pictures. Color images can be from a video system with real-time gray-scale that translates the gray tones to colors.

Translucency of the breast is dependent upon size, amount of fat, composition and optical density of skin and glandular tissues, vascular supply, and the presence and extent of fibrosis, inflammation, hemorrhage, cysts, and neoplasia. The transilluminated normal breast has a reddish yellow color with the superficial veins standing out in relief. They are smooth in outline and undulating. Marked disparity frequently exists between radiographic and optical densities. The radiographic dense breast that is difficult to evaluate by mammography may be translucent. The adjunctive use of diaphanography may provide additional information to mammography. Both benign and malignant disease can contribute to changes in shades of colors and to distortions of vascular patterns, with irregularity, dilatation, and alteration in caliber of veins. Since subtle differences in the two breasts may not be detected during diaphanoscopy, careful review of the recorded images is important. Accentuation of the red color is found in more severe grades of fibrocystic disease, while lesser degrees of the process are generally indistinguishable from the normal. Dominant nodules are best demonstrated by manipulating the breast so that

they are close to the viewed skin surface and farther from the light source. The translucent pale color of a cyst differentiates it from a solid lesion. The fibroadenoma has a brownish or deeper red color, with fair margination, and may resemble a cancer. The colors of cancers range from brown to slate to dark gray. The margins of the tumors are ill defined, and frequently the vasculature is distorted. Acute and chronic inflammations, including abscesses, are very dark; a black color signifies blood. Some abnormality may be present in three quarters of breast cancers.

Observations

Our basic work with in vitro and in vivo spectroscopy of somatic tissues, with emphasis on those of the breast, indicates profound physical problems in casting intramammary lesion shadows on the skin of the breast. Scattering of the light is a marked characteristic of transillumination of the breast. A deep lesion cannot always be maneuvered into proximity of the skin, an absolute requirement for clear borders. Subtle changes as minimal distortion of the architecture of the breast and fine structures of tiny calcifications will not be visualized. Transillumination provides an extension of physical examination of the breast but should not be a replacement for mammography.

REFERENCES

Carlsen E (1982): Transillumination light scanning. Diagn. Imag. April:28.

Cutler M (1931): Transillumination of the breast. Ann. Surg. 93:223.

Gauterie M, Gross CM (1980): Breast thermography and cancer risk prediction. Cancer 45:51.

Izard HJ, Becker W, Shilo R, Ostrum et al (1972): Breast thermography after 4 years and 10,000 studies. AJR 115:811.

9

Pathologic Study of Mammary Lesions

C. Whitaker Sewell, M. D.

GENERAL

Breast tissue has a variable component of adipose tissue that may be substantial or predominant. This fatty component defies freezing and fixation and generally requires extra fixation time compared with predominantly fibrous lesions. The urgent "need to know," which leads some clinicians to request that a specimen be rushed or processed rapidly, may, in the case of fatty specimens, result in near destruction of the tissue or, at the very least, inadequately fixed tissue that is difficult to interpret.

Similarly, adipose tissue is very difficult to cut on a frozen-section machine (cryostat). Although a pathologist may cut frozen sections of mammary neoplasms and certain benign fibrous or hyperplastic lesions with relative impunity, freezing very fatty breast lesions, particularly those containing microscopic clustered calcifications, may result in disaster. The lesion may be too artifactually distorted for interpretation, or because of the difficulty in obtaining an acceptable specimen, may lie whittled away at the bottom of the cryostat.

132

Surgeons should be mindful that the heat generated by the cautery does produce artifactual distortion of tissue, particularly the epithelium. This nearly always destroys the cells nearest the cutting edge and may, if a very thin incisional biopsy is taken entirely with the cutting cautery, totally "cook" the biopsy and prevent any histologic interpretation.

BIOPSY TECHNIQUES

Excisional and Incisional

The excisional or incisional biopsy of a palpable lesion sometimes followed by frozen-section diagnosis is a well-established procedure in breast diagnosis. A frozen-section examination is requisite if a mastectomy or other definitive procedure is to be undertaken immediately, and a well-trained surgical pathologist can be expected to make a definite diagnosis in the majority of cases. With certain lesions, a frozen-section diagnosis may properly be deferred. This particularly applies to many papillary lesions, in which it may be difficult to distinguish between a papilloma and a papillary carcinoma with certainty on a frozen-section slide. Similarly, a papillary or florid epithelial hyperplasia may occasionally undergo extensive sclerosis (the so-called radial scar lesion) and mimic the pattern of invasive ductal carcinoma. Permanent sections of paraffin-embedded, well-fixed tissue may be required to make this distinction.

Frozen section may also be helpful if a biopsy specimen is grossly suspect for carcinoma even when immediate mastectomy is not planned. This is particularly helpful in identifying malignant tissue that is to be submitted for hormone receptor studies. The practice of submitting undiagnosed random samples of mammary tissue for hormone receptor analysis is questionable.

Biopsy specimens that are not frozen should be fixed in formalin or a mixed formalin-alcohol fixative. For predominantly fibrous lesions, e.g., fibroadenoma, four to five hours of fixation prior to processing is adequate. For specimens containing a large amount of fat, overnight fixation is required.

Segmental Resection

Segmental resection is the procedure most commonly done for lesions that are identified by imaging modalities but are clinically nonpalpable. Currently these lesions are most frequently localized by wire or dye injection techniques, and the documentation of the resected lesion is achieved by immediate intraoperative x-ray of the specimen. This is done to assure the surgeon (while there is still the opportunity for further excision) that the imaged abnormality has indeed been resected. Frozen-section examination is indicated only if a definite lesion is identified on the surgeon's gross examination of the specimen and only if the lesion is of sufficient size to justify freezing; otherwise the artifactual distortion produced by freezing of a very small lesion may hinder adequate histologic interpretation of the specimen.

True microscopic lesions, such as those commonly associated with clustered calcifications, should be submitted in their entirety for histologic examination rather than partitioned for hormone receptor study. Adequate and thorough histologic examination of a microscopic lesion is far more important than any benefit derived from estrogen receptor analysis of a frozen "unknown" portion of a biopsy specimen. Sequestering and freezing a sample for receptors may forever mask the true nature of a resected lesion of microscopic size and may, for example, prevent the pathologist from ever determining whether a particular intraductal carcinoma is associated with areas of invasion.

It is sometimes helpful for the radiologist or pathologist to section serially the fresh specimen and again x-ray the slices to localize more accurately the radiographic abnormality. This assures everyone involved in the case that the imaged and resected abnormality eventually appears on a microscope slide. Serial or deeper sections of the paraffin blocks may subsequently be necessary in order to visualize adequately and diagnose the lesion. As previously indicated, adequate fixation of this tissue is essential if a confident and reliable diagnosis is to be rendered on difficult or borderline lesions. In general, unless the tissue is predominantly fibrous, overnight fixation prior to processing should be expected. The patient should be forewarned of this necessary delay so that she does not expect a diagnosis on the day following her surgery.

Collecting Duct Excision

The collecting duct excision is most often performed for nipple discharge or bleeding and is most commonly associated with either mammary duct ectasia or a papillary neoplasm within the collecting duct system. Following adequate fixation, the resected tissue is serially sectioned in a plane perpendicular to the orientation of the duct system and submitted entirely except for tissue consisting totally of fat.

Owing to the nature of the lesions expected, frozen-section examination is generally not beneficial and may be harmful to the tissue. As previously mentioned, papillary tumors may be difficult to classify by frozen-section techniques, and permanent sections are usually necessary for a definitive diagnosis. Furthermore, papillomas are delicate, friable tumors that may be damaged or even lost if unduly manipulated prior to fixation.

Fine Needle Aspiration

Fine needle aspiration techniques have been increasingly helpful in characterizing both solid and cystic lesions in the breast. The surgeon or radiologist performing these procedures should be reminded that most pathologists in the United States are comfortable in interpreting only those cells that are rapidly fixed in an alcohol solution or spray fixative. Air-dried epithelium, unlike blood cells, shows marked artifactual distortion and loss of nuclear detail. The aspirated material should be smeared onto microscope slides and rapidly (within two to three seconds) immersed in 95 per cent alcohol solution or sprayed with an appropriate fixative. This procedure is essentially the same as that used for Papanicolaou smears of the cervix. Alternatively, aspirated specimens, particularly if fluid is present, may be injected into a solution of alcohol for subsequent processing in the cytology laboratory. Aspirated material that has been mixed with fixative cannot be examined on smears but can be successfully examined using filter techniques. Formalin is never a satisfactory fixative for cytology specimens.

SAMPLING OF MASTECTOMY SPECIMENS

With the decline in popularity of and necessity for the full radical mastectomy, most current operations in which the entire breast is removed are either modified radical mastectomies or total mastectomies, the latter operation including removal of all breast tissue but only sampling of a few low axillary lymph nodes. The modified radical mastectomy resects lymph nodes from levels I and II (underneath the pectoralis minor muscle) but does not sample the few nodes in the apex of the axilla. Skeletal muscle is generally not resected in either operation unless it is necessary to include a bead of muscle beneath a deeply situated tumor. Simple mastectomies, i.e., those in which some mammary tissue remains, provide the opportunity for development of a second neoplasm in the breast.

Following mastectomy, the pathologist's responsibility is to gauge accurately the size and extent of the tumor and to search for evidence of lymphatic or vascular channel permeation. Generally, several sections are taken around the biopsy site, and the breast is thinly sliced to determine whether additional masses or lesions can be grossly detected. The number of random sections needed from the remainder of the breast should not be arbitrarily set, but rather depends on the pathologist's gross assessment of the tissue. The pathologist should be mindful that certain significant lesions, particularly lobular carcinoma in situ, are not grossly palpable lesions and are often discovered on routine or random sections.

For total mastectomy procedures that are performed for prophylactic reasons in high-risk patients or those with (noninvasive) intraductal carcinoma or lobular carcinoma in situ, numerous sections should be taken to characterize adequately the remaining breast tissue. Multifocal intraductal carcinoma is relatively common, and foci of microscopic invasion may be missed if sectioning is inadequate.

STUDY OF REGIONAL LYMPH NODES

For prognostic reasons it is important to quantitate accurately the number of axillary nodes bearing metastases. Following a total mastectomy procedure only two to four nodes from the lowest region of the axilla are usually received. A modified mastectomy theroretically contains all nodes from levels I and II and usually at least 15 nodes can be recovered. If the surgeon considers it important to distinguish between level I and level II nodes, he should place clips appropriately on the specimen to designate these levels. It is difficult for the pathologist to orient the node-bearing tissue from a modified mastectomy once it has been removed from the chest wall.

PATHOLOGY REPORT

The pathology report should include a complete gross description of the tissue resected in addition to a diagnosis and either a microscopic description or a comment detailing certain pertinent facts derived from histologic examination. The following information is considered essential.

1. Classification of the neoplasm as ductal, lobular, or other type (e.g., cystosarcoma phylloides).
2. Subclassification as medullary, colloid, comedo, and so forth, if possible.
3. Presence or absence of invasion.
4. Presence or absence of intraductal component.
5. Presence or absence of lymphatic or vascular channel permeation.
6. Number of regional lymph nodes with metastases.

Other pertinent information that is often provided includes involvement of the dermal lymphatics, nipple involvement, and differentiation of the tumor. If grading of the neoplasm is recorded, the best-differentiated lesions (tubular carcinoma, papillary carcinoma) are graded as I, whereas very poorly differentiated lesions (medullary carcinoma, invasive lobular carcinoma) are considered Grade III. Most typical scirrhous carcinomas with good gland formation would fall into the Grade II category.

10

Localization and Radiography of Biopsy Specimens

BACKGROUND

Edgar C. White, M.D., Chief of Surgery, M.D. Anderson Hospital, was a conscientious and meticulous surgeon who used great care in teaching the surgical fellows to perfect thin breast flaps in preparation for a Halsted radical mastectomy despite the usual advanced stage of the disease being treated. He then would go to the surgical lounge where this was a common sight: his sitting on a bench, head in hands, chain-smoking, and greatly dejected, being powerless to save the woman's life.

During that period as a fellow in radiology, my reporting of the mammograms done on all patients scheduled for a prebiopsy chest x-ray was without benefit of history or physical findings to try to establish whether there were any real values to the procedure. A code for benign or malignant was assigned at the time so that there would be no confusion in reviewing the results. These terse reports without use of any tentative diagnosis went onto the patient's chart prior to surgery, and apparently they were being read. About two weeks after Dr. White had begun a rotation on the breast service, he asked to see a certain mammogram, as I had missed a cancer. My response was that x-ray of the breast was no better than flipping a coin. Yet he insisted upon review of the case because he had felt a small hard lesion high in the tail of the breast. He then pointed out that in his last 14 cases my diagnosis had been histologically correct in the other 13. Such appalling news prompted a review of the previous mammograms, which revealed a few cases of proven nonpalpable carcinomas. One I had reviewed with the surgeon prior to surgery concerned a woman presenting with a left breast mass who had a small cancer in the UOQ of the right breast, detected on x-ray. Fearing some disastrous reaction from the patient, we made a trip to her room to explain that she probably would lose her right breast and not the left. Oh yes, her surgeon had already explained that to her—so great was his confidence in my mammography.

These surgeons insisted upon pushing for earlier detection by exploring less definite mammographic changes to find curable breast cancer. Dr. White even decided to biopsy fine linear calcifications in the subcutaneous fat despite my reminding him that carcinoma arose in an area of breast tissue. So anxious was he not to miss an early lesion that he was disappointed to find only foreign body reaction in an area of previous biopsy.

At first, biopsies were usually of small nonpalpable masses, which became palpable after sharp dissection into that area so that routine frozen-section diagnosis could be made. Many problems resulted for the radiologist because he had to make decisions as to what to explore and where, and he had to see that the pathologist viewed the proper area histopathologically. Every possible error resulted: Subsequent mammograms showed lesions missed by biopsy, the area in question was left in the specimen and not studied by the pathologists, cancer was thrown away, and even a small cancer was sliced away in squaring up paraffin blocks. These are the reasons for developing this meticulous approach to breast specimen radiography and practicing it without great change for over 25 years (Egan, 1962; Egan's report at the Fifth Annual Mammography Seminar in 1965). Dr. Gershon-Cohen attended the 1965 seminar and introduced our technique of localization, breast biopsy, and specimen radiography to his colleagues in Philadelphia (Berger et al., 1966).

Breast specimen radiography is, without question, a unique and most rewarding procedure: It is lifesaving; it requires the ultimate in mammography to detect early cancer changes; it has stimulated the most interest in the concept of early breast cancer; it has helped create the desire to delineate premalignant breast changes of intraductal epithelial growth patterns; and it has set the stage for and pointed out the necessity to practice the team approach in medicine.

TECHNIQUE

Mammography not only has pinpointed these problems of nonpalpable carcinoma, carcinoma in situ, certain premalignant breast lesions, and metastatic vs bilateral primary or successive primary carcinomas of the breast but also has become indispensable in proper recognition and proper treatment of these lesions. The problem usually is first to remove the questionable area at the time of surgery, and secondly, to be sure that the area in question on the mammogram is examined microscopically. When there is a definite mass on the mammograms, even though not palpable clinically in the intact breast, it usually can be found by the surgeon at the time of surgery and submitted for immediate frozen-section microscopy. The specific problem of localization encountered in using mammography in management of breast diseases is that of clustered punctate calcifications without a mass by x-ray and

without significant palpable abnormality in the breast. Many of our patients have fallen into this category of suspicious x-ray findings with no mass radiographically or clinically.

The original approach of investigating areas of clustered calcification by localization for the surgeon by mammography, removal of tissue as a biopsy specimen, and frozen-section microscopic study soon proved inadequate. Unless there was a mass noted on the mammogram associated with the calcification, the lesion would not be palpable by the pathologist even in 3 mm slices of the biopsy specimen. Calcifications seen on the microscopic sections frequently were small and associated with fibrocystic disease and could not be definitely identified with the larger 50 μ calcifications seen on the radiographs.

On gross examination, those areas that must be localized radiographically for the surgeon and pathologist usually look and feel no different than adjacent breast tissues despite precise localization on the specimen radiograph. If reliance were placed on palpation, usually an area of fibrosis would be selected for study and the area questionable by x-ray would be discarded.

Even the presence of small calcifications in the cryostat section is not proof that the proper area is being studied microscopically. Less clustered and smaller deposits of calcium, sometimes not visible by x-ray, may be what is being seen on the slides. Calcification 50 μ or larger may be seen radiographically. In slicing the usual 6 to 8 μ breast tissue preparation for staining and microscopy, such sized particles will be dislodged or fragmented by the microtome. Reliance must be placed on proper selection of the area for histopathologic study. In several instances, tissue not frozen or blocked for permanent sections was x-rayed and found to contain the mammographically suspicious calcium. In an attempt to avoid this frustration in the breast biopsies, a definite procedure has been followed for these calcifications without an associated mass on the mammograms.

The routine that has been developed as a team approach is so important that previously poorly coordinated experiences have led to the conclusion that if a breast biopsy requiring specimen radiography is not properly done and studied, it is better not to attempt the procedure. This team also includes the technologists, both x-ray and pathology, whose roles cannot be executed confidently without some knowledge of what is being attempted.

The mammograms were carefully reviewed with the surgeon for localization of the area of the breast to be removed. Often, additional views of the breast were obtained to confirm the findings. The patient was told about the procedure and a breast biopsy only was scheduled for a Monday or Tuesday. This was the original procedure so that mastectomy could be done, if necessary, on Thursday or Friday without further delay over the weekend. Fear of increased delay of definitive surgery was actually unfounded. Today we feel that a few days added to the interval between biopsy and treatment produce no increased risk with these localized carcinomas.

APPROXIMATING THE LOCATION

The area of the lesion, both the craniocaudad and the mediolateral mammographic views, is drawn or sketched (Fig. 10–1). The distances above or below and medial or lateral to the nipple are measured and recorded. This is usually adequate for the surgeon, who can visualize the shift in the breast tissue from mammographic to surgical biopsy positions. To aid him the anesthesiologist can hold up the sketches for the surgeon to see.

PINPOINTING THE LOCATION

Following localization of the lesion in relation to the nipple, the skin over it is marked and a hypodermic needle passed into the breast, with the tip aimed toward the lesion. Craniocaudad and mediolateral views are obtained to estimate the location of the needle tip in relation to the lesion (Figs. 10–2 and 10–3). If necessary, the needle is readjusted. A sketch is made of the needle and lesion and distances recorded. A small drop of 50 per cent Hypaque and Evans blue dye is injected while the needle is withdrawn. Thus, a tract of dye to the skin is injected for the surgeon to follow.

Alternative approaches include mammography over wire grids, placement of wires over the breast and radiography, insertion of a stylet containing a hooked wire, simply placing a needle into the area of the lesion and cutting the hub end off at the skin, or whatever strikes the radiologist's fancy.

BIOPSY AND SPECIMEN RADIOGRAPHY

The patient is taken to the operating room, and the biopsy specimen is obtained. The pathologist receives it and takes it intact to the mammography unit (Fig. 10–1D). Originally the radiograph was obtained with a double-loading technique: one very fine-grain film and one industrial film three times as fast, one exposure being made of the specimen on one half of the 8 × 10 inch film with the usual specimen radiographic factors and the second exposure being made with twice the mas. Developing the film that had three times greater speed at 3 min (leaving the very fine-grain film to develop for 6 min) reduced the waiting and viewing time significantly. Time is always an important factor when a patient is under general anesthesia. A mass without calcification may be better seen on radiography if the specimen is suspended in water in a radiolucent container, such as a plastic cup.

Screen-film radiography of these breast biopsy specimens may be carried out in a manner similar to that of screen-film radiography of the sliced sections of the whole breast.

When the calcifications are seen in the radiograph as in Figure 10–1E, the surgeon is informed, the biopsy wound is closed, and the patient is returned to her room. If the proper area has not been removed, the surgeon obtains additional breast tissue until the suspicious area of calcification is removed. It is mandatory that the surgeon not attempt to localize the proper site for histologic study. He cannot feel the abnormality; he disturbs the tissue by slicing erratically so that radiography is usually worthless; and he may suggest that the pathologist study the wrong area, usually a firmer area of fibrosis, and the cancer will be discarded.

In the mammography area following the initial specimen radiography, the pathologist or radiologist slices the specimen in 3 mm slices, carefully laying them on the cleared x-ray film in an orderly fashion. Proper identifying numbers are placed alongside the slices, and radiography is carried out with mas slightly decreased from that used on the intact specimen. Without disturbing the position of the slices, the radiologist reviews the specimen radiographs and indicates to the pathologist the precise area and side of each slice to be studied by him under the microscope (Figs. 10–1 and 10–2).

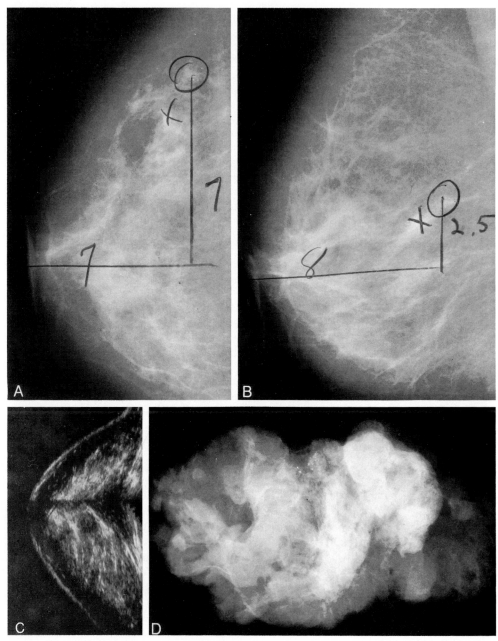

Figure 10–1. Mammogram of left breast of a 45-year-old woman as routine follow-up after biopsy of right breast for fibrocystic disease one year previously. A small cluster of calcifications was seen, poorly reproduced. The breast was still clinically normal after localization by mammography. Sketch of suspicious area in relationship to the nipple. *A*, Craniocaudad view. *B*, Mediolateral view. *C*, Sonography shows hypoechoic irregular area corresponding to the location of the calcifications. *D*, Biopsy specimen radiograph.

Illustration continued on opposite page

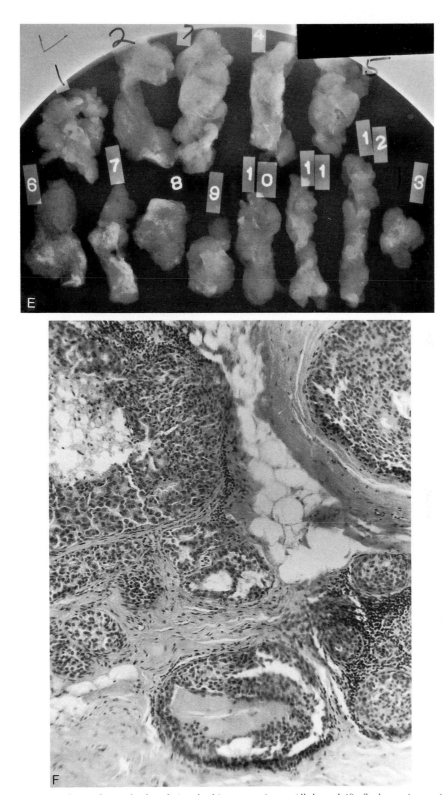

Figure 10–1 *Continued E,* Radiograph after slicing the biopsy specimen. All the calcific flecks are in specimen #6. This was the only area of intraductal carcinoma found after modified radical mastectomy. *F,* H & E preparation showing representative intraductal carcinoma bilaterally.

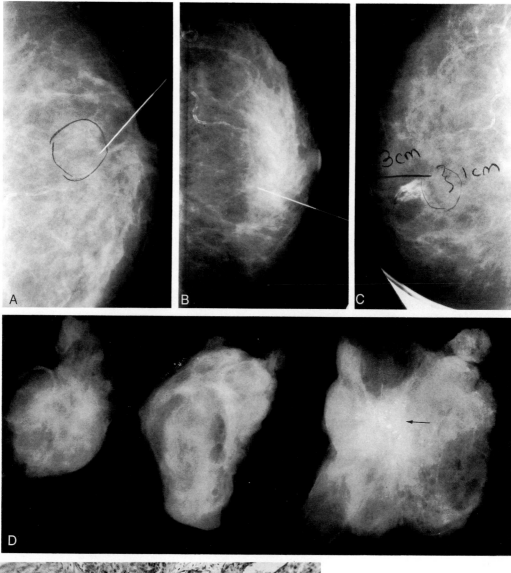

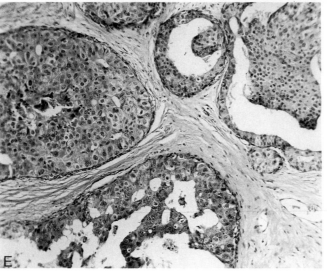

Figure 10–2. Tip of needle in area of faint calcifications. *A*, Craniocaudad view. *B*, Mediolateral view. A 36-year-old woman seen for baseline mammogram. *C*, Injection of a small amount of radiopaque material into the breast 1 cm anterior to the area containing the calcifications. *D*, Third biopsy clearly shows cluster of punctate calcifications. Two biopsies prior to this failed to reveal calcification by radiography of the specimens. Usually the proper tissue is removed with the first biopsy (2 × magnification). *E*, H & E preparation showing intraductal carcinoma.

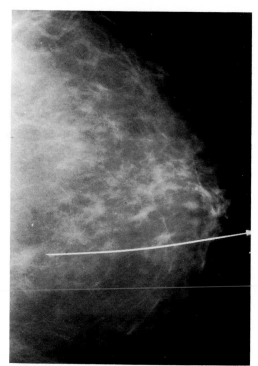

Figure 10–3. Needle localization of a nonpalpable carcinoma. A 64-year-old woman for baseline study of clinically nodular breasts. Mammography: severe ductal hyperplasia with fine and coarse coalescent nodules; one mass of 5 × 7 mm moderately invasive carcinoma containing coarse and fine calcifications. This locatization film shows placement of the tip of the needle near the mass prior to injection of radiopaque dye. Pathology: intraductal and microinvasive carcinoma. Modified radical mastectomy; all 19 axillary lymph nodes without tumor; patient alive and well two years later.

HISTOLOGIC STUDIES

Paraffin-mounted routine histopathologic studies on the areas are then carried out; this requires approximately 24 hours. This system allows the pathologist unhurried study, additional stains if needed, and consultation with other pathologists, if desired. Sometimes it is necessary to radiograph the specimen while it is still mounted in a paraffin block to see where the calcifications might be. Caution in interpretation is necessary because artifacts, present in a high percentage of the paraffin blocks, may simulate the appearance of calcification on the radiograph.

Some pathologists or surgeons may attempt to localize an area for frozen section and, if no cancer is found, resort to radiography. Seldom fruitful, this macerates the specimen to the extent that radiography is nearly impossible. In our experience, attempts of frozen-section studies of calcifications without a mass by x-ray is time consuming, causes increased anesthesia time, produces errors, and is usually quite frustrating.

RESULTS

The Emory University experience includes at least 407 nonpalpable breast carcinomas, with calcifications not associated with a mass making up slightly more than one half (Table 10–1). This number would be larger except that in many instances some palpable abnormality was present in the breast but not necessarily related to the carcinoma. All the lesions required localization for the surgeon. Almost all required specimen radiography to pinpoint the area of concern.

Use of specimen radiography for calcifications not associated with a mass reflects considerable volatility (Fig. 10–4). From the mid-1960s to the mid-1970s there was a steady increase in the number of new mammography patients with a moderate variation in the percentage having specimen radiography for calcifications only. There was a steady, but at times erratic, increase in the number of malignant biopsies. However, in the mid-1970s, at the time the wives of the President and Vice-President had highly publicized breast cancers, there was a marked increase in the number of mammography patients and fourfold increase in the number of biopsies for calcifications only, with a marked decrease in the percentage of those that were malignant.

This latter phenomenon coincided with many radiologists being forced to do mammography for the first time owing to the great public demand. Xeroradiography had been publicized as the panacea for breast imaging, the units could be leased, and the radiologists turned to the "easier and surer" method. The myriad artifacts, unexplainable to the neophyte, led to large numbers of

TABLE 10–1. Reason for Biopsy of 407 Nonpalpable Carcinomas

Number	Abnormality
214	Calcifications not associated with a mass
59	Nonpalpable mass
34	Altered architecture
16	Paget's syndrome
20	Vague changes: altered architecture, asymmetry

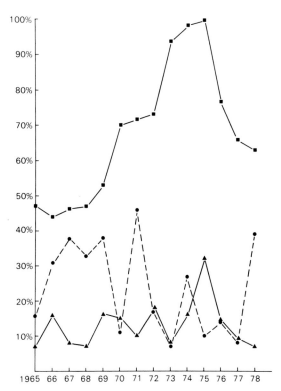

Figure 10–4. Annual new mammography patients at the Winship Clinic, the oncologic clinic of Emory University (■—■); per cent of biopsies for calcifications not associated with a breast mass that were malignant (●--●); per cent of total patients (graph expanded 10 ×) having specimen radiography for calcifications only (▲—▲).

breast biopsies with only normal tissues demonstrated. Screen-film mammography during this early phase of its use also contributed to the problems of the unwary radiologists.

After the 1976–1977 radiation scare there was a sudden and drastic drop-off in patients, with an unusually low ebb in biopsies for calcifications only but with a high percentage of these biopsies being malignant. This paralleled the period in which all seasoned mammographers noted a rapid increase in the size of cancers demonstrated by mammography.

These two events clearly demonstrate that women readily respond to sensitive issues that involve them: the female breast and cancer. Just as definite is their response, either positively or negatively, when the news media place them in a position of jurors regardless of their basis for scientific decisions.

OBSERVATIONS

If the routine described earlier is not adhered to in nonpalpable lesions and an attempt is made to localize the mammographically suspicious area by palpation, the proper area may not be removed by the surgeon. In such instances it may not be discovered until a repeat mammogram is done after a long delay; meanwhile, a false sense of security is experienced by the patient and surgeon. If palpation of the specimen by the pathologist renders a benign diagnosis, the suspicious area may be discarded, the true nature of the disease never being known unless cancer recurs in the area of biopsy.

Such efforts are justified, inasmuch as very early lesions are being demonstrated. There is limited local invasiveness with these lesions, and rarely is there spread beyond the breast. The surgeon is more confident that he is carrying out proper treatment, and the pathologist renders a more reliable opinion. Such demonstrations by mammography of cancers so small that they are nonpalpable in a 3 mm slice are stimulating physicians to cooperate in learning more about breast cancer, to the benefit of the patient.

A marked increase in the number of calcific deposits on the specimen radiograph as compared with the number of calcifications in the mammograms indicates that the lesion is almost certainly cancer. For a time the author thought that such observations could lead to the x-ray technologist's being a part of a quicker "frozen-section" process by radiography. But this proved unreliable.

Precise localization from the mammograms of the proper tissue to be removed by the surgeon is readily accomplished, and usually only one biopsy attempt is required. The surgeon must know how the patient was positioned for mammography, as there may be considerable variation from this position and the position during surgery. Visualizing change in the breast position (from mammography to biopsy) is superior to attempting localization by various metallic markers or gadgets. The nipple is the best landmark. The anteroposterior thickness of the breast in position for biopsy is markedly reduced. There are various degrees of movement of the breast on the chest wall with change in position; more importantly, there is marked variation in the way and degree that the breast moves in relation to the thorax. The pendulous, soft, and atrophic breast flows about markedly as opposed to the small firm breast.

Usually lesions lateral to the nipple tend to move farther laterally than would be expected; if the first biopsy is unsuccessful, the probability of a more successful section would be greater laterally. Conversely, lesions medial to the nipple do not tend to move as far laterally in relationship to the nipple. Lesions superior or inferior to the nipple tend to maintain that relative distance. As to depth, there is little correlation with the two positions; the only sure way is to approach the posterior capsule, but not penetrate it, and take tissue anterior to it.

Mammograms are indicated for all patients with breast complaints and/or positive physical findings. This obviously select group of patients represents a rich source of occult breast cancers. Using mammography in this manner, approximately 10 to 20 per cent of breast cancers coming to surgery are biopsied on the basis of mammographic findings. X-ray findings will influence the decision to biopsy without delay in an unknown additional number of patients—as many as 40 per cent additional cases with screening.

There are many good reasons for doing mammography in patients for whom a biopsy is indicated on clinical findings. Mammography is a valuable adjunctive diagnostic aid in breast diseases; the combined accuracy of clinical judgment and mammographic findings is over 95 per cent. This helps in scheduling the operating room and in selecting the type of anesthesia and surgical draping. Patients with a clinically suspicious mass are a fertile group for nonpalpable carcinomas, both in the opposite breast and in the same breast as the suspect lesion. Treatment planning is much improved with some knowledge of what lies in the other seven quadrants in which no biopsy is planned. A very important baseline study is established for follow-up studies of both breasts if benign, or of the remaining breast should the lesion be cancer.

Mammography has been most rewarding when a nonpalpable cancer is demonstrated that would otherwise have been missed on clinical examination.

At least 15 per cent of patients with one breast cancer have or will develop a cancer in the opposite breast, and well over 75 per cent of the second cancers will be second primaries. The second primary would probably be of such biologic nature (similar to the first primary that has allowed the patient to live long enough to develop the second breast cancer) that an excellent prognosis is expected. Mammography is proving of extreme importance in early diagnosis and mandatory vigorous treatment of the second breast. It is our only efficient means of differentiating metastatic from primary cancer of the opposite breast, so important in institution of proper treatment of the second breast.

The policy of biopsying suggestive nodules, whether elicited by palpation alone, by mammography alone, or by both, will lead to a larger number of biopsies. However, it also leads to the discovery of a larger number of cancers in the early course of their development. At Emory University, tabulation of three 5-year periods showed the ratio of malignant to benign biopsies of breast lesions to be 38, 35, and 35 per cent. During the last five-year period in which mammography was used extensively there was a definite increase in breast biopsies, but the ratio of malignant to benign remained unchanged.

Prior to mammography our incidence of bilateral simultaneous primary breast carcinomas at Emory University was less than 0.3 per cent as compared with 3 per cent during a five-year period when mammography was used. In another series of 728 patients with breast cancers having mammography and also having a 3 per cent incidence of bilateral simultaneous primary breast cancers, the presence of 18 of 21 simultaneous second primary breast cancers was unsuspected clinically but unequivocally demonstrated by mammography. Eleven of 28 successive bilateral cancers were detected by mammography on 278 patients who had had a previous radical mastectomy for proven breast cancer 1 month to 16 years previously.

Equipment for breast specimen radiography is being developed as the demand for the procedure increases. Prior to 1964, the ordinary x-ray machine for mammography was reduced to its lowest kvp, necessary mas, finest grain film, shortest object-film distance, and best collimation; controlled hand processing was required. At that time, in redesigning our x-ray unit for precise output we incorporated kvp as low as 10 kvp for specimen radiography. Historadiography required building a unit to produce 6 kvp. Radiography at lower kilovoltages would require the additional burden of a vacuum. We found our rebuilt x-ray unit with beryllium window, and removal of all added filter gave excellent specimen radiographs, with the special unit reserved for particular uses. There are now available commercial x-ray units for specimen radiography that are much more economical than the redesigning of an x-ray unit to be used for routine mammography.

These relatively inexpensive 6 to 20 kvp x-ray units may be used routinely for radiography of breast biopsy specimens, conveniently in the pathology laboratory. The units are plugged into ordinary 110 volt electrical outlets, are self-contained, and are properly protected. Their low milliamperage does require prolonged exposures and additional time for processing depending on the physical arrangement of the radiology and pathology sections. Grossly obvious cancers and certain typically benign lesions need not be radiographed prior to frozen-section study. However, all pieces of the tissue from a noncancerous biopsy should be radiographed before or after frozen-section study. An estimated 1 to 5 per cent additional cancerous or precancerous lesions will be thus identified for treatment at an extremely early stage or earmarked for close follow-up study.

The radiographic detail is so fine that both the pathologist and the radiologist will have a much clearer conception of the minute, but gross, three-dimensional manifestations of breast lesions. More and more teams will require such studies as mammography uncovers an increasing number of smaller breast cancers.

This added burden on radiology-pathology colleagues seems justified as a cooperative effort for the patient's welfare. Actually, breast specimen radiography provides the all important additional dimension to pathologic study of breast lesions just as mammography has added the third dimension to the clinical examination of the breast.

POINTS TO BE SOLVED

Is the cluster seen on both views for localization? Can it be identified as the same group by number, size, density, and configuration?

Is the cluster at nearly the same relative depth within the breast, so that one is not seeing one cluster on one view and another cluster on another view?

Is the cluster seen on the mediolateral view but not on the craniocaudal view? Is a coned-down or spot view needed? Should the view be repeated with the breast rotated medially? Laterally? Or both? Is an angled craniocaudad view needed?

Is the cluster seen on the craniocaudad view but not (not sure) on the mediolateral view? Is a coned-down or spot view needed? A lateromedial view?

Are the calcifications real and not artifacts? Are they on the skin as in a nevus or in an ointment or powder? Then can the cluster be sketched and measured out on a drawing of both the craniocaudad and the mediolateral view, so that the radiologist can confidently recommend biopsy and specimen radiography without confusion, unnecessary expense, and trauma?

ALTERNATIVE LOCALIZATION METHODS

Since the use of mammography is increasing and specimen localization and radiography are mandatory for proper removal and precise histologic examination of the mammographically suspicious area in the breast, many means and devices are being used for that purpose. Greater alterations in relationship of structures in the breast under severe compression when compared with positioning on the operating table make exact localization of an area of greater necessity. There is also a tendency to reduce breast deformity by removal of less breast tissue as a biopsy specimen.

NONINVASIVE LOCALIZATION

Several noninvasive techniques for localization of mammographically suspicious areas include: direct measurements in relation to the nipple (Egan, 1962); coordinates plotted on a diagram (Berger et al., 1966); stereo-mammography (Price and Butler, 1971); grid devices with compression (Muhlow, 1974); markers taped to the skin (Malone et al., 1975); and stereotaxis (Bolmgren et al., 1977).

INVASIVE LOCALIZATION

Invasive localization techniques include: needle insertion, adjustment dye injection (Egan, 1962); use of two needles (Simon et al., 1972; Libshitz et al., 1976); inserted needle taped to skin of breast (Threatt et al., 1974); self-retaining curved-tip wire (Frank et al., 1976).

Variations include position of patient,

amount of dye, type of dye, and interval to surgery. These variations are almost as numerous as radiologists doing the localizations.

CASE HISTORY

A 34-year-old woman was seen for routine follow-up. She was gravida 3, para 3, had nursed for a total of nine months, and had no family history of breast cancer. The left breast had been removed two years before for intraductal comedo- and microinvasive comedocarcinoma. The 17 axillary lymph nodes

found in the modified radical mastectomy were free of tumor.

Two previous mammograms of the right breast showed three faint calcifications in the same area, insufficient for biopsy because they were few and there had been no interval change. During the year prior to the present mammogram the calcifications became denser and more numerous (Fig. 10–5). There were also definite changes on breast sonography despite the changes of only intraductal carcinoma.

There was only one deposit of carcinoma in each breast, and each modified radical mastectomy contained 17 normal lymph nodes. Both breasts contained atypical ductal hyperplasia and focal papillomatosis.

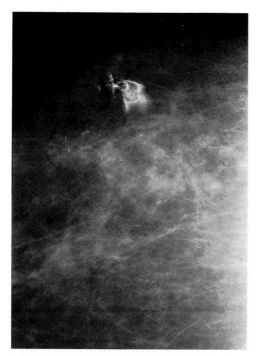

Figure 10–5. Comedocarcinoma calcifications that appear benign. Localization and biopsy: intraductal comedo carcinoma. Modified radical mastectomy, all 19 axillary lymph nodes free of tumor. The patient was free of disease two years later.

REFERENCES

Berger SM, Curcio BM, Gershon-Cohen J, Isard HJ (1966): Mammographic localization of unsuspected breast cancer. AJR 96:1046.

Bolmgren J, Jacobson B, Nordenstrom B (1977): Stereotaxic instrument for needle biopsy of the mamma. AJR 129:121.

Egan RL (1962): Fifty-three cases of carcinoma occult until mammography. Am J Roentgenol Radium Ther Nucl Med 88:1095.

Egan RL (1972): Mammography, 2nd ed. Springfield, IL, Charles C Thomas, p. 11.

Frank HA, Hall FM, Steer ML (1976): Preoperative localization of nonpalpable breast lesions demonstrated by mammography. N Engl J Med 295:259.

Libshitz HI, Feig SA, Fetouh S (1976): Needle localization of nonpalpable breast lesions. Radiology 121:557.

Malone LJ, Frankl G, Dorazio RA, Winkley JH (1975): Occult breast carcinomas detected by xeroradiography: clinical considerations. Ann Surg 181:133.

Muhlow A (1974): A device for precision needle biopsy of the breast at mammography. AJR 121:843.

Price JL, Butler PD (1971): Stereoscopic measurement in mammography. Br J Radiol 44:901.

Simon N, Lesnick GJ, Lorer WN, Bachman AL (1972): Roentgenographic localization of small lesions of the breast by the spot method. Surg Gynecol Obstet 134:572.

Threatt B, Appelman H, Dow R, O'Rourke T (1974): Percutaneous needle localization of clustered mammary microcalcifications prior to biopsy. AJR 121:839.

11

Correlated Clinical, Radiographic, and Pathologic Approach to the Study of Breast Diseases

BACKGROUND

The introduction of an adequate, safe, simple, accurate, and reproducible mammography technique in 1956 coincided with a controversial period in the history of breast cancer. There was a very high incidence of the disease, which is the most common cancer in the female, but a very low ten-year salvage rate despite improvement in extended surgery and high-voltage radiotherapy. Women were discovering 95 per cent of their breast cancers, yet the breasts were most accessible to clinical examination. Women were delaying seeking medical care owing to fear and lack of rapport with physicians; physicians were missing 25 per cent of these relatively advanced cancers on initial examination. There was no satisfactory classification of breast diseases by the pathologists despite voluminous literature on the subject. There was no uniformity in definitive or palliative treatment of the disease despite many available modalities. There was lack of knowledge of the natural history of breast cancer even though it had been recognized for centuries and had provoked much controversy. There was a minimum of rapport between the patient, the referring physician, the surgeon, the radiologist, and the pathologist despite the intimate involvement of each specialty.

In our busy tumor institution (M.D. Anderson Hospital) there was a very brief period of lack of interest following the introduction of mammography. But surgeons became keenly interested with the appearance of histopathologic diagnoses from the mammograms on the patients' charts prior to biopsy. They soon developed enough confidence to explore suspicious areas of the clinically normal breast on mammograms, which often proved to be cancers. Indeed, they were so anxious to find possibly curable breast cancer that they insisted upon my pointing out smaller and smaller lesions, fewer and fewer calcifications, and more minor breast architectural changes. This period of mutual learning and planning by the radiologist and surgeon and adaptation of radiographic procedures to breast problems was so intense that mammography passed rapidly through the stage of an x-ray laboratory procedure into a valuable routine adjunctive diagnostic procedure in patients with breast diseases.

At the end of one year of his surveillance of our work at M.D. Anderson Hospital and Tumor Institution, Lewis C. Robbins, M.D., Chief, Cancer Control Program, PHS, US DHEW, reported (1962):

We discussed the development of Egan's mammography technique with the whole team that made the breakthrough possible: the surgeons; the pathologists; the statistician who collected and analyzed the results; and the director under whose administration the study was conducted. We soon learned to respect the scientific integrity of Dr. Egan whose results are evidence of a real and tangible breakthrough.

The pathologists soon appreciated that their problems in localization and diagnosis of breast lesions were reduced when the tissues were reviewed in conjunction with the mammogram. With an unusually high accuracy of mammographic diagnosis of breast cancer, the pathologist was concerned when there was not histopathologic confirmation. As he then began studying the tissue more carefully and sought help from the radiologist, much routine breast tissue radiography followed. Very early in the clinical application of mammography it became apparent that the radiologist, surgeon, and pathologist must diagnose breast diseases as a team. Mammography was not a substitute for physical examination; the two were complementary. Nor was either a substitute for biopsy and histopathologic study.

The mammograms could record all the clinical signs of breast cancer, except heat and color, and often prior to clinical appreciation. For the first time these mammograms provided excellent radiographic detail as a permanent and graphic reduction of the three dimensions into two, thus providing a unique study of the disease processes in relation to other intramammary structures as well as those structures surrounding the breast.

The indications for mammography soon extended to almost every decision to biopsy or not biopsy a breast lesion. This collaboration by the surgeon, pathologist, and radiologist (going unnoticed by other radiologists) provided four years of unhampered routine use of mammography in a tumor institution (Egan, 1960). Customs, tenets, and procedures changed drastically, and as a radiologist I had to be prepared to meet many challenges. Surgeons had become accustomed to expect and to accept histopathologic study only on what they felt and removed from the breast; the pathologists were poorly stimulated to search the remainder of the breast more carefully or extensively. Uncomfortable discrepancies between the shadows on the mammograms and the palpatory findings were not readily reconciled, particularly when "nonpalpable shadows" proved to be serious disease processes.

Methods had to be devised to locate and biopsy nonpalpable breast lesions, to correlate palpatory findings with x-ray and histology studies, and to learn more about the natural history of breast cancer for improved treatment and prognosis. Sharp disagreements were inevitable between the specialties on this uncharted frontier.

Radiography of breast tissue specimens proved rewarding in localizing lesions seen on the radiographs but overlooked by the pathologist on his routine breast studies. The radiographic and microscopic findings of breast calcifications were widely discrepant until the pathologist realized that many calcific particles were being shattered by the microtome or dissolved in acid fixation or stains.

These slowly evolving attempts to avoid unfortunate errors in diagnosis of breast cancer led to the realization that the most satisfactory approach to the study of breast diseases was through team effort of surgeon, radiologist, and pathologist. Each could contribute facets of his specialty and stimulate the others in a more meticulous evaluation of disease processes in the breast. Thus began recognition of the necessity for correlated studies of breast tissues. Radiography of these breast specimens, both biopsy and complete or partial mastectomy, proved most useful, particularly in the following situations:

1. To determine if the proper area of the breast has been removed by the surgeon in his biopsy.

2. To ensure that the proper area of the biopsy specimen is studied by the pathologist.

3. To provide a means of improving mammography technique as a precise approach to more graphic recording of the changes of breast disease that must be eventually captured in the mammogram of the intact breast.

4. To provide finer detail on the radiographs so that earlier changes of breast diseases can be understood and searched for in diagnosis by mammography.

5. To provide additional diagnostic criteria for a more detailed study of the characteristics of breast lesions, and to investigate such findings as increased calcifications seen in a biopsy specimen, as compared with the intact breast, which are more apt to be cancer.

6. To allow the surgeon a dramatically graphic sense of the character of his clinical findings.

7. To give the pathologist further depth in the understanding of the gross and micro-

scopic changes of breast diseases in three dimensions.

8. To provide the pathologist with rapid and inexpensive "whole-organ study" of the breast (Fig. 11–1 to 11–3).

METHODS OF STUDY

The whole-breast study approach has the real advantage of combining the interest and special inclination of the various specialties of radiology, surgery, and pathology both in investigation and in evaluation of minute gross and microscopic changes of the breast. Also, radiographic pathologic techniques not only are the most rapid and economical approach to whole-organ study but also are the only true whole-organ study of the breast.

Careful study of the slicer radiographs can eliminate much tissue for study, such as complete fatty areas; eliminate the whole-slicer histologic mounts as the method of search of abnormalities; and allow precise selection of any and all areas for microscopic study. Many of these areas can be studied with small blocks that are more easily mounted, and more satisfactory preparations can be made. The greatest advantage is that radiography of the specimen allows complete study of the whole organ; many times with reliance on only the slide preparations of the whole organs, areas of interest may be discarded. Even if one attempted the impossible task of mounting all the breast for histologic preparations, much of the tissue would be lost in squaring up blocks for the microtome and only a small percentage of attempted slices would be cut and suitably mounted for staining and study. With such an approach, subserial sectioning is usually resorted to and often confined to areas that had some palpable abnormality in the intact breast. Furthermore, the task of physically handling, studying, and storing the preparations of a whole breast would be enormous.

Pathologists who have had the opportunity to review or work with us on our present radiographic-microscopic whole-organ study feel that it is a more complete approach, is more productive, is more readily accomplished, and is less expensive. Several pathologists have spent time with us observing this unique approach to the study of breast diseases and have adopted the procedure in their institutions.

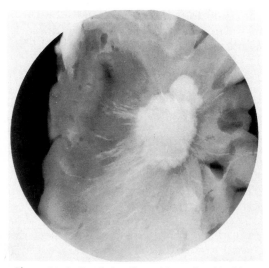

Figure 11–1. Detailed radiographic study of highly invasive breast carcinoma, infiltrating intracystic papillary carcinoma. The 4 to 5 mm thick slices of breast tissue allow use of shorter object-film distance, lower kvp, longer exposure time, finger grain film, and better collimation. Excess breast tissue is not superimposed so that finer radiographic detail is obtained for more precise evaluation of breast changes.

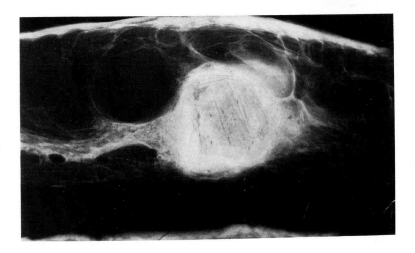

Figure 11–2. Five mm slicer section of the breast in Figure 11–1 showing another intracystic papillary carcinoma (noninvasive). Blood within the cystic portion is still frozen. Note smooth borders.

SOURCE OF MATERIAL

Traditionally, an incision or excision biopsy of a breast lesion has been followed by a frozen-section diagnosis of cancer prior to radical mastectomy. Post-mortem material was procured haphazardly, frequently was not fresh, was usually a limited subcutaneous mastectomy, had little bearing on the study

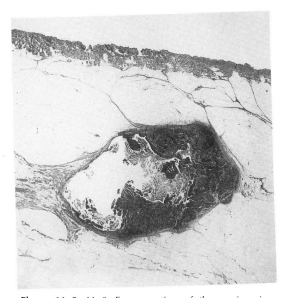

Figure 11–3. H & E preparation of the noninvasive intracystic papillary carcinoma. The blood has run out, leaving the papillary carcinoma within the thick wall. Thus, the radiographic and sonographic characteristics of these lesions are readily appreciated. Often these lesions are large; the pathologist cannot study the entire periphery microscopically and relies upon the radiologist to pinpoint the area of peripheral invasion. The fine calcifications of these lesions are usually obscured on the mammograms by the radiographically dense blood in the lesion.

at hand, and offered absolutely no information as to the future progression of the breast disease or the patient's response to the disease.

For the best radiographic studies, the specimen, whether biopsy or simple or radical mastectomy, should be intact. Partial slicing or cutting into the specimen produces air pockets and distortion of the tissues so that worthwhile radiography is almost impossible. Intact breast specimens usually are obtained following needle biopsy and diagnosis; positive axillary lymph node diagnosis with positive clinical and x-ray findings in the breast and an occasional true occult breast cancer; strong clinical and x-ray findings in the breast, especially in surgically poor-risk patients; and on some occasions simple mastectomy, prophylactic and/or diagnostic, following a radical mastectomy for cancer or prior to prosthetic implant of the breast.

PROCESSING WHOLE-ORGAN SLICES

A few days prior to mastectomy, the surgeon alerts the mammography section that a whole breast will be available for study. The mammography pathologist then receives the mastectomy specimen directly from surgery (Fig. 11–4).

The axillary nodes are dissected from the radical mastectomy specimen for routine histopathologic study so that the patient can be told in a few days whether or not radiation therapy will be given. The otherwise intact specimen is then chilled and lightly frozen overnight, being placed in the freezer compartment of the icebox at −10°C. Usually 24

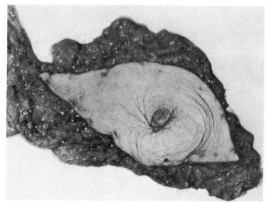

Figure 11–4. Radical mastectomy specimen of a large breast prior to removal of the axillary lymph node area. This breast contained a moderately advanced clinical and radiographic cancer that produced some retraction of the skin near the nipple.

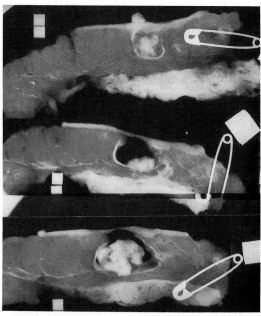

Figure 11–5. Original approach to whole-organ study of breast included chilling, slicing with hand-held knife, and identification by numbered lead strips pinned to each slice. Noninvasive portion of an intracystic papillary carcinoma. The old liquid blood has oozed out, leaving the central mass enclosed in the thick-walled cyst.

hours of chilling is the only preparation needed prior to slicing the mastectomy specimen. Keeping the specimen over the weekend in the freezer compartment is satisfactory. It is easily sliced, is easily handled, and maintains its natural color for photography and mounting of suitable slices in clear plastic. The specimen prior to chilling can be placed with the nipple downward in a funnel-shaped plastic container. The breast will then be frozen in a more normal shape and the slices will correspond more closely to the mediolateral mammogram. By thus preventing the breast from flowing over a large area prior to freezing, almost all the fibroglandular tissue can be placed on a 3¼ × 4 inch piece of glass (lantern slide size).

The breast is then sliced in the vertical plane (beginning medially and progressing laterally) into 0.5 cm thick slices, initially with a knife (Fig. 11–5) and then with a large commercial meat slicer (Fig. 11–6). A smooth sharp blade is used, not one with a serrated edge. The slicer sections are carefully laid out in numerical order on sheets of clear plastic and are identified with number tags that are visible on both photographs and radiographs (Figs. 11–7 and 11–8). An average of 25 slices are obtained from each breast. Some specimens may produce over 50 slices. Even by placement of the 5 mm slices on the sheets of plastic and not disturbing them until time of placement in a tissue fixative, the fat of the breast warms and the slices flatten out to a 4 mm thickness; handling the slices causes more thinning and produces air spaces and distortion of the structures.

Identification of each specimen radiographed is essential. The small specimens can be placed on the clear film with a small lead numeral alongside each, with the patient's number and date included. The large slices of radical mastectomy specimens may be identified with numerals punched in small

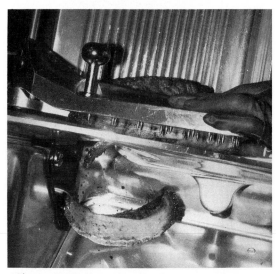

Figure 11–6. Close-up view of mastectomy specimen being sliced on heavy-duty commercial meat slicer.

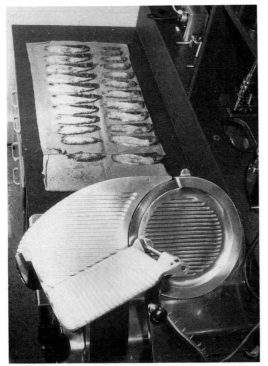

Figure 11–7. Another view of commercial meat slicer used in whole-organ breast studies. The 0.5 mm thick slices (in this case totaling 23) are carefully laid out in neat order following slicing.

lead sheets that are attached to the slices with safety pins; these can be read both on the color photographs and on the radiograph of the specimen (Fig. 11–5). We prefer an alternative identification system of punching numerals in plastic, also easily seen in the photograph or in these low kvp radiographs (Fig. 11–8). The slices for radiography are grouped in two, three, or four, which conveniently fit on one half of the 8 × 10 inch films (Fig. 11–9). The slices are then radiographed, photographed in color (Fig. 11–10), and fixed for subsequent mounting in paraffin blocks and cutting for histologic study either as whole slicer mounts or as various-sized, selected areas of interest.

A representative slice, without fixation or staining, is mounted intact in natural color in clear plastic. These preparations are thin enough for study by transillumination yet thick enough to impart the all important aspect of tridimensional display of breast tissue. The natural color of the various tissues is maintained in this plastic without deterioration over long periods of time.

RADIOGRAPHIC TECHNIQUE FOR BREAST SPECIMENS

Enumeration of precise x-ray factors is difficult, since there are ranges of thickness of the part to be radiographed, various-sized areas to be covered by the cone, and marked differences of output of various x-ray units. Some guidelines can be presented, but each mammographer must experiment with his x-

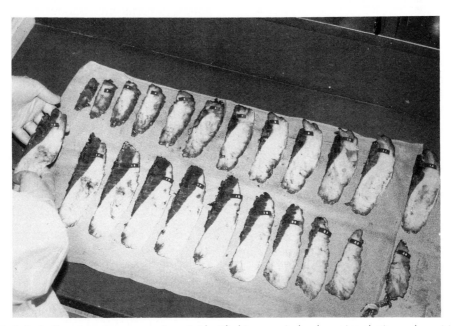

Figure 11–8. Each slice of mastectomy specimen is identified in numerical order, using plastic numbers visible both in the photograph and in the radiograph slices.

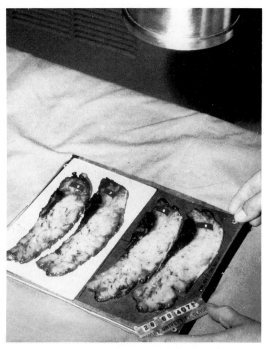

Figure 11–9. Radiographs of mastectomy slicer sections are obtained by triple loading of film. Usually only the number of slices fitting on one-half the 8 × 10 inch cardboard holder are radiographed at one time. The slices are placed on cleared x-ray film prior to study for ease in handling and prevention of distortion.

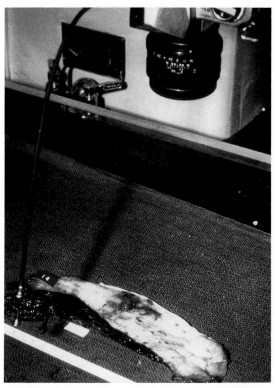

Figure 11–10. One set of radiographs of slicer sections is viewed wet for technical quality. Some indication of the specimens most likely to be interesting has been gained; these are then photographed in color while still intact.

ray unit for precise techniques; often a trial exposure must be made, the result inspected, and factors weighed accordingly. For best results, close film holder contact can be obtained by placing the specimen on a cleared sheet of x-ray film, which is also useful in handling the specimen without disturbing the relationship to markers and the protection of the film holder.

Maximum collimation is used: A 4 inch area could be covered with the cylinder cone fully extended using a 22 inch target-film distance; a 10 inch area would require the cylinder cone not extended and a 40 inch target-film distance; intermediate areas would require coning and target-film distances varied accordingly. The minimum possible filtration of the beam is used; the beryllium window tube offers a definite advantage with practically no filtration of the x-ray beam. With this degree of collimation and filtration, the lowest kvp possible is used for penetration and is compensated by mas— usually one-half the mas required for routine mammography.

Triple loading the x-ray film holder with extremely fine-grain film provides a radio-

graph for the pathologist, the patient file jacket, and the specimen film jacket. Unlike double loading in routine mammography, there will be differences in density of the three films. After the specimen radiographs are dried they are jointly reviewed by the radiologist and the pathologist for selection of study material, which includes representative slices for whole-organ routine hematoxylin and eosin stains; whole-organ or localized areas for calcification stains; whole-organ slices through the nipple, the tumor, or other interesting areas; more limited tissue for mounting; and numerous small sections for detailed microscopic study (Fig. 11–11).

PHOTOGRAPHY

Photography of each slice is carried out immediately after inspection of one set of the specimen radiographs for radiographic quality. A mounted 35 mm camera with prearranged floodlights is used to make color transparencies. Several slices may be in-

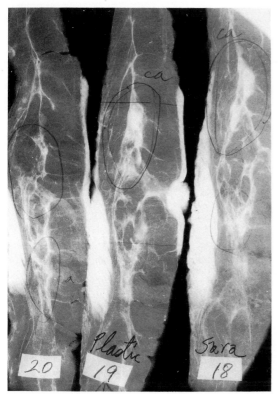

Figure 11–11. After specimen radiographs are dried, the radiologist and pathologist review them, mark areas for microscopic study, select specimen for plastic mounting, and plan overall study of specimen. The encircled areas, above, were two separate foci of infiltrating duct carcinoma.

cluded in one photograph, or a close-up of only a portion of one slice may be made. Usually only one side of the slices is photographed and in the same relationship as on the radiographs for future correlation.

An alternative approach is chilling the breast, slicing, and photographing followed by routine fixing of the slices by the pathologist prior to radiography. The slices for plastic mounting do lose their natural colors with this method.

HISTOLOGIC PREPARATIONS

Whole-organ mounts of the breast have been used variously in the past for the histopathologic study of diseases of the breast. The techniques varied because of the technical problems involved in the fixation and cutting of the specimens; the results were often not comparable and of limited value. In spite of these problems, study of properly prepared whole-mount sections of breast is

needed for the correlative histopathologic and mammographic study of breast diseases, since mammography has become a major adjunctive procedure in the early detection of cancer of the breast.

Primarily we study adjacent cuts of sections of whole breasts that are stained with the hematoxylin and eosin technique and with a modified von Kossa technique. The large sections are cut on a sliding microtome, directly mounted on 3¼ × 4 inch lantern slides (Fig. 11–12), and viewed under the microscope or used for projection on a large screen. Occasionally, whole-slice sections may require a larger glass slide for mounting.

All routine slices are cut 6 to 7 μ thick regardless of the size of the mount. Technically these are much more difficult to handle and mount, but they are far superior for light microscopy. Display sections may be cut as thick as 12 to 20 μ, but these are poor for microscopic study.

Following photography the breast slices are taken to the special mammography-pathology laboratory. The slice for plastic mounting is set aside, and certain routine sections are selected (from the wet radiographs and visual inspection of the gross material) for diagnostic purposes as well as the sections to be processed by the whole-organ mount technique.

Fixation, Embedding, and Staining

1. Place the slices for whole mount in 10 per cent formalin solution for two to three days, depending on the size of the specimen.

2. Transfer into 80 per cent alcohol and leave overnight.

3. Transfer into 95 per cent alcohol for three to four days, depending on the size of the specimen, changing the 95 per cent alcohol solution once each day.

4. Transfer into 100 per cent alcohol for two days (48 hours), changing the 100 per cent alcohol once each day.

5. Transfer into xylol; change xylol each day, until the slice becomes transparent and only the calcified areas and/or the tumor stay white and opaque. This requires one to two days, depending on the size of the specimen slice.

6. Xylol must be completely clear when the specimen slice is first put in. If the xylol turns white or cloudy, the specimen slice has to be taken back to Step 3 and left one more day in 95 per cent alcohol solution. Then continue with steps as outlined.

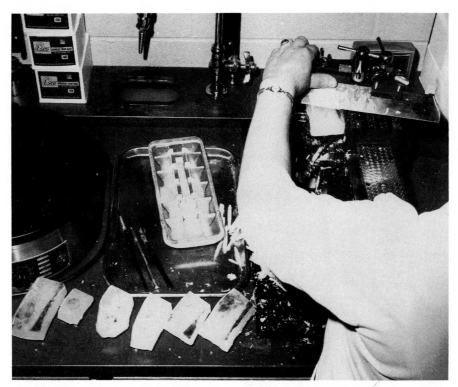

Figure 11–12. Large microtome used in preparation of whole-breast organ histopathologic studies. Also displayed are various sizes and shapes of tissues selected for microscopic study. Keeping these large knife blades sharp is a recurrent problem.

7. The specimen slice is now ready to be embedded in Paraplast. Since every specimen slice has a different shape and size, it is best to make your own embedding forms. Cardboard boxes can be used, the inside covered with glycerin. Fill with Paraplast and embed the tissue. It is very important that the tissue to be embedded is straight and flat. Use an embedding iron.

8. Cool, mount paraffin blocks on wooden blocks, and size $1 \times 1\frac{1}{2} \times \frac{3}{4}$ inch.

9. Cut sections on a large sliding microtome 6 to 7 μ thick (Fig. 11–12).

10. Float onto $3\frac{1}{4} \times 4$ inch lantern slides (available from any photo supplier—ESCO ground-edge coverglass, size $3\frac{1}{4} \times 4$ inch), and dry overnight in paraffin oven; take at least two slides for each area or depth to be studied, one for hematoxylin and eosin and one for von Kossa stain.

11. Cool, stain one slide with hematoxylin and eosin, and place coverslip (Figs. 11–13 and 11–14) (Roboz Surgical Instrument Co., Inc., 810 18th Street N.W., Washington, D.C., 20006. Coverglass thickness number 1, size 80×100.) Use 1000 ml beakers for all

staining procedures. Hang $3\frac{1}{4} \times 4$ inch lantern slides on hanger (Hanger No. 6, Kodak Sheet Film Developing Hanger).

Modified (von Kossa) Calcium Stain for Whole-Organ Mounts

The following specific steps are followed as a modification of the von Kossa stain for calcium in breast specimens, using the usual 7 μ thick tissue on the proper size glass mounts:

1. Xylol, 2 minutes each.
2. Xylol, 2 minutes each.
3. 100 per cent alcohol, 2 minutes each.
4. 100 per cent alcohol, 2 minutes each.
5. 95 per cent alcohol, 2 minutes each.
6. 95 per cent alcohol, 2 minutes each.
7. Distilled H_2O, 1 to 2 minutes.
8. 10 per cent silver nitrate solution, 15 minutes (save solution).
9. Distilled H_2O, rinse well, with constant agitation, 1 minute.
10. Distilled H_2O, rinse well, with constant agitation, 1 minute.
11. Film developer (Dektol, Kodak Developer), prepare as directed by manufacturer,

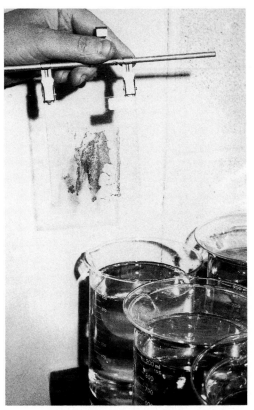

Figure 11-13. Medium-sized section of tissue mounted for staining. This single-slide holder is replaced by a specially designed plastic multiple-slide holder in staining large numbers of slides. Note the 1000 ml beakers that serve as containers for the solutions used in staining.

1 minute. The tissue will turn dark brown. Use freshly prepared solution only.

12. Distilled H_2O, rinse well, 2 minutes each.

13. Distilled H_2O, rinse well, 2 minutes each.

14. Hypo (Edwal, Quick-Fix, 1 gallon size, use undiluted). Prepare as directed by manufacturer, about 3 minutes. Use full strength until fatty tissue turns almost white; the nipple and skin will stay brown. Use freshly prepared solution only.

15. Water—several changes.

16. Distilled H_2O.

17. Nuclear fast red (Kernechtror), 1 minute. Dissolve 2 gm nuclear fast red powder in 1000 ml of 5 per cent aqueous aluminum sulfate solution with the aid of heat. Cool and filter. Add a crystal of thymol as preservative. Keep at room temperature.

18. Wash in tap water.

19. Dehydrate with two changes of 95 per cent alcohol, then 100 per cent alcohol, 2 minutes each.

20. Clear with two changes of xylol, 2 minutes each.

21. Mount with Permount.

Calcium salts stain consistently black, the nuclei orange, and the cytoplasm orange to yellow.

Preparation and Embedding Whole Breast Slices in Transparent Plastic

The following three steps are used to prepare the tissue:

1. Place fresh or fixed specimen into a 25 per cent glycerin-water solution for 24 hours.

2. Transfer specimen to a 50 per cent glycerin-water solution and allow it to remain until it sinks.

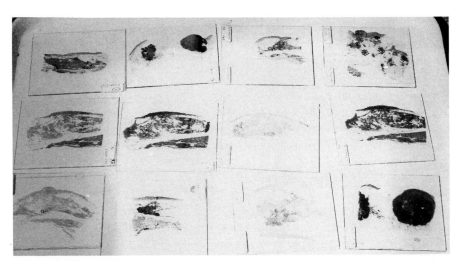

Figure 11-14. Appearance of various preparations as part of correlated radiographic-pathologic whole-organ study of a number of breasts. Black dots of India ink are frequently used to outline cancer in the specimen: upper right, numerous foci, lower left, a very tiny focus of carcinoma.

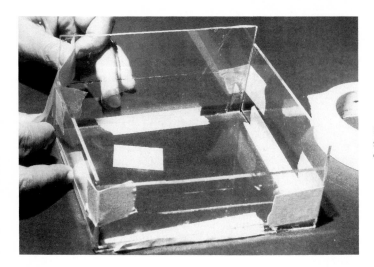

Figure 11–15. Assembled glass form used in plastic mounting of whole-organ breast slices; various sized embedding forms are commercially available.

3. Repeat Step 2 using a 75 per cent glycerin solution, followed by a 100 per cent solution, allowing specimen to remain in each solution until it sinks. Specimens may remain in 100 per cent glycerin until ready for embedding.

Forms for embedding the specimen in plastic are made from ordinary window glass. With a glass cutter, cut the base of the form according to the size of the specimen. Cut strips of glass 1 inch wide in proper lengths to form the four sides. Tape the sides to the base using Scotch masking tape to form an open tray (Fig. 11–15).

Embedding the specimen in the clear plastic is then carried out:

1. First pour a plastic base in a container and allow it to harden. Add 20 drops of catalyst to each 100 ml of plastic (Castolite Liquid Plastic with Hardener, The Castolite Co., Woodstock, IL 60098).

2. Take specimen out of 100 per cent glycerin, and place in acetone for 3 minutes. Pat specimen with paper towel until thoroughly dry.

3. Place specimen on hardened base of plastic, pour about ¼ inch of liquid plastic with catalyst over specimen. Allow to gel (almost hard), and test with glass rod.

4. Repeat Step 3 until specimen is fully embedded in plastic. There should be ¼ inch of plastic covering the specimen at the final pouring.

5. After the last layer has completely hard-

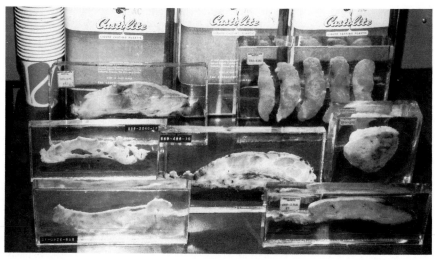

Figure 11–16. Several slices of breast mounted in clear plastic as part of a correlated clinical, radiographic, and pathologic study of the breast; note various sizes of mounts.

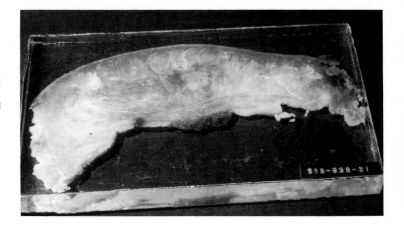

Figure 11–17. Close-up view of 0.5 cm slice of whole breast. This tissue, unfixed, retains its natural color and is thin enough for transillumination.

ened, place plastic block for 2 or 3 hours in paraffin oven to dry at 50 to 60°C.

6. Let cool at room temperature and remove from form (Figs. 11–16 and 11–17).

Display of Preparations

For demonstration of the correlation of the clinical, radiographic, and pathologic features of a breast lesion, breast histologic preparations, either hematoxylin and eosin or von Kossa stain, are mounted on one half of the 3¼ × 4 inch glass, the arrangement depending on the shape of the tissue preparation. On the other half may be mounted the actual radiograph of that particular section, or a photographic copy of the radiograph, or the corresponding colored transparency. A radiograph and colored transparency may be mounted side by side for projection and comparison. At times all three may be mounted on the same lantern slide for comparison.

For a more impressive display by transillumination, the whole-organ histologic preparations may be cut 20 μ thick and stained with hematoxylin and eosin. Series of subserial stained sections may be carefully piled in the order cut and transilluminated for a three-dimensional effect.

Historadiography and Calcifications

The more reliable method of demonstrating the tiny calcifications seen only with optimal lighting and a magnifying lens has proved to be contact radiography (placement of the thin breast specimens in close contact with the film holder containing a very fine-grain film emulsion). The calcifications that are visible under such conditions in radiographs of the specimen, even though very small, we consider to be macrocalcifications, in sharp distinction to those seen only on the stained sections under the microscope, which we consider to be microcalcifications.

To compare the calcifications seen on mammography with those seen by microscopy, a routine for historadiography has been developed. Specimens are radiographed for location of calcifications, microscopic sections are cut 5 to 10 μ thick, mounted on thin backing, and stained with a specially modified von Kossa stain. A 6 to 20 kvp x-ray machine was constructed to radiograph these stained sections. With the stained tissue (the calcium appears black) under the microscope, the location of the calcium is readily identified. Comparisons with routine histologic preparations—including whole-organ section mounts—are also done.

OBSERVATIONS

The only disadvantage of the technique of whole-mount preparations is the slightly longer preparation time required to achieve an adequate whole-organ mount. Whole-organ blocks, however, are more easily prepared and cut by this technique than by those previously described. The method permits the use of much larger blocks without tissue autolysis or shrinkage, makes cutting on a large sliding microtome much easier, and thus gives greater opportunity for more detailed study of breast diseases, especially for the correlative histopathologic studies with the mammography. The dehydration procedure described here is more efficient and yields tissue samples that stain more readily and more uniformly than after many other dehydration procedures we have tried. The improved dehydration procedure allows for more effective identification of abnormal cells and therefore enables more accurate diagnostic and statistical studies. Tissue sections stained by a modified von Kossa technique provide material suited to correlative studies of the histopathology of diseases of the breast, of the distribution of calcium deposits, and of the radiographic appearance of the calcium deposits.

Patterns of calcification in the breast can be more precisely studied. Some are almost pathognomonic of cancer, some are unquestionably benign in nature, and others are only suspiciously like cancer. Approximately one third of this last group will demonstrate proved cancer—some carcinoma in situ only, the remainder usually being severe ductal hyperplasia and/or adenosis. In this suspect cancer group there are four to ten faint, small, frequently rounded flecks of calcification in a cluster without an associated mass. There is no abnormality palpable in the biopsy specimen.

The most concerted approach to the study of breast lesions has changed some of our concepts of human breast cancer. Only 1 in 20 cases follows the usually described pattern of breast cancer of a primary mass with varying degrees of local extension with or without metastasis to the axillary lymph nodes. The carcinomas are usually multiple, are of different histologic types, and readily metastasize within the breast. Clearly defined noninvasive intraductal (in situ) carcinoma can be identified in almost every whole breast containing duct carcinoma. At times it is in close proximity with the area of invasive carcinoma, but at other times many distant areas of ductal hyperplasia noted on the radiograph of the slicer specimen must be studied to identify the in situ lesion. Many Stage I cancers require much closer study to be differentiated from in situ carcinoma.

EARLY BREAST CANCER

Definition

Early breast cancer is a nonspecific and relative term indicating the earliest recognizable phase of developing cancer.

Background

To reduce breast cancer mortality, the mammography radiologist constantly strives to bring the patient with breast cancer to earlier diagnosis and definitive treatment. On the mammograms there are certain changes that are merely variations of normal, but in a progressive manner these can be shown to proceed to proliferative epithelial changes, to metaplasia of these proliferative cells, to malignant cells still confined to the lumen of the ducts, and finally to frankly invasive cancer of the breast. Prior to the establishment of a mammographic technique with much improved radiographic detail, these changes were not often appreciated. Only occasionally was the possibility referred to in the breast by the pathologist, even though premalignant processes were strongly suspected in other parts of the body.

Cooperative studies of minute detail on the mammogram by the radiologist and corresponding areas on the histopathologic preparations by the pathologist have made possible recognition of these changes. By combined studies of many biopsy specimens, breast quadrant resection, simple mastectomy, intact breast or subcuticular mammary dissection, and radical mastectomy specimens, the pathologists have clearly shown progression of these glandular changes from normal to cancerous. Tissue preparations used for study include routine histopathologic studies, special stains, whole-specimen or whole-organ slicer sections singly and in serial sections, embedding of tissue in clear plastic for transillumination, and, very importantly, detailed radiography of the specimens. The ducts and glandular tissue can be clearly seen floating in fat in 3 to 5 mm slices that are embedded in clear plastic when transilluminated. Clearing of the adipose tissue by removal of its color also allows transillumination of thicker slices for anatomic studies of the breast structures.

The pathologist, as a member of the team concerned with the diagnosis and treatment of breast cancer, is impressed that the cancer now being studied is much smaller and has a marked reduction in the number of positive axillary lymph nodes. The pathologist now also freely uses the term "mammography breast cancer," i.e., one requiring both localization for surgical excision and biopsy specimen radiography for precise tissue selection for histopathologic study.

In certain cases there is some orderliness in progression of breast diseases to carcinomas, and in many instances it appears to be a prolonged process. Much work will be required to determine whether there is a point of irreversibility, and just what that point may be, so that treatment can be instituted at a much earlier stage of development. Ductal epithelial proliferation is at least potentially, and most likely actually, precancerous. Prognosis of a breast cancer that must be localized by radiography is much better than for the usual premammography 2 to 4 cm carcinomatous mass discovered by the woman in 95 per cent of the cases.

Detection

Discovery of a truly early breast cancer by means other than mammography is unusual. On rare occasions a small deposit of carcinoma has been found by the pathologist in breast tissue removed for a noncancerous process. I recall the considerable interest in demonstration of an unsuspected small duct carcinoma in breast tissue removed during excision biopsy of a fibroadenoma in one of the first breast surgical procedures in which I participated during the late 1940s. In our whole-organ studies many small breast cancers were demonstrated by light microscopy but usually as a result of study of an area abnormal on the radiograph of the slicer section.

However, review of these minute and subtle changes on radiographs of breast specimens re-emphasizes the necessity for mammograms of maximal detail. State-of-the-art mammograms of excellent quality are easily obtained. Under no circumstance should attempts be made to interpret those in which the quality of the examination has been sacrificed. Mammograms of poor technical quality are best not interpreted. Complementary imaging should never be attempted without first having optimal mammography.

The secondary mammographic signs of malignancy are those that are the direct result of an invasive mass. When these are present, the lesion cannot be considered early, even when nonpalpable. Primary signs may be associated either with a mass lesion or with early cancer. A most useful primary sign is the presence of calcification. Other breast diseases may be associated with discrete, punctate calcification, but the yield of carcinoma is proportionately high in patients in

whom the particles are numerous, irregular in shape, or clustered.

Other mammographic indications of early cancer are prominence of ducts, asymmetric dilatation of veins, and focal disturbances in the supportive tissue pattern. An increase in density or altered breast architecture in serial mammograms, especially in a postmenopausal patient, is a strong indication of the presence of cancer; cancers found in this way are usually early. Ductal hyperplasia, especially with a very fine nodular pattern on a fatty background, is a strong indicator of risk of breast cancer.

Mammographic vs Pathologic

The concepts of mammographically early cancer and histologically early cancer are not necessarily the same. Clustered calcifications may indicate the site of an invasive mass, which, because of general breast density, is mammographically invisible. A diffuse increase in density may result from widespread lymphatic permeation with numerous invasive nodules too small to detect; this usually produces a characteristic edematous appearance. Further study of mammography and the development of new criteria and improved techniques are vitally important; our whole-organ studies reveal innumerable mammographically invisible cancers.

To the pathologist, an early breast cancer is one that is confined to the tissue from which it is derived, such as noninvasive intraductal carcinoma and lobular carcinoma in situ. Differences in diagnostic criteria for these lesions still exist among pathologists but are smaller than differences in clinical importance of the two lesions. It is at this stage, before the breakdown of the ductal structure, that we wish to discover breast cancer regardless of the cell origin.

An occasional patient who has, upon histopathologic study, only noninvasive carcinoma will be found to have axillary metastasis. The evaluation by light microscopy of invasion in breast carcinoma is not entirely reliable. Histopathologic criteria for lethal Stage I and indolent Stage II carcinomas need elucidation.

Mammographic vs Clinical

For the clinician, whose concern is with the diagnosis of breast diseases and the responsibility for treatment, emphasis on early cancer has posed a whole set of new problems: (1) communication with and responsibility to his patients; (2) selection and utilization of modern diagnostic techniques; (3) diagnosis and treatment of a cancer that is not palpable; and (4) methods of location and removal of a lesion manifested only by a cluster of calcifications. Although the practice is not universal, many surgeons will no longer undertake breast biopsy without prior mammography. Even with tumors that are obvious on palpation, the additional information obtained is helpful in deciding on a course of therapy and in estimating prognosis. Furthermore, the initial study of the opposite breast serves as a baseline for follow-up.

BREAST RESPONSE TO CARCINOMA

Breast cancer evokes a multiplicity of tissue responses. Some of these produce specific changes on the mammograms and their meanings are clear-cut; others are less specific in their mammographic changes and their significance is less definite. The radiologist must be aware of all such tissue responses and recognize their alterations of the mammographic patterns.

Almost all breast cancers arise from duct epithelium. These epithelial cells of the ducts are capable of producing the many histologic types of breast cancer. At present we should not concern ourselves overwhelmingly with histologic types and grades of breast cancer, even though we are aware that certain types, such as mucinous and intracystic cancers, are less aggressive. Rather we should concentrate on size, growth pattern, types of tissue response, and extent of breast cancers.

Response of tissues to breast cancer observed by light microscopy and on the mammograms involves both parenchyma and supporting tissues: (1) ducts, (2) lobules, (3) intramammary connective tissue, (4) skin, (5) blood vessels, (6) lymphatics, (7) nipple, (8) probably nerves, (9) adipose tissue, and indirectly (10) immunochemical systems of the body. Our observations with their suggested significance can be accepted only for challenge. Time and expense has prevented whole-organ study of an equal number of "normal" breasts for comparison. Both breasts are under the same systemic and intrinsic influences so that the opposite breast is not a normal comparison. Further-

more, there is inherent selection of our present whole-organ material: (1) Breasts with advanced, inoperable disease are not studied; (2) very early lesions requiring specimen radiography for localization are often studied; (3) moderately advanced cancers that can be proved by needle biopsy or are clinically and by x-ray strongly suggestive of cancer are studied; and (4) the borderline dominant nodule requires excision and the whole breast is not studied.

Ductal Epithelium

The earliest change believed to be related to breast cancer is in the duct epithelium. The cells are increased in number, producing thickening of the layers of epithelial cells lining the ducts (see Chapter 16). Next is a varying degree of disorderliness of these cells accompanied by metaplasia and anaplasia of the cells. Then follows atypism of the cells, in situ or intraductal carcinoma, and finally invasive duct carcinoma.

Ductal epithelial proliferation led in two ways to our early histologic investigation of mammographic changes. A certain number of densities on the mammograms that were labeled calcifications were not proved microscopically. After introduction of mammography the pathologist did admit that there were many more breast calcifications than previously realized but at the same time proved that these faint densities confused with calcifications were ducts packed with hyperplastic epithelium seen on-end on the mammograms. In the second instance, prominence of the ducts produced a snowflake appearance on the mammogram that was so frequently associated with cancer that it was used as a secondary mammographic sign of cancer. Early histologic verification of this pattern was always ductal hyperplasia, a term used in our mammographic report. Not until whole-organ, slicer-section radiography was done, with each section studied without superimposed tissue, was it demonstrated that an identical mammographic pattern could be produced by periductal fibrosis. However, this secondary sign of cancer is just as valid in either instance.

One gets the impression that ductal epithelial hyperplasia or in situ carcinoma is more marked near sites of invasive duct cancer. This may be only because more studies are made of the cancerous sites, for ductal hyperplasia may be just as marked at great distances from the invasive lesion. Patterns of ductal hyperplasia (or in situ cancer) are varied: small, infrequent areas; entire ducts from the major ducts to the terminal ducts; alternately with normal epithelium along the same duct; or involving one or many lobules. At times the invasive carcinoma engulfs intraductal carcinoma.

Lobules

The lobules respond to cancer similarly to the ducts since they are composed of the more terminal ducts. It is convenient to think of a lobular response, as we do maintain a category of lobular in situ and lobular invasive carcinoma. The usual normal lobular patterns in the breast are poorly maintained after age 60.

Connective Tissue

The connective tissue of the breast anatomically is divided into intralobular and interlobular connective tissue. The former is periductal in location, responding as glandular tissue, and the latter is supportive. Such a definite physiologic division is not certain, since two types of fibrosis are recognized.

The periductal fibrosis occurs as a uniform but varying thickness or cuff about the ducts. Cellular structure of the fibrocytes usually can be recognized swirling about the ducts. This periductal fibrosis is extremely variable in location and degree. It may be more marked near the carcinoma or may be remote from it, about ducts containing in situ carcinoma or hyperplastic or even normal epithelium. As noted on the mammogram it may not be differentiated from ductal hyperplasia—a differential of no great significance in the mammographic diagnosis of breast cancer.

The other type of fibrosis, which we label collagenosis, occurs in a different location and has a different appearance. It is usually distributed uniformly throughout the breast, but it may be patchy and not necessarily associated with the ducts. On H & E it stains a lighter pink, has a homogeneous or wavy appearance, and is acellular. This may or may not be similar to the fibroplasia often seen with mastodynia in younger women who are below the age group at risk for cancer. It may also be only coincidental with the breast cancer.

Skin

Thickening of the skin can best be estimated in mammograms of the intact breast, especially if tangential to the x-ray beam. It is difficult to judge thickening of the skin on histopathologic preparations, as the skin has retracted and the cut may be at an angle (Figs. 11–2 and 11–3). Prior to mammography, thickened skin was seldom recognized unless there was actual invasion either by continuity of the tumor or via the lymphatics. Early skin thickening may not be recognized, but as the process advances varying amounts of collagen material appear just beneath the skin. Invasion of the skin lymphatics is a later stage.

Blood Vessels

A nonspecific response to breast cancer is increased vascularity, manifested most clearly on the mammograms by enlarged subcutaneous veins. Vessels near the cancer are seldom seen, since fat is needed to produce the necessary contrast. In a fatty breast, nearby enlarged veins may be seen. The increased vascularity perhaps represents some increased metabolic activity induced by the carcinoma; in these cases, thermography may indicate increased heat. Increased vascularity on the mammograms is considered a rather late sign of cancer.

Lymphatics

There are three generally recognized locations of the lymphatic systems of the breast: periductal, on the surface of the gland, and immediately subcutaneous. The three systems probably intercommunicate only in the subareolar region. The finding of metastatic carcinoma in a low axillary lymph node and only intraductal carcinoma on whole-organ study of the breast casts doubt on our ability to recognize lymphatics, ducts, and extraductal clumps of cancer cells. The basement membrane stain is unreliable; extraductal cancer cells could, in fact, produce a pseudomembrane, and a lymphatic packed with cells could resemble a duct containing intraductal carcinoma.

Dilated lymphatics, with or without cancer cells, may be recognized on the mammograms and verified histologically in the subdermal area.

Diffuse breast cancer occurs as (1) secondary deposits via the lymphatics from carcinoma of the other breast; (2) secondary deposits from a primary in the same breast via the periductal lymphatics; or (3) myriad primary foci of origin that spread along the ducts. Usually there is a combination of the several ways of occurrence. Thus the intramammary lymphatics play an important role in spread of carcinoma within the breast.

Nipple

Paget's disease of the breast is a syndrome of carcinoma of the breast, usually centrally located and ductal in type, with distinct morphologic changes of the epithelial cells of the summit of the nipple. The primary carcinoma in some instances is intraductal; usually the growth along the duct to the summit of the nipple can readily be demonstrated (see Chapter 25). In one of our cases, even with meticulous study, complete connection could not be demonstrated. The origin of the large pagetoid cells of the nipple is not known. These cells may be carcinoma cells or epithelial cells that have reacted to the presence of carcinoma. Similar-appearing pagetoid cells may at times be demonstrated within a duct carcinoma of the breast.

Nerves

In reviewing our breast history form, it was found that pain was an important symptom of breast cancer. Pain is a frequent complaint associated with many breast changes; it was the primary complaint in a significant number of our patients. We have not demonstrated any relationship with perineural lymphatic involvement.

Adipose Tissue

The adipose tissue of the breast may be invaded by carcinoma or replaced by carcinoma, but the only alteration noted is an edematous appearance on the mammograms with some extensive primary carcinomas or with metastatic carcinoma from the opposite breast.

Systemic Response

The systemic response to breast cancer is a highly speculative one. Our studies show that there may be no significant or massive increase in lymphocytes with a breast cancer. In one patient awaiting radical mastectomy, a discrete tumor mass regressed to one-half its size in six days. Whole-organ studies revealed almost complete liquefaction of the center of the tumor. There was no apparent alteration in blood supply.

Gynecomastia is another systemic response that, in some way, may be related to breast carcinoma or its etiology. Cancer in the male breast has been poorly studied, for it is an uncommon cancer. Relationship of breast carcinoma to gynecomastia is interesting, if purely speculative (see Chapter 15).

Growth Pattern

More and longer experience with mammographic growth patterns of breast cancers allows reliable categories for prognostication. In increasing aggressiveness these are (1) noninfiltrating, such as calcifications of the cancer type without a mass or dense smooth-bordered intracystic papillary lesions; (2) cir-

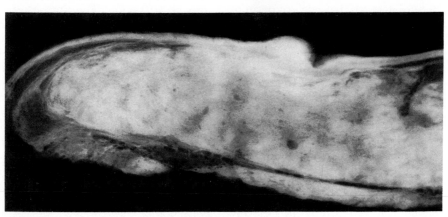

Figure 11–18. Fibroplasia. A 49-year-old woman with a self-discovered mass. There was a suspicious mass and calcifications bilaterally. Bilateral simultaneous primary intraductal carcinomas were demonstrated; all axillary lymph nodes were negative for tumor.

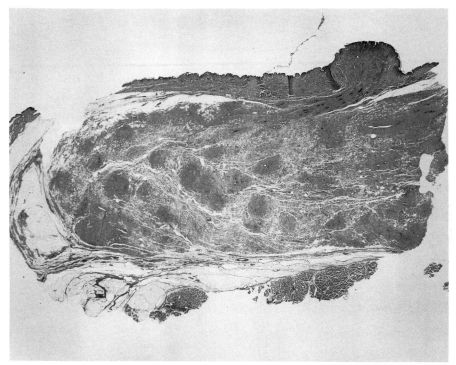

Figure 11–19. Representative whole-organ mount of both breasts shows fibrous discoid fibroglandular tissue, labeled fibroplasia. No tumor in this particular section.

Figure 11–20. Incomplete removal of the breast by a classic Halsted radical mastectomy. A 49-year-old woman with a suspicious clinical mass and positive mammogram. The operative procedure was performed by a highly competent oncologic breast surgeon.

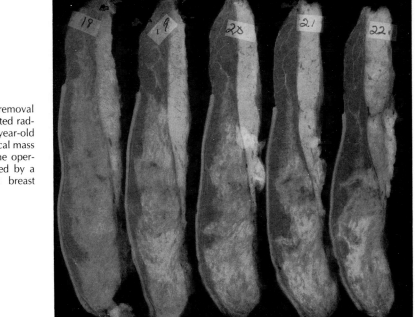

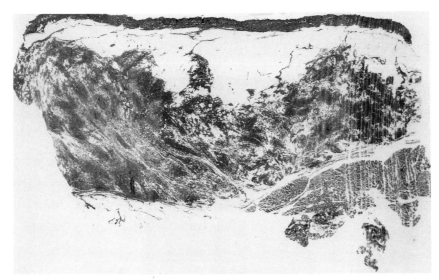

Figure 11–21. Whole mount of slicer section. Clearly illustrated is a cut through breast tissue. This was noted in slicer sections 13 through 27 of a total of 28 slices. If this much breast tissue can be left with a radical mastectomy, one wonders how much breast tissue is left following a simple mastectomy.

cumscribed, such as mucinous or medullary carcinoma with lymphoid stroma with only minimal peripheral reaction; (3) intermediate, between (2) and (4); and (4) infiltrative, as illustrated by the pathologist's category of scirrhous carcinoma.

The carcinomas studied by correlated whole-organ breast slices by radiography and light microscopy are not so readily categorized, especially the last three categories. Gallager, as pathologist, and Martin, as radiologist (1969), correlated mammograms with full-size tissue mounts of 47 breasts with infiltrative carcinoma and made tremendous contributions to this approach. They suggest the classification of (1) knobby, (2) stellate, and (3) spiculated. We recognize the patterns, but most of our cases are combined patterns that are not as neatly categorized as in Figure 11–1 and many other cases. Until some greater significance of subdivision is apparent, our four mammographic patterns will suffice.

OBSERVATIONS

With close and complete study, multiple sites of invasive carcinoma can be demonstrated in almost every breast with primary carcinoma. Also, in each case there is associated ductal hyperplasia and in situ carcinoma and in many instances similar lobular changes. Some of these changes are contiguous, and, in fact, carcinoma may surround ducts containing noninvasive cell types. Lob-

ular in situ carcinoma may be closely associated with intraductal carcinoma in the same duct system. Such close proximity can be considered a single focus. A single tumor with nearby intraductal carcinoma may have another area of carcinoma contiguous with the lymphatics and still be a single focus.

The whole-organ preparations are extremely useful in studying the background tissues in the breast, e.g., the predominant feature of fibrocystic disease (Figs. 11–18 and 11–19). The case illustrated was in the early part of our correlated studies and was unusual in that radical mastectomies were still occasionally being done for limited carcinomas.

The whole-organ correlated studies can precisely demonstrate the extent of the fibroglandular tissues of the breast. (Figs. 11–18 and 11–19). Peripherally, as it blends with the fatty tissues, the exact extent of the glandular tissues cannot be determined by palpation or inspection (Figs. 11–20 and 11–21). This case illustrates the wide anatomic extent of some breasts.

REFERENCES

Egan RL (1960): Experience with mammography in a tumor institution. Evaluation of 1,000 studies. Radiology 74:894.

Gallager HS, Martin JE (1969): The study of mammary carcinoma by correlated mammography and subserial whole organ sectioning: early observations. Cancer 23:855.

Robbins LC (1962): Purposes of the mammography reproducible study. Cancer Bull 14:102.

12

Clinical, Pathologic, and Radiographic Classification of Breast Diseases

INTRODUCTION

Simplicity of the classification of breast diseases must be maintained for the radiologist studying gross pathology. The radiologist must have some knowledge of the various physiologic processes, overgrowth patterns, diffuse fibrocystic diseases, adenosis, large cyst formations, fibroadenoma, and intraductal papillomatosis to understand the normal mammogram, normal variants, dominant benign lesions, or malignant lesions of the breast.

Despite considerable controversy among pathologists as to the exact terminology that should be applied to various disease processes in the breast, the radiologist should select a simple working classification of breast disease that encompasses the clinical findings, the surgical disease, gross and microscopic disorders, and the radiographic findings. Fortunately, a practical simplicity can be achieved by realizing that the important consideration in radiographic examination is whether an individual breast lump is carcinoma or benign disease. Radiographic diagnosis can be this exact. Our classification is not intended to be static. In practice, it has proved to be workable, concise, and acceptable to the radiologist, pathologist, and clinician. Changes in the classification are anticipated as experience is gained, and we hope that such changes will reflect advances in general understanding of the disease processes of the breast.

Prediction of histologic types of carcinoma of the breast by their mammographic appearance is not always possible. Carcinomas showing a marked infiltrative pattern on the mammograms usually are the scirrhous or mixed histologic types. The circumscribed pattern is more often produced by carcinoma simplex, medullary carcinoma with lymphoid stroma, and adenoid cystic, mucin-producing, or intracystic papillary carcinomas. The noninvasive intraductal carcinoma and lobular carcinoma in situ present less defined radiographic features. The rarer types, such as carcinoma with osseous or cartilaginous metaplasia, are recognized by the pathologist as distinct entities. The radiologic designations of massive, diffuse, and inflammatory apply to patterns of intramammary spread without attempt at histologic correlation; Paget's carcinoma is in a similar category in which nipple changes are noted radiographically.

Terms that are nonexpressive and confusing, such as "dysplasia" and "mastopathy," have been avoided. For the present it seems advantageous to avoid "dysplasia," a term sufficiently nonspecific to imply neither cause nor effect but only intermediate phenomena.

The noninvasive breast carcinomas include noninfiltrating intracystic papillary carcinoma, noninvasive intraductal or comedo carcinoma, lobular carcinoma in situ, and Paget's disease when the deep-seated primary breast carcinoma is noninvasive. These lesions may be readily demonstrated mammographically as a dense smooth cyst or as calcifications or altered arrangement of the fibroglandular tissues, but the noninvasive character cannot be predicted.

Similarly, precancerous breast lesions are not precisely diagnosed by mammography. In many instances there is close radiographic and histopathologic correlation of proliferative ductal epithelial hyperplasia into metaplasia, anaplasia, and atypism, followed by intraductal carcinoma in situ and invasive duct carcinoma. In some cases at least, there appears to be a natural history of breast cancer through a somewhat orderly progression over a long period of time through an irreversible stage into eventual carcinoma. Only since the use of mammography have pathologists been faced with early breast cancer; no one pathologist has gained enough experience with these changes to delineate clinical entities. Once these diagnostic criteria are defined, treatment of the precancerous lesions can be realistic with modalities already available.

"Medullary," meaning soft, is a term used by the pathologist for the gross appearance of soft, circumscribed carcinomas. It should be reserved for use only in this classification to indicate the specific type of cancer known as medullary carcinoma with lymphoid stroma. The softness of a lesion cannot be judged radiographically, as opacity to x-ray can only be estimated (a pure diamond is radiolucent).

Similarly, "scirrhous," meaning hard to the pathologist, should be avoided by the radiologist, as he cannot estimate the hardness of a lesion by mammography. This type of lesion is usually highly invasive by mammography.

Nonindigenous lesions of the breast, although they may have special features influenced by developmental and physiologic changes to which the breast is subject, are similar to lesions in other anatomic sites and include specific infections and benign and malignant neoplasms. Congenital anomalies and developmental variants also occur. Appropriate categories in the classification are necessary.

In contradistinction to these nonindigenous lesions are processes that arise specifically in breast tissue. Here the classifier is at once impeded by ignorance. There is simply no solid information regarding the specific causation of the various changes usually called fibrocystic disease. The difficulty is that fibrocystic disease lies in the "borderland of neoplasia," an area possibly less well understood than neoplasia itself.

Dilatation of the major ducts of the breast is a common radiographic appearance produced by intraductal papillomata, usually localized and easily recognized, or by retention of inspissated material in the ducts.

The diagnosis of breast diseases by mammography is based on alterations in the breast. However, as the radiograph of the breast is a three-dimensional permanent and graphic study of extremely fine macroscopic changes, the radiologist's opinion should contribute much to the evaluation of the breast along with the pathologist's gross and microscopic material and the clinician's physical examination. Amputation of the breast does cause anatomic distortion, and slicing of the surgical breast specimen is at times frustrating. The pathologist depends completely on the surgeon for selection of the amount and location of the tissue to be used as biopsy material. Although the breasts are most accessible to inspection and palpation, they present perplexing problems in evaluation of both the normal and the abnormal states.

Although only one organ system is recorded radiographically, the opportunity afforded for comparison with features of the opposite breast is invaluable. This contrasts with many other radiographic examinations such as that of the chest, which includes pulmonary, osseous, cardiovascular, muscular, and other soft tissue structures. Study of the breast can then quickly be made by the radiologist. Breast radiography can be adeptly performed by any radiologist once he becomes familiar with various normal and abnormal radiographic features. The period of self-training is not excessive; however, the ability to produce mammograms of good quality is sine qua non.

A single mammary duct epithelial cell has a unique propensity to produce protean clinical diseases of the breast; yet these epithelial cells are totally derived embryonically from the same invaginated ectodermal cells along the milk line.

A somewhat overlooked fact that affects the classification of breast diseases is that the breast tends to react as a whole to those diseases which are peculiar to it. Even those elements of breast that are generally regarded as supportive participate to some extent in function. An intraductal papilloma has a fibrous or myxoid stroma that keeps pace with the epithelial proliferation; carcinoma elicits varying degrees of fibrous response and lymphoid infiltration. Duct hyperplasia is a feature constantly associated with lobular carcinoma in situ. This concept of multiple tissue response is pertinent to an understanding of fibrocystic disease.

VARIATIONS IN HISTOPATHOLOGY OF BREAST DISEASES

The whole-organ, multiple tissue response is further complicated by wide variations in hormonal milieu and cyclic changes involving both the host and the breast.

Effect of Pregnancy and Lactation

Fairly uniform cyclic changes in the epithelium occur during pregnancy and lactation. The cells of the terminal ducts multiply and enlarge the end of the ducts during pregnancy in preparation for secretion of milk while lactating. Thus, one of the characteristics of an epithelial cell is uniformly producing acini and secreting milk. Even here aberrations occur, such as uncontrolled hypertrophy or failure to return to normal blunt ducts following cessation of lactation.

Cyclic Changes

Other cyclic changes occur in the epithelium during the menstrual cycle, with involvement of supporting tissues to produce yet more poorly categorized changes as in fibrocystic disease. Resultant clinical entities, such as cystic disease or fibroplasia, have encouraged clinical and pathologic confusion in classification even though the only significant components of fibrocystic disease are lobular and ductal hyperplasia. Here there are pitfalls in attempting a classification based on ductal or lobular changes, as these cells frequently are indistinguishable by light microscopy.

Host Resistance

Another nagging intangible is tumor aggressiveness vs host resistance. The extent of either is directly influenced by the other; i.e., the less the host resistance the more aggressive the tumor, while the greater the host resistance the less the aggression of the tumor. This concept perhaps applies more to the duct and lobular carcinomas, with allowances for subtypes in these groups. In a breast harboring a scirrhous duct carcinoma there may be a tubular carcinoma, with one type of carcinoma being highly aggressive in comparison with the other. Similarly, a medullary carcinoma with lymphoid stroma may be in the same quadrant as a highly infiltrative duct carcinoma. Multiplicity of sites of breast carcinoma should suggest lowered rather than increased host resistance. This is generally true of duct carcinomas, especially those with a scirrhous element, which have a high mortality rate; however, it is not true of multiple intracystic papillary carcinomas, which have a good prognosis and are found in elderly women, in whom one should expect lowered resistance.

OTHER PROBLEMS IN BREAST CANCER CLASSIFICATION

The increasing cooperative role of the surgeon, radiologist, and pathologist affects any attempt to classify breast cancer.

Multicentricity and Multiple Types of Breast Cancers

The greatest roadblock to a meaningful correlated clinical, radiographic, and pathologic evaluation of breast diseases is not the diverse histopathologic features of the single breast carcinoma, albeit they are gargantuan, but the frequent presence of multicentricity and multiple types of carcinoma in the same breast. This involves infinite numbers and groups of carcinoma to tax the pathologist, especially since the presence of many types may be unknown to him. It then does not seem remarkable or unconventional that for years I have considered each breast carcinoma as different from all others and even different from day to day.

"Minimal" Breast Cancer

Beginning almost three decades ago the surgeons, and then the pathologists, were challenged with problems in resection and in diagnosis of "mammography" breast cancers, as they were originally termed by the pathologist. Various other terms have been proposed: "nonpalpable" breast cancer, "occult" breast cancer, "early" breast cancer, and "subclinical" breast cancer. Without unanimity in definition these designations became meaningless, except that they did connote a cancer less advanced than the ones detected by the usual means without x-ray studies. After more than a decade Gallagher and Martin (1971) introduced the term "minimal" breast cancer, which became the byword.

Then arose confusion as each investigator applied his own definition. Minimal carcinoma originally included lobular carcinoma in situ, intraductal carcinoma, and "minimally" invasive carcinoma, either lobular or ductal, with a mass no larger than 0.5 cm in greatest diameter. Our criticism of the term was that it implied an assuredly curable carcinoma. This was erroneous, as 25 per cent of our lesions meeting these criteria were Stage II. This was later confirmed by Vana et al. (1981) with data from the Surveys of the American College of Surgeons indicating that 23 per cent of these "minimal" cancers presented with axillary lymph node metastasis. Some investigators suggested an upper limit of 1.0 cm in diameter, as there was no greater incidence of axillary metastasis than with tumors 0.5 cm in size. However, tumors over 1.0 cm in diameter had a significantly lowered survival. Survival and recurrence rates for even small tumors with axillary metastasis (about one fourth) suggest that size cannot be the only criterion for less advanced invasive breast carcinoma. It is hoped that this popular term could be redefined to become meaningful: all noninvasive carcinomas and invasive carcinomas 1.0 cm or less in greatest diameter with axillary lymph nodes in each instance free of metastasis.

The more curable cancer that suggests a better prognosis would be similar to a minimal carcinoma, e.g., low-grade infiltrating carcinoma; tubular, adenoid cystic, mucinous, intracystic papillary carcinomas, and cystosarcoma phylloides.

Both these data and our own suggest that Stage I of the $T_1N_0M_0$ classification should not include all tumors 2 cm or less in diameter but should be subdivided into tumors 1 cm or less and tumors 1.1 to 2 cm, for better expression of prognosis of breast cancer based on staging.

Imaging Modality Characteristics

The seemingly endless search for a more expressive classification of breast cancer, particularly duct carcinoma, may benefit from further breast imaging. Many of the contributions of radiography are well known. The complex nature of a mass (cystic and solid) may be better demonstrated by breast sonography. The degree of desmoplasia within a duct carcinoma (strongly related to prognosis) and reaction of the surrounding tissues may be better portrayed by sonography. The relative degree of oxygenation of hemoglobin within a tumor is readily displayed by near-infrared light studies. Magnetic resonance studies may well contribute to a better understanding of the biologic and physiologic properties of cancers as well as the concentration of tumor cells per unit volume of tumor. Once the various patterns of cancer activity in the intact breast are established by these modalities, better selection of a limited number of imaging procedures will then be possible.

MAMMOGRAPHIC EXAMINATION

Mammography has distinct advantages over physician examination and gross pathologic examination of the breast in depicting (1) minute, subgross, almost microscopic changes; (2) the three-dimensional view of both the lesion and the surrounding tissues; (3) the internal and external features of a lesion; (4) the reaction of the surrounding tissues; and (5) valuable diagnostic signs otherwise not available, such as calcifications, increased vascularity, and skin thickening.

Furthermore, mammography is an objective approach to the diagnosis of breast lesions. Dependable, specific, and reproducible precise changes serve as criteria of breast diseases. Physical findings are subjective and, as such, often are vague. They are only as reliable as the experience of the observer and are limited in that positive signs are few. The expertise in clinical evaluation of subtle breast changes is lost when passed from teacher to student. Mammography thus provides a permanent record for objective evaluation of these subtle changes in comparison with the less accurate and more subjective clinical evaluation.

Aims

The fundamental aims of mammography are to demonstrate the absence or presence of a lesion, to select any dominant mass or change requiring biopsy, and to determine the benignity or malignancy of a lesion when possible. The structures of the breast or the lesion are often so clearly outlined in fine detail that much information is derived as to the character of the changes in the breast, the histologic type of malignancy, or the histologic diagnosis of the benign lesion.

Much information on prognosis is usually available.

The radiologist makes a real contribution to the clinical and pathologic classification in terms of not only the thoroughness and completeness of the study of each breast but also the three-dimensional study of the tumor itself and the response of the tissue in the intact breast. In the first instance he may alert the pathologist to the presence of a second separate primary carcinoma or an intramammary lymph node. The radiologist may better judge the aggressiveness of the tumor or an increased acoustic impedance to a tumor. Since the radiologist notes differing contours of the mass at different parts of the periphery and seldom sees a true knobby or pure stellate lesion, as is seen on a histologic preparation of a single slice through the lesion, he becomes aware that contour is often complex and nonspecific and may be as varied as the pathologist's diverse classification of infiltrating duct carcinomas.

Criteria

Mammography is the study of gross pathology of the breast despite its resolution of 50 μ particle size compared with resolution of 2 to 3 mm particle size in general chest radiography. Radiographic studies of thin tissue slices at 12 kvp is a bridge between gross surgical pathology and light microscopy. Rather than attempt to define a fine line where gross pathology of the radiologist ends and microscopic study of the pathologist starts, the two approaches should be combined. This philosophy allows the radiologist more freedom of inquiry and broadens the pathologist's role in breast studies.

Although we do not encourage evasive mammographic diagnoses, the radiologist must be allowed a small percentage of examinations as an indeterminate group. Such studies would include the technically difficult examinations, lesions presenting with equivocal findings (a dominant benign mass with some irregularity of its borders or a circumscribed carcinoma), or the unusual situation in which the highly reliable secondary signs of carcinoma are associated with a benign process. Our philosophy of aggressiveness is far more rewarding, i.e., convincing a clinician that a borderline lesion requires investigation rather than temporizing with a potential cancer. This approach produces few unproductive biopsies, as 90 per cent of our positive diagnoses are cancer while a large number of Stage 0 and Stage I carcinomas are biopsy proved. The clinician has no quarrel with a one-in-three carcinoma biopsy rate with borderline calcifications not associated with a mass.

BENIGN BREAST DISEASES

Description of the transition from the normal breast into benign breast disease is an exercise in fine semantics and judgment of the variations of normal breast anatomy. For example, the syndrome of fibrocystic disease encompasses lymphocytic infiltration, fibrosis, duct dilatation and cyst formation, ductal epithelial hyperplasia, and lobular hyperplasia. Varying degrees of these changes occur in all normal breasts. There is no sequence of their appearance, and although a preponderance of one change may suggest some special form of fibrocystic disease, all five elements are still present to some degree. Thus, this process is hardly a disease and does not represent true neoplasia. A cyst is a collection of fluid within what was a duct; epithelial hyperplasia is an increased number of normal cells; and lobular hyperplasia, or adenosis, is only an overgrowth pattern.

In an attempt to impose some order on the benign diseases they will be considered as discrete or diffuse breast changes—intraglandular, extraglandular, or subareolar in location and cystic or noncystic in nature (Table 12–1). They will be classified with the full knowledge that at present many of the lesions cannot be differentiated. Dichotomy into cystic and noncystic lesions will be helpful in breast sonography.

MALIGNANT BREAST DISEASES

The sole purpose of breast studies is to detect cancers in a curable stage. To date mammography has proved to be the only reliable method to detect breast cancer prior to signs and symptoms. Yet mammography has two inadequacies: A small percentage of palpable lesions are not demonstrated by x-ray, and an unknown percentage of prevalent breast cancers are overlooked on mammography as well as on physical examination. The former cases are those of academic concern to the diagnostic radiologist. He may be chagrined, but the proper treatment is still

TABLE 12–1. Benign Breast Lesions

Discrete benign intraglandular lesions
  Noncystic
    Fibroadenoma
    Adenolipoma
    Lactating fibroadenoma
    Juvenile fibroadenoma
    Giant fibroadenoma
    Cystosarcoma phylloides, benign
    Miscellaneous
  Cystic
    Cysts of fibrocystic disease
    Galactocele
    Intracystic papillary lesions
  Altered architecture
    Fat necrosis
    Biopsy
    Radial scar

Discrete extraglandular (in skin and subcutaneous area)
  Noncystic
    Lipoma
    Scleroderma morphea
    Nevus
    Hematoma
  Cystic
    Sebaceous (epidermal) cyst
    Apocrine gland hyperplasia
    Hematoma

Discrete subareolar
  Noncystic
    Inverted nipple
    Subareolar fibrosis
    Abscess
    Intraductal papilloma
    Sweat gland adenoma
    Miscellaneous
  Cystic
    Dilated ducts
    Intraductal papilloma in dilated ducts

Diffuse
  Noncystic
    Fibrocystic disease
      Predominantly cystic
      Predominantly fibrous
      Ductal or lobular hyperplasia
        Ductal hyperplasia
        Lobular hyperplasia
      Sclerosing adenosis
    Mixed
    Fibroadenomata
    Intraductal papillomata
    Miscellaneous
  Cystic
    Cystic fibrocystic disease

Benign male breast disease
  Gynecomastia

carried out. In the latter, however, lies a potential for improvements in breast imaging.

Over 90 per cent of breast cancers arise from ductal epithelial cells. It is here that emphasis should be placed in determining which cellular activity is of importance and which is premalignant. Ductal hyperplasia is readily recognized on mammography, and it carries a four- to sevenfold increase in risk of malignancy. This pattern can be appreciated but is less apparent on breast sonography than on mammography. These same ductal epithelial cells are capable of producing the acini of lobules; they are the forerunners of lobular hyperplasia; and as they proceed into malignancy they retain many of the characteristics of the mother cells, such as the ability to secrete milk and calcium. Also, since the pathologist cannot always recognize the fine distinction between individual ductal and lobular cells, if one exists, there is little point in going to great extremes to separate lobular and duct carcinoma. We noted in our whole-organ studies that "lobular" carcinomas were associated with intraductal carcinoma or invasive duct carcinoma. The supposedly diagnostic features of lobular carcinoma, such as Indian filing, also occur with invasive duct carcinomas. Yet we still include lobular lesions in our classification of breast malignancies.

The classification of malignant diseases of the breasts that we devised for the National Reproducibility Study of Mammography in the early 1960s has proved acceptable to the clinician, radiologist, and pathologist. The essential features are retained here.

Basically this classification considers noninvasive and invasive carcinomas, special histologic types of carcinomas, bilateral carcinomas, multicentric carcinomas, sarcomas, and metastatic tumors (Table 12–2). Breakdown of the components has been suggested to better explain the growth pattern and thus the changes on breast studies.

Noninvasive Carcinoma

The main feature in the radiographic diagnosis of intraductal carcinoma is calcification; of intracystic papillary carcinoma, a cystic component; and of lobular carcinoma in situ, nonspecific lobular or diffuse change.

Intraductal

There is a continuum of progression of normal ductal epithelial cells into hyperplasia, into atypical forms of cells, into metaplasia, into intraductal carcinoma, and finally, breaching the basement membrane of the ducts, into invasive carcinoma. In the past few years a body of pathologists, but by no means all pathologists, have established and

TABLE 12–2. Classification of Malignant Breast Diseases

Noninvasive carcinoma
  Intraductal
    Solid
    Comedo
    Papillary
      Solid
      Intracystic papillary
    Tubular
    Lobular

Invasive carcinoma
  Duct
  Comedo
  Scirrhous
  Simplex—not otherwise specified (NOS)
  Adenocarcinoma
  Lobular
  Medullary with lymphoid stroma
  Tubular
  Solid Papillary
  Mucin-producing
  Intracystic

Special types of carcinoma
  Paget's
  Carcinoma with metaplasia
  Inflammatory
  Bilateral primary
  Multicentric
  Male

Sarcoma
  Cystosarcoma phylloides
  Mesenchymal (lipo-, neuro- angio-, fibro-)

Metastatic cancer
  From opposite breast
  From distant foci

agreed on specific criteria for the diagnosis of intraductal carcinoma based on ductal epithelial cell changes. All criteria may not be clearly present, leaving many gray areas in diagnosis. Most students of breast disease consider intraductal carcinoma as (1) having already broken through the basement membrane, although not in the area of histologic study; or (2) having an extremely high potential for metastasis. Also, all duct carcinomas arise from ductal epithelial hyperplasia even though all ductal hyperplasia does not proceed to intraductal carcinoma.

Intraductal carcinoma is envisioned as being associated with calcifications. This stems from the usual discovery of fine stippled calcifications on mammography. Study of a large number of whole-organ breast preparations bore out the association of intraductal carcinoma with calcifications as paralleling that of invasive duct carcinoma: 60 per cent of intraductal carcinomas had calcification on mammography; 80 per cent on thin breast section radiography; and at least 90 per cent on histopathologic study. Of course, calcifications on 7 μ thick preparations were not the same as those recognized on radiography. Fifty μ sized particles seen by x-ray would be shattered by the microtome blade except, at times, for the softer large calcifications of comedo intraductal carcinoma that would be cut by the blade.

The concept of considering two types of intraductal carcinoma provides (1) a distinction of less aggressive comedo intraductal carcinoma from more aggressive solid intraductal carcinoma; (2) an association of calcifications and types of calcifications with breast carcinoma; and (3) an explanation for formation of calcification in the breast by at least two means.

Solid Intraductal. The "solid" intraductal carcinomas are those distended ducts with closely packed viable cancer cells. A cribriform pattern is often present. A variant is arrangement of these cells in a pattern that reminds one of "Roman bridges" and "flippers of dolphins." These ducts may be surrounded by thick cuffs of periductal fibrosis and/or lymphocytes, hypothetically a defense mechanism. Light microscopy of H & E stains may fail to show carcinoma cells beyond the ducts, while electron microscopy may readily demonstrate such a bridge of the basement membrane (Ozello, 1971). Also, with light microscopy only a small portion of this diffuse multifocal disease is studied and, with an occasional axillary lymph node metastasis, it is best to consider this process invasive. Some of these deposits of carcinoma do not demonstrate calcification.

Intraductal Comedo. Intraductal comedocarcinoma is characterized by distention of the ducts with thick grumous material containing a large amount of calcification. This is a more indolent tumor and may fill a quadrant or most of the breast with no or minimal invasion. In most cases there are multiple sites of tumor in multiple lobes, and bilaterality is frequent. This suggests a large area or base for formation of the carcinoma rather than diffuse spread of tumor from a single site via the ducts. This carcinoma is often associated with Paget's disease of the breast, as it has the propensity to grow along the ducts, the path of least resistance, to reach the summit of the nipple. This prolonged process may require years to become clinically evident, since Paget's disease of the nipple may be present for years before a palpable mass in the breast is noted.

Papillary and Tubular Intraductal. Variations in the pattern of intraductal carcinoma occur in papillary and tubular forms. There are no charactertistic gross changes. Both tend to be less aggressive than the solid intraductal carcinoma.

Invasive Carcinoma

No intraductal carcinoma produces a gross breast mass until infiltration occurs. In these lesions calcification and only vague changes in the architecture can be anticipated. Once invasion occurs, a wide range of changes are seen in the breast to explain the many diverse responses. In distinction from the benign mass expanding, pushing breast tissue aside and maintaining a smooth border, the border of the malignant invasive mass is always irregular, as these cells penetrate the surrounding tissue. The reaction of these tissues to the invading malignant cells determines this border. It may range from the relatively smooth border of the medullary carcinoma with lymphoid stroma, pushing tissue aside while invading and creating only a mild response of lymphocytes, to the gamut of massive fibrosis, scarring, and contraction of scirrhous carcinoma.

In many breast carcinomas there is not always clear-cut histologic distinction of cell types or gross morphology. The common mother cell is capable of producing any of these epithelial tumors. There are subtle shifts in progression into different characteristics, tumors of distinctly different histologic types may be present, and multicentric foci are common and manifest different histologic types.

Duct

Invasive duct carcinoma, a general term, may be envisioned as a basic, or "root," type upon which variations may be superimposed, e.g., desmoplasia of scirrhous carcinoma or calcification pattern of comedocarcinoma. In the use of this term, these variations are recognized while their predominance is discounted.

In this classification, invasive duct carcinoma is the extension of the purely cellular, or solid, intraductal carcinoma. These features may be retained even though the lesion manifests highly invasive elements. The distinction of this finer classification provides the opportunity to recognize wider variations in all duct carcinomas. It constituted 26 per cent of our total carcinomas.

Comedocarcinoma

The invasive comedocarcinoma is an extension of the intraductal comedocarcinoma and in its early phase of invasiveness may excite very little reaction from the breast tissue. In this stage it made up 6 per cent of our total carcinomas.

In long-standing lesions, comedocarcinoma can proceed to a phase of highly invasive carcinoma with a preponderance of scirrhous changes, the comedo element being barely recognizable except for areas of the calcification pattern. These calcifications are still considered as being produced by the comedocarcinoma. At this stage the sonographic pattern, the x-ray appearance, and prognosis are the same as with any highly invasive duct carcinoma. The comedocarcinoma with scirrhous elements made up 6 per cent of the total carcinomas in our series.

With such a predominant highly invasive scirrhous element superimposed on the comedocarcinoma it could be postulated that two distinct carcinomas are present: one arising as a comedo variety and the other as a nearby solid variant.

Scirrhous

Scirrhous breast carcinoma does not represent a special cell type. The term connotes a degree of desmoplastic reaction to cancer cells regardless of the cell type. Since there is fibrotic reaction to all breast carcinomas of all cell types, this diagnosis is subjective. Usually it is reserved for moderately severe to severe desmoplasia (fibrosis). Our whole-organ studies strongly bore out that the more severe the scirrhous elements, the worse the prognosis. Scirrhous carcinoma produces the most marked changes within the breast. The changes are directly related to the degree of fibrotic response. The scirrhous element was seen in an additional 15 per cent of the invasive duct carcinomas. This represents a scirrhous component in 35 per cent of all comedo and invasive duct carcinomas.

Carcinoma Simplex

This term is reserved for those invasive duct carcinomas that cannot be specifically classified histologically. The histologic appearance is usually of uniform cells without attempt to produce any specific structure. These cancers tend to be only moderately aggressive and may merge into or with other cell types of carcinoma. The lesion is also labeled not otherwise specified (NOS).

Adenocarcinoma

Since most breast carcinomas arise from lining epithelial cells, they are true adenocarcinomas. Yet this term is reserved for those invasive duct carcinomas that have a great tendency to produce acini or glandular structures. They are not common breast carcinomas, are usually circumscribed, and have a relatively better prognosis. They have no characteristic features that could differentiate them from other moderately circumscribed breast carcinomas. They tend to occur in women younger than the usual age for invasive duct carcinoma.

Lobular

The diffuse nature of lobular carcinoma makes the gross description nonspecific. On x-ray there may be only vague asymmetry in density and architecture, or there may be a distinct localized density suggestive of a true mass. The histologic appearance of infiltrative cells in Indian-file fashion is common, but such cell arrangements also occur with invasive duct carcinoma. The changes range from a vague disturbance in architecture to a dense solid mass. The lesion is uncommon and exhibits a severe prognosis similar to other highly invasive duct carcinomas. This perhaps is related to its advanced stage upon recognition.

Medullary Carcinoma with Lymphoid Stroma

The medullary carcinoma with lymphoid stroma is associated with premenopausal or menopausal age, is rather well circumscribed, and carries a better prognosis than most invasive duct carcinomas. Histologically the tumor is made up of closely packed, structureless, uniform cells. Varying numbers of lymphocytes are found within the tumor, hence the term "medullary carcinoma with lymphoid stroma." A similar tumor without lymphoid stroma is also recognized; it is not included by us with medullary carcinoma with lymphoid stroma, but instead as a form of duct carcinoma.

Tubular

The relative nonaggressiveness of the tubular carcinoma makes this usually only a histologic lesion. However, with sufficient invasion and tissue response the lesion will produce varying degrees of infiltrative changes of a malignant mass.

Solid Papillary

The solid papillary carcinomas have no distinguishing radiographic features. These tumors also are less aggressive.

Mucin-Producing

Special mucin stains will demonstrate some mucin in almost all breast carcinomas. The term "mucin-producing carcinoma" is reserved for those lesions with abundant mucin with clumps or nests of carcinoma cells floating in pools of mucin. This rather uncommon tumor is well circumscribed and occurs in older women. Mucoid and mucinous are appropriate names, but colloid is not.

Intracystic Papillary

This uncommon breast carcinoma occurs in older women, who are most likely to have fatty breasts; with its blood content, it produces an almost opaque rounded shadow on mammography. A papillary tumor arises in a duct, blocks the duct, and with its friable hemorrhagic tendency bleeds and produces a blood-filled cyst. The inner wall is lined with projections of tumor into the cyst, adding to the thickness of the wall. Repeated hemorrhage increases the concentration of hemosiderin. Even though the carcinoma is still confined to the cyst, surrounding breast tissues respond to produce nearby altered architecture that contributes to the irregularity of the boundary of the lesion.

Upon breakthrough of the cyst wall and infiltration of the breast, a highly invasive tumor is produced. Thus, at this stage a contiguous poorly demarcated cyst and highly invasive mass is demonstrated.

Special Types of Carcinoma

Paget's

Paget's disease of the breast is a syndrome of a breast carcinoma that extends along the ducts onto the nipple, producing pagetoid changes in the epithelium of the summit of the nipple. Almost all cell types of carcinoma have been a part of Paget's syndrome, although the majority are the comedo type.

Carcinoma with Metaplasia

The carcinoma cells of invasive duct carcinoma may show histologic changes of metaplasia as epidermal carcinoma, osteogenic sarcoma, or chondrosarcoma. Usually these metaplastic cells are in small clumps seen only by light microscopy. However, on rare occasions a large mass of tumor may be present in areas of invasive duct carcinoma, with enough calcifications in bone or cartilage to be seen on the mammograms. Chondrosarcoma would be the first to produce such a change; then, osseous tissue may or may not be superimposed.

Inflammatory Carcinoma

Inflammatory carcinoma of the breast is a clinical syndrome with the carcinoma associated with all signs of inflammation: redness, heat, swelling, and pain. The carcinoma is usually a diffuse highly invasive duct carcinoma. The radiologist can see an extensive carcinoma and the pathologist may even find cancer cells in the dermal lymphatics, but neither can recognize heat, pain, or color by radiography or light microscopy.

Bilateral Primary Breast Cancer

The problem of bilateral carcinomas, the second primary, and metastasis of a carcinoma from the opposite breast has long been an enigma. Histologic criteria for the differential diagnosis of the second primary breast cancer are not always absolute. Mammography has contributed greatly to this important distinction.

Multicentric and Diffuse Carcinoma

Multiple foci of cancer are frequently present. Spread through the ducts for considerable distances occurs with formation of satellite nodules, or several duct systems may be involved with similar or different histologic cell types of carcinoma. Metastatic carcinoma from the opposite breast spreads diffusely throughout the lymphatics and can be superimposed on a primary focus.

Male Breast Carcinoma

The same changes are seen in male breast cancer, including calcifications, as are seen in the female.

Sarcomas

Although infrequent, sarcomas of all mesenchymal cell types occur in the breast as fat, nerve, smooth muscle, blood vessels, fibrous tissue, and so forth. There are no distinguishing features on breast imaging.

One lesion, cystosarcoma phylloides, will be encountered occasionally. These are usually benign but can be malignant. Histologic diagnosis is not reliable unless actual invasion is demonstrated. Usually the clinical course of recurrence or metastasis establishes the diagnosis of malignancy.

Metastatic Carcinoma

Opposite Breast

Metastatic breast carcinoma from the opposite breast is a diffuse process without gross mass formation. The changes of edema, increased breast density, and diffuse skin thickening are produced and are nonspecific.

Distant Foci

Almost all malignant diseases have produced metastatic foci in the breast. The more common are melanoma and lymphoma. A mass with a gross appearance of a fairly well circumscribed breast carcinoma is formed in contradistinction to the diffuse deposits from a carcinoma of the opposite breast.

CLINICAL CORRELATION

Rapport between the radiologist and the clinician responsible for the patient's care must be established, since errors in mammography are inevitable. The report of the mammograms must convey the full value of the study: (1) An unequivocal malignant lesion must be reported so that delay in treatment will be avoided; (2) the absence of a lesion must be indicated so that the patient can be reassured or the search for a primary malignant lesion directed elsewhere; (3) benign disease must be clearly described so that it can be treated accordingly; (4) the presence of a dominant nodule must be indicated; or (5) changes in the breast or the quality of the mammograms that indicate an indefinite diagnosis must be emphasized. Even with a procedure of high diagnostic accuracy, the radiologist must repeatedly point out the limitations of mammography.

In interpretation of the shadows on the mammograms obtained for diagnosis of benign or malignant lesions there should be constant search for changes that aid in predicting a relationship of benign processes to malignancy and findings that aid in better treatment planning.

Combining clinical findings with radiographic findings for final evaluation of the

studies has merit. Clinical examination by the radiologist assures that the patient is seen by a physician and the position of the palpable nodule in the breast is known. From the inception of our mammographic program requiring research and evaluation of the procedure, it was necessary to be as objective as possible in the interpretation of the examinations and to evaluate the mammograms without benefit of history or clinical findings.

The radiologist perhaps should take a different approach to mammography from our own for controlled clinical studies in an institution where each patient is assured evaluation by highly competent breast examiners. A clinical examination carried out on each patient having mammography should be combined with gross and histopathologic study of all tissue removed. Only then will mammography provide the maximal experience to the radiologist and the greatest benefit to each patient.

HISTOPATHOLOGIC CORRELATION

Regarding the diagnosis of breast disease, a few rather informal remarks by a tumor pathologist who had performed pathologic diagnoses of breast diseases as a daily routine for a number of years may be apropos. According to Gallager (1963), there are a certain number of irreducible errors in pathologic diagnosis of breast diseases. Specifically with frozen-section diagnosis there is an estimated 5 to 10 per cent range in which the diagnosis is not reliable. This includes not only those confusing cases such as papillary lesions, sclerosing adenosis, and plasma cell mastitis but also certain cases of medullary carcinoma that may be confused with Hodgkin's disease. In a complete pathologic study with an indefinite number of sections from the entire breast prepared under optimal circumstances with access to all special stains and unlimited time to examine all the material, the error rate should fall to 1 or 2 per cent. For a time the resident placed excised bits of breast tissue in his hand in such a way that he could not see the specimen and then by palpation alone made a diagnosis. He proved correct in predicting whether the lesion was benign or malignant 80 to 85 per cent of the time.

After nearly 30 years, with wider acceptance of mammography and the growing confidence of women and their physicians in its ability to detect breast cancer, the milieu has changed for the pathologist. The decline in size of breast cancers makes the gross pathologic diagnosis less evident; with detection of more Stage 0 and early Stage I carcinomas by mammography the pathologist is challenged frequently by borderline and questionably invasive lesions.

CHALLENGE: CLASSIFICATION OF HYPERPLASTIC PROCESSES

Breast cancer mortality could be reduced by recognition of benign changes in the breast that are regularly followed by carcinoma. Such lesions could even justify systematic prophylactic mastectomy. Epithelial hyperplasia, ductal or lobular, as a component of fibrocystic disease may be such a lesion. With our present knowledge we cannot identify either radiographically or histopathologically precisely which hyperplastic process will proceed to invasive carcinoma, so we cannot justify such an aggressive approach as prophylactic mastectomy. The patient with these epithelial changes does deserve the most meticulous observation.

Frequent physical examinations and annual mammograms are indicated, and the appearance of the slightest asymmetry is an absolute indication for investigation. Sparing the scalpel whenever physical examination or a mammogram raises the question of a developing cancer should now be history.

We are living in an era of transition in the understanding of breast cancer. More changes are yet to come. Implicit in this environment is a challenge to push forward the frontiers of diagnostic capability until we can reliably and reproducibly detect noninvasive cancer of the breast and define effective and minimally hazardous ways of treating it.

REFERENCES

Gallagher HS (1963): Personal communication.
Gallager HS, Martin JE (1971): An orientation to the concept of minimal breast cancer. Cancer 28:1505.
Ozzello L (1971): Ultrastructure of the human mammary gland. In Sommer SC (ed): Pathology Annual 1971, New York, Appleton-Century-Crofts.
Vana J, Bedwanie R, Mettlin C, Murphy GP (1981): Trends in diagnosis and management of breast cancer in the U.S.: From surveys of the American College of Surgeons. Cancer 48:1043.

Benign Breast Diseases

BACKGROUND

Benign breast lesions are of great interest to the radiologist because there is at times difficulty in differentiating the breast with benign disease from the one with malignant disease. Of even greater difficulty is differentiation of the benign processes from normal breasts. The breast considered normal to palpation and mammography frequently has a tissue diagnosis of disease. Microscopic study of the breast tissue following biopsy, amputation, or post-mortem examination rarely indicates an entirely normal gland.

An etiologic classification of the extremely diverse benign breast diseases that is acceptable to the clinician, radiologist, and pathologist is elusive. The proposed one has been acceptable for a number of years and represents a grouping of more value to the radiologist, as it is one that follows a descriptive pattern, aids in differentiating one benign process from another, and segregates the benign from the malignant lesions. Familiar uncomplicated precise nomenclature is retained. A slight modification of the classification to include cystic and noncystic lesions accommodates breast sonography (see Table 12–1).

The groupings of the various disease processes are not absolute but do serve to indicate the likelihood of a single or more localized process as opposed to multiple or diffuse

177

processes. Also, the location of the disease process within the breast often is of value to establish the etiology of the changes produced on the mammograms.

DISCRETE INTRAGLANDULAR LESIONS

Noncystic

There are certain radiographic features common to the isolated discrete benign nodule of the breast. These well-circumscribed masses are smooth bordered, oval, rounded, or lobulated. They are noninvasive. As they expand nearly equally in all directions fat is pushed aside, producing a thin radiolucent line about the periphery. This line may be seen in its entirety or may be obscured in some portions of the periphery by overlying dense tissue. Benign nodules are rarely accompanied by secondary changes in the breast. The calcification of a benign lesion is relatively coarse and of a more uniform density compared with cancer calcification. Very

frequently a lesion may be simply labeled benign without histopathologic identity. In the fatty atrophic breasts of elderly women care must be exercised, as a circumscribed carcinoma may mimic the benign breast nodule.

Fibroadenoma

In women of childbearing age the fibroadenoma is by far the most common solid benign tumor. Breast carcinoma is rare before the age of 20 years and uncommon before the age of 30 years. The mere possible existence of breast carcinoma during those ages and the frequency of fibroadenomata make this a problem lesion clinically. Also, during pregnancy and lactation a fibroadenoma may reach an enormous size, often referred to as a lactating fibroadenoma, making the patient bedfast. Differentiation from a potentially malignant cystosarcoma phylloides produces another clinical problem.

Only approximately 25 per cent of fibroadenomata are large enough to be seen grossly or to be imaged. The balance are seen only microscopically. Histologically there are a

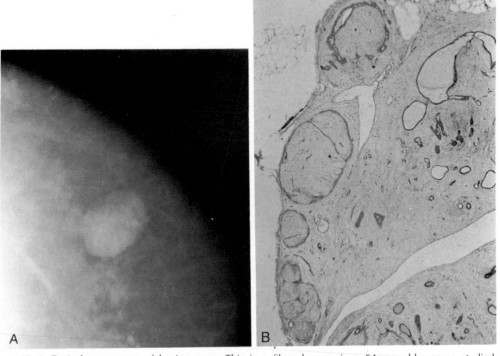

Figure 13–1. Typical appearance of benign mass. This is a fibroadenoma in a 54-year-old woman studied for a questionable nodule in the breast. *A,* The homogeneous, smooth-bordered, rounded lesion with a radiolucent rim pushing the normal breast tissue aside fulfills the criteria for a benign lesion. There is a small notch posteriorly. *B,* Photomicrograph demonstrating intracanalicular type.

number of distinct patterns of fibroadenomata with consequent variation in appearance on breast imaging. All are composed of a compact mixture of fibrous and glandular elements. Adipose tissue is only incidental.

Since the fibrous and epithelial elements are subject to the same stimuli as the remaining fibroglandular tissues, a carcinoma could possibly form within the fibroadenoma. Presumably there is no higher risk of this happening than in an equivalent amount of nearby breast tissue. The mean age of discovery of a fibroadenoma is between 30 and 35 years. At least one fifth of the patients will have multiple lesions, which often will be bilateral. In rare instances fibroadenomata will continue to be formed as long as fibroglandular tissues remain. At Emory University, one-half as many fibroadenomata are biopsied as the number of cancers. Also, 80 per cent of the clinically recognized fibroadenomata are demonstrated on breast sonography (see Chapter 7).

Fibroadenomata may be solitary or multiple, unilateral or bilateral, varying in size from several millimeters to filling almost the entire breast and pushing the normal glandular tissue into a portion of the periphery of the breast. Fibroadenomata less than 3 cm in diameter are usually homogeneous, are only slightly denser than the surrounding glandular tissue, and have a paucity of adipose tissue. They may be identified only by the presence of a homogeneous density surrounded by a thin layer of fat. Often a small notch may be distinguished at the periphery of the lesion (Figs. 13–1 to 13–3). The periphery may have a wavy, bosselated, or lobulated appearance.

Characteristic coarse calcifications may be identified in a high percentage of the older fibroadenomata (Fig. 13–4). These may be a single, central, heavy, amorphous deposit or multiple, fairly coarse calcifications, distributed near the periphery (Fig. 13–5). As the menopause nears, complete dissolution of the soft tissue element of a fibroadenoma may result without a residual density on the mammogram (Fig. 13–6). After reaching a certain stage of growth, the fibroadenoma may remain static for a period, followed by apparent degeneration within the lesion and appearance of calcifications in the soft tissue mass (Figs. 13–7 and 13–8). Microscopic study may reveal only amorphous calcific material without a soft tissue component. Some of these calcifications reach 2 cm in size and produce the densest structures seen on mammograms. Infrequently regrowth may begin apart from the older calcified portions of the fibroadenoma, with a soft tissue component separating the calcifications by this increase in soft tissue component (Fig. 13–9). The usual homogeneous density of the

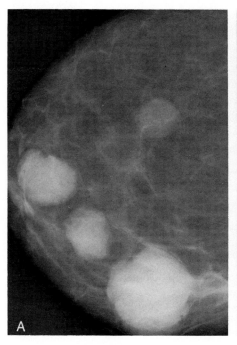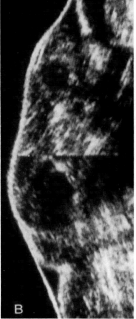

Figure 13–2. Multiple fibroadenomata. A 22-year-old woman with lumps in both breasts. Clinically: multiple, moveable masses bilaterally with some bulging of the skin. A, Mammography: smooth-bordered, homogeneous, lobulated masses, four on the right and five on the left (not shown). B, Sonography: well-demarcated, lobulated masses, low-level internal echoes, very slight increased through-transmission. Pathology: bilateral fibroadenomata.

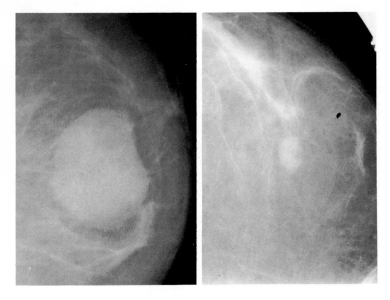

Figure 13–3. Typical notches in fibroadenomata. Two women aged 29 and 36 years.

soft tissue component of the fibroadenoma may be interrupted by radiolucent areas of adipose tissue that have been incorporated within the capsule.

The calcifications remaining in breasts of women approaching menopause or later in life are frequently noted on the mammogram, indicating that this lesion is far more common than clinically suspected. There are no data to suggest how many unsuspected fibroadenomata do not calcify.

When a discrete, rubbery, firm, freely mov-

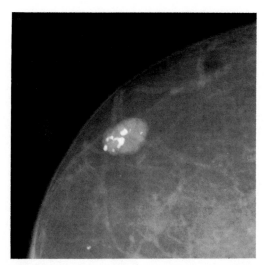

Figure 13–4. Fibroadenoma containing coarse flecks of calcium. This 61-year-old woman only recently discovered the nodule that was clinically highly suspicious for cancer. The coarse amorphous calcification in the benign lesion, despite the age of the patient, clearly indicates a histopathologic diagnosis of fibroadenoma.

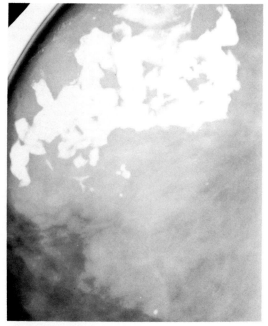

Figure 13–5. Large calcifying fibroadenoma. One large heavily calcifying fibroadenoma and numerous smaller, partially calcifying fibroadenomata are shown in a 90-year-old woman who had masses in her breast for "a long time." Clinically: 4 × 5 cm and 2 cm masses, carcinomas. Biopsy revealed fibroadenomata.

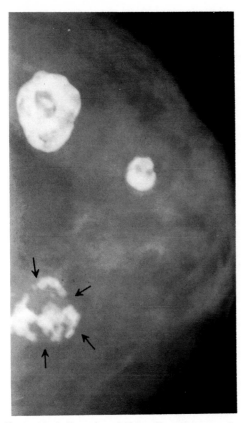

Figure 13–6. Densely calcifying fibroadenomata in the breast of a 78-year-old woman. The upper two are central calcifications; the soft tissue component of the lesion has been resorbed. In the lower lesion the calcification is more peripheral and a remnant of a soft tissue mass is still present at the edges (arrows).

able mass is present in a dense virginal breast without a demonstrable mass on the mammogram, the diagnosis of fibroadenoma is practically absolute. As the fibroadenoma is composed of proliferating glandular tissue and may therefore be of the same density as a normal glandular tissue, it may not be identified on the mammogram as a discrete mass until encapsulation occurs. Also, there is very little adipose tissue in the young breast. Frequently only a portion of the periphery of a lesion can be noted, or its presence may be recognized only by its more homogeneous appearance. A thin rim of fat about all or part of the periphery of a lesion or encroachment on the scanty subcutaneous tissue may lead to the diagnosis.

Many cysts and fibroadenomata may not be differentiated by mammography, but the characteristics, as outlined in Table 13–1, usually are sufficient clues to the diagnosis.

Small peripheral calcifications in a fibroadenoma may be arranged so that stippled calcification of carcinoma is suggested. Careful study of mammograms of both views of the breast, however, indicates that the calcifications are in the periphery, more certainly identifying the lesion as fibroadenoma. Fibroadenomata are frequently encountered on the mammograms; one should not be distracted by their presence but should search the remainder of the mammogram carefully for the presence of carcinoma. There is little

TABLE 13–1. Characteristics and Gross Appearance of Fibroadenomata and Cysts on Mammograms

Characteristic	Fibroadenoma	Cyst
Size	Small, or may enlarge breast	Variable, less tendency to large size
Shape	Variable, may be rounded or ovoid	Often enlongated with long axis perpendicular to chest wall; less variable; rounded or ovoid
Borders	Smoothly lobulated or bosselated; may have a distinctive notch	Smooth, equally distended in all directions; appearance of being under great tension
Calcifications	Central: heavy, amorphous; peripheral: coarse, sharp, intermittent, frequent	Occasional faint eggshell type in periphery; small flecks about periphery in glandular tissue; infrequent
Density	Similar to surrounding glandular tissue	Denser than surrounding (usually) more atrophic glandular tissue
Number	One, few, more separate discrete masses	Tendency to be numerous; coalescence; may be single
Texture	Lobulations transversely, less dense at notch; may be homogeneous	Homogeneous regardless of size
Stroma	Normal glandular tissue of young adult	Involuting—older type, usually associated with diffuse fibrocystic disease
Patient age	Young adult	Premenopausal into postmenopausal group
Needle aspiration	Solid tumor	Withdrawal of slightly discolored fluid causes disappearance of lesion; injected air outlines smooth inner wall

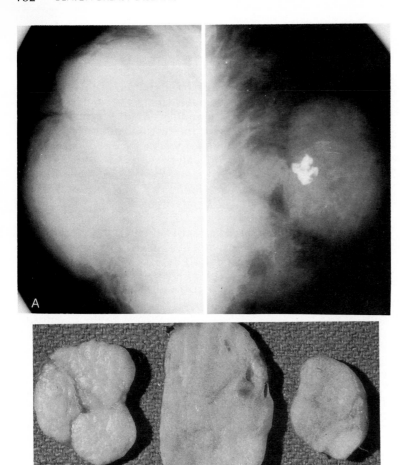

Figure 13–7. Calcifying and noncalcifying fibroadenoma. A 33-year-old woman, gravida 3, para 2, no nursing, with sore breasts. Clinically numerous bilateral fibroadenomata. *A,* Mammography: Fibroadenomata fill most of both breasts with one calcifying on the left. *B,* Gross photograph of three of the typical lesions after slicing. Pathology: fibroadenomata, intracanalicular type.

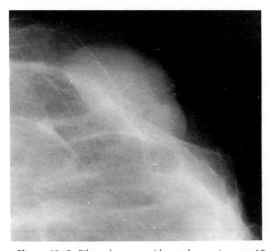

Figure 13–8. Fibroadenoma without change in over 15 years. A 42-year-old woman with a breast mass being followed by her physician. Clinically a well-circumscribed fibroadenoma. Mammography: 2.2 × 3.6 cm lobulated, noncalcifying fibroadenoma bulging into the subcutaneous tissues. She elects to keep it intact.

chance that even a rather large fibroadenoma will mask a carcinoma. Study of the two views of the breast will show the carcinoma to be separate so that each lesion can be observed individually.

Adenolipoma

A variant of the fibroadenoma is the adenolipoma with a variable amount of fat within the capsule. Histologically the lesion has islands of adipose tissue in areas of fibroglandular tissue. Mammographically there are two general types—probably similar processes but with different appearances at different ages.

In our patients aged 19 to 40 years with adenolipomas, the mammographic appearance was similar to that seen in Figures 13–10 to 13–13. The history and clinical findings are those of an ordinary fibroadenoma.

In one 75-year-old woman with a history

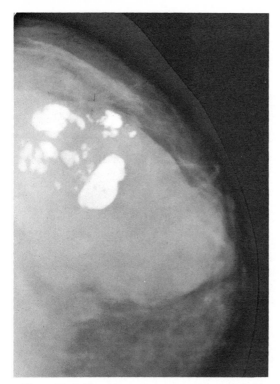

Figure 13–9. Fibroadenoma vs cystosarcoma phylloides. A 39-year-old white female, gravida 3, para 3, with a slowly growing mass in the breast for six months. Clinically: 9 × 5 cm hard lesion with an area of skin fixation. Mammography: 9 × 6 cm lobulated fibroadenoma; old calcified portion posteriorly, re-established growth anteriorly. Pathology: large lactating fibroadenoma or cystosarcoma phylloides. A 9 cm recurrent mass nine months later after histopathologic study following simple mastectomy indicated probable malignant cystosarcoma phylloides. There was no recurrence during a two-year follow-up.

of gradually enlarging mass of the breast for many years, the adenolipoma had a different mammographic appearance: a large encapsulated tumor, smoothly outlined, not quite so radiolucent as fat, that contained gross amorphous irregular plaquelike and linear calcifications similar to those seen in old fibroadenomata.

Lactating Fibroadenoma

The lactating fibroadenoma may become so large that it will not project onto a 14 × 17 inch film, producing a bedridden patient. This lesion occurs in young women, often black, and is associated with pregnancy. Histologically the mass contains acini filled with pink-staining (on H & E) secretion similar to milk. There are no radiographic or sonographic specific features (Figs. 13–14 and 13–15). The general pattern of fibroadenoma and the clinical setting must be relied on for the suggested diagnosis.

Juvenile Fibroadenoma

Even in the adolescent and teenage female patients, over 90 per cent of the fibroadenomata were of the adult or conventional types. The occasional one with a more cellular stroma and florid glandular pattern resembles to some extent the giant fibroadenoma. Clinical differentiation from cystosarcoma phylloides is difficult. Not too many breast tumors are studied radiographically in this very young age group. We studied one with sonography (Fig. 13–16).

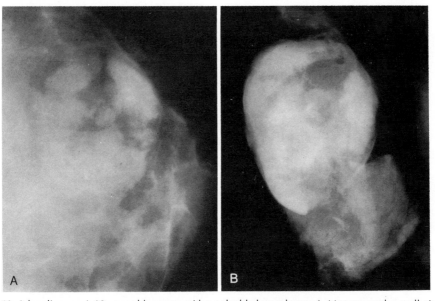

Figure 13–10. Adenolipoma. A 19-year-old woman with a palpable breast lump. *A,* Mammography: well-circumscribed, lobulated, nonhomogeneous mass on a background of dense fibroglandular tissue, characteristic of an adenolipoma. *B,* Specimen radiograph shows the benign nature of the mass with a fatty component.

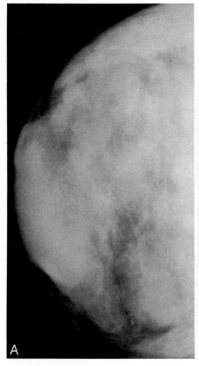
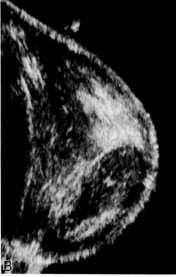

Figure 13–11. Adenolipoma. A 33-year-old woman with gradually enlarging right breast. Clinically: breasts soft and nodular, right larger than left. *A,* Mammography: large bosselated mass, filling most of the anterior medial breast, containing fat; adenolipoma. *B,* Sonography: medial half of breast replaced by a benign tumor containing markedly nonhomogeneous internal echoes, suggesting a variant of fibroadenoma or cystosarcoma phylloides. Pathology: adenolipoma.

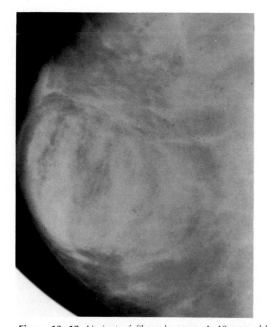

Figure 13–12. Variant of fibroadenoma. A 40-year-old white female with carcinoma of the sigmoid colon. Clinically: 3 × 3 cm cystic lesion of the breast. Mammography: 6.5 × 4.5 cm benign lesion, lobulated like a fibroadenoma but with bands of radiolucent tissue within the capsule. Pathology: adenolipoma.

Giant Fibroadenoma

The "giant" fibroadenoma is histologically an enlarged fibroadenoma that may fill a large part of the breast and can be distinguished only by the relative size (Figs. 13–17 and 13–18). These massive true fibroadenomata are more common in black females, predominantly in teenagers. A clinical distinction from cystosarcoma phylloides can be made, as the latter tumors occur in later decades.

Cystosarcoma Phylloides, Benign

The cystosarcoma phylloides may be any size up to that filling most of the breast. It too is a well-circumscribed mass found in relatively young women (mean age about 45 years). There is no distinguishing radiographic feature from the fibroadenoma except for the tendency not to calcify. It is composed of masses or sheets of dense fibroglandular elements separated by gelatinous, viscid material (Fig. 13–19). The name is derived from phylloides (leaf), a cystic component, and sarcoma (active one cell tissue). The sarcoma appellation is a misnomer

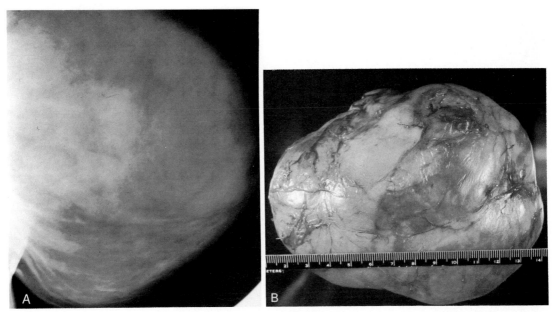

Figure 13–13. *A,* Large, lobulated, nonhomogeneous adenolipoma. A 20-year-old black female with an enlarging breast since normal delivery ten months before. Clinically: mass with symmetric breast enlargement. Mammography: 10 × 13 cm, smoothly circumscribed, lobulated, benign lesion, which may be adenolipoma, giant fibroadenoma, or cystosarcoma phylloides. Pathology: giant lobular fibroadenoma. *B,* Photograph of gross specimen.

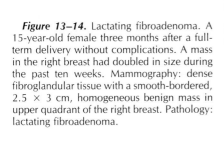

Figure 13–14. Lactating fibroadenoma. A 15-year-old female three months after a full-term delivery without complications. A mass in the right breast had doubled in size during the past ten weeks. Mammography: dense fibroglandular tissue with a smooth-bordered, 2.5 × 3 cm, homogeneous benign mass in upper quadrant of the right breast. Pathology: lactating fibroadenoma.

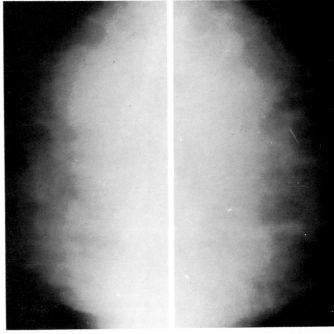

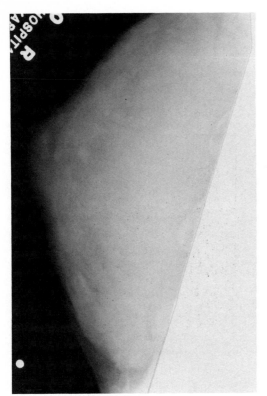

Figure 13–15. Lactating fibroadenoma. A 21-year-old black female, gravida 1, para 1, with a mass in the breast for four months, appearing in the last week of pregnancy. Clinically: 6 × 7 cm cystic mass. Mammography: 4.5 cm, rounded, dense, benign tumor centrally, in an almost homogeneous lactating breast, either fibroadenoma or cyst. Pathology: lactating fibroadenoma.

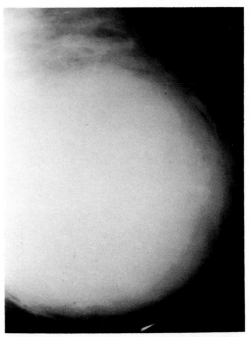

Figure 13–17. Large fibroadenoma mimicking a cystosarcoma phylloides. A 21-year-old nulliparous woman with an enlarging breast for four to six months, or "a long time." Clinically: most likely cystosarcoma phylloides. Mammography: homogeneous, encapsulated, smooth-bordered 9.5 × 10 cm benign-appearing mass pushing the breast tissues into the superior portion of the breast. Pathology: intracanalicular fibroadenoma.

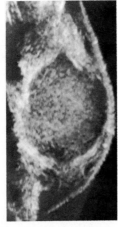

Figure 13–16. Juvenile fibroadenoma. A 12-year-old female with a breast lump for several months. Clinically: large, firm, movable mass. Sonography: a well-demarcated, slightly lobulated mass filling most of the breast. There are numerous homogeneous high-level internal echoes. Pathology: juvenile fibroadenoma.

because only a small percentage of these lesions become malignant. Histologic distinction of benign vs malignant is sometimes unreliable. Recurrence or metastasis establishes the presence of malignancy.

The basic histologic structure is that of a fibroadenoma with added cystic clefts and the sarcomatous appearance of monotonous cellular stroma, usually benign in appearance. Metaplasia may occur, suggesting fibrosarcoma or liposarcoma. In Haagensen's series of 84 cases there were cystosarcomas at ages 14, 15, 16, and 18 years (Haagensen, 1971). He reported four cases of bilaterality from the literature that were quite unlike fibroadenoma; in other reported series, all containing fewer than 100 cases, as many as 17 per cent metastasized and death occurred. Even in these lethal tumors histologic criteria were unreliable. The postulation was that in these massive tumors the truly small malignant areas were not seen. Yet, in other clinically benign tumors the whole lesion has appeared highly malignant.

The pathologist must decide whether the lesion is merely a giant variant of a fibroad-

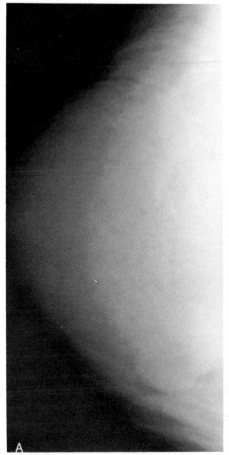

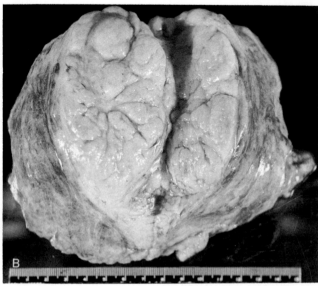

Figure 13–18. A, Fibroadenoma in a dense breast. A 19-year-old black female with painless enlargement of the breast for one year. Clinically: central breast mass. Mammography: 6 × 8 cm smooth homogeneous lesion, either giant fibroadenoma or cystosarcoma phylloides. B, Photograph of gross specimen. Pathology: (simple mastectomy): 9 × 7.5 cm giant fibroadenoma.

enoma and is entirely benign or whether some are malignant and are truly sarcomas. The radiographic differentiation of a cysto-sarcoma phylloides and a large fibroadenoma is not made with any degree of certainty (Fig. 13–20). Even though the lesion fills most of the breast, it still possesses the characteristics of a benign lesion (Fig. 13–19).

New growth of an old solid benign lesion may be an interesting observation but does not necessarily indicate malignancy. With evidence of invasion of some portion of the periphery, the lesion will be definitely malignant, this at times will be indistinguishable from a large intracystic papillary carcinoma showing invasive characteristics. At times mammography may aid in selection of the proper area of histopathologic evaluation for malignancy.

A common feature of cystosarcoma phylloides is symmetric enlargement of the breast. This finding, coupled with a large breast mass without other secondary changes, allows a reliable diagnosis clinically.

In our experience, the majority of lesions with a histopathologic diagnosis of cystosarcoma phylloides had apparent cure with simple mastectomy. However, a few recurred locally and even fewer produced distant metastases.

Miscellaneous Lesions

Other benign discrete solid breast lesions encountered may include adenoma (Fig. 13–21), granular cell myoblastoma, neuroma, hemangioma (Fig. 13–22), fibroma (Fig. 13–23), intraglandular hematoma (Fig. 13–24), and lipoma (Fig. 13–25). These lesions, oc-

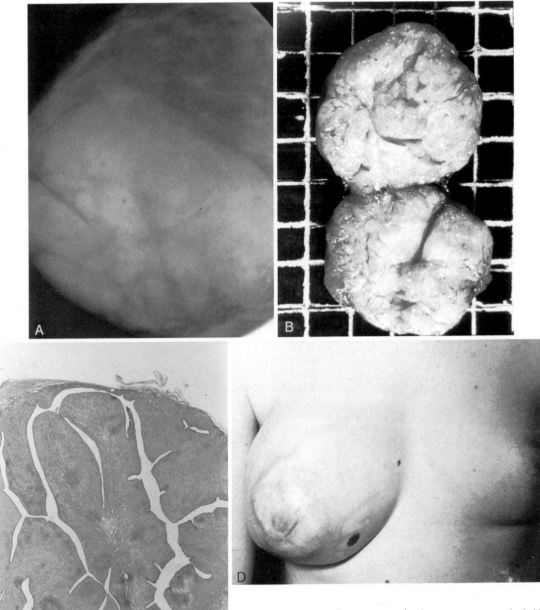

Figure 13–19. Nonhomogeneous benign cystosarcoma. *A*, A 10 × 13 cm mass is shown that still retains the characteristics of benignity. The name, cystosarcoma phylloides (leaflike), is illustrated by a cavity filled with cauliflower-like masses of solid tissue (or cystadenoma) floating in semiliquid material. Sarcoma is a reference to its fleshy nature rather than an indication of malignancy. *B*, Photograph of sliced specimen. *C*, Low-power field characteristic of leaflike protrusions of neoplastic stroma into cystic spaces. The stroma showed only rare mitotic figures, indicating a benign lesion. *D*, Photograph of the breast with characteristic symmetric enlargement by the cystosarcoma phylloides.

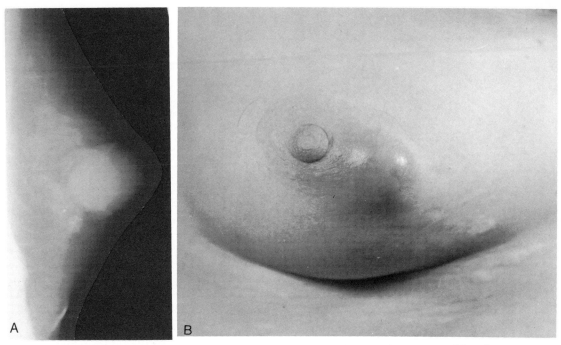

Figure 13–20. Cystosarcoma phylloides. A 57-year-old white female with benign lesion removed from breast 14 years before and lump beneath areola for one and one-half years, increasing in size over past three months. Clinically: 2 cm cystic mass bulging the skin with 4 × 5 cm underlying mass. A, Mammography: 2 × 3 cm smooth mass; also nearby lesion with coarse calcification, either fibroadenoma with subareolar cyst or two fibroadenomata. B, Photograph of lesion that shows bulging and discoloration of the skin. Pathology: (simple mastectomy): cystosarcoma phylloides with cystic areas and focal calcifications.

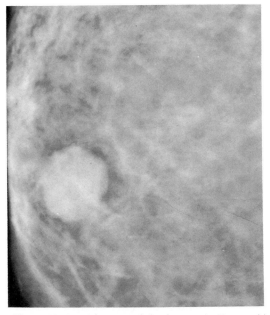

Figure 13–21. Adenoma of the breast. A 40-year-old white female with a breast lump for three weeks. Clinically: 3 cm carcinoma. Mammography: one 2 cm and two 0.5 cm fibroadenomata. Pathology: three adenomata, 2 cm, 0.6 cm, and 0.5 cm, with fibrocystic disease.

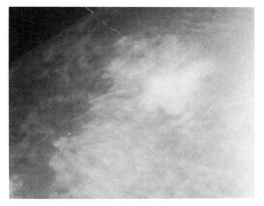

Figure 13–22. Hemangioma of the breast. A 79-year-old woman who had a mass in her breast several days before. Over 20 years ago she had had a breast biopsy in the same general area for benign disease. Clinically: 2 × 1.5 cm dominant nodule, carcinoma. Mammography: 1.5 × 2 cm intermediate growth pattern of cancer. Pathology: cavernous hemangioma.

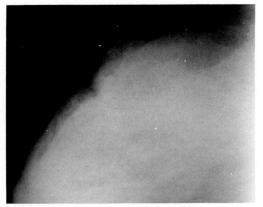

Figure 13–23. Fibrous tumor of Haagensen. A 64-year-old woman with a lump UOQ of the breast with a biopsy in the area two months before. Clinically: "tumor still there." Mammography: large, poorly outlined homogeneous and lobulated tumor in upper hemisphere of the breast pressing the fibroglandular tissues inferiorly. Pathology: 5 × 2 × 3 cm tumor of dense fibrous tissue with interspersed fat; extensive stromal fibrosis, atrophy of the glandular tissue, and remote hemorrhage into the collecting ducts, consistent with the fibrous tumor of Haagensen. No malignancy.

curring in the glandular portion of the breast, usually have no identifying characteristics. Each will usually be designated a benign lesion, most frequently mistaken for a fibroadenoma. All are infrequently encountered.

A discrete mass within the fibroglandular tissue of the breast without surrounding altered architecture may be produced by an intramammary lymph node. It may be too small for recognition even when it contains a metastatic deposit of breast carcinoma. The usual clue to its presence on the mammogram is a rounded nodule with a notch with a nearby, or distant, invasive carcinoma (see Chapter 17).

Cystic

Cysts of Fibrocystic Disease

Simple cysts associated with fibrocystic disease occur in all breasts and vary in size from microscopic collections of fluid in the ducts to large, clinically discernible masses. They are multiple and bilateral. Clinically or sonographically there may be only one detectable cyst, or both breasts may be honeycombed with innumerable cysts. Cysts peak in frequency at 35 to 50 years of age. They occur most frequently in premenopausal and menopausal women. Cysts are clinically of interest only if they are palpable. The palpable mass alarms the patient and arouses concern of differential diagnosis in the clinician. Cysts may become quite large before they become palpable.

In breasts of a density comparable with

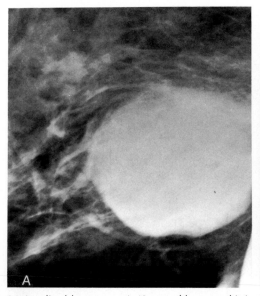
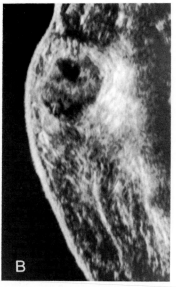

Figure 13–24. Localized hematoma. A 42-year-old woman hit in the breast two weeks before. A mass was apparent clinically. *A,* Mammography: 3.5 × 4.5 cm dense, homogeneous, smooth, lobulated benign mass. *B,* Sonography: large well-demarcated area containing nonhomogeneous internal echoes, except anechoic central area, with increased through-transmission, a complex mass. Bloody fluid was aspirated and the mass slowly disappeared.

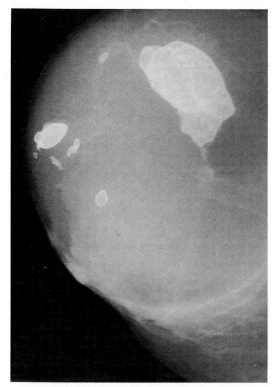

Figure 13–25. Calcifying lipoma. An 80-year-old female with advanced arteriosclerotic degenerative disease of the brain and with breast mass present "long, long time and getting bigger." Clinically: hard as a rock, reddened skin and areola, large superficial vein; carcinoma. Mammography: 14 cm lipoma that appears under marked tension; scattered islands of calcification measuring up to 2.5 × 5 cm. Pathology: lipoma with large calcified areas.

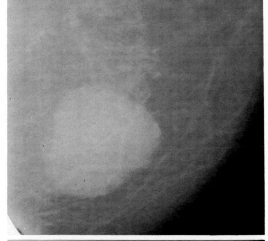

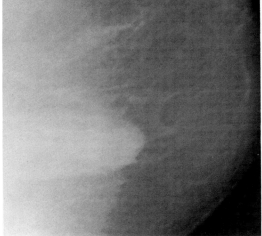

Figure 13–26. Single dominant cyst. A 46-year-old female with a breast lump for two months that was clinically movable. Mammograms: more spherical on craniocaudad view (upper); ovoid on mediolateral view with long axis perpendicular to chest wall (lower). Various configurations of the cyst are produced from pressure on the walls by supporting structures. Pathology: cyst associated with fibrocystic disease.

those containing fibroadenomata, the cystic disease lesion is almost as difficult to outline. Because cystic disease is associated with the less dense breasts of the older age group, the cyst appears more opaque on the mammograms. Comparison with a cyst on one mammogram with a fibroadenoma on another mammogram made with similar radiographic factors reveals no significant difference in density of the two lesions. The cysts may be solitary or may occur in clumps. The borders are often sharp and clear, suggesting that the contents are under great tension. There may be associated fibrotic disease. The process is limited to the fibroglandular tissue without arising in the subcutaneous adipose tissue. The trabeculae coursing toward the nipple prevent equal expansion of the cyst in all directions and produce more frequently an ovoid shape with the long axis perpendicular to the chest wall (Fig. 13–26).

The anterior surface of the large cyst is almost invariably clear, as there is less over-

lying tissue toward the apex of the coned-shaped breast. Its posterior aspect may be less well defined. Well-coned views with better penetration may be required to study the posterior portion of some cysts (Fig. 13–27). Very rarely, the wall of a cyst may calcify in a faint eggshell fashion, or flecks of calcium may be closely apposed to the wall. Increase in size of the cyst may cause extension of the cyst into subcutaneous tissue and actual bulging of the skin, but without skin thickening.

The cyst as a dominant nodule may appear to have unclear borders but, with close study, a thin radiolucent line is revealed in some portion of the periphery. Apparent indis-

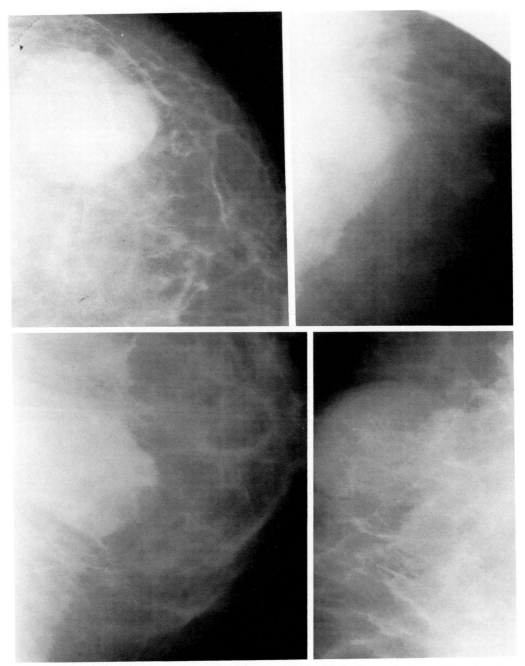

Figure 13–27. Single palpable cysts in four different breasts. Characteristically they tend to be ovoid, outlined by a thin rim of fat, and occurring in fibroglandular breasts where the tissue obscures the posterior border. If there is any concern, compression with increased collimation and mas will also delineate the posterior border.

tinctness of the cyst border is produced by trabeculae passing in front of or behind the lesion and is accentuated by an increase in fibrous tissue as well as numerous small, ill-defined cysts that are frequently associated (Fig. 13–28). The cyst may displace or distort the superimposed trabeculae, but these trabeculae are clearly seen traversing the tumor as opposed to the increased density of the mass and retraction of the trabeculae toward the malignant mass.

A rather striking demonstration of its character results from aspiration of the cyst contents with the introduction of air to outline the extremely smooth inner walls. This is not necessary to exclude carcinoma, as the lining of the cyst does not undergo malignant degeneration.

Clinical examination followed by needle aspiration of clear (nonbloody) fluid permits not only the diagnosis but also the treatment. If the mass disappears completely, the incident is closed. However, if a mass persists, the lesion must be investigated further or followed closely.

One must develop one's own philosophy about aspiration of nonpalpable cysts under sonographic control. The sonographic appearance of a cyst is characteristic. Breast

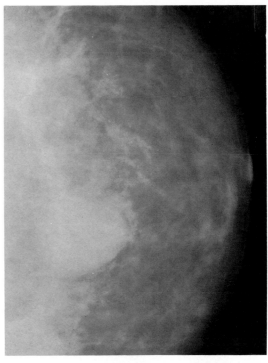

Figure 13–28. Usual appearance of a dominant cyst in fibrocystic disease. A 29-year-old white female who discovered a lump in her breast. Clinically: dominant nodule. Mammography: fibrocystic disease with a 2.5 × 3 cm discrete cyst. Pathology: fibrocystic disease, large cyst.

Figure 13–29. Cyst in dense glandular breast. A 51-year-old woman with nodular breasts. *A,* Mammography: dense, nodular, almost homogeneous fibroglandular tissue without fat for contrast. *B,* Sonography: large, simple cyst. After localization the surgeon could feel it for aspiration. In this case ultrasound only caused additional trauma.

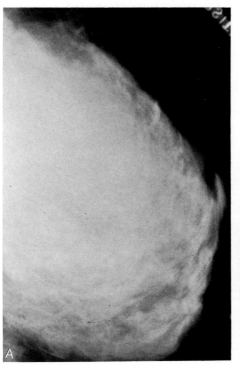

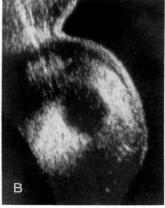

sonography provides assurance that the mass is cystic, can aid in directing the needle properly, and can help determine whether all the fluid has been aspirated. Breast sonography demonstrates many nonpalpable cysts and many with dense fibrocystic disease that are not delineated on the mammograms. This has proved to be an area in which breast sonography excels (Figs. 13–29 to 13–31).

A localized single major duct may present as a cystic lesion. Usually the duct is an elongated structure, but many appear somewhat rounded. The usual cause of dilatation

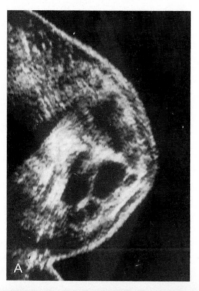

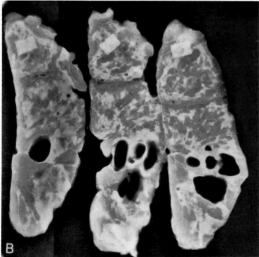

Figure 13–30. Multiloculated cyst. A 45-year-old woman who had needle aspiration of the breasts five times bilaterally two weeks before. *A*, Sonography: numerous multiloculated cysts at numerous levels in both breasts. *B*, Whole-organ slicer sections representative of both breasts.

is inspissated grumous material in the duct that may produce internal echoes on sonography. On occasion a similarly dilated duct may be produced by a papilloma bleeding into and distending the duct to produce a cyst. This duct would contain blood and if the papilloma is sufficiently large would produce internal echoes. Cysts may resemble fibroadenomata and may calcify, (Figs. 13–32 to 13–35).

At times radiologists are amazed to find numerous very large cysts in both breasts that may produce some vague nonspecific palpatory findings. Apparently cysts must enlarge gradually, perhaps during some menstrual cycles, distending the capsule repeatedly. The fluid is not under very great tension and is similar to water in a balloon that feels soft. Overnight, or over a short period of time, however, 1 to 2 ml of additional fluid is secreted into the cyst, producing tension within the cyst. The patient then notices a fullness or pain in her breast, feels a lump, and then presents to her physician with a firm cystic mass.

Galactocele

To reach a mammographic diagnosis of galactocele, a cystic structure containing radiolucent material must be seen (Fig. 13–36). The galactocele is formed in relationship to pregnancy and lactation but may perist past cessation of lactation.

Depending on the percentage of fat in its milklike content, on mammography (1) it may not be radiolucent, appearing as a simple cyst; (2) it may be radiolucent with its thin wall clearly outlined; or (3) there may be layering of the fat over the milk (Figs. 13–36 to 13–39). The fluid consistency is similar to condensed milk.

Colostrolipocele

Even less frequent is the colostrolipocele, a variant of galactocele (Fig. 13–40). This cyst contains large cells (Donné cells) and is packed with droplets of fat identical to that of colostrum (hence its name). The consistency of the contents is almost that of toothpaste.

On breast sonography both variations will appear as a well-demarcated benign mass. It may be anechoic, with simple cyst type increased through-transmission, or, with increased lipid content, there may be internal echoes. Needle aspiration confirms the diagnosis.

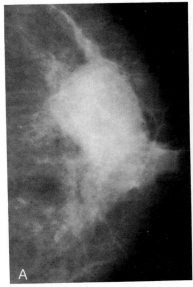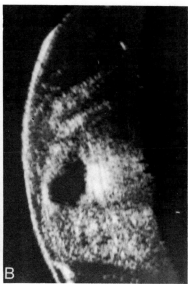

Figure 13–31. Use of sonography in cyst aspirations. A 51-year old woman on estrogens. Mass, aspirated one week earlier, re-filled. *A,* Mammography showed a homogeneous 3 cm mass with indistinct borders that could represent circumscribed carcinoma but by history was a cyst refilled and surrounded by hematoma and/or edema. *B,* Sonography: well-demarcated rounded lesion, thickened walls surrounded by high-level echoes, increased through-transmission, and lateral refractive edges.

Intracystic Papillary Lesions

Intracystic papillomata contain blood and produce extremely dense masses. This is not a common lesion. It is seen in the older patient (usually 65 years or older) and stands out sharply against the fatty, atrophic radio-lucent tissues (Figs. 13–41 to 13–43). The relative density of these lesions allows easy recognition; they are less dense than the amorphous calcification of a degenerating fibroadenoma and usually are denser than most carcinomas, particularly mucin-producing carcinoma. The papillary growths within the cyst bleed, producing a concentration of blood pigments. The content is a dirty black liquid filling the spaces between the degenerating fronds of the papillary lesion. Intracystic papillomata may reach great size, filling almost the entire breast as does cystosarcoma phylloides.

Frequently, only one area of the periphery reveals invasiveness on the mammograms; this must be searched for and the pathologist alerted. Only with sections through the invasive portion of the cyst wall will the pathologist be assured of a correct diagnosis of intracystic papillary carcinoma. In many instances, the pathologist has had difficulty in establishing the diagnosis of carcinoma and the lesion has recurred in the same area. This may be sufficient reason for considering all intracystic papillary lesions to be malignant. Intracystic papillomata located deep in the breast differ in gross appearance and behavior from intraductal papillomata recognized in a more immediate subareolar area; the two lesions may be considered separate radiographic entities. Perhaps the difference is tenuous, as either intracystic papilloma or intraductal papilloma may occur in the subareolar area, but the malignant potential of

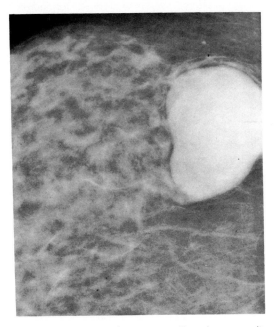

Figure 13–32. Cyst that suggests fibroadenoma radiographically. A 54-year-old woman with a questionable lump in the breast. Mammography: smooth-bordered, homogeneous mass with notches of a fibroadenoma. Sonography demonstrated a simple loculated cyst. Aspiration confirmed the diagnosis of cyst.

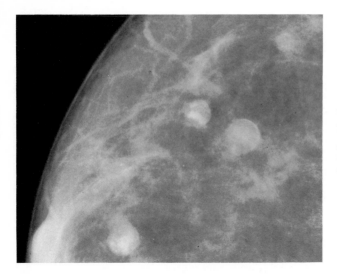

Figure 13–33. Calcifying inflamed inclusion cysts. A 60-year-old woman seen for a checkup. Mammography: four rounded lesions, the largest being 7 mm in size, with calcifications in the walls suggestive of calcifying cysts. Pathology: epidermal inclusion cysts with surrounding dermal fibrosis.

intracystic lesions makes the clinical differentiation of value (see Chapter 22).

Altered Architecture

Fat Necrosis

An area of traumatic fat necrosis may have little in the way of mammographic distinguishing characteristics from carcinoma or little difference in appearance from hyperplastic fibrosis associated with fibrocystic disease. To be recognized by sonography, a high level of echoes with some attenuation of the sound beam would be required.

The mammogram is rarely of reliable help in differentiating fat necrosis from carcinoma. Short of histologic study, there is no way to exclude carcinoma when this lesion is present

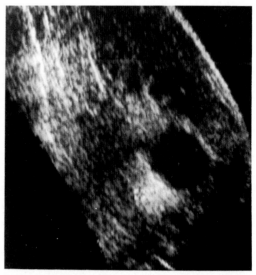

Figure 13–35. Ruptured cyst. A 52-year-old woman with a soft breast lump. Aspiration produced a small amount of fluid. Mammography showed a 3.5 × 4 cm homogeneous circumscribed mass containing coarse flecks of calcification (not shown). With its indistinct borders, a medullary carcinoma could not be excluded. Sonography: rather well-demarcated oval mass with slightly irregular borders, lateral refractive edges, nonhomogeneous high-level internal echoes; most likely medullary carcinoma. Pathology: putty-like mass containing a cyst; cystic disease. Comment: leakage of cyst material with fibrotic and histiocytic reaction; mild ductal hyperplasia.

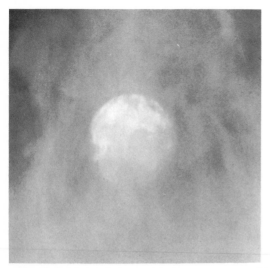

Figure 13–34. Calcified cyst of the breast. A 47-year-old woman seen for baseline mammography. The cyst contained amorphous dark brownish material; the calcification is in the walls.

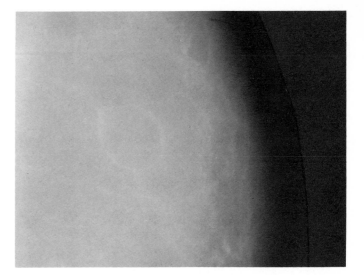

Figure 13–36. Galactocele. A 46-year-old white female, gravida 1, para 1. Clinically: lump in the breast. Mammography: 1.5 × 2 cm, thick-walled, cystic structure with radiolucent center. Pathology: circumscribed, 1.5 × 2 cm cystic structure containing fatty fluid, compatible with galactocele.

in the breast. Breast carcinoma occurs at least 40 to 50 times as frequently as fat necrosis; many women who present with an invasive carcinoma recall trauma to their breast. One is simply playing for very poor odds with an x-ray or ultrasound diagnosis of fat necrosis. This is despite knowing that one third of the lesions occur in the subareolar region and many are just beneath the skin. Fat necrosis may mimic abscess, also a differential lesion with carcinoma.

Histologically, for a diagnosis of fat necrosis we prefer that all the following changes be present: fibrosis, multinucleated giant cells, fatty acid crystals, blood pigments, and oily deposits—all in an area that is densest at its center. Paraffin injected to enlarge the breast has produced a similar pattern but is no longer used.

Biopsy

Breast studies immediately following a biopsy (usually for benign disease, as the

Figure 13–37. Galactocele. The smooth-walled oval lesion is readily visible owing to its radiolucency, approximately that of adipose tissue (single arrow). This 27-year-old woman, in her ninth month of her third pregnancy, had been aware of a difference in her breasts for at least two months. After needle aspiration, the lesion recurred, and, following delivery, it was surgically excised. Note the width of the vein during pregnancy (opposing arrows).

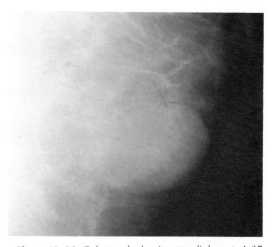

Figure 13–38. Galactocele that is not radiolucent. A 37-year-old female, gravida 3, para 3, seven months post partum. Clinically: 3 × 4 cm cyst. Mammography: 3 × 4.5 cm benign lesion, most likely a cyst. Pathology: a cyst containing thin, fatty fluid; a galactocele.

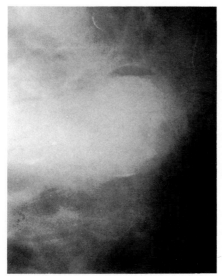

Figure 13–39. Galactocele. A 48-year-old woman with a poorly defined subareolar nodule on the left for an indefinite time, gravida 3, para 3; nursed a total of 18 months; last delivery at age 33 years. Mammography: 2.1 × 2.3 cm smooth, rounded, mostly homogeneous, benign mass. A fluid level was noted in the erect mediolateral view but not in the craniocaudad view. No recent aspiration attempts. Pathology: galactocele containing the usual milky fluid with many histiocytes. Parts of the capsule were calcified. The diagnosis would not have been suggested without the erect view.

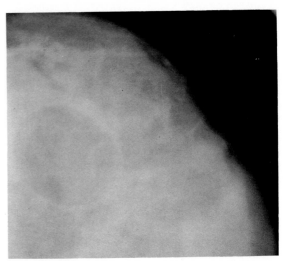

Figure 13–40. Colostrolipocele. A six-month pregnant, 32-year-old female presenting with a painless lump in the breast. Clinically: 4 cm, hard, movable mass. Mammography: galactocele. Aspiration revealed thick fluid, milky in appearance. The cyst refilled and was surgically removed. The specimen was a 5 × 3 × 2 cm cyst; analysis of the contents revealed Donné cells, high fat content similar to colostrum, and no lactose.

Figure 13–41. Intracystic papilloma. A 72-year-old woman presented with a 4 × 5 cm mass noted in her breast for over six months. *A,* Mammograms show the very dense 4 × 4.5 cm homogeneous rounded lesion, smooth anteriorly, but with indistinct borders posteriorly, radiographically diagnosed as intracystic papillary carcinoma. *B,* Histopathologic study revealed a benign lesion without demonstrable carcinoma.

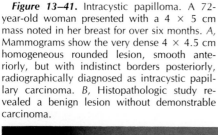

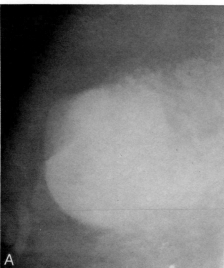

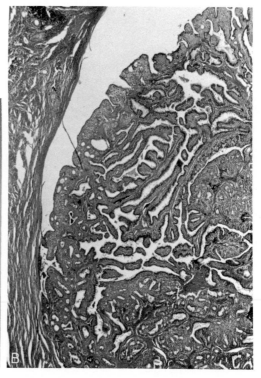

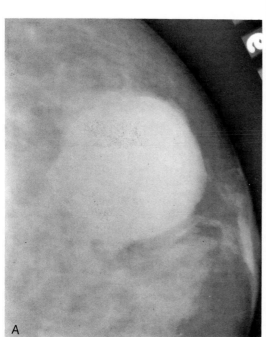

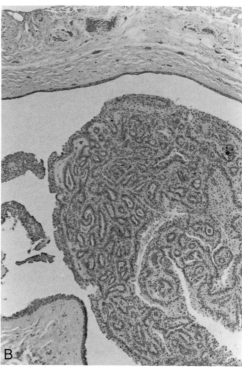

Figure 13–42. Intracystic papilloma. An 85-year-old white female with a lump in the breast for 18 months. Clinically: 6 × 7 cm mass. *A,* Mammography: 4 cm intracystic papillary carcinoma (coded on the basis of density and irregular borders posteriorly). Pathology: 4 cm cystic mass containing a 3 cm polypoid growth, probably malignant; later interpreted as intracystic papilloma and fibrocystic disease, shown on photomicrograph (*B*).

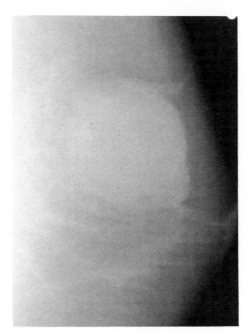

Figure 13–43. Intracystic papilloma. A 54-year-old white female with a lump in the breast for three months. Clinically: 2 cm mass adherent to the skin; carcinoma. Mammography: 4 cm dense cyst, intracystic papilloma, without definite demonstrable invasion (coded as malignant on basis of density of the cyst). Pathology: 4.8 × 2.6 × 1.7 cm intracystic papilloma; cyst filled with reddish brown fluid.

breast remains intact) may produce an ill-defined and noncircumscribed alteration, not unlike an infiltrating carcinoma, depending on the degree of hemorrhage and tissue reaction

The healing biopsy may show varying degrees of changes within the glandular tissues depending upon the amount of tissue removed, hemorrhage, infection, and/or foreign body reaction. No local change may be apparent, or there may be severe changes indistinguishable from carcinoma. The skin usually shows some deformity of flattening or retraction, possibly thickening (more often on sonography than on mammography), requiring a rather precise tangential view. All scars should be recorded prior to interpretation of breast imaging (see Chapter 32).

Radical Scar

The nonspecific fibrotic appearance of the radical scar has no distinguishing diagnostic characteristics. This pattern, which may simulate an invasive duct carcinoma, is usually caused by extensive sclerosis of papillary or florid epithelial hyperplasia. This lesion, like traumatic fat necrosis, will require histologic study for differentiation from a malignant process.

DISCRETE EXTRAGLANDULAR LESIONS (IN SKIN AND SUBCUTANEOUS AREA)

Extraglandular benign breast tumors are not indigenous to the breast and are similar to the same lesions that occur elsewhere in the body. The usual radiographic features of benignity apply. There is little that identifies their histologic nature except perhaps location.

Noncystic

Lipoma

The recognition of lipomas on mammograms depends on a discrete radiolucent mass in the fibroglandular tissues, outlined on both views of the breast by heavier than normal trabeculae that are sharply displaced by the mass of adipose tissue (Fig. 13–44).

Fatty tissues entrapped by Cooper's ligaments may produce a discrete, fairly firm tumor clinically. On breast imaging it will appear normal or, perhaps, with prominent Cooper's ligaments. Upon biopsy and severance of the these confining ligaments the "tumor" becomes a soft mass of adipose tissue. True lipomas are rarely found in the subcutaneous fat.

The internal echoes of the lipoma on sonography are disorganized, a characteristic of adipose tissue. The lesion would be recognized with difficulty in a fatty breast on sonography. In a rather dense fibroglandular breast a localized area of fatty tissue may be recognized. This can usually be identified as it changes shape with changes in scan level and merges with other fatty areas. The diagnosis of lipoma by mammography requires the presence on both views of a radiolucent area with distinct borders.

Scleroderma Morphea

Localized plaques of thickened skin may be produced by scleroderma morphea without specific characteristics (Fig. 13–45). There is also some degree of associated fibrosis in

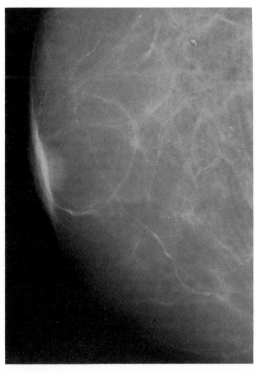

Figure 13–44. Lipoma. A 55-year-old white female with carcinoma of the uterine cervix; mass in the breast noted on admission. Mammography: 3 cm lipoma (trabeculae also displaced in other view). Pathology: 2.5 × 3 cm lipoma. The lesion must be clearly outlined in both mammography views.

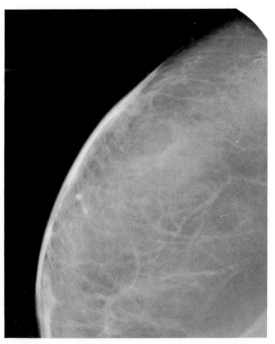

Figure 13–45. Scleroderma morphea. A 51-year-old white female with swelling of the breast for nine months and recent tenderness. Clinically: 4 × 6 cm area of hardened skin, mottled light pink hue, no underlying mass. Mammography: localized thickening of skin, minimal fibrosis beneath, no tumor, benign. Pathology: scleroderma morphea.

the skin and subcutaneous tissue, with flattening of the skin that may be apparent on the mammogram. On breast sonography disorganized echoes and/or some degree of attenuation of the beam may be produced. Since the underlying subcutaneous and glandular tissues are only slightly altered in appearance, the lesion is not confused with the local skin changes of carcinoma.

Nevus

A nevus may be sufficiently large to appear on mammography. It may appear on both views. A view tangential to the x-ray beam is helpful for a radiographic diagnosis. Usually air around the nevus can be recognized for the diagnosis of the dense discrete mass. On occasion nevi produce a stippled fine calcification pattern that must be differentiated from the calcifications of carcinoma. Nevi are characteristically denser than the skin and project above the skin (Fig. 13–46). They do not invade the subcutaneous tissue as one would expect with a melanosarcoma of the skin.

The location of all nevi should be known prior to interpretation of imaging studies.

Scar (Keloid)

A small linear scar of the breast may not be recognized on mammography. Yet even a small scar on a breast studied by sonography without compression may be readily apparent with the breast hanging loose in the water tank. This depends on the amount of subcutaneous fibrosis and shortening of the Cooper's ligaments and the depth of which this fibrosis extends into the breast. The fibrosis, in turn, depends to some degree on whether there had been some associated infection. Keloids may be associated with similar subcutaneous fibrosis as well as piling up the scar tissue itself to several millimeters in thickness. Their importance relates to the differentiation of secondary changes associated with carcinoma (see Chapter 19).

In these skin lesions, any attentuation of the beam will extend from the skin into the subcutaneous tissue and breast as a helpful differential point.

Cystic

Sebaceous (Epidermal) Cyst

The sebaceous cyst may become large enough to be demonstrated on breast imaging. As a benign skin appendage tumor it is

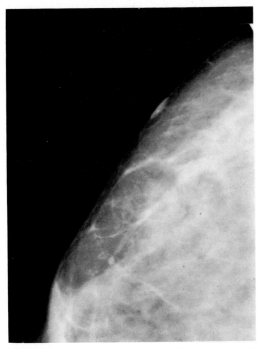

Figure 13–46. Nevus. A 55-year-old woman seen for routine checkup. Clinically: nodular breast with a nevus. Mammography showed only nodular breast and a nevus. Sonography: bulging of skin, marked attenuation by the nevus.

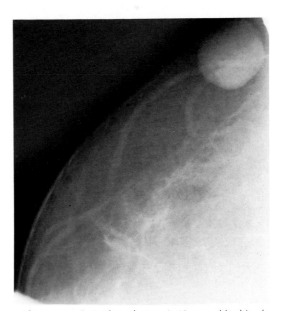

Figure 13–47. Epidermal cyst. A 40-year-old white female with a breast nodule present for one year. Clinically: 4 × 2.5 cm firm nodule. Mammography: 2.3 cm smooth, homogeneous, benign lesion, not related to breast tissue, located near the skin; a skin appendage cyst. Pathology: 3.8 × 2.5 cm epidermal cyst.

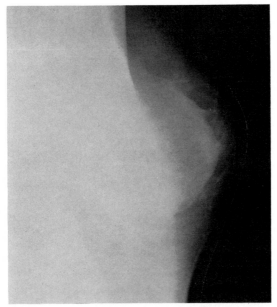

Figure 13–48. Epidermal cyst. A 48-year-old white female with a mass in the breast for an indeterminate number of years. Clinically: 10 × 5 cm hard, nodular, movable mass; no retraction or nodes. Mammography: 5 cm benign lesion, atypical fibroadenoma. Pathology: 4.5 × 4.2 × 4.0 cm cyst filled with white, amorphous, friable material; cyst wall 2 mm thick; epidermal cyst. (An unusually large cyst.)

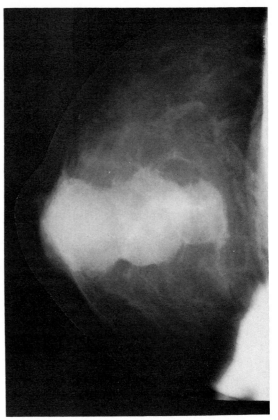

Figure 13–49. Bilateral apocrine gland hyperplasia and cyst formation. A 58-year-old white female with masses in both breasts for six months. Clinically: 4 × 4 cm carcinoma left breast; 5 × 5.5 cm carcinoma right breast, bilateral axillary metastases, Paget's disease of both nipples. Mammography: smoothly margined densities, subareolar in location; thickening and deformity of the overlying skin; bilateral carcinomas (right only shown). Pathology: bilateral apocrine gland hyperplasia with numerous cysts ranging in size from 10 mm to 45 mm.

in the subcutaneous area, its most distinguishing feature (Figs. 13–47 and 13–48). It is perhaps the only rounded, well-demarcated, homogeneous cystlike lesion seen in this location. Despite the presence of internal echoes, the cystic nature of the mass will be evident on sonography.

Aprocrine Gland Hyperplasia

Aprocrine gland hyperplasia of any significant degree is usually associated with cyst formation. It is located in the subcutaneous area of the breast and in the region of the areola, where glandular tissue is scant. The glands most commonly involved are those about the areola, suggesting the etiology (Fig. 13–49). The cysts usually elevate and thin the overlying skin. The cysts arising from the areolar skin may extend into the underlying breast tissue. Again, a rounded, well-demarcated cystlike lesion in this area suggests the diagnosis.

Hematoma

A localized hematoma consists of a local cystic dilatation of a subcutaneous vein with blood. It presents as a circumscribed round or oval mass (Fig. 13–50). The tip-off will be the rather small cyst, its location along a vein on mammograms, recent trauma, and perhaps residual ecchymosis.

Despite the frequent history of trauma to the breast, hematomas are not often seen. A hematoma or hemangioma may produce a discrete, smoothly outlined lesion in the subcutaneous adipose tissue. The hematoma is usually associated with a history of trauma and ecchymosis of the overlying skin. A subcutaneous vein may be traced into the mass (likened to a vessel into a cavernous lake in the skull) and away from it, suggesting the diagnosis.

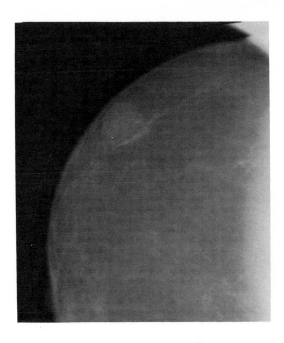

Figure 13–50. Hematoma that subsequently resorbed. A 53-year-old white female who bumped her breast seven days previously noted ecchymosis two days later. Clinically: no mass but disturbing ecchymosis. Mammography: 11 × 15 mm smooth lesion, from its location a sebaceous cyst. Normal study three weeks later (not shown); the ecchymosis had disappeared. Follow-up at three years showed no clinical or radiographic abnormality.

DISCRETE SUBAREOLAR LESIONS

Noncystic

Inverted Nipple

Nonspecific shortening of the major ducts or a congenital deformity may produce varying degrees of nipple retraction and actual inversion (Fig. 13–51). The dense fibrous tissue of the nipple may appear as a mass with attenuation of the sound beam. If there is any question on sonography, the patient can be examined clinically. An air pocket at the inverted nipple can be avoided by filling the space with petroleum jelly.

Subareolar Fibrosis

In the region of the subareolar ducts an increase in density is such a frequent finding

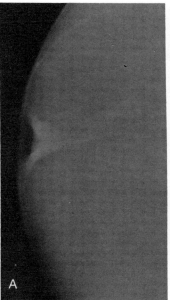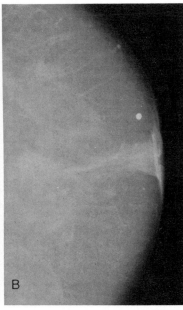

Figure 13–51. *A,* Congenital retraction of the nipple. A 55-year-old white female with bilateral nipple retraction as long as she could remember (examined because of a mass in the opposite breast, a carcinoma, with the same degree of nipple retraction). Clinically: confusing, since there was a carcinoma in the other breast. Mammography: nonspecific nipple retraction. No change during four-year follow-up. *B,* Nonspecific nipple retraction. A 65-year-old white female with nipple retraction for six weeks. Clinically: retraction of the nipple only. Mammography: nonspecific retraction of the nipple. No change in subsequent four years.

on the mammogram that it can be difficult to assess its exact significance. Dilated ducts and intraductal papillomata often produce increased subareolar density, but when uncomplicated by periductal inflammatory changes, the ducts are sharply outlined even when dilated and tortuous. Such dilated ducts are usually soft, without production of a palpable mass. Even after a radiologist has seen a number of mammograms he will be unable to judge when the normal dilatation has extended into the abnormal. Usually it is of no concern unless the etiology of a subareolar mass or nipple discharge must be explained. Description of the normal mammogram is almost as difficult as describing the normal mucosal pattern of the colon.

There is a definite pattern of development from normality to subareolar fibrosis that is readily appreciated if a series of mammograms in various stages of the process are examined. As dilatation in the ampullary portion of the ducts progresses, the dilated portion of duct may extend beyond the periphery of the areola or deep into the breast substance. The duct wall becomes less distinct owing to the periductal inflammatory reaction, usually noted first in the subareolar area but extending progressively deeper into the glandular tissue. At this stage, there is some shortening of the ducts with minimal nipple retraction (Fig. 13–52). The outlines of the large ducts are lost as the result of fibrosis. A homogeneously dense, poorly defined mass, roughly triangular in shape and with the apex at the nipple, becomes evident beneath the areola and extends several centimeters into the breast tissue (Figs. 13–53 and 13–54). Sharp, coarse calcifications may be seen; these are usually located in the area of the density beneath the areola but may be scattered throughout the breast (Fig. 13–55). This type of calcification is usually associated with secretory disturbances of the breast. The thin radiolucent line just beneath the skin extends its normal course toward the base of the nipple, an invaluable differential point from carcinoma in this site.

Carcinoma arising from the subareolar area does not differ from carcinoma elsewhere in the breast; it is not symmetrically placed in relation to the nipple and produces definite skin changes when of comparable size. Subareolar fibrosis is usually bilateral, with one breast more involved by ductal dilatation and fibrosis than its mate. In cases of well-advanced subareolar fibrosis there may be some hesitation in dogmatically excluding carcinoma (Fig. 13–56) (see Chapter 20).

Abscess

Breast abscesses range from a mild periductal inflammatory process, through a pus-filled necrotic pocket with marked peripheral

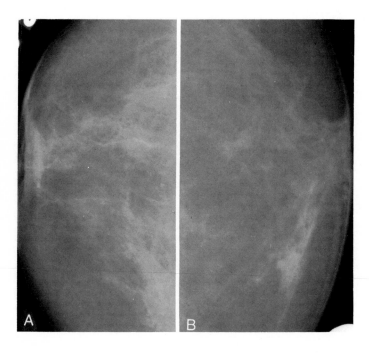

Figure 13–52. *A,* Composite density of dilated ducts as beginning subareolar fibrosis. A 44-year-old white female with breast pain and bleeding nipple for seven years. Clinically: dilated ducts with serosanguineous nipple discharge. Mammography: dilated ducts. Pathology: cystic dilatation of ducts with moderate hyperplasia. *B,* Dilated ducts with nipple retraction as progression. A 45-year-old female admitted because of retracted nipple of unknown duration. Clinically: carcinoma with Paget's disease of the nipple. Mammography: dilated ducts with early subareolar fibrosis. Pathology: dilated terminal ducts containing desiccated material and thick gray secretions with periductal nonspecific inflammatory changes.

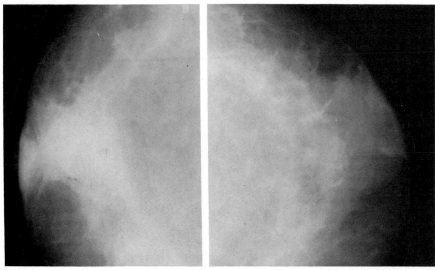

Figure 13–53. Bilateral nature of subareolar fibrosis. A 47-year-old black female with right nipple discharge for two months. Clinically: bilateral dilated ducts and clear nipple discharge on the right. Mammography: bilateral dilated ducts with subareolar fibrosis more marked on the left. Pathology: (left breast only): dilated ducts with inspissated material, cystic dilatation of the ducts, nonspecific inflammatory changes.

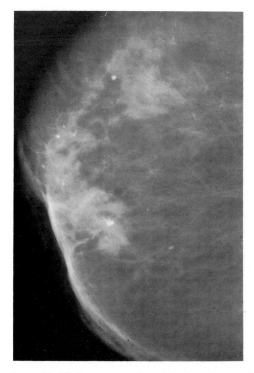

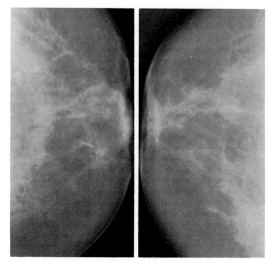

Figure 13–54. Subareolar fibrosis, bilateral. Mammograms were made of both breasts of a 62-year-old patient, gravida 5, para 5, with gradual retraction of both nipples over the past six to eight years. Clinically: retracted, fixed nipples; ill-defined bilateral subareolar thickening. Mammography: bilateral density beneath both nipples, shortened prominent ducts, and retracted nipples with one side more advanced than the other.

Figure 13–55. Asymmetric advanced subareolar fibrosis. This 67-year-old woman noted progressive nipple retraction for two to three years; at one time she was bothered by a nipple discharge. Clinically: invasion of the nipple and retraction of the skin of the areola with a 4 cm hard, fixed mass beneath the nipple. Mammograms: 2 cm poorly circumscribed subareolar mass, coarse and fine sharp calcifications, marked nipple retraction, and overlying skin thickening and retraction; subareolar carcinoma. Pathology: 1.5 × 2.5 cm mass of chronic inflammatory tissue with marked fibrosis.

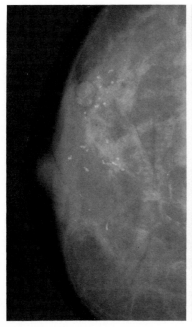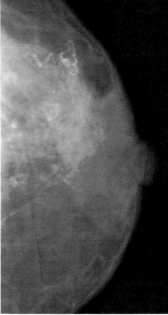

Figure 13–56. Advanced subareolar fibrosis to the degree of plasma cell mastitis. A 57-year-old white female with a lump deep to the right nipple and nipple discharge. Clinically: watery nipple discharge on the right; also, firm subareolar mass with nipple retraction; left breast, no abnormality. Mammography: advanced subareolar fibrosis bilaterally, more marked on the right, with scattered coarse calcifications, verruca; faint calcifications on the left. Pathology (right breast only): duct dilatation, surrounding severe fibrosis with calcifications, nonspecific inflammatory changes.

fibroglandular reaction, through a chronically draining process, to fibrotic replacement and residual scarring. The acute abscess and the chronic abscess may mimic carcinoma radiographically (Figs. 13–57 and 13–58). They may also be hard retractive masses clinically, or they may produce skin edema and reddening, suggesting inflammatory carcinoma.

Since the place of entry for the bacteria in most breast abscesses is in the vicinity of the nipple, most of the changes are in the subareolar area. Infectious processes usually involve ducts containing inspissated material; extension along these dilated ducts does occur. There may be spontaneous discharge of material through the nipple: A localized abscess may form, which either drains spontaneously or produces satellite abscesses, or incision and drainage is done. Usually a fistula is formed, with slow healing of the abscess accompanied by reinfection and exacerbation. A chronic breast abscess then ensues (Fig. 13–59). On occasion, an infected cyst is encountered.

Early involvement of the ducts will appear simply as a dilated duct, with possible indistinctness of its margins. As an acute abscess is formed there may be increased vascularity, overlying skin thickening, and indistinct, infiltrative density. At this stage, differentiation from a subareolar carcinoma is difficult. The associated clinical signs are the same as

the first manifestations of inflammatory carcinoma. The distinct spiculation of carcinoma is not seen, and there is no characteristic calcification within the abscess. Laminated

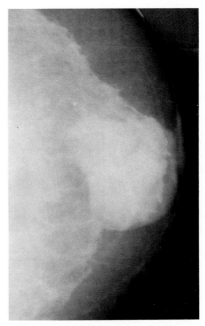

Figure 13–57. Early abscess formation. A 64-year-old white female with a breast lump for one week. Clinically: 3 × 2 cm carcinoma deep to the nipple. Mammography: 3 × 4 cm density, smooth anteriorly, irregular posteriorly; carcinoma. Pathology: acute and subacute mastitis with abscess formation.

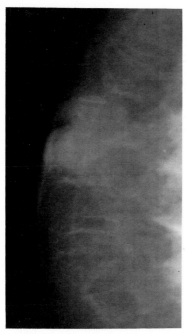

Figure 13–58. Chronic recurring breast abscess. A 36-year-old white female, gravida 5, para 5, with repeated subareolar infections requiring incision and drainage, following the birth of her last child five years before. Clinically: 4 cm indurated mass above level of nipple with pus exuded through a small ulceration. Mammography: 2 cm density, infected cyst with thickening of overlying skin. Pathology: localized, 2 cm chronic breast abscess.

thickening of the skin is seen occasionally over the abscess; this has not been observed in carcinoma and may prove a useful differential point in diagnosis.

The chronic breast abscess lacks the symmetry of density beneath the areola, the homogeneous density, and the coarse flecks of calcification of subareolar fibrosis (Fig. 13–59). Clinical information is of little value in differentiation of carcinoma from abscess, especially when chronic granulomatous tissue has developed in the infectious process. In only half the breast abscesses was differentiation from carcinoma made with any degree of certainty by mammography. This is not particularly discouraging, as many of the abscesses require surgical treatment in the form of excision so that tissue will be available for microscopic study.

Many breast abscesses will require additional radiographic evaluation and often follow-up of their clinical course and response to antibiotics. If enough skin changes of reddening and edema are present to suggest inflammatory carcinoma, that breast is already inoperable and a short course of antibiotic therapy will cause no harm.

Granulomatous lesions occur (Fig. 13–60).

Intraductal Papilloma

To be seen on breast images the intraductal papilloma must produce localized dilatation of a duct (Figs. 13–61 and 13–62). Rarely does the intraductal papilloma contain the distinguishing mulberry configuration of tiny calcifications—usually so small that they are obscured by the surrounding tissues. Diffuse

Figure 13–59. A, Chronic breast abscess. A 40-year-old white female with a slowly growing breast mass for four months. Clinically: 3 cm mass, definitely fixed, dimpling of the skin, retraction of the nipple; carcinoma. Mammography: 1 cm subareolar mass with retraction and thickening of areola; carcinoma (in retrospect, subareolar fibrosis would be a better choice of diagnosis by mammography). Pathology: 2.8 × 2.5 × 2.4 cm mass due to chronic breast abscess. B, Chronic granulomatous tissue resulting from a breast abscess. A 48-year-old white female, para 13, with a small lump above the areola for one year; three months ago it was swollen, red, and tender and drained spontaneously. Clinically: ill-defined central mass with retraction; carcinoma. Mammography: skin changes without definite mass, chronic breast abscess. Pathology: chronic granulomatous inflammatory tissue.

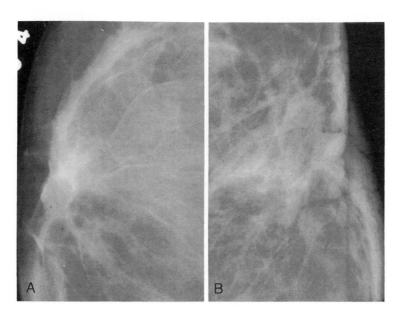

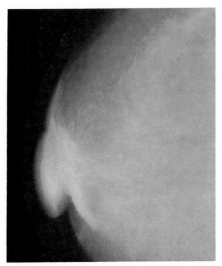

Figure 13–60. Granuloma of the nipple area. A 67-year-old black female. Clinically: subareolar mass. Mammography: subareolar dense abscess with localized skin and nipple thickening. Pathology: granuloma of the nipple area suggestive of tuberculosis.

subareolar papillomata may produce an appearance similar to that of duct dilatation with inspissated material. An isolated papilloma may be some distance from the ampulla, may produce cystic dilatation up to several centimeters with repeated hemorrhage, and cannot be differentiated from an intracystic papilloma. Usually the intraductal papilloma alone produces an intermittent bloody nipple discharge, since it does not completely block the ducts as the intracystic papillary lesion often does.

Contrast studies may outline the papilloma but at times will show only a nonspecific obstruction or filling defect (Fig. 13–62*B*). Many papillomata calcify (Fig. 13–63) or become sclerotic (Fig. 13–64).

Sonographically there may be nonspecific diffuse or local duct dilatation. If a cystic lesion is formed in the breast, it will manifest the signs of a cyst but may retain internal echoes (Fig. 13–65).

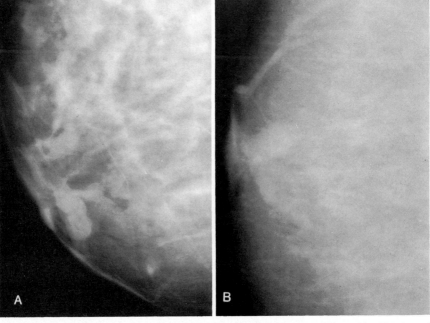

Figure 13–61. *A,* Intraductal papilloma. This 58-year-old woman had noted intermittent bleeding from this nipple for four months. Clinically: Several drops of blood could be expressed; no mass. Mammography: 1.2 × 0.7 cm lobulated mass just beneath the inferior portion of the areola associated with at least two dilated ducts; benign, but etiology not definite. Pathology: 1.5 × 0.5 cm intraductal papilloma. *B,* Intraductal papilloma associated with ductal epithelial hyperplasia. This 55-year-old woman had been aware of an intermittent nipple discharge for several years; recently the nipple became sore. Clinically: vague subareolar mass, clear nipple discharge, excoriation of the nipple. Mammography: poorly defined 1 cm density beneath the nipple and moderately increased vascularity (compared with opposite breast). Papilloma was histopathologically proved.

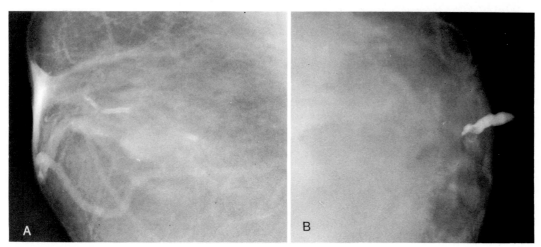

Figure 13–62. A, Discrete intraductal papilloma. A 69-year-old white female with bloody nipple discharge for four months. Clinically: bloody nipple discharge, 0.5 cm nodule. Mammography: 1 cm smoothly rounded benign lesion; intraductal papilloma despite nonspecific retracted nipple and increased vascularity. Pathology: 1 cm intraductal papilloma. B, Contrast study of an intraductal papilloma. A 41-year-old white female with annoying bloody discharge for one month. Clinically: bloody nipple discharge. Mammography: dilated ducts. Contrast mammography: dilated ducts with small irregular obstructing lesion; intraductal papilloma. Pathology: intraductal papilloma.

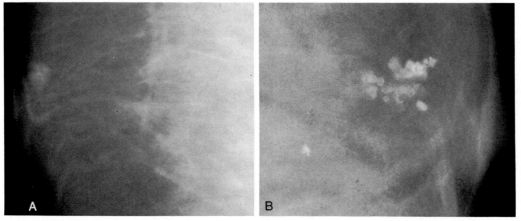

Figure 13–63. A, Calcifying intraductal papilloma. A 56-year-old white female with a sore breast and nipple discharge. Clinically: 4 mm nodule or dilated duct, clear nipple discharge. Mammography: 6 × 9 mm nonmalignant subareolar mass containing calcification; either intraductal papilloma or dilated duct. Pathology: 5 × 7 mm intraductal papilloma. B, Coarse calcifications of a large duct papilloma. A 62-year-old woman who had a previous biopsy of the breast. Clinically: large pendulous breasts. Mammography: fatty breast, periareolar skin distortion from the previous biopsy, and a cluster of large calcifications probably related to the major ducts. Pathology: old degenerated intraductal papillomata with heavy amorphous calcifications. These are unlike the fine mulberry calcifications usually associated with a papilloma.

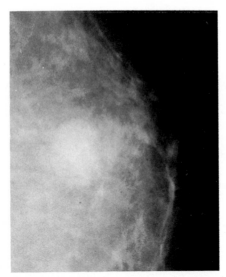

Figure 13–64. Intraductal papilloma. An 83-year-old woman with a firm subareolar breast mass. Mammography: 1.2 × 1.4 cm circumscribed mass that probably is associated with the major duct system. Pathology: a sclerotic papilloma.

Sweat Gland Adenoma

Sweat glands are normally found in the areola and skin of the breast. Neoplasms rarely arise from these sweat glands. If so, they are benign and produce no specific changes except for location. They usually start as a "pimple" and may enlarge to ulceration.

Miscellaneous Subareolar Lesions

For appraisal of nipple retraction, each mammogram must be obtained with the nipple in exact profile. Some degree of nipple retraction is frequently encountered, espe-

cially in the involuting breast. Even with rather marked nipple retraction, few abnormal densities may be noted. Congenital nipple retraction is nonspecific on the mammograms. It is well to remember carcinoma can occur in a patient with congenital nipple retraction.

Nonspecific granulomatous infections are usually indolent, long-standing, and fairly well circumscribed on the mammograms. The usual fungi and pathogens are grown in cultures. Many of the lesions are merely academic, since their ominous clinical nature eventually leads to removal of tissue to establish the diagnosis.

Cystic

Dilated Ducts

Ducts dilated with inspissated material, when the dilatation is limited to the major ducts, cannot always be differentiated from ductal dilatation resulting from intraductal papillomata and/or ductal hyperplasia (Figs. 13–66 and 13–67). In almost all breasts there is some degree of ductal enlargement. This occurs first in the region of the ampulla, and the dilation may extend progressively deeper into the glandular tissue (Figure 13–68); several ducts may be involved. As dilatation progresses elongation of the duct occurs, with the resultant wormy appearance on the mammogram beneath the areola; the scanty periductal fat beneath the areola becomes displaced; and the composite shadow of numerous dilated ducts produces a homogeneous density, usually triangular, beneath the areola. This finding is usually bilateral, and more advanced in one breast than the other.

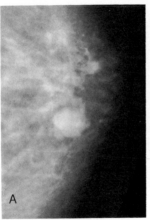
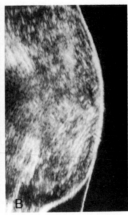

Figure 13–65. Papilloma. A 54-year-old woman seen for checkup. Clinically the breasts were normal. *A,* Mammography: ductal hyperplasia, lobular subareolar benign mass; dilated duct vs papilloma. *B,* Sonography: hypoechoic subareolar area. Pathology: intraductal papilloma.

Figure 13–66. *A,* Dilatation of major ducts, duct ectasia. This 51-year-old woman had bloody discharge of the nipple for at least six weeks. Clinically there was a serosanguineous nipple discharge, flattening of the nipple, and an ill-defined subareolar mass, probably carcinoma. Mammograms revealed no evidence of malignancy. Histopathologic study demonstrated markedly dilated ducts with inspissated grumous material. *B,* Cystic dilatation of ducts. A 51-year-old black female with breast lump for one week. Ill-defined thickening deep to the areola. Mammography: smoothly dilated ducts. Pathology: cystic dilatation of the ducts containing amorphous grumous material.

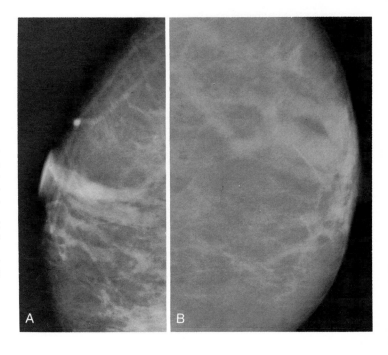

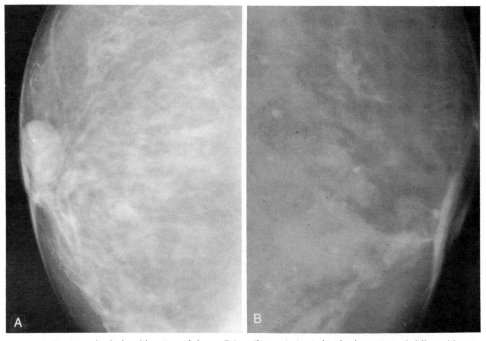

Figure 13–67. Cystic and tubular dilatation of ducts. Primarily cystic in *A,* but both cystic and diffuse dilatation in *B.*

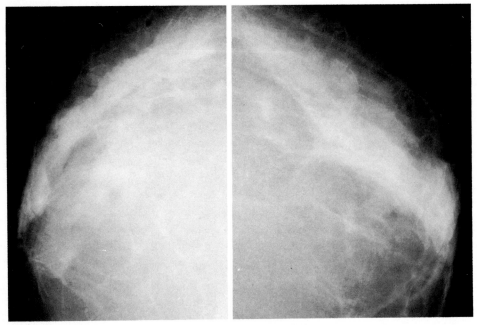

Figure 13–68. Bilateral dilatation of major ducts. A 67-year-old woman for checkup. The enlarged ducts extend from the subareolar area deep into the breasts.

An intraductal papilloma more often involves one duct and may be more deeply located in the breast substance, deeper than the ampullary region where nonspecific duct dilatation begins. Extensive ductal hyperplasia also involves numerous ducts, but the less smoothly outlined branching ducts are easily traced deep into the breast substance. The dilated duct may become secondarily infected, causing abscess formation with the production of secondary signs of infection: reaction about the duct, increased vascularity, and thickening of the overlying areola. Fibrosis may result (Fig. 13–69).

There may be inspissation of material in a duct after lactation, producing the appearance of a dilated duct. Once the grumous material is extruded, the appearance of the mammograms returns to normal.

Intraductal Papilloma in Dilated Ducts.

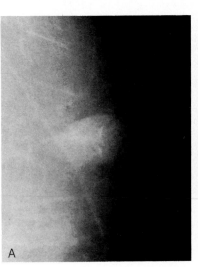
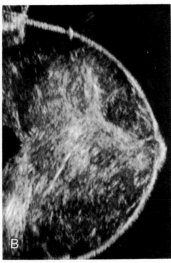

Figure 13–69. Mass of duct ectasia and periductal fibrosis. A 67-year-old woman seen for baseline mammogram. *A,* Mammography: 0.8 × 1.2 cm indistinct mass with slightly lobulated borders. *B,* Sonography: prominence of Cooper's ligaments and distortion of breast architecture. No malignancy upon biopsy.

Intraductal papilloma in dilated ducts will have no identifying characteristics except as a compound lesion on sonography.

DIFFUSE INTRAGLANDULAR LESIONS

The approach of grouping similar mammographic appearances has resulted in excellent correlation of certain wide-field views on mammograms. With selected areas for histopathology study, some groupings show promise with further study and other groupings are less promising. There are distinct and recognizable patterns of diffuse, usually bilateral, radiographic changes in the breast that allow categorization. Certain patterns reflect distinct entities, but most frequently the patterns are mixed and overlapping.

Noncystic

Fibrocystic Disease

Fibrocystic disease is a highly descriptive term for certain gross changes in the breast, and it is most adaptable to the radiologist's terminology. The term "fibrocystic disease"

is intended to encompass all those processes that are characterized by cyst formation, duct dilatation, lobular or ductal hyperplasia, and stromal fibrosis of varying degree and in varying combinations. For convenience in describing the mammograms, fibrocystic disease may be separated into three types: (1) predominantly cystic, (2) predominantly fibrous, and (3) ductal or lobular hyperplasia. (Lymphocytic infiltration is a feature of fibrocystic disease that is not recognized on the mammograms.)

PREDOMINANTLY FIBROUS DISEASE

A radiographically recognizable form of fibrocystic disease, similar in appearance to the fibrous component of the fibrocystic disease with identifiable cysts, may be identified in many breasts in which discrete cyst formation is absent. No specific dominant nodule is outlined on the mammograms, but confluent deposits may produce a clinically palpable nodule (Figs. 13–70 and 13–71).

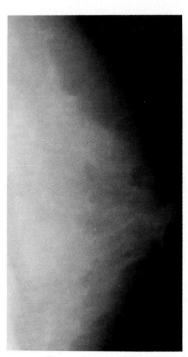

Figure 13–70. Fibrotic element of fibrocystic disease. A 2 × 3 cm dominant nodule was palpable in this breast of a 38-year-old woman. The mammograms indicate a generalized increased density of the breast without a demonstrable nodule. Histologic study of the nodule provided diagnosis of fibrosis and fibrocystic disease.

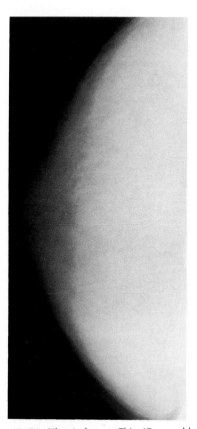

Figure 13–71. Fibrotic breast. This 47-year-old woman had lumps in both breasts for one year. Clinically she had several masses in both breasts; the largest mass was in the upper outer quadrant of this breast and at biopsy was 0.5 cm. Histologic study revealed severe fibrosis.

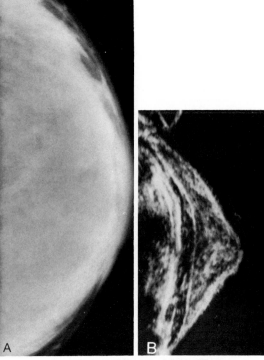

Figure 13–72. Fibroplasia, a form of fibrocystic disease. A 25-year-old woman with lumpy breasts. *A,* Mammography: dense, almost homogeneous breast tissue with a paucity of fat in both the subcutaneous and the glandular portions of the breasts. *B,* Sonography: high-level echoes with a distorted architectural pattern; no visible subcutaneous fat. The pectoral muscle development suggests an athletic woman.

FIBROPLASIA

In the breasts of some women approaching menopause, near-homogeneity of the breast on mammography is maintained (Figs. 13–72 and 13–73). From the radiographic appearance, these could easily be regarded as pubertal or young adult breasts. These women have persistent mastodynia; the breasts remain firm, are difficult to examine clinically, and often contain vague nodularities. Difficulty arises in deciding whether such breasts are normal variants or are diseased. The pathologist's description of extreme fibroplasia led us to consider this mammographic appearance as a distinct entity, a diffuse form of fibrocystic disease of fibrous type.

DUCTAL OR LOBULAR HYPERPLASIA

There are two distinct forms of hyperplastic types of fibrocystic disease that may be recognized by mammography. Usually each is more commonly associated with the premenopausal type of breast, in which consid-

erable glandular tissue remains, the breast is relatively firm, and that breast still retains moderate radiographic density. Both may be present to varying degrees in the same breast, but both are bilateral.

Ductal Hyperplasia. Rather prominent major ducts may be traced into the breast to a greater extent than is normally seen. The ducts may be distinctly outlined in continuity into the third or even fourth arborization. They then become apparent as numerous ill-defined 2 to 3 mm densities that resemble snowflakes (Figs. 13–74 and 13–75). As a rule, these densities do not interfere appreciably with the x-ray study of the breast. Ductal hyperplasia is a strong secondary sign of carcinoma mammographically (see Chapter 16).

Lobular Hyperplasia. Numerous densities scattered throughout both breasts, often with one breast slightly more involved than the other, may be recognized. The densities are

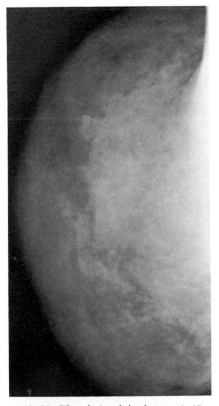

Figure 13–73. Fibroplasia of the breast. A 45-year-old white female with painful breasts and a lump present for three days. Clinically: 3 × 4 cm mass, possible carcinoma; nodularity in both breasts. Mammography: diffuse, dense glandular tissue; fibrocystic disease; no malignancy. Pathology: diffuse fibrocystic disease with extreme fibrosis; fibroplasia.

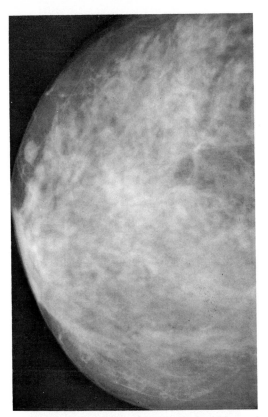

Figure 13–74. Fibrocystic disease with ductal hyperplasia. A 46-year-old white female with injury to the breast four days before. Clinically: subareolar nodule with superficial ecchymosis. Mammography: ductal hyperplasia; the small subcutaneous benign lesion above the nipple proved to be a hematoma. Pathology: fibrofatty tissue containing old hemorrhage; ductal hyperplasia.

of lobular or segmental distribution. Some opacities are quite large and dense, obscuring overlying trabeculae and producing homogeneous areas. Their outlines mimic the irregular borders of certain cysts; other lesions with clear margins may suggest fibroadenomata. Some have almost straight edges as though restrained by the supporting ligaments (Fig. 13–76). Less typically, the densities due to hyperplasia or adenosis may be sparse. Thus, it is difficult to differentiate among areas of hyperplastic fibrosis, ill-defined areas of conglomerate cyst formation, and fat necrosis.

SCLEROSING ADENOSIS

Some areas of sclerosing adenosis may be microscopic in size or may exist in variably sized, ill-defined patchy densities on the mammogram; they may be diffuse, with or without coalescence of densities on the mammograms. Specific radiographic delineation

of the specific density that will be labeled sclerosing adenosis by the pathologist is not possible with any degree of certainty. The association of sclerosing adenosis with calcification patterns is discussed in Chapter 27.

The radiologist may be overwhelmed by the multiplicity of densities in the breast (Fig. 13–77); this need not occur, as he can study each area and each nodule of each breast, initially and upon follow-up studies, pinpointing areas of concern.

MIXED TYPES

Most breasts show a mixture of the types of fibrocystic disease (Fig. 13–78).

Fibroadenomata

Fibroadenomata are usually solitary or few in number. On occasion, numerous fibroadenomata may be identified throughout one or, more often, both breasts (Figs. 13–79 to 13–81). In the very young dense breast only one or two may be identified, and these only with difficulty. As additional adipose tissue is deposited in the breast, numerous lesions may be identified by the characteristic ap-

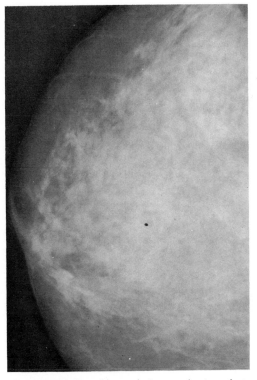

Figure 13–75. Ductal hyperplasia as predominant feature of fibrocystic disease. This 47-year-old woman presented with a lump in the opposite breast that proved to be an area of fibrosis associated with ductal hyperplasia.

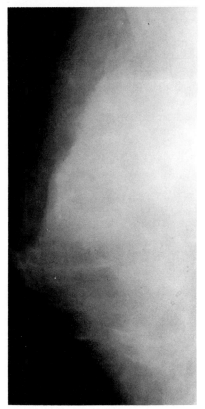

Figure 13–76. Lobular hyperplasia. The mammogram shows a nonspecific increase in density. Clinically a dominant nodule was present that proved on biopsy to be lobular hyperplasia. Note the smooth border anteriorly, sometimes diagnostic of adenosis.

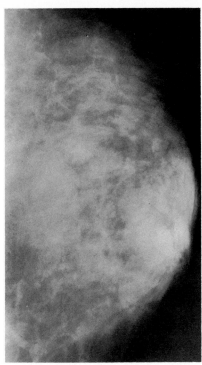

Figure 13–78. This mammographic mixed pattern of fibrocystic disease is the more frequently encountered, particularly in patients around menopausal age. This 47-year-old woman complained of slightly tender, lumpy breasts.

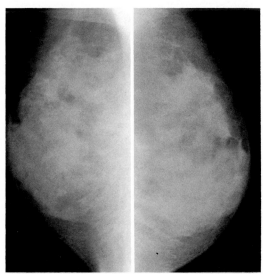

Figure 13–77. Fibrocystic disease, sclerosing adenosis. A 42-year-old white female with a mass in the left breast for two years, similar mass in the right breast of almost the same duration; nipple discharge. Clinically: 4 × 2.5 cm mass, left breast, without skin fixation. Mammography: (left and right): 4 × 2 cm mass deep to each areola, subareolar fibrosis; fibrocystic disease. Pathology: (left breast only): fibrocystic disease, sclerosing adenosis, intraductal papillomata.

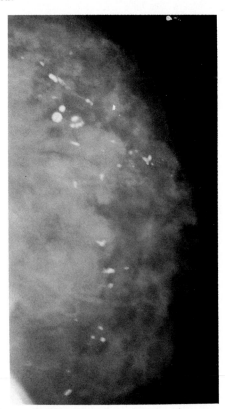

Figure 13–79. Fibroadenomatosis. The numerous masses, calcifying and noncalcifying, are fibroadenomata. This 89-year-old woman had masses in both breasts for many years. Clinically, bilateral carcinoma was suspected.

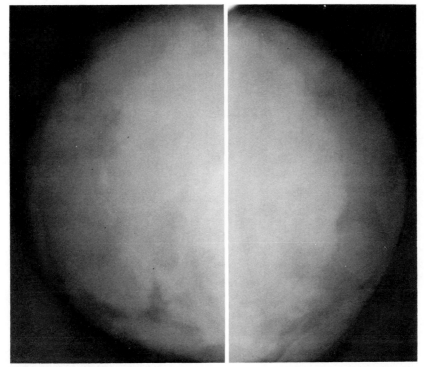

Figure 13—80. Bilateral large fibroadenomata. This 18-year-old student had been aware of lumps in her breasts for two to three years. More recently, some of them were enlarging. Several were removed.

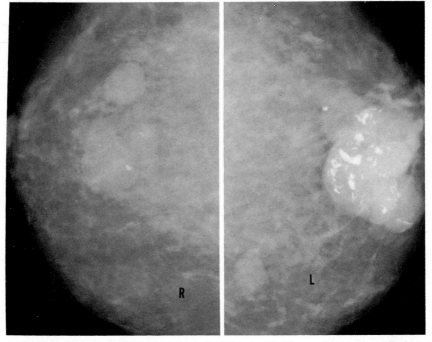

Figure 13—81. Numerous lobulated fibroadenomata in both breasts. A 53-year-old woman with clinically diagnosed malignancy in left breast and normal right breast. Centrally there were 2.5 and 5 cm masses palpable in the left breast. Mammography reveals many more fibroadenomata than were suspected clinically and also indicates the masses of calcifications in the lesions.

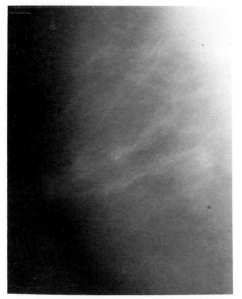

Figure 13–82. Intraductal papillomata. These ill-defined densities proved on histologic study to be intraductal papillomata. This 49-year-old woman complained of vague breast pain and and intermittent serous nipple discharge.

pearance or by the presence of coarse calcification. Diffuse fibroadenomata may pose a differential diagnostic problem with cystic disease or adenosis.

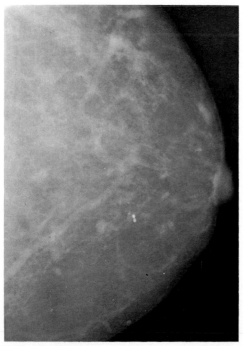

Figure 13–83. Papillomatosis. A generous subareolar biopsy revealed numerous papillomata. Most of the other ill-defined densities are probably also papillomata. The patient, a 51-year-old woman, presented with a serosanguineous nipple discharge.

Intraductal Papillomata

Intraductal papillomata may be diffusely scattered throughout the glandular tissue and at some distance from the major ducts, just as with multiple fibroadenomata. Since the solid or cystic character of these small discrete nodules cannot be determined by their appearance on the mammograms, it is impossible to arrive at a histologic diagnosis (Figs. 13–82 to 13–84). Sonography may be helpful, however.

Miscellaneous Diffuse Intramammary Lesions

Areas of traumatic fat necrosis and of hyperplastic fibrosis may be diffuse in nature and have little in the way of distinguishing radiographic characteristics. In practice, they

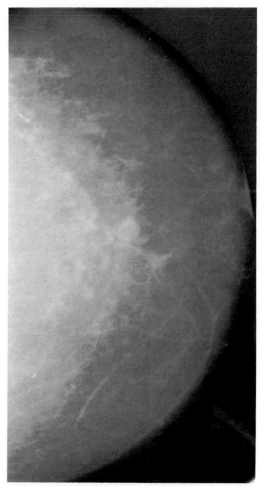

Figure 13–84. Intraductal papillomata, diffuse. A 70-year-old woman with carcinoma of the opposite breast. Clinically: vague nodules in the breast. Mammography: discrete benign nodular deposits measuring up to 1 cm in diameter; fibrocystic disease. Pathology: multiple intraductal papillomata.

no doubt would be placed in a diagnostic category with fibrocystic disease, fibrous type.

Lactating mastitis produces increased diffuse, nearly homogeneous density in the already dense lactating breast and may be difficult to evaluate on the mammogram. Localized or diffuse bacterial mastitis may be encountered (Figs. 13–85 to 13–87). Tuberculosis also produces a diffuse increase in density throughout the breast (Fig. 13–88). Diffuse hemorrhage into the breast, usually following surgical exploration, produces a rather characteristic appearance. The area of hemorrhage is homogeneous and denser than a pubertal breast, owing to the diffuse deposition of hemosiderin (Fig. 13–89).

The breasts are subject to all types of trauma, including self-inflicted injury (Figs. 13–90 and 13–91). Foreign bodies in the breast are frequently encountered (Fig. 13–92). Ointments and medication on the skin of the breast sometimes produce confusing shadows on the mammograms; metallic compounds suspended in ointment may appear

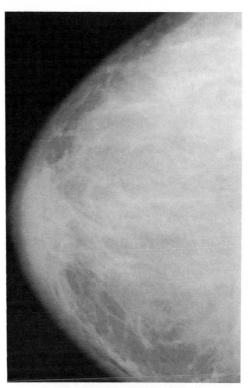

Figure 13–86. Diffuse bacterial mastitis. This 54-year-old woman noted rapid development over the past five days of a large painful mass in the lower inner quadrant of the breast. Upon needle biopsy, foul-smelling purulent material was obtained. Microscopic study showed acute inflammation with pus cells; no malignancy.

as tiny flecks of calcification. With views of the breast in profile these densities will be on the skin and not in the breast substance. Abnormal growth patterns are often diffuse (Fig. 13–93).

Calcifications

Breast calcifications are, on one end of the spectrum, unequivocally benign and, on the other end, unequivocally malignant. The central gray area is a problem to all mammographers. This has been referred to in the section on specimen radiography.

Cystic

Cystic Fibrocystic Disease

Many cysts dispersed throughout the breast frequently are encountered and produce a honeycombed appearance to the breast grossly. Sonographically and mammographically these cysts have the same characteristics as single cysts.

A simple cyst that is a discrete lesion in an

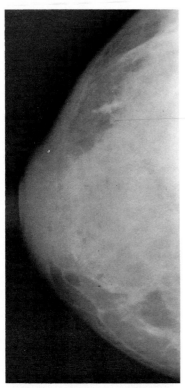

Figure 13–85. Localized mastitis of subareolar portion of breast. A mammogram was performed on a 43-year-old woman after biopsy in the area seven days earlier for fibrocystic disease. There is diffuse density, thickening of the skin lateral to the nipple, and a few small residual air pockets.

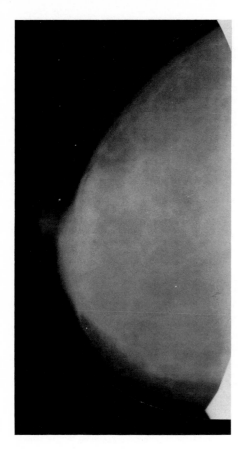

Figure 13–87. Postlactating mastitis. A 43-year-old black female, gravida 12, para 10; breast mass for one month; cessation of lactation five months previously. Clinically: diffuse mass, skin edema, positive axillary node; carcinoma. Mammography: diffuse density in breast, localized areolar skin thickening, no underlying mass; carcinoma. Pathology: chronic mastitis.

Figure 13–88. Diffuse tuberculosis of the breast. A 67-year-old white female with enlarging breast for an indefinite period. Clinically: diffuse enlargement and turgidity of the breast; skin edema; carcinoma. Mammography: diffuse density throughout the breast without demonstrable mass but with diffuse skin thickening; carcinoma. Pathology: tuberculosis of the breast.

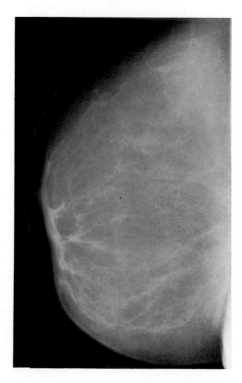

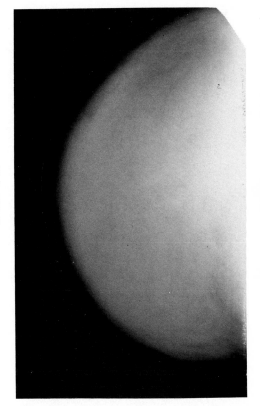

Figure 13–89. Diffuse breast hemorrhage. Hemorrhage occurred in a 38-year-old woman following a biopsy nine days previously for fibrocystic disease. Clinically: A large mass was felt, but upon biopsy there were only changes of fibrocystic disease and marked hemosiderin deposits in the glandular tissue. Mammography shows diffuse increased density in the breast.

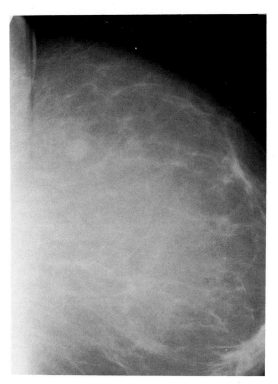

Figure 13–90. Breast caught in wringer. A 54-year-old black female who presented with osteolytic metastases and a history of having caught her breast in a washing machine wringer several months previously. Clinically: carcinoma of the breast. Mammography: localized, slightly laminated, thickened skin, without underlying mass; benign. Post-mortem studies two months later: small primary bronchogenic carcinoma; benign thickening of the skin of the breast.

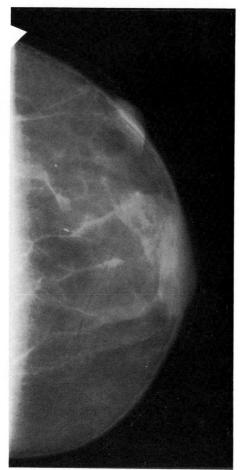

Figure 13–91. Second-degree burn. A 66-year-old white female with subareolar inflammatory changes and axillary lymph node enlargement. Application of a hot water bottle to the breast resulted in a second-degree burn; note blister on the skin.

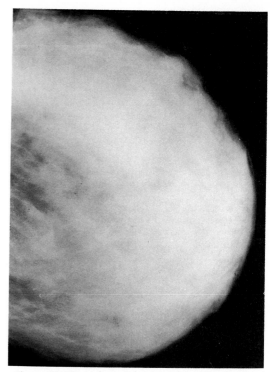

Figure 13–93. Malignant hypertrophy of the breast. A 30-year-old woman with breasts swollen three times normal size. Three years ago her breasts had swelled but not so badly. Biopsy at the time indicated a benign process. The patient had been on one month of therapy for rheumatoid arthritis prior to the initial x-ray study on 5-11-82. She had been off drugs for the second study on 7-1-82. Mammography: 5-11-82: dense fibroglandular tissue throughout both breasts with only minimal edema of the subcutaneous fat. Marked diffuse skin thickening extending outward from the areola. 7-1-82: resolving parenchymal density and skin changes. Sonography: high-level nonhomogeneous echoes throughout both breasts; thickened skin around the areola. The second study shows partial resolution. Pathology: malignant hypertrophy with apparent excessive growth of glandular tissues, connective tissue, and fat, with an unremarkable appearance. After a three-month regimen of progesterone the breasts had returned to almost the previous size.

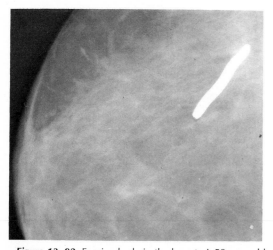

Figure 13–92. Foreign body in the breast. A 58-year-old white female with a questionable nodule in the breast. Mammography: normal breast except for presence of a metallic foreign body. The patient could not recall how it arrived there.

otherwise normal breast is an infrequent finding. Usually the overall appearance is that of multiple cysts with accentuation of the intervening glandular and connective tissue pattern (Figs. 13–94 and 13–95). There generally is one large dominant cyst—on occasion possibly two or more discrete cysts—as well as numerous smaller cysts, producing shadows that cannot be differentiated from masses of hyperplastic tissue. Numerous cysts are seen symmetrically distributed throughout the glandular tissue, and the smaller the cysts, the more numerous they are. The cysts are round or ovoid, or their shape may be determined by the pressure exerted on their walls by surrounding

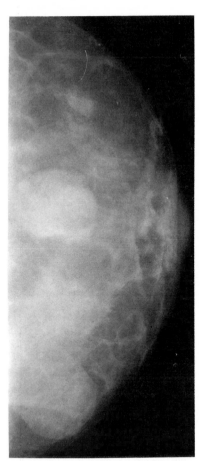

Figure 13–94. Numerous cysts as dominant feature of fibrocystic disease. Some of the cysts are clearly outlined; some are partially obscured by dense surrounding tissue. This 20-year-old woman had been aware of lumps in both breasts for several months.

evaluation. Experience indicates that the radiologist rarely overlooks carcinoma in such breasts if the mammograms are satisfactory.

OBSERVATIONS

In Table 13–2 the nomenclature of the pathologist for benign breast biopsy cases overlaps, but generally hyperplastic or overgrowth patterns producing increased density on the mammogram or fibrosis and scarring were found in most of the x-ray false positive diagnoses. Many descriptive diagnostic terms were often used to refer to the same breast and to the same lesion, but only the single most appropriate one was used in the table. In the large number of breasts containing clustered calcifications not associated with a mass, a malignant lesion was found in only 25 to 33 per cent of the biopsies. Since these calcifications occur with a wide range of the pathologists' diagnoses, they are scattered throughout the table, not just under adenosis and ductal hyperplasia.

supporting structures. The disease is bilateral. Only rarely is a single cyst identified—a reliable differential point from single fibroadenoma.

The breast containing numerous cysts may be confusing and difficult to evaluate clinically. Frequently, the clinician feels a nodule in the less involved breast and reports the severely involved breast normal, or he may single out a small, radiographically insignificant cyst and completely overlook large cysts in other areas of the breast. Apparently such large, nonpalpable cysts enlarge so gradually that they do not have sufficient tension to be firm and hence feel like the surrounding tissue. Over a short time a small increase in fluid may increase the tension within the cyst making it uncomfortable and causing the patient to feel the mass.

Even with the increased overall density of these breasts and the many cysts present, mammography is proving an aid in clinical

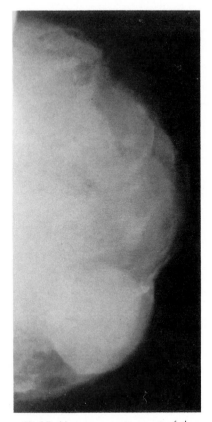

Figure 13–95. Numerous cysts, most of them poorly outlined. This 44-year-old woman had several cysts removed, others aspirated. Mammograms revealed bilateral cysts which were proved by needle aspiration of clear amber fluid.

TABLE 13–2. Various Benign Histopathologic Diagnoses, Their Radiologic Diagnoses, and Those Lesions Most Frequently Confused with Carcinoma

Benign Lesion with Biopsy	Total	Benign X-ray Diagnosis	Coded as Malignant
Fibrocystic disease	2136	1933	203
Fibroadenoma	1181	1046	135
Sclerosing adenosis	168	112	56
Ductal hyperplasia	110	80	30
Adenosis	104	80	24
Abscess	89	43	46
Fibrosis	88	53	35
Intraductal papilloma	80	64	16
Gynecomastia	63	63	0
Duct ectasia	48	46	2
Lipoma	31	31	0
Fibrous mastopathy	24	23	1
Duct papillomatosis	22	20	2
Cystosarcoma phylloides	21	16	5
Lymph node, benign	18	18	0
Duct hyperplasia with atypia	16	6	10
Sebaceous cyst	16	16	0
Blunt duct adenosis	12	6	6
Duct papilloma with atypia	12	10	2
Scar tissue	12	11	1
Fat necrosis	11	2	9
Mastitis	11	10	1
Apocrine metaplasia	8	6	2
Cystic disease cysts	8	8	0
Focal calcifications only	7	2	5
Cystic dilatation	6	6	0
Terminal duct hyperplasia, atypia	6	2	4
Lobular hyperplasia, atypia	6	5	1
Hematoma	6	4	2
Radial scar	5	5	0
Fibrous hyperplasia	4	3	1
Scleroderma morphea	3	2	1
Fatty infiltration	3	3	0
Lobular atypia	3	1	2
Dilated ducts	3	3	0
Tuberculosis	2	1	1
Neurofibroma	2	2	0
Ectopic breast	2	2	0
Periductal mastitis	2	2	0
Cystic hyperplasia	2	2	0
Radiation changes (prior treatment)	2	1	1
Masoplasia	1	0	1
Granulomatous tissue	1	0	1
Granular cell myoblastoma	1	1	0
Subtotal	4356	3750	606
Cyst aspiration	2006	1911	95
Total	6362	5661	701

Encountered in 55,157 consecutive mammograms at Emory University.

The rate of fibroadenoma biopsy would have been higher in this series except that in very young women mammography was not routinely used prior to breast biopsy, inasmuch as they went directly to surgery. It was in the older women of cancer age that mammography was more frequently used prior to biopsy. In a number of these patients, mammography, confirmed by sonography, revealed the presence of a solid dominant nodule; without identifying amorphous calcifications, the diagnosis of fibroadenoma was not definite by x-ray.

Considering the total number in this series of 4356 benign and 2077 malignant biopsies, the overall rate of benign biopsies labeled malignant by x-ray was 9.4 per cent. If cyst aspiration was considered a diagnostic procedure, and the cyst was suspicious in 95 mammograms, that false positive rate was 8.3 per cent.

REFERENCE

Haagensen CD (1971): Disease of the Breast, 2nd ed. Philadelphia, W.B. Saunders, p 235.

Malignant Breast Lesions

14

BACKGROUND

Mammograms depict all the significant changes in breast diseases, except heat and color, that are detectable on clinical examination. The mammogram records the obvious changes often seen on photographs of the breasts used as a diagnostic procedure. Radiography is a better controlled and more valuable method than transillumination or ultrasound for evaluation of the relative density of breast masses. Mammography encompasses the diagnostic features of infrared photography as well, with finer delineation of more veins. Mammography contains the salient features of the various approaches to diagnosis of lesions in the intact breast, demonstrates changes more clearly and accurately, and provides a detailed study of a mass in its environment.

The clinically freely movable carcinomatous nodule lacks secondary changes and cannot be precisely differentiated from a single benign mass or distinguished from other movable benign nodules in the same breast. In contrast to the paucity of primary clinical signs of carcinoma of the breast, several valuable local signs appear on the mammograms, some of which are almost pathognomonic. More than one such sign is often present in the same lesion. The same signs utilized for the clinical diagnosis of carcinoma of the breast frequently are appreciated much earlier on the mammogram.

In most breast lesions a single glance at the mammogram suffices for the diagnosis of a mass. If scrutiny of the mass on the mammogram is not sufficient for a diagnosis, study of the complete breast must be made, including nipple, areola, skin, glandular structures, subcutaneous tissues, retromammary space, vascularity, and axilla.

The typical malignant tumor of the breast not only produces localized changes at the primary site of the lesion but also may excite diffuse alterations in some or all of the breast structures at a distance from the lesion. The appearance of the mass itself is primarily a result of its capacity for infiltration of the surrounding tissues and replacement of normal structures. Some of the diffuse and distant changes in the breast cannot be explained so readily.

RADIOGRAPHIC SIGNS OF CANCER

The radiographic diagnosis of malignant breast diseases depends on local and distant changes produced by the disease. At times more than one sign of breast cancer will be present and one sign will be frequently associated with another sign, e.g., skin retraction and skin thickening or a highly infiltrative mass and increased vascularity. Yet it is considered most appropriate to present each sign separately.

The changes on the mammograms indicating the diagnosis of cancer of the breast may be conveniently thought of as local, or primary signs, and distant, or secondary signs, as follows:

I. Primary mammographic signs of cancer
  A. Density of the lesion
  B. Relative size of the lesion
  C. Shape of the lesion
  D. Calcifications
II. Secondary mammographic signs of cancer
  A. Nipple and areolar changes
  B. Skin thickening
  C. Skin retraction
  D. Increased vascularity
  E. Ductal hyperplasia
  F. Asymmetry
    1. Distortion of breast architecture
    2. Straightened trabeculae
    3. Increased stromal density
  G. Nonspecific duct prominence
  H. Axillary lymph nodes
  I. Intramammary lymph nodes

Primary Mammographic Signs of Cancer

The malignant lesion to some extent displaces and compresses structures; to a much greater degree the lesion actually infiltrates the surrounding tissue and produces destruction and distortion of the trabeculae. In the peripheral zone of the carcinoma, clumps or strands of malignant cells excite irregular fibrosis with retraction and reactive edema. Consequently, the periphery may be composed of clear, distinct, fine linear strands extending irregularly outward from a central mass; there may be a blur or halo from marked edema; or there may be varying combinations of each kind of reaction (Figs. 14–1 to 14–8).

The primary signs of mass and calcifications of breast cancer are so important and sufficiently overlap the changes of benign diseases that separate chapters (18 and 27) are devoted to mass and calcifications.

The primary radiographic signs of carcinoma are related to the tumor mass and include its density, clinical vs x-ray size, shape, borders, and calcification content. The actual size of the tumor makes little difference in diagnosis. In the fatty breasts, regardless of how pendulous and difficult to

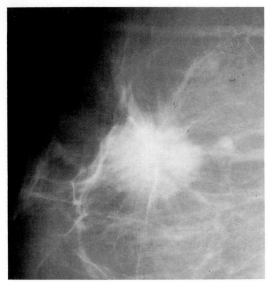

Figure 14–1. Highly infiltrative breast carcinoma. The patient, a 70-year-old woman, presented with a lump in her breast. Such advanced carcinomas are readily diagnosed either clinically or by mammography. Clinically the mass was 4.5 × 5 cm; on the mammograms it measured 2 × 2.5 cm.

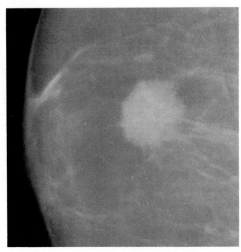

Figure 14–3. Slightly less infiltrative carcinoma than that seen in Figure 14–2. There is less retraction of the ducts and nipple and less reaction about the periphery of the mass. This 62-year-old woman had noted a breast lump for three weeks.

examine clinically, carcinomas less than 0.5 cm are readily diagnosed. However, these may be difficult to detect in glandular breasts by mammography and palpation even at the time of open biopsy. Large, clinically evident lesions may be obscured by increased density of the skin and edematous breast tissues. Spiculated masses as small as 2 × 3 mm in size may be easily diagnosed if a few flecks

of calcification are present. The frequency of carcinoma calcifications is suggested in Table 14–1.

Secondary Mammographic Signs of Cancer

Approximately 80 to 85 per cent of localized breast cancers will be readily diagnosed by the x-ray appearance of the mass; in the remaining cancers the presence or absence of very reliable secondary signs must be used for diagnosis. Secondary signs of malig-

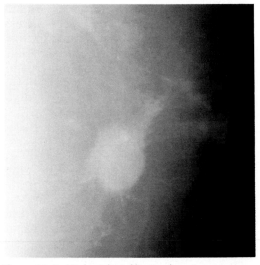

Figure 14–2. Moderately infiltrative breast carcinoma. The patient, a 57-year-old woman, had noted "drawing in" of the nipple for two months. Several major ducts are stretched into prominence, and there is nipple flattening.

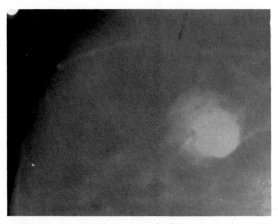

Figure 14–4. Well-circumscribed carcinoma in a 67-year-old woman with no complaint. Spicules may be seen in some parts of the periphery, however. Routine follow-up for mastectomy performed on the opposite breast five years before.

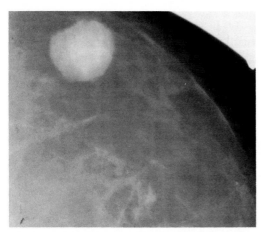

Figure 14–5. Well-circumscribed carcinoma that almost appears benign. There is no real fat line; close scrutiny shows very fine spicules arising from several points on the periphery. This 80-year-old woman had noted a lump for two months. Clinically, the 2.5 × 1.5 cm firm mass with questionable skin changes suggested carcinoma. X-ray: 1.5 cm circumscribed carcinoma. Pathology: 1.5 cm medullary carcinoma with lymphoid stroma; axillary lymph nodes free of metastases.

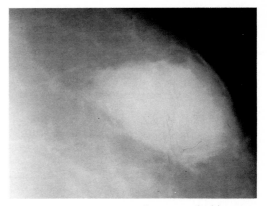

Figure 14–7. Moderately well-circumscribed breast carcinoma. In a portion of the periphery there is a suggestion of an incomplete fat line. There are faint calcifications, skin changes, and increased vascularity to indicate the diagnosis radiographically. This 57-year-old woman had been aware of breast changes for at least eight months.

nancy, even though elusive at times, occur in such a high percentage of these lesions that the diagnosis is even more definite in the majority of carcinomas. In reference to mammographic detail, it is far more desirable to have excessive complementary criteria than to have insufficient data for a sound diagnosis.

The mammographer must first become fa-

miliar with the classic secondary signs of breast carcinoma in order to appreciate the finer, more subtle changes of early breast cancer. The first 126 consecutive carcinomas that I studied, in the first clinical application of mammography, are used to demonstrate the frequency of the secondary radiographic signs of carcinoma, even though technically these studies were superior in quality to our present-day screen-film mammography. Although many of these carcinomas were ad-

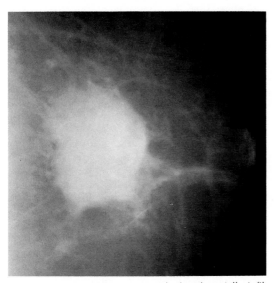

Figure 14–6. Partially circumscribed and partially infiltrative mass of carcinoma. This 63-year-old woman had noted the presence of a lump in her breast for over six months.

Figure 14–8. Faint mass of highly infiltrative carcinoma. Some carcinomas apparently spread so widely and rapidly that there is little chance for production of a solid mass. This central carcinoma in a pendulous clinically normal breast was found on routine follow-up after opposite radical mastectomy four years previously.

TABLE 14–1. Frequency of Typical Calcification Associated with Carcinoma of the Breast and the Area of Calcification in 126 Consecutive Carcinomas Studied by Mammography

Carcinoma Calcification (Area-Diameter)	Number
None	50
Less than 1 cm	12
1–2 cm	35
2.0–5 cm	27
Over 5 cm	2
Total	126

vanced both clinically and radiographically, they do display the secondary signs of carcinoma of the breast. Unfortunately, these signs are still encountered today.

The secondary radiographic signs of carcinoma are nonspecific but extremely valuable nonetheless. They include nipple and areolar changes, skin retraction, skin thickening, increased vascularity, ductal hyperplasia, distortion of breast architecture, increased stromal densities, nonspecific duct prominence, axillary lymph nodes, intramammary lymph nodes, and invasion of the retromammary space.

The relationship of the cancer to the breast and the response of the breast tissues is poorly understood but is complex. The altered physiology associated with the abnormal tumor-host situation is varied and poorly coordinated with the histologic type of cancer or its size and location. A small primary breast carcinoma may evoke a multiplicity of marked breast changes, such as increased vascularity, increased heat, collagenosis, diffuse skin thickening, distant fibrotic response, prominence of the ducts, retractive phenomena, signs of inflammation, and distant metastasis. Yet a very large breast cancer may have an indolent growth pattern with very little secondary response from the surrounding tissues. One individual may respond with breast enlargement and signs of

inflammatory cancer, yet another's response to the presence of cancer will be atrophy or shrinking of the breast with thickened, cool skin.

Only prolonged and meticulous investigation of whole-organ studies will yield valid data that can be used to understand the varied host responses and the growth patterns of breast carcinomas. These secondary radiographic signs of breast cancer need not be completely explained to be useful whenever necessary in arriving at the proper diagnosis.

Nipple and Areolar Changes

Nipple retraction is a nonspecific sign but can occur with carcinoma (Table 14–2). The degree of retraction is subjective, and the exact relationship to the carcinoma cannot always be judged with certainty.

Nipple and areolar changes associated with carcinoma will be seen repeatedly throughout this series of cases. Without the demonstration of a carcinoma, the finding of nipple retraction is of little importance radiographically; in the clinical presence of nipple retraction, however, the mammogram may allay the anxiety of the clinician. Complete inversion of the nipple is frequently associated with a benign process; despite the stronger and more numerous attachments of the ducts and trabeculae to the nipple, carcinoma aggressive enough to produce nipple inversion has often produced fixation of the nipple by edema. A breast with nonspecific nipple retraction (Fig. 14–9) or with congenital retraction may develop an unrelated carcinoma. Other illustrations are shown in Chapter 20.

Skin Thickening

Localized thickening of the skin immediately overlying the carcinoma is a valuable secondary sign of carcinoma, frequently appreciated on the mammograms before it is apparent clinically. The frequency of this finding (Table 14–3) refers to the routine

TABLE 14–2. Frequency of Nipple Retraction, Increased Vascularity, and Distant Fibrotic Exposure to Cancer in the First Consecutive 126 Cancers Studied by Mammography

Degree	Nipple Retraction	Increased Vascularity	Distant Fibrotic Tissue Response
None	84	68	87
Minimal	9	9	—
Moderate	28	42	23
Marked	5	7	16
Total	126	126	126

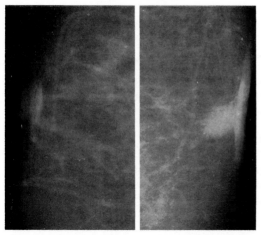

Figure 14–9. Nipple retraction—only sign of carcinoma. A 75-year-old woman who was treating her slowly retracting left nipple with hot soaks and petroleum jelly. No mass clinically. Mammograms: retraction of nipples, with an underlying density on left, but no mass. Upon biopsy of this area there was noncalcifying intraductal comedocarcinoma and microinvasive papillary carcinoma. After modified radical mastectomy all 24 axillary lymph nodes were free of tumor. Five years later the patient was free of disease.

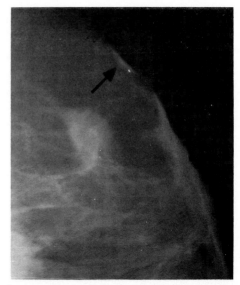

Figure 14–10. Localized skin retraction by carcinoma. A 70-year-old woman with soft 2 cm breast nodule clinically without skin changes. The 1.5 cm moderately invasive carcinoma clearly shows skin retraction and thickening.

mammographic views; with careful positioning to project the skin adjacent to the lesion in profile, a higher incidence of skin thickening can be demonstrated.

There is unusually a limited area of skin thickening associated with the localized area of skin retraction overlying the carcinoma. (Figs. 14–10 to 14–12). Clinically, local skin changes about the areola are appreciated only with difficulty. A carcinoma in this location usually produces some retraction of the niple, flattening of the areola, and thickening of the areolar skin.

As clinical findings of plateau formation, dimpling, or retraction become more obvious, progressive thickening of the skin with involvement of a larger area of the skin overlying the carcinoma occurs. This is more marked the more superficial the location of the carcinoma. While local thickening pro-

gresses there is next seen an area inferior to the nipple that begins to thicken as part of diffuse skin thickening. This quickly involves the skin of the whole breast as a diffuse thickening (see Chapter 19).

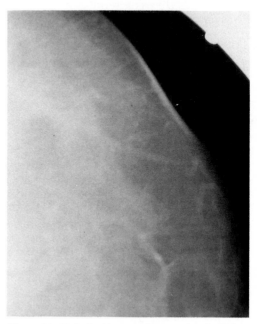

Figure 14–11. Early skin retraction associated with breast carcinoma. This is probably apparent only in thickening of the skin due to retraction. Such early flattening of the skin may be appreciated on the mammograms prior to clinical recognition. The patient, a 63-year-old woman, presented with a mass that proved to be infiltrating duct carcinoma with one positive low axillary lymph node.

TABLE 14–3. Frequency of Local Skin Thickening Associated with Carcinoma of the Breast in 126 Consecutive Carcinomas Studied by Mammography

Local Skin Thickening (Area-Diameter)	Number
None	77
Less than 2 cm	10
2–4 cm	29
Over 4 cm	10
Total	126

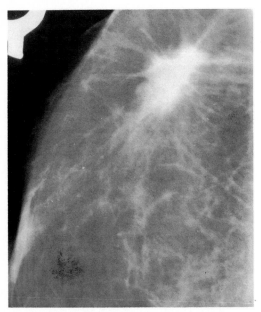

Figure 14–12. Local skin change not recognized clinically. A 71-year-old woman being treated for adenocarcinoma of the uterus. Vague breast complaints led to discovery of a 3 cm soft breast mass. A 2 × 1 cm carcinoma is producing early skin changes.

Skin Retraction

Usually localized skin retraction is adjacent to the carcinoma (Figs. 14–10 to 14–12). Some retractive strands may be seen extending from the carcinoma to the skin, but this is not always so. Whether the overlying skin is always thickened or merely is retracted to produce an apparent thickening cannot be judged with certainty (compare Figs. 14–11 and 14–12). Skin retraction over the tumor as well as retraction of the nipple may be located some distance from the mass. Frequently the localized areas of skin retraction cannot be appreciated clinically, even by experienced observers with optimal lighting, yet they are clearly evident radiographically (Fig. 14–12). Evidence of skin retraction or thickening in

an area not in profile on the mammogram may be indicated by a bandlike density, similar to a wrinkle in the skin of the breast. When necessary, the skin overlying the lesion may be studied more thoroughly with additional tangential views. A more detailed discussion of skin retraction and thickening is found in Chapter 19.

Vascularity

Increased vascularity, when present, is a useful secondary sign of a malignant lesion, but carcinomas do occur in breasts without increased vascularity and, on occasion, benign lesions produce an increase in vein size. The relative increase in size of subcutaneous veins of the breast is of aid in studying breasts containing malignant disease. On the mammograms, the diameter of the veins may become four times as great in the presence of carcinoma. Table 14–4 indicates how frequently this sign was present in the group of 126 carcinomas. Increased vascularity may be the only diagnostic aid with circumscribed carcinomas and is never lightly regarded. In our experience a mass of any type associated with increased vascularity was malignant 75 per cent of the time.

The presence of a poorly defined small carcinoma may be indicated by an increase in the caliber of the veins. On the mammograms, the size of the veins, rather than their number, is important (Figs. 14–13 to 14–15). There is a rather surprising symmetry of the veins, both in distribution and in size in the normal breast. There is great variation from individual to individual, however—so much so that mammograms of the uninvolved breast are needed for comparison. If there is an increase in vascularity about the lesion itself, these plexuses are indistinct; the small individual vessels probably contribute only to the haziness at the periphery of the carcinoma (Figs. 14–14 and 14–16). Increased vascularity is a less reliable sign of the presence

TABLE 14–4. Vein Diameter Ratio (VDR) as Measured for 101 Consecutive Mammography Cases*

Disease (Proved by Pathology)	No. of Cases	No. of True Positives	No. of True Negatives	No. of False Positives	No. of False Negatives
		VDR (1.2 × or Greater)			
Cancer	27	14 (51.8%)	—	5 (18.5%)	8 (29.5%)
Benign	54	—	26 (48.3%)	25 (51.7%)	—
		VDR (1.4 × or Greater)			
Cancer	27	10 (37.3%)	—	1 (3.7%)	16 (59%)
Benign	54	—	44 (81.5%)	10 (18.5%)	—

*Of the total, 20 cases were not suitable for measurement and 17 cases were previous radical mastectomy patients.

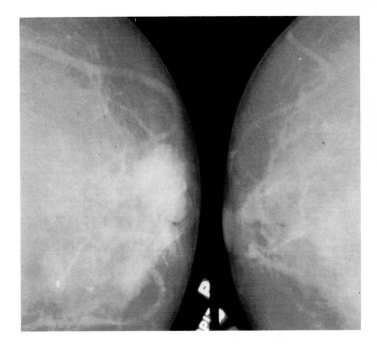

Figure 14–13. Increased vascularity associated with subareolar carcinoma (left). It is the caliber of veins that is increased, not necessarily the number. The veins visualized are usually subcutaneous; note the symmetric distribution.

of carcinoma than thickened skin, since prominent veins may be associated more frequently with benign conditions.

During the mid- to late 1950s, precise evaluation of increased vascularity in a breast with cancer was attempted. Biostatisticians at M. D. Anderson Hospital analyzed a group of consecutive mammography patients with breast cancer. Increased vascularity was judged present if veins in comparable views of one breast appeared larger in both the craniocaudad and the mediolateral views.

Enlargement was judged by visual inspection. There was increased vascularity in slightly less than 50 per cent of the patients with breast cancer. Approximately 25 per cent of benign lesions manifested increased vascularity. If a nodule was present on the mammograms and there was increased vascularity, that nodule had to be considered cancer.

The conclusions were that if increased vascularity were present along with other findings, it was most helpful; if increased vas-

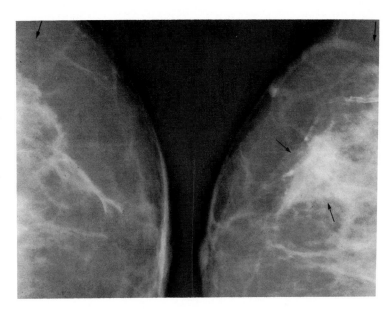

Figure 14–14. Carcinoma with increased vascularity. A 64-year-old woman with a suspicious breast nodule. Mammography: poorly defined mass with hazy borders due to local vascularity (arrow) with marked diffuse increased vascularity. Pathology: Stage II duct carcinoma.

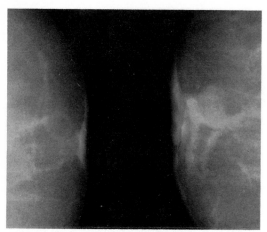

Figure 14–15. Occult carcinoma with increased vascularity. Search mammography (following proven metastasis to "egg-sized" axillary lymph node): subareolar mass with marked increased vascularity; primary breast carcinoma. Pathology: duct carcinoma.

cularity was the only finding, carcinoma was excluded only after careful study. Increased vascularity was a sign of relatively advanced cancer and had real prognostic significance: Without increased vascularity the prognosis for breast cancer patients for one- and five-year salvage was 87 and 67 per cent, respectively; with increased vascularity the prognosis for one- and five-year salvage was 74 and 11 per cent, respectively.

Recently, at Emory University a more sophisticated evaluation of the importance of increased vascularity in the diagnosis of breast cancer was attempted. Comparable veins, usually in the mediolateral mammographic view, were designated between two grease-pencil marks. Two engineers independently measured the width of the veins between the pencil marks using a 7-power microscope. The results of their measurements agreed completely on 101 consecutive mammography patients. The vein diameter ratios (VDR) of 1.2 and 1.4 were selected for analysis (Table 14–4). Fifty-two per cent of the carcinomas had a VDR of 1.2 or greater; also 52 per cent of the breasts with normal or benign disease had a VDR of 1.2. In 18 per cent of the patients with cancer, the normal breast unexpectedly had a VDR of 1.2 or greater. From Table 14–4 it is readily seen that use of a VDR of 1.4 reduced markedly the number of false positive diagnoses but also reduced the number of true positives.

From this study it was found that the eye readily judges a VDR of 1.2 and usually 1.1; a vein in one view may appear enlarged but in the other view may appear larger in the opposite breast. Visual inspection of the veins for increased vascularity in both views was superior to accurate measurement of the diameters in a single set of comparable views.

At times, increased vascularity is a most valuable secondary diagnostic sign of carcinoma and will lead to the proper diagnosis (Fig. 14–16 and 14–17). An infected cyst or breast abscess may produce increased vascularity. This can be observed in less specific processes, such as fibrocystic disease, or even in normal breasts (Fig. 14–18). When an increase of three to four times the usual size is noted in the caliber of the veins, carcinoma can be excluded only after careful analysis. Increased vascularity of the breast should

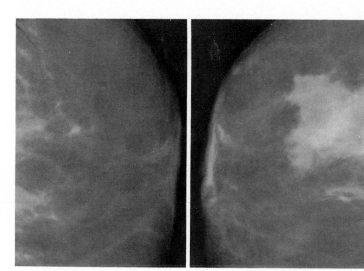

Figure 14–16. Infiltrative duct carcinoma. The nonspecific density projected just above the left nipple can be readily interpreted as carcinoma with use of the secondary signs of areolar skin change and increased vascularity. This infiltrative duct carcinoma was found in a 58-year-old woman who had had a breast lump for over eight months.

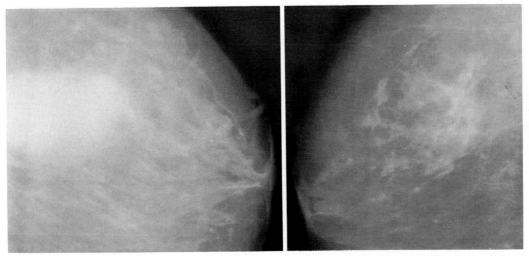

Figure 14–17. Appearance of lesion in the right breast strongly suggests an oval cyst against a background of diffuse fibrocystic disease. There is a suggestion of a fat line. The definite increase in vascularity is the key to the differential diagnosis of this well-circumscribed carcinoma from a cyst. The increased overall density of the breast is also an aid. The patient, a 63-year-old woman, had a 3 × 5 cm medullary carcinoma with lymphoid stroma.

alert the radiologist to inspect the mammograms carefully to be sure that the entire gland is recorded on the films. The exclusion of carcinoma should be considered only after excellent studies are obtained.

Ductal Hyperplasia

Ductal epithelial hyperplasia occurs so frequently with breast carcinoma that it can be considered a secondary sign, as described in Chapter 16.

Breast Asymmetry

Comparison of radiographs of paired organs for asymmetric changes is one of the oldest forms of diagnostic radiology, e.g., the lung in the intercostal interspaces, the renal calyces, or un-united epiphyses. Thus, in 1956 with the institution of mammography it was natural to compare the two breasts. Two things became apparent: (1) There was an extremely wide variation in the appearance of the breasts of different women; and

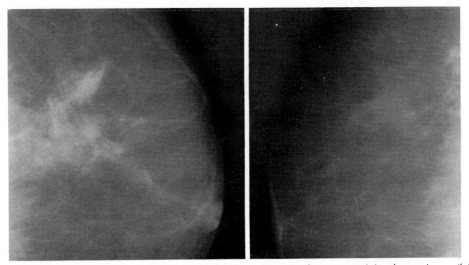

Figure 14–18. Moderate increase in vascularity in the right breast opposite the one containing the carcinoma (left breast). This is not usual but does occur on occasion, particularly if the carcinoma is small and only moderately invasive, as is this duct carcinoma in a 48-year-old woman studied for pain in the opposite breast. There are additional vague densities and nipple retraction, but this breast with increased vascularity has remained normal for over five years.

(2) the two normal breasts were highly symmetric. Meticulous care was exercised to obtain corresponding views of each breast in a similar fashion. In repositioning the breast to accomplish this it became readily apparent that a density in one view could be changed markedly by slight variation in positioning or technical factors. This was a strong reason that compression was avoided as much as possible. The two craniocaudad and the two mediolateral views were placed on the viewbox as mirror images of both breasts for interpretation of the studies.

These maneuvers together with close inspection of the mammograms revealed the most subtle variations in the two breasts. It was later, as women began returning for their comparative or follow-up mammograms that the policy of viewing older studies with newer ones in the same manner was adopted.

Other than the obvious asymmetry of masses, clusters of calcifications, and increased vascularity there emerged a more refined comparative study of distorted breast architecture, straightened trabeculae, fibrotic response, increased stromal density, nonspecific duct prominence, and any other asymmetry.

Distortion of Breast Architecture. Because most carcinomas of the breast occur in older patients with involuting fatty breasts, the carcinoma is readily demonstrated against this homogeneous adipose tissue. Breasts will frequently contain numerous ill-defined or somewhat discrete opacities in addition to the dominant nodule of carcinoma. This increase in density is best appreciated by comparison with the opposite breast (Fig. 14–13, 14–16, 14–17, and 14–19 to 14–22). In such cases the pathologist, after what he considers a careful study, may assure us that carcinoma was demonstrable only in the actual mass. Densities in the other breast as well as the thickened skin and increased vascularity in the breast with cancer may be due to the presence of carcinoma and not to its invasion of these areas. The secondary changes of the breast stroma with carcinoma are associated with an overall increase in density of the gland. Changes of fibrocystic disease are constantly bilateral, often with one breast more involved than the other, but without overall increase in density of the organ. These densities in the stroma associated with carcinoma may be indistinguishable from numerous foci of lobular carcinoma or at times from satellite nodules of carcinoma; however, either ap-

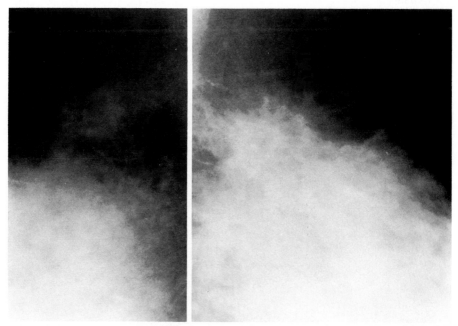

Figure 14–19. Asymmetric density signals breast carcinoma. A 54-year-old woman with a thickening in the UOQ of the right breast. Close inspection of this asymmetry revealed ducts packed with cells and extremely minute calcifications between the benign-appearing visible ones. Biopsy and modified radical mastectomy: abundant intraductal comedocarcinoma plus infiltrating duct carcinoma over an area of 3 × 2 × 1.8 cm; extensive lymphatic permeation and areas of vascular involvement; 0 of 18 low and 2 of 9 midaxillary lymph nodes contained metastases. The patient was free of disease three years later.

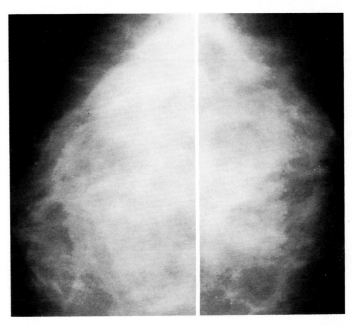

Figure 14–20. Altered architecture producing asymmetry in the right breast. A 44-year-old woman seen for checkup; previous biopsy 20 years before. No mass was noted but some background stranding of ducts was suggested. Sonography confirmed the altered architecture. Biopsy revealed intraductal and duct carcinoma with a scirrhous element. All 18 nodes recovered from the modified radical mastectomy were free of tumor. Three was no evidence of disease two years later.

pearance helps to substantiate the diagnosis of malignant disease. Closer and more complete whole-organ studies are demonstrating such changes to be the cause of these previously poorly understood densities. Another explanation that appears feasible is the overly marked collagenosis associated with some breast carcinomas.

Satellite nodules of carcinoma of the breast cannot be differentiated from additional primary carcinomas on the mammograms. Small deposits of carcinoma, in a breast containing a larger carcinoma, may be considered satellite nodules. No real significance is attached to the differentiation of multiple primaries, satellite nodules, and distant fi-

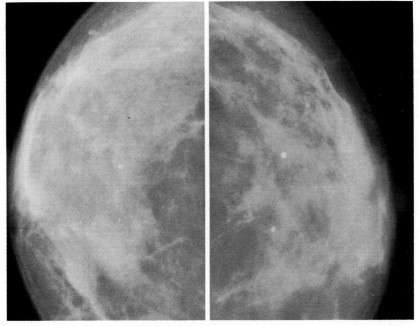

Figure 14–21. Asymmetry in fatty breasts. This 64-year-old woman had a checkup as she was still taking hormones following oophorectomy many years previously. The asymmetry, with increase in density on the right, slightly inner quadrant, is doubly suspicious when coupled with the increase in vascularity. A Stage I (11 nodes negative for tumor) duct carcinoma.

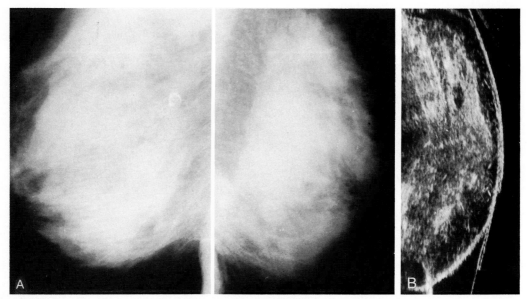

Figure 14–22. Sonography is an aid in cases of vague asymmetry. A 62-year-old woman; no family history; left breast biopsy 29 years before. *A,* Mammography: right breast larger with more fibroglandular tissue; asymmetric area on the left, straightening of Cooper's ligaments well above the nipple, increased vascularity. *B,* Sonography; persistent irregular hypoechoic area with nonhomogeneous internal echoes; disruption of the surrounding architecture; small cyst at a distance. Pathology: 1.5 × 2 × 3 cm hard mass of intraductal and duct carcinoma with scirrhous component; ductal hyperplasia. Modified radical mastectomy; 3 of 18 axillary lymph nodes with metastases.

brotic response; each finding indicates poor prognosis.

Distant fibrotic response to the presence of a carcinoma in the breast is often a subjective evaluation, best appraised by comparison with the mammogram of the opposite breast (Fig. 14–23). Even with a minimal or questionable finding the tissue was considered abnormal unless readily explained (e.g., by a previous biopsy). Such a change has been diligently searched for and explains the high incidence of this finding (Table 14–2). This finding may be the first change noted on serial mammograms rather than increase in density of the carcinoma per se.

Increased Stromal Density. Asymmetry of the supporting structures may be noted on the mammograms and may be a reflection of

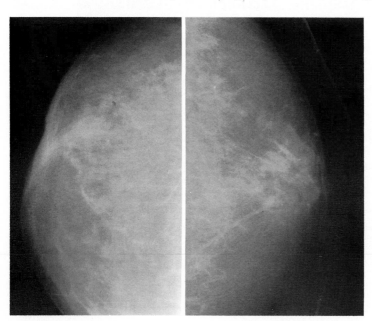

Figure 14–23. Ominous asymmetry produced by a papillary intraductal carcinoma. This 82-year-old woman was studied for a red right nipple discharge of one week's duration. No masses were present. Mammograms: a poorly defined subareolar mass, flattening and thickening of the areola, increased density in the breast, and increased vascularity. Although there was wide ramification within the duct system by the papillary carcinoma, no invasion could be demonstrated.

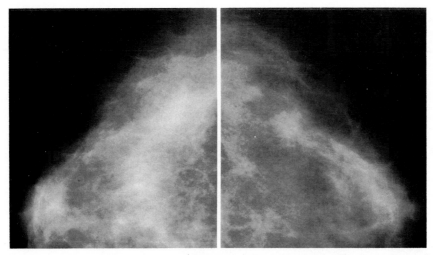

Figure 14–24. Asymmetry in nodular breasts. A 36-year-old woman with nodular fibrocystic disease for evaluation. Mammography: ductal hyperplasia with islands of fibroglandular tissue, increased asymmetrically on the right upper and middle portions of the breast. On such a background this asymmetry is viewed with suspicion, although coalescent fibroglandular tissue is possible. Pathology: duct carcinoma; modified radical mastectomy; 19 axillary lymph nodes free of tumor. Sixteen years later no evidence of disease.

a carcinoma. Numerous ill-defined or even somewhat discrete opacities may be present in addition to the dominant nodule of carcinoma. Void of carcinoma cells or glandular tissue upon microscopic study, these scattered fibrotic opacities in association with a dominant nodule are secondary signs of carcinoma.

Nonspecific, poorly defined increased stromal density in one breast often is the clue to a serious abnormality. No actual mass will be outlined, and typical stippled calcification will not be present to identify the lesion. The changes may be localized and limited to one quadrant of the breast or one area (Fig. 14–24). A mass may be suggested (Figs. 14–25 and 14–26). Even more difficult is recognition of one area in many of coalescent fibroglandular tissue as being of greatest importance (Fig. 14–27). The disturbing asymmetric increase in stromal density may involve a large portion of the breast, or even the entire breast (Figs. 14–28 to 14–30).

This extremely important aspect of subtle changes of early breast cancer cannot be overemphasized. Recognition and keen eval-

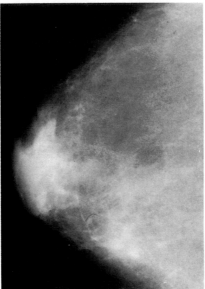
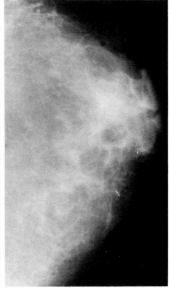

Figure 14–25. Asymmetry of carcinoma in the young. A 35-year-old woman whose physician felt a lump in the breast. Mammography: 5 × 7 × 8 mm irregular density in inner quadrant on the right breast with overlying skin flattening and increased vascularity in the area. Pathology: duct carcinoma. All 16 axillary lymph nodes found in the modified radical mastectomy were free of tumor. The patient was free of disease four and one-half years later.

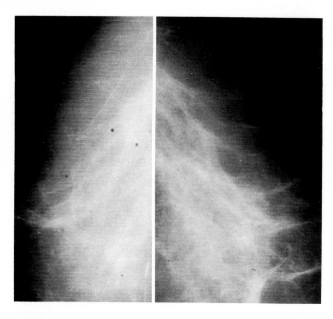

Figure 14–26. An obvious asymmetric small carcinoma. A 59-year-old woman with a right breast lump for two weeks. Clinically the mass was 1 cm in diameter. Radiographically and on gross pathology this Stage I duct carcinoma measured 7 × 8 mm in size. No evidence of disease five years later. The grid lines resulted from a stationary mammography grid being evaluated at the time.

uation of these subtle alterations cause no excess breast biopsies but assuredly do save women's lives.

Straightened Trabeculae. The trabeculae arise from a large area in the posterior aspect of the breast and are always more widely separated the greater the distance from the

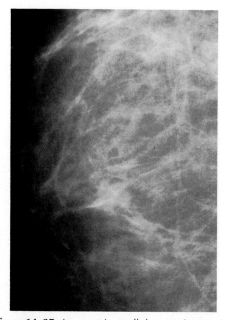

Figure 14–27. Asymmetric small duct carcinoma. A 48-year-old woman seen for a checkup of nodular breasts. The small density just slightly below the nipple called attention to this area of a 4 × 6 mm poorly defined mass that otherwise resembled other areas of coalescent fibroglandular tissues. This proved to be a moderately infiltrative duct carcinoma; all axillary lymph nodes without tumor. No evidence of disease 12 years later.

nipple. Separation of the trabeculae as they approach the nipple does not occur normally. Also, as these trabeculae course smoothly through arcs of all planes they are seen for only short distances. Whenever the straightened trabeculae are noted, great care must be used in search of this area.

Another variation of this trabecular straightening is the fibrillary retractive phenomenon, a less well-developed sign of retraction about the carcinomatous mass. It is most often appreciated in the subcutaneous adipose tissues, where the fine fibrils—the magnitude of a spider's web—are straightened from a normal smooth curving course to become rectilinear and visible for some distance (Fig. 14–31). This sign is particularly valuable in the dense glandular breast, where the actual carcinoma may be almost completely obscured by glandular tissue. This finding is of particular importance when the mass is seen with great difficulty; straightening of a single strand of suspensory breast tissue or Cooper's ligaments may be significant (Figs. 14–32 to 14–34).

Nonspecific Duct Prominence

Prominence of one or several ducts leading into the vicinity of a mass may be helpful in distinguishing a cancer. These changes usually are part of an altered architecture, such as straightening of trabeculae and nodulation at the periphery of the cancer. The ductal changes may be categorized as (1) dilated duct or ducts, usually more prominent anterior to the mass (Fig. 14–2); (2) ducts

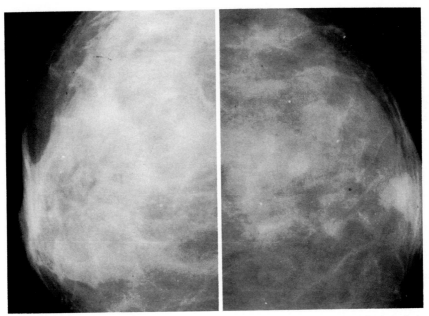

Figure 14–28. Asymmetric density of breast cancer. A 60-year-old woman who complained of a right breast mass that clinically was "poorly defined." Mammograms: increase in density of the central portion of the right breast. Minute inspection of the tissue projective just above the right nipple reveals faint stranding, signaling the presence of carcinoma. Pathology: highly infiltrating, poorly outlined duct carcinoma. Nodes were negative. After four years no evidence of disease.

stretched into prominence (Fig. 14–9); (3) ducts filled with cancer (Fig. 14–16); (4) ducts stretched and/or filled with cancer (Fig. 14–2); or (5) ducts retracted irregularly about the periphery of the cancer (Fig. 14–6). (See Chapter 20.)

Axillary Lymph Nodes

Demonstration of axillary lymph nodes is of diagnostic value (Figs. 14–35 to 14–38). Since normal axillary lymph nodes are dem-

onstrated on occasion, it is necessary to differentiate them from lymph nodes containing metastatic cancer. A small axillary node heavily calcified from some previous inflammatory disease offers no problem. This rough rule is suggested: If a mass on the mammograms is compatible with carcinoma of the breast, and axillary nodes are demonstrated, the lesion is likely to be carcinoma and the nodes to contain metastatic disease. If no mass is present in the breast and the nodes

Figure 14–29. Asymmetry of intraductal carcinoma. A 45-year-old-woman seen for a baseline mammogram; normal breasts clinically. Mammography: The density on the left is homogeneous and practically structureless; on the right is an asymmetric 1 × 1.5 cm irregular density centrally with a suggestion of coarse spiculation; highly suspicious. Pathology: intraductal carcinoma with no evidence of microinvasion. Modified radical mastectomy; all 16 axillary lymph nodes free of metastasis; six years later the patient was free of disease.

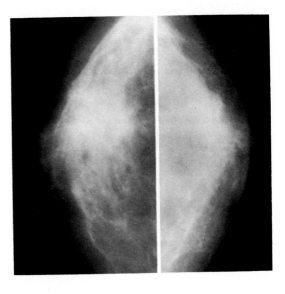

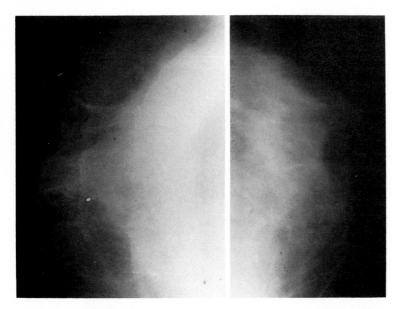

Figure 14–30. Increased breast density poorly explained. A 50-year-old woman with bilateral fibrocystic disease and a cyst (right) clinically noted for at least two months; two paternal aunts with breast cancer. Mammography: diffuse increased density on right, scattered small calcifications, increased prominence of the trabeculae centrally. All findings individually nonspecific but together are quite suspicious. Pathology: intraductal comedo and duct carcinoma, estimated to be 3 to 3.5 cm in size; adenosis and sclerosing adenosis also in area of neoplasm. Modified radical mastectomy; 3 of 18 Level I and 0 of 3 Level II axillary lymph nodes with metastases. The patient was free of disease seven years later.

are less than 1 cm in size, they probably do not represent regional metastasis; if the nodes are greater than 1 cm in diameter, they are probably pathologic, either as part of

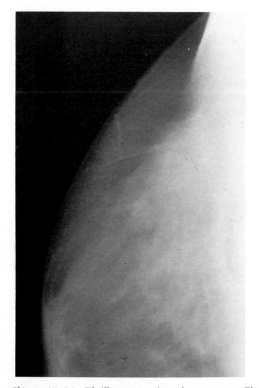

Figure 14–31. Fibrillary retractive phenomenon. The straightened fine fibrils extending from the skin across the subcutaneous fat and into the mass indicate the presence and location of this partially obscured carcinoma. This 38-year-old woman had noted vague changes in her breast for three weeks. The carcinoma was obvious clinically.

generalized lymphadenopathy or as the result of some local etiologic factor. Partial replacement of a lymph node by fat indicates that the node is probably normal. In addition, stippled calcifications similar to breast cancer may be seen in the nodes and indicate metastasis. Usually the cancer calcification seen in the nodes is fairly coarse, since higher kvp is not the optimal energy range for demonstration of fine flecks of calcification. As with increased vascularity, this secondary sign of carcinoma adds to the diagnostic accuracy of mammography.

The higher voltage needed to penetrate the axilla does not result in optimal detail for study of the breast but does outline the axillary lymph nodes embedded in the axillary fat. Several small, rounded, discrete densities may occasionally be seen in the upper outer quadrant of the breast associated with carcinoma of the breast. These usually represent low axillary lymph nodes. When the entire axilla is filled with carcinomatous lymph nodes that have ruptured and become matted, the entire axilla and tail of the breast on the mammogram are homogeneously dense owing to replacement of the fat by carcinoma.

Masses in the axilla are often confusing on clinical examination. Mammography may be of value in deciding whether a carcinoma in the breast is present to account for axillary lymph node metastases. Mammography may demonstrate a palpable lesion in the breast to be a benign mass and indicate that the clinician should search elsewhere for the

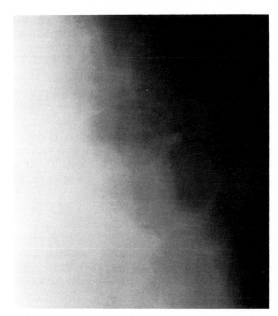

Figure 14–32. Combined secondary signs of ductal hyperplasia and fibrillary retraction. A 33-year-old nulliparous woman with large painful breasts. Clinically: nodular breasts, difficult to examine, no dominant nodule. Mammography: The careful examination of technically good mammograms required of severe dense ductal hyperplastic breasts led to scrutiny of this area in the left breast. There was a fleck of coarse calcification usually causing detailed search for smaller particles; a nearby vein was clearly visible and a single straightened trabecula led into a localized area of coalescent tissues. Two more strands toward the skin were probably straightened, and possibly one posteriorly. The clinician then explored this pinpointed area in a problem breast. A 5 × 6 mm duct carcinoma with fibrosis was demonstrated; nodes were normal, and there is no evidence of disease three years later.

cause of enlarged nodes. Frequently, the clinician is unable to determine whether a mass in the axilla is due to axillary lymph node enlargement or primary carcinoma in the tail of the breast. If the mammograms clearly show a spiculated mass in the region of the tail of the breast with normal breast tissue extending around the mass, the diagnosis of carcinoma of the tail of the breast is clear. The demonstration by mammography of a carcinoma in the tail of the breast is of great clinical help.

In early mammography, advanced cancer was a frequent finding. Of a group of 252 patients having mammograms prior to a radical mastectomy as the primary treatment for carcinoma of the breast (no previous biopsy or irradiation), 179 had microscopic evidence of axillary lymph node metastasis. Positive axillary lymph nodes were also diagnosed by mammography in 144 of these 179 cases. Thus, the finding of axillary nodes on the mammograms was a useful secondary radiographic sign of carcinoma of the breast in 80 per cent of these cases.

Today, after many years of the routine use of mammography and its influence on early detection, study of the axilla by x-ray contributes very little. In our referral patients who have been screened and had removal of obvious disease, the best examination is of the exposed axilla carried out by palpation during surgery in an attempt to locate any possibly enlarged diseased nodes.

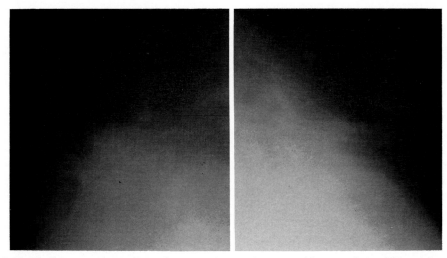

Figure 14–33. Fibrillary retraction points to breast carcinoma. A 55-year-old woman being followed for questionable lump in very nodular breasts. Mammography: slight increase in density UOQ left, with stranding of trabeculae. One clinician then felt a "5 to 10 cm" mass in area. Biopsy revealed highly invasive comedocarcinoma with 6 of 18 axillary lymph nodes with tumor. Widespread disease appeared shortly thereafter.

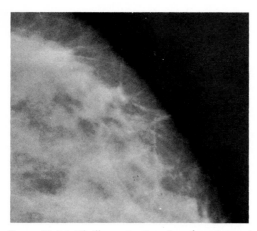

Figure 14–34. Fibrillary retractive sign of carcinoma in a very dense breast. A 39-year-old woman, gravida 3, para 1, no nursing, no family history, with a breast lump for six weeks in clinically nodular breasts. Mammography: stretching of a Cooper's ligament into prominence as a fibrillary retractive sign. The vein in the area was increased in size. After attention was focused on this area some increased thickening could be felt. Pathology: intraductal and a 1 cm duct cell carcinoma with fibrosis. Modified radical mastectomy; 0 of 4 nodes Level I and 2 of 14 nodes Level II had metastatic deposits. The distribution of recovered axillary lymph nodes was unusual. There was a background of severe ductal hyperplasia, sclerosing adenosis, papillomatosis, and varied mammary "dysplastic" changes. The patient was living and well eight years later.

Various unusual and often unexpected lesions may be spotted in the surrounding tissues included in the axillary view (Fig. 14–39).

Intramammary Lymph Nodes

Intramammary lymph nodes occurred in 25 per cent of our whole-organ breast studies. Typically, in the vicinity of the malignant mass or toward the upper outer quadrant from the primary carcinoma will be seen one or several discrete well-circumscribed densities that are suggestive of benign solid or cystic masses and measure up to 1.5 cm in diameter. Axillary nodes may or may not be present. The opposite breast may contain no such deposits. The intramammary nodes containing carcinoma are easily differentiated from the irregular satellite nodules or the ill-defined deposits of distant fibrotic response to carcinoma (see Chapter 17).

Retromammary Space Obliteration

Although cancers near the posterior breast capsule may produce relatively early reaction about the deep layer of superficial fascia with disruption of the retromammary space, obliteration of this space usually indicates ad-

vanced disease. The involvement of the retromammary space may be evident from local obliteration of the thin fat line or may be present as obliteration of the retromammary space in its entire extent into the axilla. Deep fixation may not be present clinically even though obliteration of the retromammary space has occurred radiographically. Edema of the areolar tissue of the retromammary space precedes actual invasion and fixation of the breast to the chest wall.

Several of these secondary radiographic signs of cancer have been deemed sufficiently important for emphasis. Thus, chapters are devoted to subareolar (including nipple) changes of carcinoma, ductal epithelial hyperplasia, skin changes, intramammary lymph nodes, and differentiation from alterations produced by surgery and radiotherapy.

HISTOLOGIC AND CLINICAL TYPES OF BREAST CANCER

The separation of histologic types of breast cancer for breast imaging can be simplified as (1) noninvasive, or in situ lesions; (2)

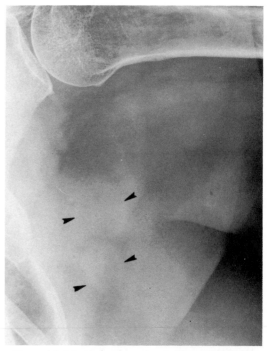

Figure 14–35. Cropped routine axillary view to show several axillary lymph nodes, 2 to 3 cm in diameter. These nodes (arrowheads) contained metastatic carcinoma from an infiltrative duct cell carcinoma of the ipsilateral breast.

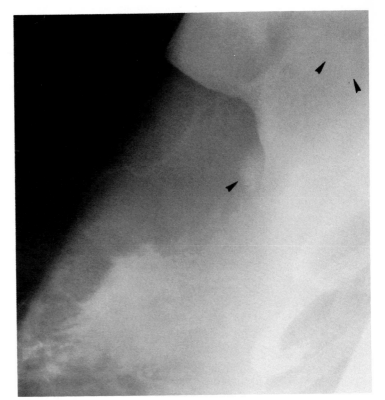

Figure 14–36. Variation of axillary view in attempt to show entire breast, massive carcinoma, and axillary contents fill the 8 × 10 inch film. Low nodes (single arrow) and middle nodes (double arrow) are shown but not the apex of the axilla. This compromise, although inclusive of a large area, demonstrates all structures poorly.

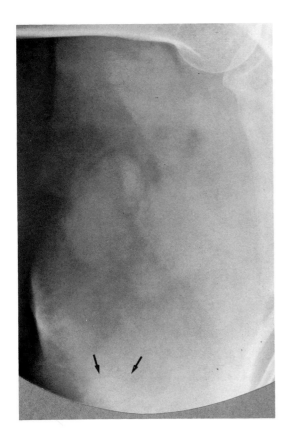

Figure 14–37. Massive axillary lymph node metastases in a 69-year-old woman with a highly invasive duct carcinoma. The nodes are numerous and very large but remain discrete.

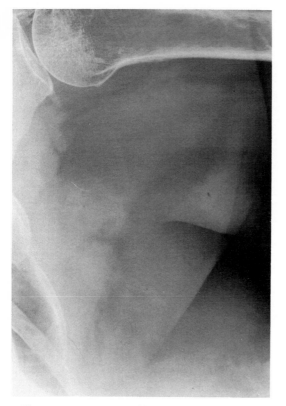

Figure 14–38. A 73-year-old woman with a long history of breast mass and breast retraction from an infiltrating duct carcinoma. The borders of the nodes posteriorly and superiorly are indistinct, indicating rupture of the carcinoma outside the nodes into the axillary fat.

However, the histologic nomenclature used is sufficiently universal that each type considered will be recognized. Too, this represents one pathology department's approach to a daily working routine. Breakdown may give better insight into the complex group of breast cancers. Certain types, locations, and clinical situations require separate chapters.

Noninfiltrating Carcinoma

The noninfiltrating carcinomas (intraductal, in situ) that are most frequently recognized in the breast are those that produce calcifications (noninfiltrating duct and intraductal comedo) or a mass (intracystic papillary). Those that produce a pseudomass without calcifications or altered architecture are recognized only with difficulty. The latter include lobular carcinoma in situ and varied noncalcifying carcinomas, such as papillary and tubular. These are most often studied when found in breast tissue that has been excised for some other reason.

Almost all histologic types of breast carcinoma are manifested as an intraductal carcinoma or by an intraductal component. Medullary carcinoma with lymphoid stroma does not have a recognizable intraductal phase. Metaplasia in breast carcinoma occurs in its infiltrative portion. Intracystic papillary carcinoma arises in the duct and although it

invasive carcinomas that are predominantly ductal in type (comedo, duct, lobular); (3) variants of duct carcinoma (scirrhous, tubular, apocrine, papillary, medullary without lymphoid stroma, metaplastic); (4) special histologic types (medullary with lymphoid stroma, mucinous, intracystic papillary); (5) clinical syndromes (Paget's, inflammatory); (6) sarcoma; and (7) metastasis.

Certain histologic types of breast carcinoma tend to produce (although not necessarily) certain growth patterns and changes mammographically. There are also specific clinical syndromes associated with breast cancer. Many are sufficiently characteristic that the histologic diagnosis or clinical syndrome may be recognized from the mammogram.

No attempt is made to substantiate strict criteria for these histopathologic types of carcinomas. Not all pathologists would agree with this arbitrary breakdown of duct carcinoma but instead would consider all such lesions simply as infiltrating duct carcinoma.

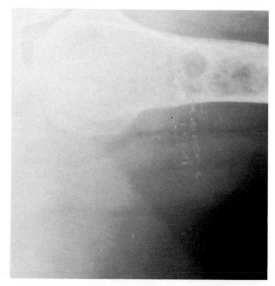

Figure 14–39. Multiple myeloma. Mammograms of a 63-year-old woman during a diagnostic work-up revealed normal breasts, but peculiar cystic lesions of the humerus were suggestive of multiple myeloma, which they proved to be.

may dilate the duct beyond a recognizable structure, it is still intraductal until the capsule is breached. Sarcomas and metastases, from the opposite breast or a distant site, have no intraductal element.

At least 90 per cent of all breast cancers arise from duct epithelium; it is neither difficult nor unusual to assume a phase confined to the epithelium. Just as in squamous carcinoma of the uterine cervix, there are demonstrable changes in the ductal epithelium of epithelial proliferation, dysplasia, atypia, metaplasia, anaplasia, and carcinoma in situ. Although precancerous lesions of the breast are not precisely demonstrated by mammography, there is excellent histopathologic correlation of many phases of epithelial hyperplasia. Close cooperative studies by radiologists and pathologists have rekindled interest in breast cancer. At what precise stages the disease is irreversible, is neoplastic, or is invasive is not easily determined. There are many subtle changes in the epithelial cells prior to the recognition of obvious cancer cells that have broken through the basement membrane of the ducts and into the surrounding tissue. The basement membrane of the duct is not a constantly demonstrated structure histopathologically. The pathologist may assume its presence when, actually, it has been altered and breached by cancer cells.

The radiologist can arouse suspicion as to the presence of noninfiltrating breast cancers. There is a stage in which intracystic papillary carcinoma is not confined within the cyst; in Paget's disease, even at the stage of nipple involvement, there also may be limited or no demonstration of cancer cells outside the ducts.

There are two noninfiltrating breast cancers that are diagnosed either by blind biopsy (usually breast tissue removed in a biopsy for other purposes) or by investigation of clinically unsuspected findings on the mammograms. These lesions are intraductal carcinoma in situ and lobular carcinoma in situ.

The intraductal carcinoma in situ is a carcinoma that is confined entirely within ducts and has no invasive components. The pathologist usually prefers the term "intraductal carcinoma." That intraductal carcinoma is used to indicate noninfiltrative duct carcinoma or carcinoma in situ is a paradox to many people. Carcinoma means not only abnormal cells but also those cells in an abnormal location. If carcinoma-like cells are still within the ducts, only one half of the definition is fulfilled. The diligence of the pathologist influences this diagnosis to a certain degree, as illustrated by one of our patients presenting with axillary lymph node metastasis. This required radiography of slicer sections of the entire breast, preparation of 64 blocks for histologic analysis, and three months for demonstration of one point of invasion in the breast. This stage of preinvasive cancer may persist for years, during which it presents no abnormality to palpation even when observed in the 2 to 4 mm breast slicer sections. Ultimately, the basement membrane is breached and cancer cells invade the immediate periductal tissues. The intramammary lymphatics closely follow the ducts, which explains how a microinvasive carcinoma may metastasize. A mass may be demonstrated by mammography or an abnormality palpated in the slicer sections only after there is infiltration beyond the duct into the surrounding breast tissue.

Prior to formation of a mass, the appearance on the mammogram is that of ductal hyperplasia; only in the presence of calcifications can the radiologist suspect carcinoma or carcinoma in situ. The fine intraductal type of carcinoma calcification may be seen in clumps throughout the densities or diffusely sprinkled throughout a large portion of the breast. (The difficulty of precisely differentiating the flecks of calcification of cancer from benign processes such as fibrocystic disease is stressed in Chapter 27.) It is most difficult to be certain what percentage of intraductal carcinoma in situ contains calcifications on mammograms, since this finding is the usual reason for biopsy. In this series, calcifications have been identified in practically all cases. The lesion may be confined to a limited area in one duct, one lobule, or several lobules or may extend diffusely throughout the breast.

There are advantages to considering two variants of intraductal carcinoma, comedo and solid types. This provides a distinction between the ducts filled with pasty, grumous material of desquamated epithelial cells and detritus and the solidly arranged matrix of viable epithelial cells (despite fenestrations and cribriform pattern). The more indolent comedo type tends to grow along ducts, to produce calcifications in the detritus of the ducts, and to proceed slowly into diffuse, poorly marginated comedocarcinoma. The solid type is more aggressive, is more apt to

TABLE 14–5. Features of Intraductal Comedocarcinoma

Path. Type Cancers	Number	Patient Age (Years)				Detection				Axillary Lymph Nodes*			Tumor Path. Size (cm)					Path. Sites		
		<40	40–50	51–60	60+	X P +–	X P ++	X P –+	X P ––	None	Low	All Levels	0	<1	1–2	2.1–5	>5	1	2–5	6+
One	32	6	7	13	6	23	5	0	4	28	1	1	19	3	3	3	7	27	2	3

X = x-ray; P = physical examination; + = positive; − = negative.

produce a mass of infiltrating duct carcinoma, and produces calcifications by active cellular secretion. Both types are recognized primarily on x-ray by calcifications (see Chapter 27).

Intraductal Comedocarcinoma

Clinical Features. Noninfiltrating comedocarcinoma was diagnosed 32 times as a single histologic type of carcinoma, for an incidence of 1.4 per cent of the total primary operable cancers (Table 14–5). The average age was 51.9 years, with the oldest patient being 81 and the youngest 24 years old. It was associated with all cases of infiltrating comedocarcinoma as well as with many intraductal and infiltrating duct carcinomas. Twenty-five cases were found by mammography alone, and no lesion was biopsied on the basis of clinical findings alone. Although the intraductal comedocarcinoma per se was not palpable, five women had some vague palpable abnormality in the breast that was not related to the lesion. Most of the women were asymptomatic or had complaint unrelated to the carcinoma.

Radiographic Features. The most common cause of investigation was the presence of radiographic clustered calcifications not associated with a mass (Figs. 14–40 and 14–41). Usually when the widespread (or numerous deposits of) typical variegated flecks of calcifications were present radiographically, the pathologist was able to demonstrate some area of invasion. At times there was sufficient reaction about the lesion to cause increased density or pseudomass (Fig. 14–42). This occurred ten times, and in four instances diagnostic calcifications were not noted in the radiographicaly suspicious mass. This, however, is much less common than with the solid form of intraductal carcinoma. An

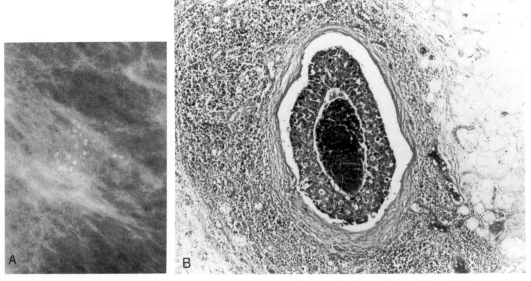

Figure 14–40. Intraductal comedocarcinoma. A 71-year-old woman being followed after mastectomy for carcinoma 14 years before. Clinically normal breast. A, Mammography: cluster of coarse and intermingled fine calcifications without mass; LOQ on a background of ductal hyperplasia. Sonography was normal. Pathology (localization, biopsy, specimen radiography): intraductal comedocarcinoma without demonstrable microinvasion. B, High-grade malignant cells are within the ducts dilated with characteristic central necrosis with periductal inflammatory response. Modified radical mastectomy; marked epithelial hyperplasia and foci of atypia; no further carcinoma. Remaining breast normal after two years.

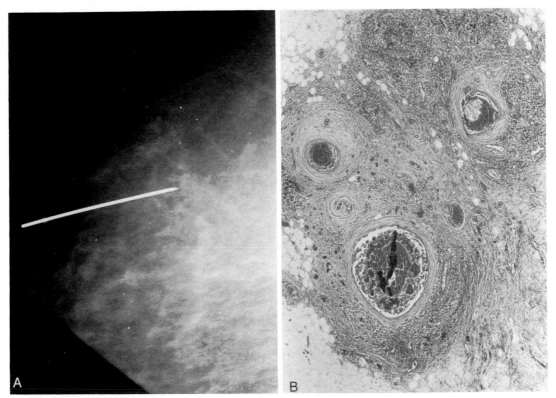

Figure 14–41. Pseudomass of intraductal comedocarcinoma. A 74-year-old woman postmastectomy for Stage I duct carcinoma two years before. No clinical abnormality. *A,* Mammography: severe ductal hyperplasia with coalescent fine nodularity, cluster of fine calcifications with slight increase in density (near needle tip). Pathology (localization, biopsy, specimen radiography): intraductal comedocarcinoma without evidence of mass or microinvasion. *B,* The ducts are expanded by malignant cells undergoing central necrosis. There is calcification of the necrotic material within the ductal lumen. Large numbers of lymphocytes surround the ducts with periductal reactive fibrosis producing a pseudomass. Modified radical mastectomy; 18 lymph nodes negative; no abnormality after four years.

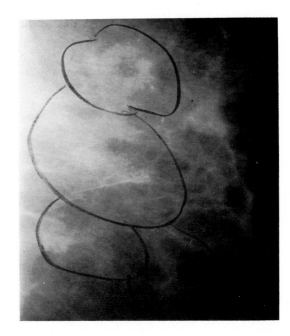

Figure 14–42. Multiple sites of intraductal comedocarcinoma. A 59-year-old woman with soreness in the left breast for two years; no abnormality clinically. Mammography: four sites of clustered calcification of comedocarcinoma type without associated mass, in the left breast only. Pathology (localization, biopsy and specimen radiography): intraductal comedo without evidence of microinvasion. Modified radical mastectomy; all four sites proved to be intraductal comedocarcinoma; 20 axillary lymph nodes free of metastasis. The patient was free of disease four years later.

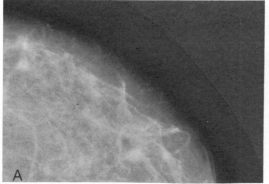

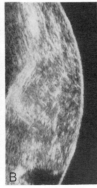

Figure 14–43. Noninvasive comedocarcinoma. A 70-year-old woman seen for checkup. *A*, Mammography: innumerable calcifications UOQ following ducts to nipple. *B*, Sonography: no abnormality but a background of ductal hyperplasia. Pathology: intraductal comedocarcinoma; modified radical mastectomy; 0 of 19 nodes positive; patient alive without disease two years later.

anechoic area on sonography is seldom produced (Fig. 14–43). Intraductal comedocarcinoma occurred 18 times in fatty breasts or with fatty ductal hyperplasia, four additional times with ductal hyperplasia, and ten times in glandular or coarsely nodular breasts (see Chapter 27).

Clinical Course. Five lesions had two or more distinct sites in the breast and three had more than six sites, indicating that multiplicity of sites is to be expected (Fig. 14–42). There were six bilateral lesions, two simultaneous, and four nonsimultaneous. Bilaterality is more often proved in the invasive form.

Treatment consisted of radical mastectomy (1), modified radical mastectomy (21), complete mastectomy (8), and tumorectomy (2). Whole-organ studies were done on two breasts. There were only three deaths related to breast cancer, two of these being in the six women who had opposite breast primary infiltrative carcinomas and one woman who developed an infiltrative duct carcinoma following tumorectomy only for an intraductal comedocarcinoma (Table 14–6). Corrected survival for this lesion per se was 100 per cent.

Solid Intraductal Carcinoma

Clinical Features. The most frequent ocurrence of solid intraductal carcinoma was in association with infiltrating duct carcinoma, where it could be found in the vicinity of the main mass of tumor and usually with additional distant foci. As a single histologic type of carcinoma it was demonstrated 97 times, for an incidence of 4.4 per cent of the total primary operable cancers (Table 14–7). The average age was 51.6 years, the oldest patient being 84 and the youngest 25 years. This lesion was found primarily by mammogra-

phy, and that was usually following localization and specimen radiography for clustered calcifications without a mass (Fig. 14–44). At times it could be demonstrated in breast tissue for some unrelated finding. A complaint related to this lesion per se was unusual. Solid intraductal carcinoma was demonstrated 65 times by mammography alone and eight times by results of clinical examination; five lesions developed under observation. In Table 14–7 the gross pathologic size refers to an estimate of the area of involvement, not true mass size.

Radiographic Features. By the time that myriad diagnostic calcifications occurred, the lesion was most likely invasive. Borderline calcifications without a mass was the usual finding (Fig. 14–44). This occurred 78 times. These calcifications tended to be finer, sharper, and of more nearly equal density than those of comedocarcinoma. Unlike the intraductal comedocarcinoma, this solid type produced sufficient peripheral reaction to form a pseudomass in ten cases, five of which contained calcifications (Fig. 14–45). This could be apparent on sonography despite the absence of invasiveness demonstrated by his-

TABLE 14–6. Follow-up of 32 Intraductal Comedocarcinomas Occurring as a Single Histologic Type of Carcinoma

	Number	% Alive
Patients treated 5 years ago	13	
Alive	8	62
Dead, breast cancer	2	
Dead, not breast cancer	3	
Patients treated 10 years ago	9	
Alive	4	44
Dead, breast cancer	1	
Dead, not breast cancer	4	

One death from breast carcinoma more than 20 years after tumorectomy for intraductal comedocarcinoma.

TABLE 14–7. Features of Solid Intraductal Carcinoma

Path. Type Cancers	Number	Patient Age (Years)				Detection				Axillary Lymph Nodes*			Tumor Path. Size (cm)					Path. Sites		
		<40	40–50	51–60	60+	X P + −	X P + +	X P − +	X P − −	None	Low	All Levels	0	<1	1–2	2.1–5	>5	1	2–5	6+
One	97	9	25	29	34	65	19	8	5	84	4	2	66	18	5	8	0	75	17	5

X = x-ray; P = physical examination; + = positive; − = negative.

topathology. In whole-organ studies for infiltrating duct carcinoma, separate foci of solid intraductal carcinoma were common. The lesion occurred 50 times in fatty breasts or with fatty ductal hyperplasia, 17 additional times with ductal hyperplasia, and 30 times in glandular or coarsely nodular breasts (see Chapter 27).

Clinical Course. Seventeen lesions had two or more distinct sites in the breasts, and five had more than six sites, demonstrating frequent multiplicity. There were six bilateral lesions, two simultaneous, and four nonsimultaneous. Treatment consisted of radical mastectomy (7), modified radical mastectomy (62), total mastectomy (18), and tumorectomy (10). Ten breasts had whole-organ studies. The five-year survival rate was 80 per cent and corrected survival was 97 per cent (Table 14–8). Four deaths were associated with bilateral carcinomas.

Observations. Intraductal carcinoma must be considered a mammographic carcinoma. Prior to this study the diagnosis was practi-

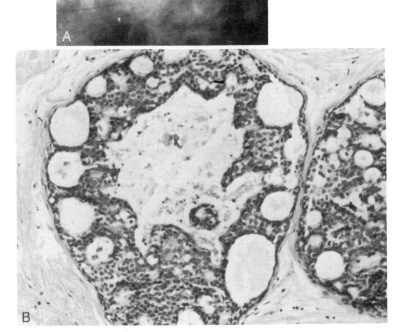

Figure 14–44. Intraductal carcinoma and atypical lobular hyperplasia. A 53-year-old woman seen for baseline study. *A,* Mammography: a focus of several small calcifications near the needle tip. Pathology (biopsy and localization in specimen): several small foci of intraductal carcinoma. *B,* The typical pattern of solid (rigid) cribriform intraductal carcinoma. Modified radical mastectomy; no further tumor but multifocal areas of atypical lobular hyperplasia. All nodes free of tumor; no evidence of disease two years later.

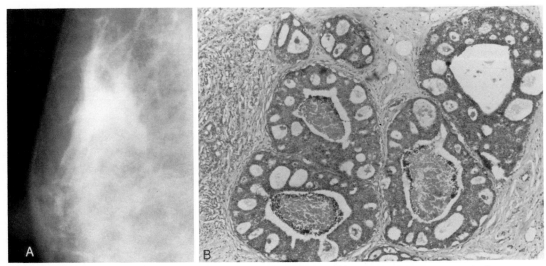

Figure 14–45. Intraductal carcinoma with lobular extension. A 48-year-old woman, 10 years post surgical menopause, gravida 2, para 1, no family history, with an enlarged "milk duct." Clinically: mild thickening, UOQ of the breast. *A,* Mammography: 1.5 cm mass, increased vascularity, altered architecture, fine calcifications. Pathology: intraductal carcinoma, solid type, with lobular extension. *B,* This cribriform pattern with central necrosis shows the rigid holes or fenestrations seen in many intraductal carcinomas. *B,* This cribiform pattern with central necrosis shows the rigid holes or fenestrations seen in many intraductal carcinomas. Modified radical mastectomy; all 14 axillary lymph nodes free of tumor. No disease five years later.

cally nonexistent and, at best, highly controversial. This lesion has stimulated more interest by far in breast diseases, their pathology, and their natural history than most other breast lesions combined.

It is not known how often solid intraductal carcinoma occurs without calcification, as the calcifications are usually the reason for investigation. On whole-organ studies we did know that the noncalcifying form existed. In these 97 cases there were ten radiologic masses or pseudomasses, and only five contained suspicious calcifications. In the remaining 87 without a mass, nine did not contain radiographic calcifications. This leads one to suspect that an unknown, but probably significant, number of these noninfiltrating carcinomas are being overlooked.

TABLE 14–8. Follow-up of 97 Solid Intraductal Carcinomas Occurring as a Single Histologic Type of Carcinoma

	Number	% Alive
Patients treated 5 years ago	35	
Alive	28	80
Dead, breast cancer	1	
Dead, not breast cancer	6	
Patients treated 10 years ago	23	
Alive	10	43
Dead, breast cancer	5	
Dead, not breast cancer	8	

Axillary lymph node metastasis does occur with solid intraductal carcinoma, usually an occasional node or a few low nodes only. In our two cases with all levels of nodes involved there was a highly invasive duct carcinoma in the opposite breast. Similarly, the cancer deaths were associated with invasive duct carcinomas of the opposite breast.

Papillary Intraductal Carcinoma

Clinical Features. Noninfiltrating papillary carcinoma was demonstrated 48 times as a single histologic type of breast carcinoma, for an incidence of 2.2 per cent of all primary operable carcinomas (Table 14–9). The average age was 54.8 years, with the youngest patient being 24 and the oldest 92 years. Over one half, 29 cases, were found by mammography alone. Four lesions were biopsied on the basis of clinical findings; some palpable abnormality was present in 12 other breasts but was not necessarily associated with the carcinoma. Almost all the women were seen for routine work-ups or had minimal symptoms.

Radiographic Features. Twenty-five of the lesions had associated calcifications. A suggestion of a mass or an area of increased density was present in 20 cases. Thirty of the lesions were in fatty breasts or in fatty ductal hyperplasia, five additional ones in ductal hyperplasia, and 13 in glandular or coarsely

TABLE 14–9. Features of Intraductal Papillary Carcinoma

Path. Type Cancers	Number	Patient Age (Years)				Detection				Axillary Lymph Nodes*			Tumor Path. Size (cm)					Path. Sites		
		<40	40–50	51–60	60+	XP +−	XP ++	XP −+	XP −−	None	Low	All Levels	0	<1	1–2	2.1–5	>5	1	2–5	6+
One	48	3	8	10	27	29	12	4	3	43	0	0	30	7	9	2	0	36	9	3

X = x-ray; P = physical examination; + = positive; − = negative.

nodular breasts. There are no specific identifying radiographic diagnostic criteria, except for the presence of calcifications and asymmetry or vague mass (Fig. 14–46).

Only three lesions developed under observation over a long follow-up. This could suggest rather frequent recognition by mammography; alternatively, comparison of the infiltrating papillary carcinoma data shows that many go unrecognized and proceed to infiltrative lesions, as 17 such carcinomas were found under observation.

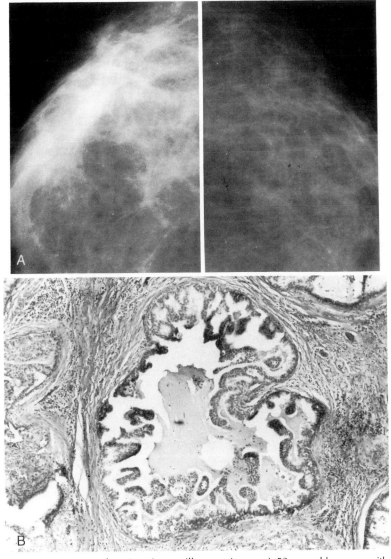

Figure 14–46. *A* and *B*, Asymmetry of noninvasive papillary carcinoma. A 52-year-old woman with a breast lump for one year considered to be nodular fibrocystic disease. Mammography: increase in density in right upper quadrant without a definite mass. Atypical calcification in left lower quadrant. Pathology, right upper quadrant: papillary intraductal carcinoma without any foci of invasion. Modified radical mastectomy; all lymph nodes free of tumor. After six years no evidence of disease and no change in the calcification in the left breast.

TABLE 14–10. Follow-up of 48 Intraductal Papillary Carcinomas Occurring as a Single Histologic Type of Carcinoma

	Number	% Alive
Patients treated 5 years ago	21	
Alive	20	95
Dead, breast cancer	0	
Dead, not breast cancer	1	
Patients treated 10 years ago	9	
Alive	7	78
Dead, breast cancer	0	
Dead, not breast cancer	2	

Clinical Course. Nine lesions had more than two sites in the breast, and three had more than six sites, indicating frequent multiplicity (Table 14–9). Bilaterality of noninvasive papillary carcinoma was not demonstrated.

Treatment consisted of modified radical mastectomy (26), radical mastectomy (1), complete mastectomy (11), and tumorectomy (5). Whole-organ studies were carried out on five breasts. No positive axillary lymph nodes were found in the 43 specimens studied. There were no deaths from the disease, although the 92-year-old patient died after four years and another death occurred eight years after treatment; both women were free of disease (Table 14–10).

Tubular Intraductal Carcinoma

Although there were 16 cases of infiltrating tubular carcinoma, frequently with an intraductal component, there was no single histologic type case of noninfiltrating tubular carcinoma. Even the infiltrative form is detected with difficulty both clinically and by x-ray. There is some solace: This is an infrequent lesion with very good prognosis.

Lobular Carcinoma in Situ

Another noninfiltrating breast cancer is lobular carcinoma in situ. The origin of this lesion is the epithelium of the acini or blunt duct in the mammary lobules. The involved lobules enlarge and the acinar lumens are obliterated by proliferating cells, but the overall configuration of the mammary lobules is maintained.

Lobular carcinoma in situ of the breast may have consistently precise interpretation by some pathologists; some pathologists' criteria may be less consistent; and some pathologists may allow variable subjectivity to enter

into their interpretation of this lesion. The histopathologic appearance is fairly consistent, with the greatest variable being the degree of change. There are larger than normal epithelial cells distending terminal ducts, some degree of acinar formation, and hyperplasia of the lobules with coalescent increased cellular activity to produce the area of lobular carcinoma in situ. These uniformly enlarged individual cells, lacking strict cytologic criteria of malignancy, have a clear, pale-pink cytoplasm, round nucleus, and normal nuclear-cytoplasmic ratio, without significant granularity to the chromatin.

Breasts with lobular carcinoma in situ do develop invasive carcinoma. The invasive lesion is often ductal in origin rather than lobular and is like an invasive duct carcinoma. Lobular changes are progressive and may be compared in this respect with ductal epithelial changes. Parallel ductal changes introduce the distinct possibility that the invasive lesion may be of ductal epithelial origin. In many instances our lobular carcinomas in situ proved, upon many deep sections, to be intraductal carcinomas growing down into the terminal or blunt ducts.

Surgeons are aware that the widest divergence of opinion of pathologists relates to the earliest phases of carcinoma. Lobular carcinoma in situ of the breast may not be found on the limited material subjected to frozen-section study but later may be demonstrated on additional deep paraffin studies. Surgeons may become reluctant to accept the frozen-section diagnosis of lobular carcinoma in situ. Since the significance of this interpretation by the pathologist is not clear, there is little uniformity of approach to treatment. Some surgeons prefer to follow the patient closely than to reoperate.

To introduce further confusion, there are extremely wide differences geographically in the incidence of lobular carcinoma in situ of the breast. At Memorial Hospital in New York City, the largest series thus far followed for the longest period of time has been reported. Hutter (1970) has indicated that in this series of patients with lobular carcinoma in situ followed for 20 years, 35 per cent developed an invasive carcinoma. There is almost 100 per cent cure if the lesion is treated at a noninfiltrating stage but only 40 per cent five-year survival if it is treated at an infiltrating stage—a worse prognosis than with ductal carcinoma. Almost half of these in situ lesions are bilateral; all do not progress

TABLE 14–11. Features of Lobular Carcinoma in Situ

Path. Type Cancers	Number	Patient Age (Years)				Detection				Axillary Lymph Nodes*			Tumor Path. Size (cm)					Path. Sites		
		<40	40–50	51–60	60+	XP +−	XP ++	XP −+	XP −−	None	Low	All Levels	0	<1	1–2	2.1–5	>5	1	2–5	6+
One	55	4	24	18	9	32	3	2	18	43	1	0	48	4	3	0	0	40	12	3
Two	73	11	18	21	23	26	32	8	7	50	10	11	19	12	20	22	0	37	29	7
Three	5	1	1	2	1	2	1	1	1	3	1	1	0	0	1	3	1	3	1	1
Total	133	16	43	41	33	60	36	11	26	96	12	12	67	16	24	25	1	80	42	11

X = x-ray; P = physical examination; + = positive; − = negative.

to infiltration, as some are arrested and some regress.

This New York series is very similar to ours in which whole-organ studies were carried out. There is overlap of intraductal carcinoma growing into the ducts and lobular carcinoma growing along the ducts. One area of the breast may show primarily lobular and another intraductal carcinoma. Most of the invasive carcinomas that develop are ductal.

Clinical Features. Lobular carcinoma in situ was encountered 133 times as a distinct histologic type of breast carcinoma for an incidence of 6.0 per cent of all primary operable breast cancers (Table 14–11) but 88 were associated with other cancers. The average age was 51.9 years, with the oldest patient being 73 and the youngest 26 years. At the initial study, 60 (45 per cent) of the cases were biopsied on the basis of mammography and 11 for clinical reasons alone. A large percentage (20 per cent) went undetected on the initial examination. Only 47 had a clinically palpable area, 76 had a definable area on gross pathology, and 58 had some suggestion of mass or increased density by x-ray. Symptoms could rarely be related to the tumor.

Radiographic Features. The background stroma may be similar in both breasts, but one breast must be more extensively involved to allow recognition on the mammograms. The conglomerate, rounded, fluffy, or streaky densities arouse suspicion; the appearance is not unlike fibrocystic disease or ductal hyperplasia (Fig. 14–47). The changes in the breast may be diffuse or localized to a quadrant or to one or several lobules. The process in many cases has been shown to be indolent, possibly leading to invasive lobular carcinoma. On the mammograms there is no way to detect the noninvasive character of the lesion that is suggestive of carcinoma. Flecks of calcification do occur in breasts with lobular carcinoma in situ (Figs. 14–48 to 14–50) but may be outside the area of cancer, in

contrast to intraductal cancer; the presence of these calcifications may be the red flag to attract attention to this problem breast. A high incidence of bilaterality (Fig. 14–51) has been proved by a limited number of surgeons by routine blind upper outer quadrant biopsies in the breast opposite the cone containing the lobular carcinoma in situ. Also, these changes have been demonstrated in breasts containing intraductal carcinoma in situ, sclerosing adenosis, papillomatosis, and/or invasive cancer of the opposite breast (Fig. 14–50).

In our series calcifications were present in 22 of the 58 masses by x-ray and in 44 of the 75 cases without mass. Forty-nine of the lesions occurred in fatty breasts or with fatty ductal hyperplasia, 19 additional ones were with ductal hyperplasia, and 65 (one half) occurred in glandular or coarsely nodular breasts, making recognition most difficult.

Clinical Course. Forty-two cases had two or more distinct sites in the breast, and 11

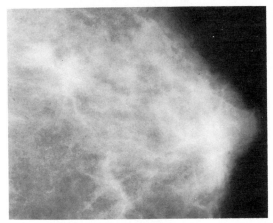

Figure 14–47. Lobular carcinoma in situ. A 67-year-old woman with a lump in the right breast. Clinically: nodularity bilaterally without a dominant area. Mammography: asymmetric, poorly defined 1 cm density containing three flecks of coarse calcification; highly suspicious. Sonography showed only mild architectural distortion in the area. Pathology (needle localization and biopsy): lobular carcinoma in situ. No further surgery. Eight years later no evidence of disease.

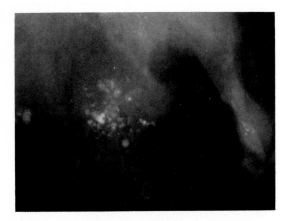

Figure 14–48. Lobular carcinoma in situ. A 49-year-old woman with nodular breasts. Mammography: fibroglandular breasts with three sites of clustered calcifications, two shown in specimen (after localization and removal). Pathology (biopsy specimen): lobular carcinoma in situ, severe ductal hyperplasia, atypia, papillomatosis. With these severe changes, mastectomy was deemed necessary. The study of the breast did show three more sites of lobular carcinoma in situ only. Lymph nodes were free of tumor. No problem with the opposite breast 12 years later.

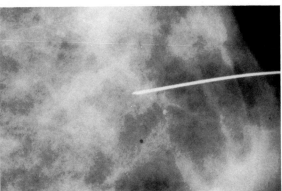

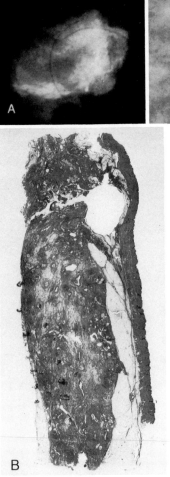

Figure 14–49. Lobular carcinoma in situ with calcification in nearby sclerosing adenosis. A 45-year-old woman with bilateral dark nipple discharge, breast biopsy two years before, clinically normal breasts. *A,* Mammography: scattered calcifications both breasts, small cluster near needle tip. Sonography: duct ectasia. *B,* Pathology of specimen: lobular carcinoma in situ. The calcifications were in sclerosing adenosis. Three years later no apparent disease. The numerous foci of lobular carcinoma in situ were located between the India ink dots on the whole-organ slicer section.

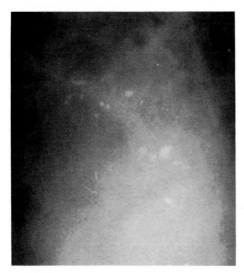

Figure 14–50. Lobular carcinoma as second nonsimultaneous bilateral primary carcinoma. A 50-year-old woman post mastectomy, left breast for ductal and comedo carcinoma, multiple sites of both types, Stage II, four years before. Mammography, right breast: five separate areas of suspicious clustered calcifications. Pathology (simple mastectomy): epithelial hyperplasia, papillomatosis, atypia with only one site of lobular carcinoma in one area of calcification. The patient died from disseminated carcinoma nine years following second mastectomy.

had six or more sites. At Emory University blind biopsy of the opposite breast is not routine. Assessment of bilaterality of lobular carcinoma in situ from our material may be misleading. Treatment policy also may be misleading, as there was a time when this lesion was so poorly understood that in early years treatment policy was vague. Treatment consisted of radical mastectomy (20), modified radical mastectomy (24), complete mastectomy (30), and biopsy and observation (13). Forty-six breasts were studied by whole-organ preparations, which contributed to the frequency with which this lesion was demonstrated. Lobular carcinoma in situ occurred with a second histologic type of malignancy 73 times and with two types 5 times. The in situ lesion was usually an incidental finding, contributing little to the findings in Table 14–11. The second lesion was duct carcinoma in 72 instances and intracystic papillary carcinoma in the other case. It was found with duct carcinoma and sarcoma one time, with duct and intracystic papillary carcinoma one time, with duct and medullary carcinoma with lymphoid stroma two times, and with duct and mucinous carcinomas one time.

The eight deaths from Table 14–12 were unrelated to lobular carcinoma in situ as the single histologic type; the seven and five suggestions of mass in this group were of questionable validity on pathology grossly and clinically; and the one positive low axillary lymph node is not readily explained.

Observations

The subtle changes on the mammograms due to noninvasive cancer demand exquisite

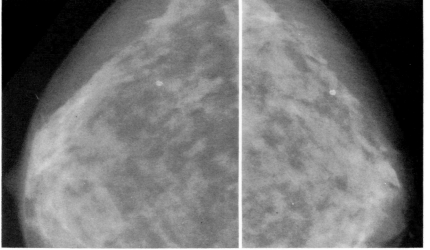

A   **B**

Figure 14–51. Bilateral nonsimultaneous lobular carcinoma in situ. A 75-year-old woman who had the left breast removed 17 years before for lobular carcinoma in situ. Mammography: *A,* Thirteen years following left mastectomy, severe ductal hyperplasia without localizing density or calcification. *B,* Four years later (reversed for comparison) breast smaller, more intense ductal hyperplasia, increase in tissue into UOQ, a definite interval change. Pathology (biopsy): lobular carcinoma in situ, question of invasion in one area, much atypia, identical to the studies of the left breast 17 years before. Two-year follow-up without apparent disease.

TABLE 14–12. Follow-up of 133 Lobular Carcinomas in Situ Alone or Associated with One Other Histologic Type of Carcinoma

	One Type		Two Types		Total	
	No.	% Alive	No.	% Alive	No.	% Alive
Patients treated 5 years ago	29		57		86	
Alive	26	90	44	77	70	81
Dead, breast cancer	3		11		14	
Dead, not breast cancer	0		2		2	
Patients treated 10 years ago	18		40		58	
Alive	10	56	18	45	28	48
Dead, breast cancer	8		20		28	
Dead, not breast cancer	0		2		2	

Of five patients with triple histologic types, four died of cancer prior to 20 years and one survived past 20 years.

radiographic detail for recognition, and differentiation is not possible with coarse-grained film techniques. Fine stippled calcification, straightened fine trabeculae, distorted trabeculae indicating altered architecture, or a small faint nodule may be the only clue and requires not only meticulous technique but also careful scrutiny under a hand lens and a bright light. There must be mutual understanding and complete cooperation of each member of the team of clinician, surgeon, radiologist, and pathologist. Rich rewards accompany these efforts; there will be nearly 100 per cent ten-year salvage rate of women so brought to proper treatment if there is adequate follow-up care of the opposite breast. Unfortunately, these localized cancers do not lend themselves to ready detection by the usual rapid and less well-controlled mass screening methods.

Radiologists often have difficulty identifying lobular carcinoma, and pathologists at times have similar difficulty with intraductal carcinoma in situ. In one case diffuse carcinoma was confidently diagnosed on the mammograms, but in the amputated breast carcinoma in situ only was demonstrated histologically; despite the lack of evidence of invasion, axillary nodes contained metastatic carcinoma of the breast. This is one lesion above all others in which the pathologist and radiologist should cooperate closely; another is the intracystic papillary carcinoma.

Predominantly Duct Carcinoma

Almost all the carcinomas being considered have their origin in the epithelial lining cells of the ducts. For clarity, comedo, infiltrating duct, and lobular carcinomas will be considered the primary duct carcinomas, with others being variants. Then several specific histologic types will follow.

Comedocarcinoma

Infiltrating comedocarcinoma is maintained in the scheme of the present classification of duct carcinomas to indicate the progression of intraductal comedocarcinoma. Again, it is advantageous to separate the infiltrative phase, as there are often distinct differences from the more common infiltrating duct carcinomas. The comedocarcinoma tends to be less aggressive, occurs in multiple sites in a more widespread area of the breast, and tends to be bilateral. However, this tumor does become highly invasive and lethal. It occurs frequently with the solid duct carcinoma, and in this setting it is convenient to assume its presence to explain its more variegated calcifications associated with the single carcinomatous mass.

Clinical Features. It is difficult to categorize comedocarcinoma, given its highly variable modes of presentation. Almost the entire breast may be filled with diffuse typical calcifications, with only scattered areas of increased density visible on the mammogram, while the woman is asymptomatic without any clinical breast abnormality. The presentation extends to the massive, highly infiltrating, inoperable breast carcinoma with fixed axillary lymph nodes. In the latter, one tends to incriminate associated solid duct carcinoma, but this is not always proved. Comedocarcinoma occurred as a single histologic type 234 times, for an incidence of 10.6 per cent of our total primary operable breast cancers (Table 14–13). The average age of the woman was 55.8 years, with the oldest being 86 and the youngest being 21 years. Biopsy was based on x-ray findings in 82 cases and on clinical findings alone in 11 cases; nine lesions were detected under observation. Thus, on initial examination, one third of the comedocarcinomas were detected by mammography alone in women without

TABLE 14–13. Features of Comedocarcinoma

Path. Type Cancers	Number	Patient Age (Years)				Detection				Axillary Lymph Nodes*			Tumor Path. Size (cm)					Path. Sites		
		<40	40–50	51–60	60+	XP +–	XP ++	XP –+	XP ––	None	Low	All Levels	0	<1	1–2	2.1–5	>5	1	2–5	6+
One	213	20	63	60	70	74	122	9	8	135	30	41	48	17	66	72	10	141	53	19
Two	21	1	9	5	6	8	10	2	1	13	4	2	3	2	3	11	2	10	9	2
Total	234	21	72	65	76	82	132	11	9	148	34	43	51	19	69	83	12	151	62	21

X = x-ray; P = physical examination; + = positive; – = negative.

related symptoms. The lack of an x-ray mass in 108 women suggests that additional cases were also probably clinically unsuspected. On gross pathology, 95 of the lesions were greater than 2 cm in diameter, with 12 of these being greater than 5 cm. In comedocarcinoma, area of lesion and size of mass are not synonymous.

Radiographic Features. The heterogeneous type of calcification of comedocarcinoma is produced with or without infiltrative masses (Figs. 14–52 to 14–54). These may be obscured on x-ray by large dense masses of tumor (Fig. 14–55). The calcifications frequently occur in many clusters throughout the breast (Fig. 14–56) or diffusely with less marked clustering (Fig. 14–57). These calcifications usually indicate indolence, but the tumor may become more aggressive with actual mass formation (Fig. 14–58) or highly infiltrative with much of the calcification obscured by mass, density, and desmoplasia (Fig. 14–59). It is suspected at this stage of development that solid duct carcinoma constitutes much of the mass, as duct carcinoma

often accompanies the later stage of comedocarcinoma (Fig. 14–60). If uninterrupted, comedocarcinoma can proceed to a stage with poor prognosis (Figs. 14–61 to 14–64).

Of the 126 x-ray masses, 94 contained calcification; in 108 lesions without mass, calcifications were seen in 88. Vague densities and asymmetry were often helpful in diagnosis, especially in the opposite breast being followed closely for the appearance of a bilateral primary carcinoma. Comedocarcinoma occurred in fatty breasts and with fatty ductal hyperplasia 122 times, in ductal hyperplasia an additional 30 times, and in glandular or coarsely nodular breasts 82 times.

Clinical Course. In 62 breasts there were two or more distinct sites of comedocarcinoma, with 21 of these having more than six sites. A second histologic type of carcinoma

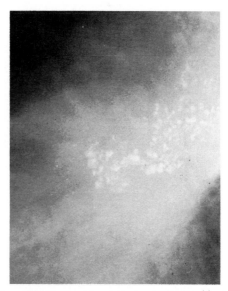

Figure 14–53. Comedocarcinoma. A 50-year-old woman with a breast lump for over four months. Clinically: 3 × 4 cm malignancy. Mammography: 1.7 × 2.3 cm homogeneously dense, moderately invasive carcinoma containing comedocarcinoma type calcifications centrally. Pathology: excision biopsy (lumpectomy): 2 × 2 × 2 cm duct carcinoma, mostly comedo in type. The patient returned to her home state for herbal treatments. No follow-up in three years.

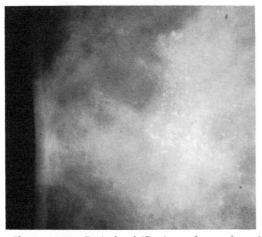

Figure 14–52. Typical calcifications of comedocarcinoma. A 59-year-old woman with a firm breast lump for three years. The calcifications covered a 1 × 2 cm area. Pathology: intraductal and comedo carcinoma; 0 of 24 nodes positive. The patient was living seven years later free of disease.

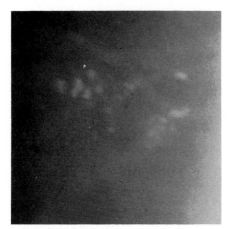

Figure 14–54. Coarse pattern of comedocarcinoma calcification. A 58-year-old woman seen for a checkup. This blowup shows small, faint, suspicious calcifications. Localization and biopsy led to a diagnosis of primarily Stage 0 comedocarcinoma; although there was no mass by x-ray, there were areas of microinvasion. The patient was free of disease 21 years later.

occurred: medullary with lymphoid stroma, 3; mucinous, 5; lobular, 8; intracystic papillary, 1; tubular, 3; and duct, 1 (the last being completely disassociated from comedocarcinoma). Bilateral primary carcinomas occurred 37 times, with 14 being simultaneous and 23 nonsimultaneous. Treatment consisted of radical mastectomy (48), modified radical mastectomy (163), complete mastectomy (13), and tumorectomy (10). Twenty breasts had whole-organ studies.

The apparent indolence of the individual intraductal comedocarcinoma and its tendency to microinvasiveness only are offset by its bilaterality, multiplicity of sites, and large areas of involvement. As far as possible, lesions combined with frank solid infiltrating duct carcinoma were removed from the comedocarcinoma classification and included with the duct carcinomas. Except for the eight lobular carcinomas, the presence of the other histologic types of carcinoma in the same breast did not connote a particularly severe prognosis. Based on this review the clinical problems with comedocarcinoma are great: Only 82 lesions were nonpalpable; 77 had axillary lymph node metastasis (43 to all levels); nearly half the tumors were over 2 cm in size pathologically; and only 88 patients were alive at five years, with 46 having died within that time, for an absolute survival rate of 66 per cent and corrected to 68 per cent (Table 14–14). Of the total 234 women with comedocarcinoma, 44 (19 per cent) died of cancer; 37 of those deaths occurred within five years of diagnosis. However, with women subjected to five or more years of follow-up, the longer-term prognosis appears improved (Table 14–15).

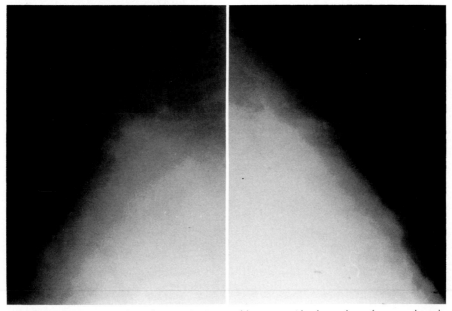

Figure 14–55. Comedocarcinoma in dense breasts. A 55-year-old woman with a breast lump for several weeks. Clinically: 5 to 10 cm mass. Mammograms: left UOQ, increased density, stranding, coarse calcifications, fibrillary retraction, appearance of teenage breasts. Pathology: 5 cm comedocarcinoma with 6 of 24 axillary lymph nodes with metastatic tumor. Death five years later from widespread disease.

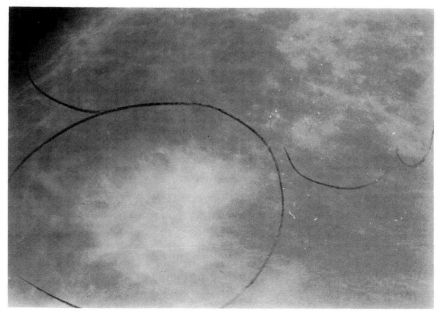

Figure 14–56. Multiple comedocarcinomas. A 57-year-old woman with bloody nipple discharge in otherwise normal breasts. One daughter had bilateral breast cancers. Mammography: numerous clusters of comedo type calcifications, some associated with increased breast density. Pathology: many areas of comedocarcinoma, some microinvasive; modified radical mastectomy; all 22 axillary lymph nodes free of tumor. The patient was alive without disease four years later. A poorly defined mass is within the largest circle.

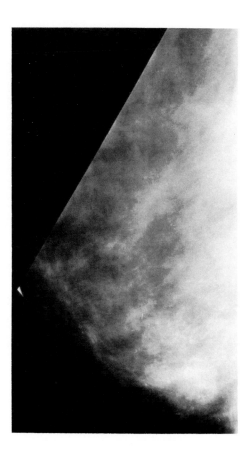

Figure 14–57. Diffuse comedocarcinoma. A 52-year-old woman with fullness of the breast. Clinically: nodularity of both breasts. Mammograms: comedocarcinoma type calcifications throughout most of the lower half of the breast. Pathology: comedo and comedo intraductal carcinoma; modified radical mastectomy; all 18 lymph nodes free of tumor. The patient was alive and well 11 years later.

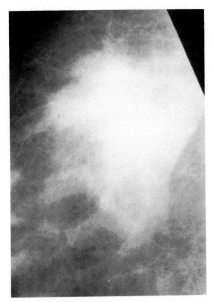

Figure 14–58. Moderately invasive comedocarcinoma. A 50-year-old woman with a suspicious breast lump for three months. Mammograms: 1.2 × 2 cm irregular mass containing comedo type calcifications associated with edema, skin thickening, and increased vascularity. Pathology: intraductal and infiltrative comedo (with reactive fibrosis) carcinoma; modified radical mastectomy; 13 of 17 Level I and 0 of 2 Level II axillary lymph nodes contained tumor. The patient was free of disease four years later.

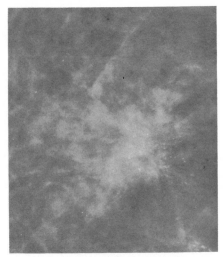

Figure 14–60. Comedo and duct carcinoma. A 65-year-old woman with a 3.5 cm hard mass in the UOQ of the breast. Mammography: 2 × 2.5 cm carcinoma above the nipple, centrally fine punctate calcifications of comedocarcinoma, peripherally spiculated and fading into the fatty background. This would represent more aggressive duct carcinoma with a moderate degree of desmoplasia. Sonography (not shown): almost anechoic mass, irregular borders, surrounding architectural changes, marked shadowing, a moderately invasive carcinoma. Pathology: intraductal and invasive comedo and duct carcinoma. Modified radical mastectomy; all 20 nodes free of tumor. The patient was alive without disease two years later.

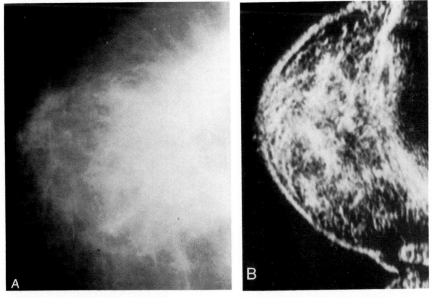

Figure 14–59. Highly invasive comedocarcinoma. A 60-year-old woman, whose mother had breast cancer, presented with a breast lump and nipple retraction. A, Mammograms: 3 × 4.5 cm highly invasive comedocarcinoma, suspect superimposed scirrhous duct carcinoma, nipple and subareolar changes. B, Sonography: large area of distorted architecture containing heterogeneous echoes, hypoechoic areas, overlying skin thickening, and distortion. Pathology: intraductal and infiltrative comedocarcinoma with marked fibrotic reaction; modified radical mastectomy; 4 of 19 low axillary lymph nodes contained tumor. Three years later, the patient developed distant metastases.

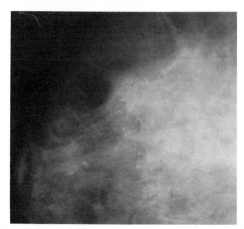

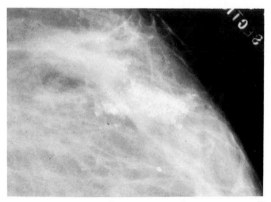

Figure 14–63. Comedocarcinoma with metastases to all levels of axillary lymph nodes. A 63-year-old woman with a breast mass; an area of overlying skin discolored and hot. Mammograms: poorly defined mass, comedo type calcifications, adjacent skin thickening. Pathology: intraductal comedo and comedocarcinoma; radical mastectomy, 8 of 13 low, 3 of 5 mid-, and 2 of 5 high axillary lymph nodes with metastatic carcinoma. Death occured three years later with widespread disease.

Figure 14–61. Diffuse comedocarcinoma. A 58-year-old woman with a breast lump for one week. Clinically: increased fullness of the breast in the area of a suspicious mass. Mammograms: myriad diffuse small calcifications UOQ, increased density UOQ, and increased vascularity. Pathology: intraductal comedo and infiltrative comedocarcinoma with 4 of 25 low axillary lymph nodes positive for metastases. Modified radical mastectomy: patient alive with metastases four years later.

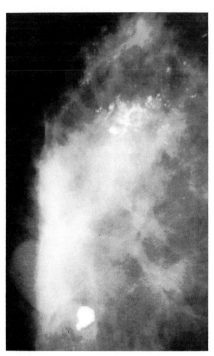

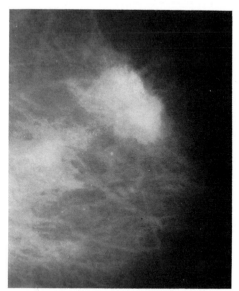

Figure 14–64. Markedly aggressive comedocarcinoma. This 65-year-old woman had heaviness in her breast for six months. There was fixation of the tissues in the subareolar area. Mammography: The area of the upper portion of the carcinoma outlined by coarse and fine calcification appeared more indolent, but as it progressed toward the nipple the appearance was more consistent with scirrhous duct carcinoma. Pathology: large area of comedocarcinoma and infiltrating duct carcinoma with scirrhous elements; no Paget's disease of the nipple. Modified radical mastectomy; four of nine low and two of eight midaxillary lymph nodes contained carcinoma. Two years after radiotherapy and chemotherapy, the patient was living without disease.

Figure 14–62. Comedo and duct carcinoma with numerous foci of intraductal comedocarcinoma. A 57-year-old woman with a rubbery breast mass. Mammograms: main mass of tumor 2 × 1 cm, the upper portion more circumscribed with comedo type calcifications; several separate areas of intraductal comedocarcinoma. Pathology: comedo and scirrhous duct carcinoma; separate foci of noninfiltrating comedocarcinoma; modified radical mastectomy; 4 of 13 axillary lymph nodes with metastatic deposits. Known metastasis two years later.

TABLE 14–14. Follow-up of 234 Comedocarcinomas Alone or Associated with One Other Histologic Type of Carcinoma

	One Type		Two Types		Total	
	No.	% Alive	No.	% Alive	No.	% Alive
Patients treated 5 years ago	122		12		134	
Alive	81	66	7	58	88	66
Dead, breast cancer	37		4		41	
Dead, not breast cancer	4		1		5	
Patients treated 10 years ago	61		8		69	
Alive	16	26	3	38	19	28
Dead, breast cancer	40		4		44	
Dead, not breast cancer	5		1		6	

Duct Carcinoma

Infiltrating duct carcinoma is an encompassing term for breast carcinoma, but for this presentation of our data the term is reserved for the progression of the solid type of intraductal lesion previously considered as a noninfiltrating carcinoma (thus excluding many variants of duct carcinoma). Even so, its manifestations are protean.

Clinical Features. The variability of this carcinoma includes degree of invasiveness, growth pattern, spread, and prognosis. Infiltrating duct carcinoma occurred as a single histologic type 551 times, for an incidence of 25.0 per cent of our total primary operable breast cancers (Table 14–16). The average age was 56.5 years, with the oldest woman being 92 and the youngest being 23 years. Biopsy was based on x-ray findings alone in 106 cases and on clinical findings alone in 55 cases. Thirty-eight occurred under observation. Clinical abnormality was present in 77.6 per cent of the cases, this being the most frequently suspected cancer. On gross pathology, 43 per cent of the lesions were greater than 2 cm in diameter, with only 15 having no measurable-sized mass.

Radiographic Features. Duct carcinomas present with myriad radiographic appearances and may be well circumscribed in portions of their periphery (Fig. 14–65) or have a finely spiculated border (Fig. 14–66). Usually this carcinoma is more readily detected clinically owing to the marked surrounding reaction, but it may be nonpalpable (Fig. 14–67). Radiography can at times be more informative as to the degree of fibrosis compared with light microscopy (Fig. 14–65). The tumor may appear rather large, over 1 cm in diameter, without metastasis (Fig. 14–65). Even the more aggressive lesions may have a good prognosis (Fig. 14–66) but often have a poor prognosis (Fig. 14–77 and 14–78). A good estimate of the prognosis will be gained by observation of the infiltrative nature of the borders as the tumor progresses into the scirrhous type with the worst prognosis. However, size and border are not absolute (Fig. 14–74 and 14–76).

It is difficult for the radiologist to appreciate the pathologist's concern about "stellate," "multinodular," and "circumscribed" lesions of the breast based on limited study of the periphery of a tumor. The radiologist has the opportunity to observe the reaction about the

TABLE 14–15. Five- to Ten-Year Follow-up of 92 Comedocarcinomas Alone or Associated With One Other Histologic Type of Carcinoma

	One Type		Two Types		Total	
	5 Years	10 Years	5 Years	10 Years	5 Years	10 Years
Alive						
Single breast	49	17	1	2	50	19
1st of bilateral	5	1	0	0	5	1
2nd of bilateral	6	0	1	1	7	1
Lost to follow-up	3	0	0	0	3	0
Dead, not breast cancer	1	1	0	0	1	1
Dead, breast cancer						
Single breast	4	0	2	0	6	0
1st of bilateral	0	0	1	0	1	0
2nd of bilateral	0	0	0	0	0	0
Total	68	19	5	3	73	22

TABLE 14–16. Features of Infiltrating Duct Carcinoma

Path. Type Cancers	Number	Patient Age (Years)				Detection				Axillary Lymph Nodes*			Tumor Path. Size (cm)					Path. Sites		
		<40	40–50	51–60	60+	XP +–	XP ++	XP –+	XP ––	None	Low	All Levels	0	<1	1–2	2.1–5	>5	1	2–5	6+
One	551	56	140	142	213	83	347	48	33	305	98	103	12	71	215	226	27	484	49	18
Two	61	7	20	16	16	34	7		4	34	16	13	3	7	22	25	4	38	17	6
Three	5	1	0	2	2	1	3	0	1	4	0	1	0	0	2	2	1	3	1	1
Total	617	64	160	150	223	106	424	55	38	343	114	117	15	78	239	233	32	525	67	25

X = x-ray; P = physical examination; + = positive; – = negative.

entire periphery and through the entire breast tissues. This massive tissue response is more important than simply the type of border of the lesion. The reliance upon these histologic criteria was clearly demonstrated when we were attempting to evaluate the response to ultrasound of masses in the breast. Assessment of the aggressiveness of a duct carcinoma could best be judged by radiographic criteria.

Calcifications were present in 147 of 268 radiographic masses and in 63 of 71 lesions without a mass. Infiltrating duct carcinoma occurred in fatty breasts and with fatty ductal hyperplasia 233 times, an additional 71 times with ductal hyperplasia, and in glandular or coarsely nodular breasts 163 times.

Clinical Course. In 67 breasts there were two or more distinct sites of infiltrating duct

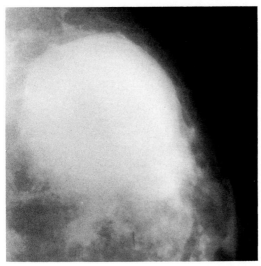

Figure 14–65. Circumscribed duct carcinoma. A 50-year-old woman with a breast mass for an indefinite time. Clinically: hard mass, probably carcinoma. Mammography: 4.5 × 5 × 5.3 cm circumscribed carcinoma; suspect medullary carcinoma at this age; there may be a second lesion of duct type anteriorly. Pathology: Grade III duct carcinoma with productive fibrosis and necrosis with extension into the lactiferous ducts; islands of intraductal comedocarcinoma are within the mass. Modified radical mastectomy; 12 axillary lymph nodes free of tumor. The patient was free of disease four years later.

carcinoma, with 25 more having six or more separate sites of tumor. A second histologic type of carcinoma occurred in 61 breasts: lobular, 35; medullary with lymphoid stroma, 7; mucinous, 14; intracystic papillary carcinoma, 3; and other, two. Two other types of carcinoma were present five times: lobular and mucinous, 3; lobular and intracystic papillary, 1; and lobular and medullary with lymphoid stroma, 1. There were 107 instances of bilateral primary carcinomas, 81 nonsimultaneous and 26 simultaneous.

Treatment consisted of radical mastectomy (173), modified radical mastectomy (287), complete mastectomy (21), and tumorectomy with radiotherapy and chemotherapy (33); whole-organ studies were done on an additional 53 radical mastectomy specimens. Nearly two thirds of the patients had involvement of the axillary lymph nodes, with one half of these being at all levels. The five-year survival was 65 per cent and corrected was 68 per cent (Table 14–17).

Lobular Carcinoma

Invasive lobular carcinoma may occur with lobular carcinoma in situ or in its absence. In our 68 cases of lobular carcinoma as a single histologic type of carcinoma, lobular carcinoma in situ occurred 28 times and was not demonstrable 40 times. In the more thorough whole-organ studies these two lesions were frequently accompanied by solid intraductal and infiltrative duct carcinomas. This occurred in seven of ten whole-organ studies. From our data one could readily pursue either of two inferences: (1) Lobular carcinoma is a distinct histologic entity that may or may not have some association with lobular carcinoma in situ but is frequently present in breasts harboring intraductal or infiltrative duct carcinoma, or both; or (2) it is a syndrome progressing in a manner similar to solid ductal carcinoma into a highly infiltrative pattern with "Indian filing" and fibrosis, not unlike scirrhous duct carcinoma. The frequent association with distinct deposits of

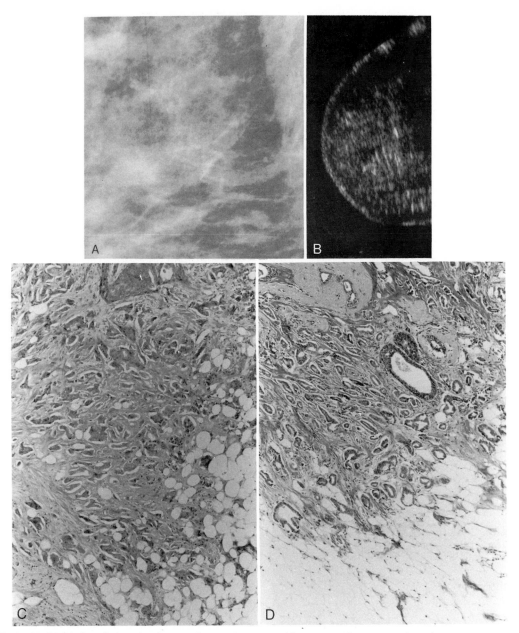

Figure 14–66. Moderately invasive duct carcinoma. A 76-year-old woman with a mass at the inframammary crease for two months. *A,* Mammography: 9 × 12 mm moderately invasive carcinoma; free margins at chest wall and inframammary skin for resection. *B,* Sonography: irregular hypoechoic mass with attenuation of the sound beam. Pathology: duct carcinoma; modified radical mastectomy; all 12 axillary lymph nodes free of tumor. The patient was alive and well four years later. *C,* One area showed rather marked desmoplastic traction. *D,* Another area showed less desmoplasia and well-formed ducts.

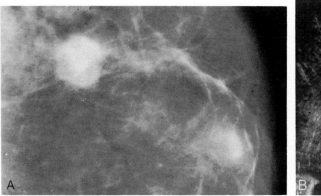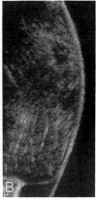

Figure 14–67. Nonpalpable advanced duct carcinoma. A 61-year-old woman complaining of a breast lump. Clinically: large breast ("can't feel a lump"). *A*, Mammography: 1.3 × 1.4 cm carcinoma, moderately invasive. Nipple is out of profile owing to problems of positioning this large breast. *B*, Sonography: irregular hypoechoic mass, nonhomogeneous internal echoes, minimal attenuation. Pathology: duct carcinoma with productive fibrosis. Modified radical mastectomy; all 24 axillary lymph nodes free of metastasis. Three years later the patient was free of disease.

duct carcinoma, even on routine pathologic studies, must be explained in some manner.

Clinical Features. Invasive lobular carcinoma also presents in a highly variable pattern, e. g., diffuse disease with vague clinical findings or discrete tumor with characteristics of the garden variety carcinoma. This tumor occurred as a distinct histologic type 112 times, for an incidence of 5 per cent of our total primary operable breast cancers (Table 14–18). The average age was 55.7 years, with the oldest patient being 86 and the youngest being 32 years. With the 68 carcinomas of single histologic type present, biopsy was based on x-ray findings alone in 18 cases and on clinical findings alone in 5 cases, while 11 developed under observation. On gross pathology, over one third of the carcinomas were greater than 2 cm in diameter.

Radiographic Features. A radiographic mass was present in 41 cases, 13 of which

were associated with calcifications. In 27 cases without a true mass by x-ray, 11 were associated with calcifications. These calcifications may have been only the red flag, without being an integral part of the developing invasive lobular carcinoma. Lobular carcinoma may produce a localized mass on the x-ray with secondary changes (Fig. 14–68) or present as a masslike area (Fig. 14–69). The changes may be in any part of the breast (Fig. 14–70). Often the changes are diffuse and poorly delimited (Fig. 14–71). Duct carcinoma may accompany the lobular carcinoma (Fig. 14–72), and the tumor may be associated with calcifications (Fig. 14–73). Lobular carcinoma occurred in fatty breasts and with fatty ductal hyperplasia 49 times, with ductal hyperplasia an additional 9 times, and with glandular or coarsely nodular breasts 54 times.

Clinical Course. In the 68 breasts with only lobular carcinoma there were 18 cases with

TABLE 14–17. Follow-up of 617 Infiltrating Duct Carcinomas Alone or Associated with One or Two Other Histologic Types of Cancer

	One Type		Two Types		Three Types		Total	
	No.	*% Alive*	*No.*	*% Alive*	*No.*	*% Alive*	*No.*	*% Alive*
Patients treated 5 years ago	337		50		4		391	
Alive	219	65	34	68	2	50	255	65
Dead, breast cancer	104		14		2		120	
Dead, not breast cancer	14		2		0		16	
Patients treated 10 years ago	262		36		3		301	
Alive	100	38	15	42	1	33	116	39
Dead, breast cancer	138		19		2		159	
Dead, not breast cancer	24		2		0		26	

Three patients lived past 20 years without disease.
One patient died with breast cancer after 20 years.

TABLE 14–18. Features of Lobular Carcinoma

Path. Type Cancers	Number	Patient Age (Years)				Detection				Axillary Lymph Nodes*			Tumor Path. Size (cm)					Path. Sites		
		<40	40–50	51–60	60+	X P +−	X P ++	X P −+	X P −−	None	Low	All Levels	0	<1	1–2	2.1–5	>5	1	2–5	6+
One	68	11	17	19	21	18	34	5	11	41	5	13	12	12	19	16	9	50	11	7
Two	42	2	15	15	10	12	18	4	8	27	8	5	3	8	10	19	2	28	10	4
Three	2	0	0	1	1	1	1	0	0	1	0	1	0	0	1	0	1	1	1	0
Total	112	13	32	35	32	31	53	9	19	69	13	19	15	20	30	35	12	79	22	11

X = x-ray; P = physical examination; + = positive; − = negative.

more than two distinct sites of tumor and in seven of these, more than six sites. A second type of histologic carcinoma occurred: with duct 40 times; with mucinous one time; and with papillary one time. Lobular carcinoma was associated with bilateral primary carcinoma 34 times, 19 nonsimultaneous and 15 simultaneous.

Treatment consisted of radical mastectomy (19), modified radical mastectomy (78), complete mastectomy (3), and tumorectomy (12). Whole-organ studies were done on ten breasts.

Of the 112 lobular carcinomas subject to five years' review, there were 38 patients alive without evidence of disease and 16 dead with disease, for a survival rate of 68 per cent (Table 14–19).

Variants of Duct Carcinoma

Scirrhous Carcinoma

Scirrhous carcinoma is not a specific histologic type of breast carcinoma but a pattern

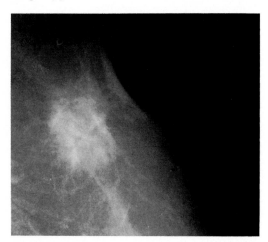

Figure 14–68. Lobular carcinoma with local skin retraction. A 70-year-old woman whose examining physician noted a breast lump with skin dimpling. Mammography: unusual-appearing spiculated 1 × 1.5 cm carcinoma with local skin retraction and thickening. Pathology: moderately invasive lobular carcinoma. Modified radical mastectomy; all 11 axillary lymph nodes free of disease. The patient was free of disease two years later.

of growth—an infiltrating duct carcinoma, irregular in shape, associated with productive fibrosis. This is the classical crab of cancer, the starburst or stellate appearance, as opposed to the well-marginated carcinoma. The irregular serrated periphery is seen by the pathologist as strands of malignant cells invading the surrounding tissues. This is accentuated on the mammograms by fibrosis and shortening of the supporting structures.

Age and Incidence. Scirrhous carcinoma was diagnosed 430 times as a single histologic type of carcinoma, for an incidence of 19.4 per cent of the total primary operable breast cancers (Table 14–20). The average age at diagnosis was 58.8 years, with the youngest patient being 25 and the oldest 88 years.

Clinical Features. The chief complaint was breast mass in 349 cases; in 59 cases the lesion was detected solely by mammography; and in 22 cases the carcinoma became evident under observation. In 35 cases, biopsy was based on clinical findings.

Radiographic Features. The masses of carcinoma were judged radiographically as moderately to highly invasive (Figs. 14–74 to 14–77). Secondary signs of adjacent and distal retraction were common as well as increased vascularity. The question of borderline operability based on radiographic criteria arose at times, especially with some of the large, more highly invasive lesions (Figs. 14–78 and 14–79). The diagnosis of scirrhous carcinoma, or carcinoma with productive fibrosis, was based on the density of the mass and its highly spiculated and infiltrative appearance (Figs. 14–75 to 14–79). Calcifications were seen within the mass in 176 cases (41 per cent). In many instances the fibrotic mass was so dense radiographically that the calcifications were obscured. These became readily apparent if studied on radiography of the specimen or whole-organ tissue slices.

The carcinomas occurred 248 times in fatty breasts or with fatty ductal hyperplasia, an additional 53 times in ductal hyperplasia, and

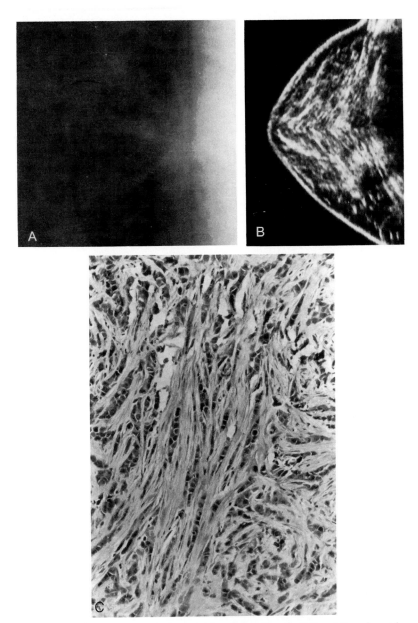

Figure 14–69. Infiltrating lobular carcinoma. A 48-year-old woman with a suspicious 1.5 cm breast lump for two weeks. *A*, Mammography: highly infiltrating carcinoma at the chest wall, approximately 8 × 10 mm in size. *B*, Sonography: irregular hypoechoic mass with shadowing near the pectoral muscles. Pathology: 8 mm lobular carcinoma. *C*, This reveals the typical pattern of invasive lobular carcinoma cells in Indian file, producing a dense mass. Modified radical mastectomy; all 19 axillary lymph nodes free of metastases. The patient was living without disease two years later.

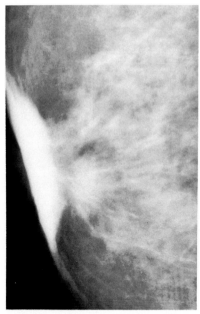

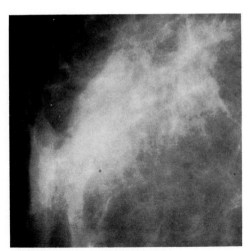

Figure 14–70. Small mass of lobular carcinoma. A 72-year-old woman with areolar changes, clinically suspicious. Normal mammograms 19 years before. Mammography: 6 × 8 mm highly invasive carcinoma producing flattening and retraction of the areola. Pathology: lobular carcinoma infiltrating the dermis and nipple. The wide field shows a diffuse pattern with lobular involvement; the malignant cells infiltrate in an Indian file pattern.

Figure 14–72. Lobular and duct carcinoma in same area. A 76-year-old woman with inverting nipple for the past three months. Clinically: ill-defined mass behind the inverting nipple; carcinoma. Mammography: 2 × 3.5 cm poorly defined asymmetric area causing nipple retraction and fixation with early diffuse skin thickening; a highly infiltrative carcinoma. Pathology: invasive lobular and duct carcinoma. Modified radical mastectomy; 8 of 14 low and midaxillary nodes contained metastases. Distant metastasis 20 months later.

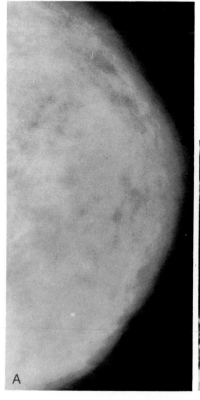

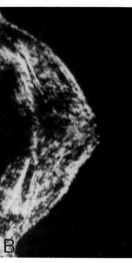

Figure 14–71. Lobular carcinoma not demonstrable by x-ray. A 45-year-old woman with nodular breasts clinically; both grandmothers and two aunts had breast cancer. A, Mammography: dense, almost homogeneous fibrocystic disease bilaterally. B, Sonography: persistent large irregular hypoechoic area with strong attenuation, surrounding disrupted architecture. Pathology: infiltrating lobular carcinoma. Modified radical mastectomy; all 18 axillary lymph nodes free of disease. The patient was alive and well three years later.

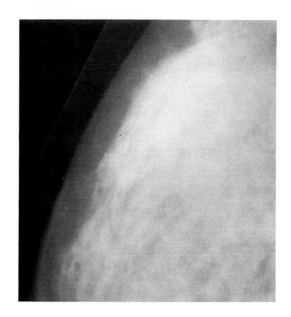

Figure 14–73. Lobular carcinoma associated with calcifications. A 58-year-old woman with a breast lump for eight months. Clinically: 3 × 4 cm suspicious area of thickening. Mammography: 2 × 2.3 cm poorly defined asymmetric area with stippled fine and coarse calcifications and increased vascularity. Pathology: 3 cm area of coalescent lobular carcinoma with extensive intramammary vascular and lymphatic involvement. Modified radical mastectomy; one of six nodes Level I and two of three nodes Level II positive for metastatic neoplasm, papillomatosis. Chest wall recurrence less than three years later.

TABLE 14–19. Follow-up of 112 Lobular Carcinomas Alone or Associated with One or Two Other Histologic Types of Carcinoma

	One Type		Two Types		Total	
	No.	*% Alive*	*No.*	*% Alive*	*No.*	*% Alive*
Patients treated 5 years ago	31		25		56	
Alive	19	61	18	72	37	66
Dead, breast cancer	11		5		16	
Dead, not breast cancer	1		2		3	
Patients treated 10 years ago	24		21		45	
Alive	6	25	9	43	15	33
Dead, breast cancer	15		8		23	
Dead, not breast cancer	3		4		7	

One patient with two types of carcinoma lived beyond 20 years.

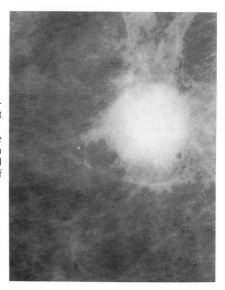

Figure 14–74. Scirrhous carcinoma presenting as circumscribed by x-ray. A 61-year-old woman 23 years postsurgical menopause with a breast lump for one week that was clinically suspicious. Mammography: 1.8 × 1.9 cm coarsely spiculated moderately invasive carcinoma. Veins in the left breast were equally prominent. Pathology: 2 cm duct carcinoma with productive fibrosis. Modified radical mastectomy; the intramammary and 15 axillary nodes were all free of disease. Five years later no evidence of disease.

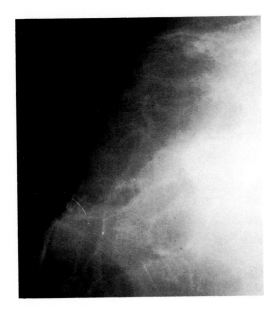

Figure 14–75. Moderately invasive duct carcinoma. A 63-year-old woman with a suspicious breast mass. Mammography: 1.4 × 1.6 cm central carcinoma with stretching of the major ducts, flattening of the areola, and increased vascularity. Pathology: modified radical mastectomy; intraductal and duct carcinoma; all 23 axillary lymph nodes free of tumor as well as the 3 × 4 mm intramammary lymph node above the tumor. No evidence of disease four years later.

TABLE 14–20. Features of Scirrhous Carcinoma

Path. Type Cancers	Number	Patient Age (Years)				Detection				Axillary Lymph Nodes*			Tumor Path. Size (cm)					Path. Sites		
		<40	40–50	51–60	60+	XP +–	XP ++	XP –+	XP ––	None	Low	All Levels	0	<1	1–2	2.1–5	>5	1	2–5	6+
One	380	33	87	111	149	50	281	28	21	188	73	98	9	57	155	138	20	211	34	13
Two	49	2	6	19	22	9	35	4	1	21	15	13	1	5	13	27	3	29	15	5
Three	1	0	1	0	0	0	0	1	0	0	0	1	0	0	0	0	0	1	0	0
Total	430	35	94	130	171	59	316	33	22	209	88	112	10	62	168	166	23	241	49	18

X = x-ray; P = physical examination; + = positive; − = negative.

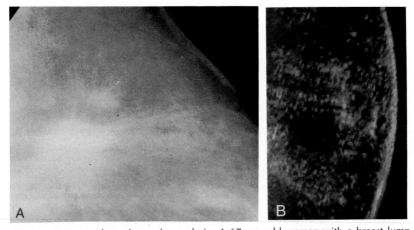

Figure 14–76. Duct carcinoma with moderate desmoplasia. A 67-year-old woman with a breast lump producing skin dimpling. Mammography: 1.5 × 1.5 cm markedly spiculated mass producing retraction of the overlying skin. Sonography: irregular, hypoechoic area; surrounding architectural distortion, extending to the skin; attenuation. Pathology: 1.5 cm duct carcinoma with moderate desmoplasia. Modified radical mastectomy; no metastases in 21 axillary lymph nodes. The patient was free of disease one year later.

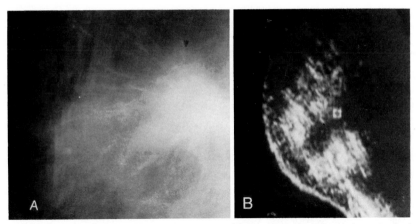

Figure 14–77. Highly invasive duct carcinoma. An 88-year-old woman with a breast lump and nipple retraction. Clinically: 2.5 cm hard mass with nipple retraction. Mammography: 1.3 × 1.5 cm highly invasive spiculated carcinoma with fixation of the nipple and areola. Pathology: duct carcinoma, scirrhous type. *B,* Sonography: highly irregular, hypoechoic area, distorted architecture, marked shadowing; highly infiltrative carcinoma. Modified radical mastectomy; 4 of 12 low and 2 of 6 midaxillary lymph nodes with metastases. The patient died two years later of "old age" but with widespread metastases.

129 times in glandular or coarsely nodular breasts.

Clinical Course. There were two or more foci of carcinoma in 49 cases and six or more sites in 18 cases. Nonsimultaneous bilateral primary carcinomas occurred in 48 women, and there were 11 cases with bilateral simultaneous primary carcinomas. In 49 instances the scirrhous duct carcinoma was accompanied by another histologic type of carcinoma: lobular, 32; mucinous, 10; medullary with lymphoid stroma, 3; tubular 3; and intracystic papillary carcinoma, 1. One breast contained scirrhous duct, medullary with lymphoid stroma, and lobular carcinomas.

Treatment consisted of radical mastectomy (154), modified radical mastectomy (241), complete mastectomy (14), and biopsy with radiotherapy (21). Whole-organ studies were done on 37 breasts. At five years there was a crude survival rate of 69 per cent and at 10 years 28 per cent, corrected to 72 per cent and 31 per cent (Table 14–21).

Tubular Carcinoma

Tubular carcinoma histologically is a well-differentiated tumor of an orderly character, with tubules lying in rather dense fibrous tissue. It can be so innocuous in appearance that it may be confused with sclerosing ad-

Figure 14–78. Highly invasive spiculated duct carcinoma. A 56-year-old woman with pain in the left breast; nipple inverted. Clinically: movable mass with nipple retracted; suspected carcinoma. *A,* Mammography: 2 × 3 cm highly invasive carcinoma with nipple retraction. *B,* Sonography: poorly defined irregular hypoechoic mass with distortion of central architecture; attenuation. Pathology: 3 cm duct carcinoma with fibrosis, with lymphatic and blood vessel permeation. Modified radical mastectomy; 1 of 15 axillary lymph nodes with metastasis. Despite vigorous chemotherapy, distant metastases appeared within a year.

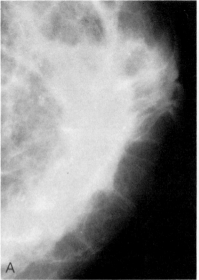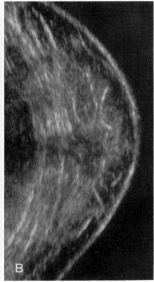

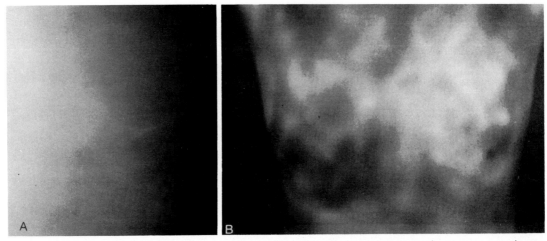

Figure 14–79. Duct carcinoma with fibrosis. A 53-year-old woman, five years post surgical menopause; mother and maternal aunt with breast cancer; breast lump for several years. Clinically the mass was cancer. *A,* Mammography: fatty breast, highly invasive 2 × 3 cm central carcinoma, poorly defined, stretching of trabeculae. *B,* Thermography: diffuse increase in heat of the breast (white is hot). Pathology: duct carcinoma with fibrosis, many scattered areas of intraductal carcinoma, ductal hyperplasia. Radical mastectomy; 36 axillary lymph nodes were free of tumor, but all showed hyperplasia. Death from widespread metastases seven years later.

enosis. Until recently it has been considered an unusual carcinoma, but Carstens (1978) reported a series of 42 tumors seen within one year, with an incidence of 10.3 per cent of all infiltrating carcinomas; he also reported an incidence of 9 per cent axillary lymph node metastasis.

Clinical Features. Tubular carcinoma was diagnosed 16 times as a single histologic type tumor, for an incidence of 0.7 per cent of our total primary operable cancers (Table 14–22). In no single instance was it confined to an intraductal (noninvasive) stage. The average age of the patients was 51.4 years, with the oldest being 77 years and the youngest being 28 years. A mass or palpable abnormality was present in 11 women. Three cases were detected by mammography alone, four were

biopsied on the basis of physical findings only, and two developed under observation. Thus, in two thirds of the cases a clinical finding was sufficiently abnormal for biopsy.

Radiographic Features. In 11 cases a radiographic mass was present (Fig. 14–80); two of these contained calcifications, and in an additional case (under observation) calcifications without a mass was the x-ray finding. There are no specific radiographic diagnostic criteria for tubular carcinoma—only a nonspecific mass, an asymmetry, or the occasional cluster of calcifications. Ten of the lesions occurred in fatty breasts or with fatty ductal hyperplasia, an additional one in ductal hyperplasia, and five in glandular or coarsely nodular breasts.

Clinical Course. Multiple sites of tubular

TABLE 14–21. Follow-up of 430 Scirrhous Carcinomas Alone or Associated with One or Two Other Histologic Types of Carcinoma

	One Type		Two Types		Total	
	No.	*% Alive*	*No.*	*% Alive*	*No.*	*% Alive*
Patients treated 5 years ago	261		41		302	
Alive	178	68	29	71	207	69
Dead, breast cancer	72		7		79	
Dead, not breast cancer	11		5		16	
Patients treated 10 years ago	187		32		219	
Alive	50	27	11	34	61	28
Dead, breast cancer	121		15		136	
Dead, not breast cancer	16		6		22	

Four patients survived over 20 years free of disease.
One patient died after 20 years with breast cancer.
One patient with triple types (medullary and lobular) died of cancer at eight years.

TABLE 14—22. Features of Tubular Carcinoma

Path. Type Cancers	Number	Patient Age (Years)				Detection				Axillary Lymph Nodes*			Tumor Path. Size (cm)					Path. Sites		
		<40	40–50	51–60	60+	X P +−	X P ++	X P −+	X P −−	None	Low	All Levels	0	<1	1–2	2.1–5	>5	1	2–5	6+
One	15	2	5	3	5	3	6	4	2	13	2	0	3	4	7	1	0	13	2	0
Two	1	0	0	1	0	0	1	0	0	0	0	1	0	0	1	0	0	0	0	1
Total	16	2	5	4	5	3	7	4	2	13	2	1	3	4	8	1	0	13	2	1

X = x-ray; P = physical examination; + = positive; − = negative.

carcinoma were found in three breasts; one was associated with a mucinous carcinoma (whole-organ study). Twelve patients were treated by modified radical mastectomy, three by radical mastectomy, and one by complete mastectomy. Three had whole-organ studies. The one patient with two types of carcinoma had axillary lymph node metastasis at all levels and died of disease within five years. Two of the remaining 15 had only low axillary node disease. All remain free of disease, 14 less than five years and one over 16 years.

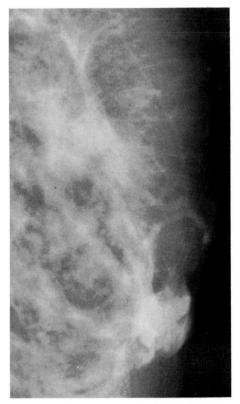

Figure 14—80. Duct carcinoma with a tubular pattern. A 67-year-old woman with a clinically suspicious breast lump. Mammography: 1.5 cm spiculated carcinoma with nipple and areolar retraction. Pathology: duct carcinoma with a focal tubular pattern and stromal elastosis. Modified radical mastectomy; 1 of 14 axillary lymph nodes contained metastasis. The patient was free of disease two years later.

Papillary Carcinoma

This group of papillary carcinomas is completely exclusive of intracystic papillary carcinomas (see Chapter 22). The papillary structure is maintained with projections into glandular spaces but grossly is a more solid tumor, as opposed to the predominantly large hemorrhagic cystic structure containing varying amounts of papillary growths along the cyst wall. A true cyst is not recognized on mammography, nor is it demonstrated by sonography.

Clinical Features. This more solid type of infiltrating papillary carcinoma occurred 145 times in our series, for an incidence of 6.6 per cent of the total primary operable carcinomas (Table 14–23). The average age was 54.8 years, with the oldest patient being 90 years and the youngest being 25 years. A mass, or some palpable abnormality, was present in 86 patients. Biopsy was based on x-ray findings alone in 37 cases and on clinical findings alone in 10 cases; in 22 cases the lesions were found under observation. Thus, in only 76 cases was the diagnosis suspected initially both by x-ray and by clinical examination. There was no mass in 34 cases, but on gross pathology in 47 cases the mass was greater than 2 cm in diameter.

Radiographic Features. Radiographically there was no mass in 61 cases, but of these lesions, 31 had suspicious calcifications. There were also calcifications in 26 of the 79 radiographic masses (Fig. 14–81). In the other cases, increased density or asymmetry called attention to the lesions. The papillary carcinomas occurred in fatty breasts or with fatty ductal hyperplasia 77 times, an additional 29 times in ductal hyperplasia, and 38 times in glandular or coarsely nodular breasts.

Clinical Course. In 46 breasts there were two to five distinct deposits of tumor and in five, more than six sites (Figs. 14–82 and 14–83). In 18 cases an additional histologic type of carcinoma occurred: with lobular, ten; with intracystic papillary, four; with mucinous, two; and with tubular, two. There were 12

TABLE 14–23. Features of Papillary Carcinoma

Path. Type Cancers	Number	Patient Age (Years)				Detection				Axillary Lymph Nodes*			Tumor Path. Size (cm)					Path. Sites		
		<40	40–50	51–60	60+	XP +−	XP ++	XP −+	XP −−	None	Low	All Levels	0	<1	1–2	2.1–5	>5	1	2–5	6+
One	127	13	14	40	60	32	71	7	17	98	14	13	29	20	36	38	4	85	39	3
Two	18	1	7	4	6	5	5	3	5	15	1	1	5	1	7	3	2	9	7	2
Total	145	14	21	44	66	37	76	10	22	113	15	14	34	21	43	41	6	94	46	5

X = x-ray; P = physical examination; + = positive; − = negative.

cases of simultaneous bilateral primary carcinomas and 30 cases of nonsimultaneous bilateral primary carcinomas. Treatment consisted of radical mastectomy (18), modified radical mastectomy (107), complete mastectomy (17), and tumorectomy (3). Five-year survival was 83 per cent and corrected survival was 88 per cent (Table 14–24). This tumor can be aggressive (Fig. 14–81).

Medullary Carcinoma Without Lymphoid Stroma

This rather vague group of tumors was separated out primarily to prevent contamination of the true medullary carcinomas with lymphoid stroma, and secondly, for any possible contribution to the understanding of breast cancer. Histologically the tumor is similar to medullary carcinoma with lymphoid stroma without the lymphocytic infiltration (Fig. 14–84).

Clinical Features. The medullary carcinoma without lymphoid stroma occurred 27 times, for an incidence of 1.2 per cent of the total primary operable cancers (Table 14–25). The average age was 48.6 years, with the oldest patient being 82 and the youngest 30 years. Two cases were detected by mammography alone and three by physical examination alone. Seven occurred under observation. Mass was the most frequent complaint and clinical finding. On gross pathology the mass was greater than 2 cm in diameter in over half the patients.

Radiographic Features. Of 19 radiographic masses, only one was associated with calcifications. In eight cases no true mass was noted (only increased density or asymmetry),

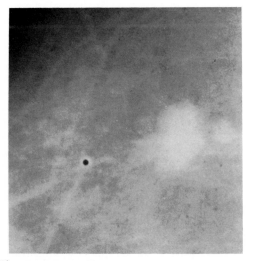

Figure 14–81. Papillary intraductal and microinvasive carcinoma. A 63-year-old woman seen for a checkup. Breasts pendulous but normal clinically. Mammography: 1.2 × 1.5 cm moderately invasive carcinoma containing stippled calcification, probably a small satellite nodule, and diffuse comedo type calcification, all on a background of coalescing ductal hyperplasia. Pathology: 1 × 1.5 cm papillary carcinoma with widespread intraductal papillary carcinoma with microinvasion. Modified radical mastectomy; all 21 axillary lymph nodes negative for metastasis. Six years later, no evidence of disease.

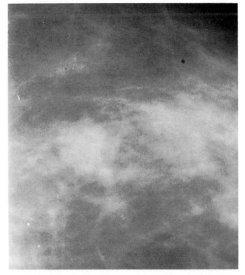

Figure 14–82. Multiple sites of papillary carcinoma. A 56-year-old woman seen for checkup. Mammography: three areas of carcinoma UOQ left breast: posterior one, 8 × 9 mm, circumscribed; anterior one, 4 × 5 cm, rather invasive; middle one, intermediate in size and aggressiveness. Pathology: four distinct sites of papillary carcinoma, much intraductal but at all sites microinvasive tumor. Modified radical mastectomy, all 19 axillary lymph nodes free of tumor. No evidence of disease three years later.

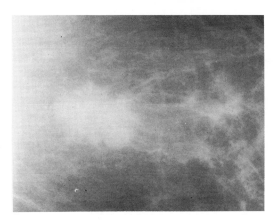

Figure 14–83. Infiltrating and intraductal papillary carcinoma with fibrosis. A 39-year-old woman with a breast lump for six weeks. Mammography: 1.8 × 3 cm carcinoma with variable borders, with areas finely and coarsely spiculated and circumscribed protuberances. Pathology: papillary intraductal and infiltrative carcinoma with fibrosis. Modified radical mastectomy; 10 of 22 nodes positive at Levels I and II. The patient was alive and free of disease almost two years later.

TABLE 14–24. Follow-up of 145 Papillary Carcinomas Alone or Associated with One Other Histologic Type of Carcinoma

	One Type		Two Types		Total	
	No.	*% Alive*	*No.*	*% Alive*	*No.*	*% Alive*
Patients treated 5 years ago	72		8		80	
Alive	60	83	6	75	66	83
Dead, breast cancer	7		2		9	
Dead, not breast cancer	5		0		5	
Patients treated 10 years ago	30		0		30	
Alive	10	33	0		10	33
Dead, breast cancer	12		0		12	
Dead, not breast cancer	8		0		8	

TABLE 14–25. Features of Medullary Carcinoma Without Lymphoid Stroma

Path. Type Cancers	Number	Patient Age (Years)				Detection				Axillary Lymph Nodes*			Tumor Path. Size (cm)					Path. Sites		
		<40	*40–50*	*51–60*	*60+*	*X P + −*	*X P + +*	*X P − +*	*X P − −*	*None*	*Low*	*All Levels*	*0*	*<1*	*1–2*	*2.1–5*	*>5*	*1*	*2–5*	*6+*
One	26	12	5	2	7	2	14	3	7	17	4	4	0	1	10	14	1	25	1	0
Two	1	0	0	0	1	0	1	0	0	1	0	0	0	0	0	0	1	1	0	0
Total	27	12	5	2	8	2	15	3	7	18	4	4	0	1	10	14	2	26	1	0

X = x-ray; P = physical examination; + = positive; − = negative.

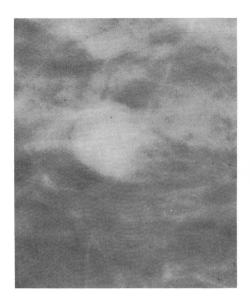

Figure 14–84. Circumscribed duct carcinoma classified as a medullary carcinoma without lymphoid stroma. A 44-year-old woman with carcinoma in skin nodules seen for routine work-up for unknown primary lesion, no palpable breast mass. Mammography: 1.5 cm mass with posterior borders smooth, anterior borders indistinct, in a large breast. Pathology: duct carcinoma, monotonous cellular structure with small cells, adjacent ductal hyperplasia with atypia. Excisional biopsy only.

TABLE 14–26. Follow-up of 26 Medullary Carcinomas Without Lymphoid Stroma Alone or With One Other Histologic Type of Carcinoma

	One Type	
	No.	% Alive
Patients treated 5 years ago	18	
Alive	13	72
Dead, breast cancer	5	
Dead, not breast cancer	0	
Patients treated 10 years ago	12	
Alive	6	50
Dead, breast cancer	6	
Dead, not breast cancer	0	

One occurred with a lobular carcinoma in situ; free of disease at 4 years.

but one of these exhibited calcifications. The carcinomas without lymphoid stroma occurred 15 times in fatty breasts or with fatty ductal hyperplasia, four additional times with ductal hyperplasia, and eight times in glandular or coarsely nodular breasts.

Clinical Course. In 25 cases there was a single focus of tumor; in one there were two foci, and in one case there was one focus of medullary tumor and one focus of lobular carcinoma in situ. In one patient there were simultaneous bilateral primary carcinomas, and in two patients there were nonsimultaneous bilateral primary carcinomas. Nine patients were treated by radical mastectomy, 14 by modified radical mastectomy, two by complete mastectomy, and one with tumorectomy (axillary lymph nodes not studied). One breast had whole-organ studies. Crude five-year survival was 72 per cent, and ten-year survival was 50 per cent (Table 14–26).

Comparison with medullary carcinoma may be made by reference to Chapter 23.

Duct Carcinoma With Metaplasia

Duct carcinoma with metaplasia occurred only four times in this series, for an incidence of 0.2 per cent of the total primary operable breast cancers (Table 14–27). The ages were 47, 48, 65, and 76 years. One lesion was found by x-ray alone and one by clinical examination alone. All produced breast

masses, three being over 2 cm in diameter by gross pathology (Fig. 14–85). Two contained calcifications. Three were in fatty breasts or with fatty ductal hyperplasia, and one was in a coarsely nodular breast. All four were treated by modified radical mastectomy. Each produced one focus of tumor; one had low axillary node metastasis. All these patients were alive and free of disease three to five years after diagnosis.

Apocrine Carcinoma

Apocrine carcinoma is another nonspecific radiographic tumor. It is composed of large apocrine cells with pale pink cytoplasm that tend to grow within dilated ducts, producing papillary projections. Snouts produced by these lining cells are the means by which their cytoplasm is extruded into the gland lumen. Other areas may show a glandular arrangement. The prognosis of apocrine carcinoma is not improved over that of duct carcinoma (Frable and Kay, 1968).

Clinical Features. In our series apocrine carcinoma occurred only nine times, for an incidence of 0.4 per cent of the total primary operable breast cancers (Table 14–28). The oldest woman was 80 years, the youngest 51 years, with an average age of 62.6 years. A mass was palpable in seven patients. Twice, biopsy was based on mammographic findings alone and twice on physical findings alone.

Radiographic Features. A mass was demonstrable seven times, with calcifications being present in four of these (Figs. 14–86 to 14–88). Suspicious calcification not associated with a mass was seen in one breast. Four lesions occurred in fatty breasts or in fatty ductal hyperplasia, another two in ductal hyperplasia, and three in glandular or coarsely nodular breasts.

Clinical Course. In one breast multiple distinct sites of carcinoma were demonstrated (Fig. 14–89). No bilateral lesions were seen. All nine patients underwent modified radical mastectomy. Two women had axillary lymph node metastasis. None died during

TABLE 14–27. Features of Duct Carcinoma With Metaplasia

Path. Type Cancers	Number	Patient Age (Years)				Detection				Axillary Lymph Nodes*			Tumor Path. Size (cm)				Path. Sites		
		<40	40–50	51–60	60+	X P +−	X P ++	X P −+	X P −−	None	Low	All Levels	0	<1	1–2	2.1–5	>5	1	2–5	6+
One	4	1	0	1	2	1	2	1	0	3	1	0	0	0	1	2	1	4	0	0

X = x-ray; P = physical examination; + = positive; − = negative.

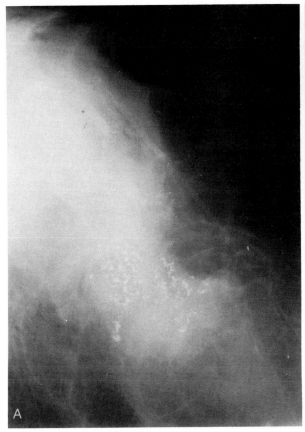

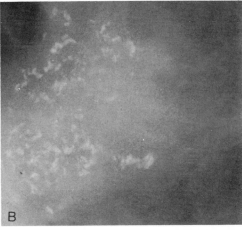

Figure 14–85. Duct carcinoma with chondroid metaplasia. A 58-year-old woman with a 3 mm breast mass UOQ left breast; mother had breast cancer. Mammography: *A*, 2.5 × 4 cm poorly defined mass, course calcifications, increased vein size. *B*, A coned-down view shows the calcifications to be irregular, plaquelike, and bizarre; could be comedocarcinoma type but more suggestive of chondromatous origin. Pathology: infiltrating duct carcinoma with widespread chondromatous metaplasia; no osseous element identified. Modified radical mastectomy; all 14 lymph nodes free of tumor. Three years later the patient was free of disease.

TABLE 14–28. Features of Apocrine Carcinoma

Path. Type Cancers	Number	Patient Age (Years)				Detection				Axillary Lymph Nodes*			Tumor Path. Size (cm)					Path. Sites		
		<40	40–50	51–60	60+	X P + −	X P + +	X P − +	X P − −	None	Low	All Levels	0	<1	1–2	2.1–5	>5	1	2–5	6+
One	9	0	1	2	6	2	5	2	0	7	0	2	2	1	3	2	1	8	0	1

X = x-ray; P = physical examination; + = positive; − = negative.

Figure 14–86. Apocrine breast carcinoma. A 62-year-old woman with a firm mass UOQ right breast; one maternal aunt had breast cancer. Mammography: 1.2 × 1.5 cm moderately invasive carcinoma, upper quadrant of the right breast, against a background of ductal hyperplasia; subareolar fibrosis on the left. Pathology: apocrine carcinoma varying from well differentiated to poorly differentiated; 18 lymph nodes free of tumor; modified radical mastectomy. The patient was free of disease six years later.

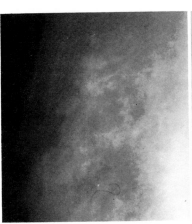

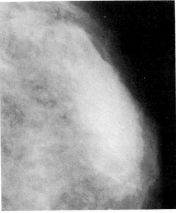

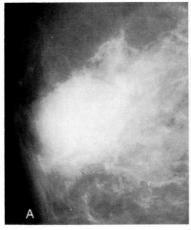

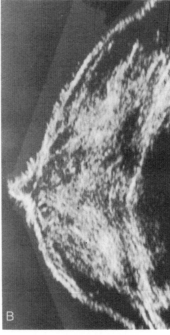

Figure 14–87. Apocrine carcinoma. A 74-year-old woman with a breast lump for one month. Suspicious mass clinically. *A,* Mammography: circumscribed subareolar carcinoma with bizarre calcifications. *B,* Sonography: slightly irregular (almost well-demarcated) mass with complex internal echoes, distorted architecture, no attenuation, skin changes. Pathology: apocrine carcinoma, invasive in type, with 2 of 18 axillary lymph nodes found containing metastases following modified radical mastectomy. The patient was free of disease 18 months later.

follow-up; no distant metastasis was demonstrated, but only one woman was subject to a ten-year follow-up.

Miscellaneous Carcinomas

Certain unusual breast carcinomas may be specific entities, whereas others simply do

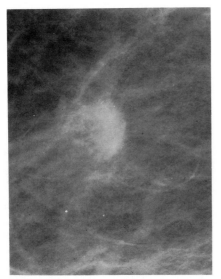

Figure 14–88. Apocrine carcinoma. A 75-year-old woman with a breast lump for one year; one sister had breast cancer. A suspicious mass was palpable. Mammography: 1.2 × 1.5 cm circumscribed carcinoma containing faint stippled calcifications. Pathology: apocrine carcinoma. Modified radical mastectomy; one Level I lymph node and one Level II node of 16 nodes contained metastatic tumor. At two-year follow-up, no evidence of disease.

not fit a neat histopathologic classification. An example of the first would be a carcinoid or lipid-rich carcinoma having specific characteristics; others would fit more nearly such growth patterns as "anaplastic" or "pleomorphic," often depending on the inclinations of the pathologist. Examples of the latter would be carcinoma simplex (not otherwise specified) or adenocarcinoma (with a tendency to acinar formation).

Experience is usually so limited that the radiographic criteria cannot be comfortably established.

Carcinoid Tumor

Two carcinoid type tumors were demonstrated in women aged 61 and 67 years. Both had symptoms unrelated to the tumor, and the tumors were demonstrated solely by mammography in breasts with fatty ductal hyperplasia. Both masses were only moderately invasive and less than 1 cm in diameter (Fig. 14–90). No radiographic calcification was present. Each produced only one site of tumor; only one had axillary lymph node metastasis. One patient was treated by radical mastectomy and one by modified radical mastectomy. Both were free of disease one and three years after diagnosis. By electron microscopy both had argyrophilic-positive granules. In neither woman was there evidence of systemic effect of a carcinoid tumor.

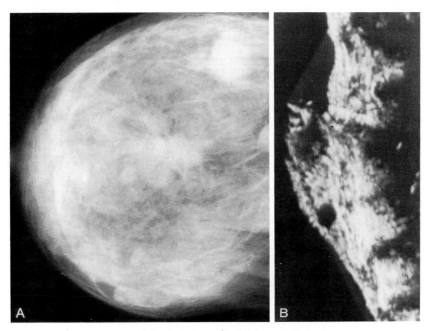

Figure 14–89. Multiple duct carcinomas, apocrine type. A 71-year-old woman with a mass in the UOQ of the right breast for two months. *A,* Mammography: seven masses ranging up to 12 × 15 mm in size, mostly well circumscribed, that suggest intracystic papillary carcinomas. *B,* Sonography: numerous fairly well-demarcated solid tumors, one cystic. Pathology: eight discrete masses of duct carcinoma; one contained central hemorrhage. Modified radical mastectomy; metastases to all axillary lymph node levels (5 of 13). The patient died of a stroke shortly after surgery.

Anaplastic Carcinoma

In three cases the carcinoma was considered unusually anaplastic, occurring in women aged 38, 46, and 56 years. Two were in a fatty breast and one in a glandular breast. Only one breast was clinically abnormal, with two lesions being found by x-ray alone. In no case was there any x-ray calcification or mass. One woman had a modified radical mastectomy without axillary lymph node metastasis and was alive and free of disease three years after diagnosis. The other two had biopsy with radiotherapy, with death occurring from disease within two years.

Pathologists describe breast carcinoma with squamous differentiation. These lesions have no special mammographic appearance.

Twenty-five cases of primary breast carcinoma were placed into this "miscellaneous" category because they did not fit into the listed histologic types. Eighteen were single lesions in one site in the breast. Six occurred with a duct carcinoma and one with a duct and lobular carcinoma. The average age of these women was 50.7 years, with the oldest

Figure 14–90. Primary carcinoid of the breast. A 61-year-old woman studied for hyperkeratosis of the right nipple. Mammography: 8 × 10 mm moderately invasive carcinoma of the UOQ of the right breast. Pathology: on localization and biopsy, a duct carcinoma with 10 of 21 axillary lymph nodes with metastases; radical mastectomy; neurosecretory granules suspected by light microscopy. Electron microscopy: Argyrophil-positive granules, 275 to 350 mm in size, in Grimelius-stained sections confirmed histogenesis of breast carcinoid. One year later, the patient was free of disease. Clinical work-up failed to demonstrate systemic effect of a carcinoid tumor.

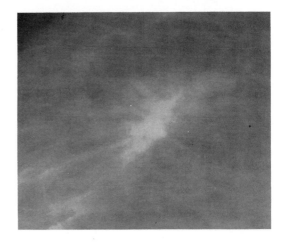

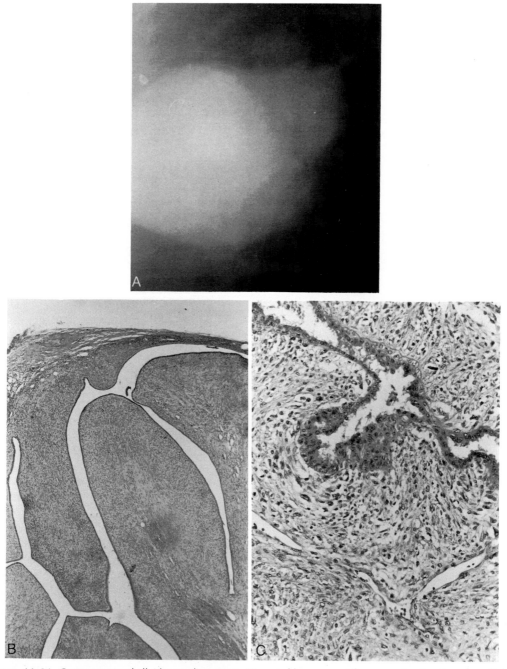

Figure 14–91. Cystosarcoma phylloides, malignant. A 63-year-old woman with a mass for two months, clinically suspicious. *A,* Mammography: 4.1 × 4.8 cm circumscribed lobulated carcinoma against chest wall; operable. Pathology: malignant cystosarcoma phylloides. *B,* Low-power field shows typical clefts and fronds. *C,* Malignant cells in the high-power field, demonstrating marked stromal cellularity and mild hyperplasia of the ductal epithelium. Estimation of the malignant potential is based primarily on the degree of mitotic activity. Modified radical mastectomy; 0 of 18 nodes positive; the patient was alive and well 11 years later.

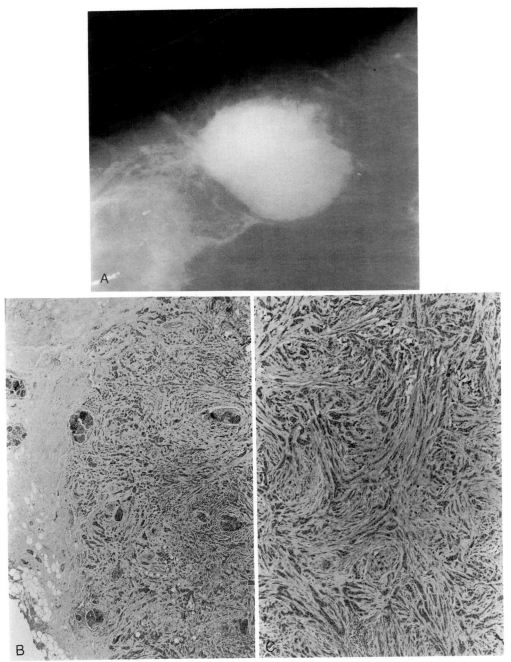

Figure 14–92. Malignant cystosarcoma phylloides. A 76-year-old woman fell eight months before and a breast mass appeared. Clinically: suspicious mass. Mammography: 4.2 × 5.2 cm circumscribed lobulated carcinoma; increased vascularity. Pathology: cystosarcoma phylloides, malignant. Modified radical mastectomy, all 21 axillary lymph nodes free of tumor. The patient was alive without disease ten and a half years later. *B*, Low-power field shows a relatively circumscribed periphery. *C*, Higher power shows swirls of malignant cells.

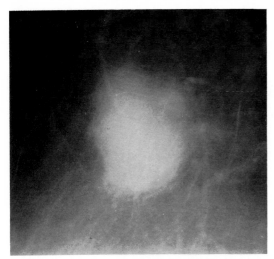

Figure 14–93. Malignant cystosarcoma phylloides. A 69-year-old woman with a "cyst" in her breast for months. Clinically: hard mass of cancer. Mammography: 2.5 × 3.1 cm lobulated circumscribed carcinoma; lobulation suggests cystosarcoma phylloides. Pathology: cystosarcoma phylloides, malignant; modified radical mastectomy; 0 of 16 nodes positive. The patient was alive and free of disease 12 years later.

being 79 and the youngest 26 years. Seven tumors were detected solely by mammography and one by clinical examination. Seven patients were treated by biopsy and radiotherapy, the remaining receiving mastectomy. Only eight cancer deaths occurred (seven in those patients without mastectomy). Exclusive of these, the prognosis was good.

Specific Histologic Types

Medullary carcinoma with lymphoid stroma, mucinous carcinoma, and intracystic papillary carcinoma are treated in separate chapters.

Clinical Syndromes

Paget's disease, inflammatory carcinoma, multiple carcinomas, and bilateral carcinomas are dealt with in their respective chapters. Also, carcinomas in the immediate subareolar area are not frequent but do occur often enough to require differentiation from the many benign subareolar densities. The clinician finds this superficial area difficult to evaluate. At times the radiologist cannot differentiate subareolar fibrosis from cancer (see Chapter 20). Lesions in the extreme periphery of the breast are discussed in Chapter 21.

Sarcoma

All the mesenchymal supporting tissues of the breast, including vascular and lymphatic tissues, can produce intramammary sarcomas. Such lesions are uncommon and usually

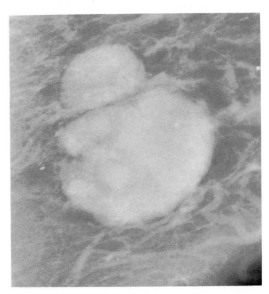

Figure 14–95. Malignant cystosarcoma phylloides. An 80-year-old woman who bruised her breast; a mass had been present for nine months. Splenectomy 17 years previously for Hodgkin's disease. Clinically: most likely cancer. Mammography: 2.8 × 3.2 cm bilobed circumscribed homogeneous mass with irregular protuberances; increased vascularity. Pathology: cystosarcoma phylloides, malignant. Modified radical mastectomy; all 16 axillary lymph nodes free of tumor. The patient was alive and well two years later.

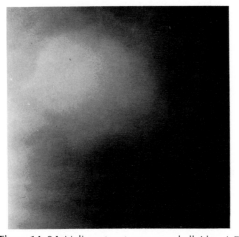

Figure 14–94. Malignant cystosarcoma phylloides. A 75-year-old woman who clinically had a breast cyst. Mammography: 2.7 × 3.3 cm circumscribed lobulated carcinoma. Pathology: malignant cystosarcoma phylloides. Modified radical mastectomy; 0 of 16 axillary lymph nodes positive. The patient was alive and well 14 years later.

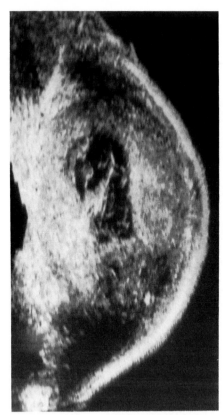

Figure 14–96. Malignant cystosarcoma phylloides. A 23-year-old woman with an enlarging breast for the past three weeks following trauma. Clinically: ecchymosis and mass, a pectoral muscle rupture and hemorrhage. Mammography before admission showed a very dense enlarged breast. Sonography: lobulated, demarcated complex mass, with irregular internal material, increased through-transmission suggesting a cystic component. Suspected a circumscribed carcinoma as medullary that is most likely to have a necrotic center. Pathology: malignant cystosarcoma phylloides with necrosis and hemorrhage. Modified radical mastectomy; 0 of 21 nodes positive. The patient was alive and well three years later.

have no specific radiographic characteristics. Two of the more common, but still infrequent, lesions are cystosarcoma phylloides and primary lymphoma of the breast.

Cystosarcoma Phylloides

Malignant cystosarcoma phylloides occurred eight times, for a 0.4 per cent incidence of our total primary operable breast cancers, indicating an infrequent tumor. Yet this lesion provokes lengthy discussion owing to its terminology and inconsistent degree of malignancy. The gross appearance on sectioning suggests the origin of the name: sarcomatous with cystic or cleftlike spaces of myxoid fluid; prolongations of tissue, like leaves, seem to float in this gelatinous fluid.

This cannot be confused with the cysts of fibrocystic disease; a benign cystosarcoma phylloides (benign sarcoma) is a misnomer. Based on size alone, a radiographic diagnostic clue was suggested years ago by the author to separate the benign and malignant versions, e.g., a giant fibroadenoma to represent benign and a cystosarcoma phylloides to represent malignant. This also is not reliable, as the smaller of the two may be malignant. For the purposes of this discussion, a malignant cystosarcoma phylloides is histologically malignant, and in the benign category it is histologically benign.

Differentiation of the benign and malignant cystosarcoma phylloides cannot be made by mammography with confidence (Fig. 14–91 to 14–96). The lesion may be so large that minute study of its borders for infiltration is impossible. The diagnosis of malignant cystosarcoma phylloides is made on a cellular basis by the pathologist. At times an area of invasion may be seen on the mammograms; the pathologist may then be directed to the proper area for histologic investigation and thus establish the diagnosis of malignant cystosarcoma phylloides.

Of our eight cases, six occurred as single deposits of tumor in the breast. On gross pathology, five were 2 to 5 cm in size and three were greater than 5 cm in diameter. One tumor occurred with a duct carcinoma and one with a duct and lobular carcinoma.

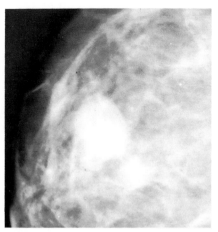

Figure 14–97. Melanoma metastatic to the breast. The patient was a 36-year-old woman with a four-year history of melanoma of the lower leg, and metastases to inguinal nodes and to the lungs bilaterally. A nodule was palpable in the breast; mammograms showed distinct nodules (above) and questionable nodules in the opposite breast. Postmortem three months later showed many melanotic nodules in both breasts measuring up to 3.5 cm.

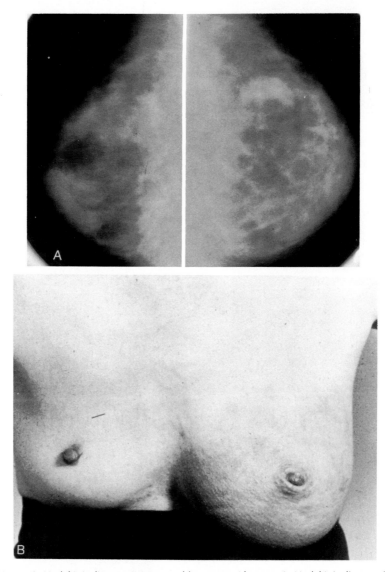

Figure 14–98. Metastatic Hodgkin's disease. A 24-year-old woman with systemic Hodgkin's disease. Clinically: bilateral axillary lymph nodes, suspicious mass in left breast. *A,* Mammography: 2 × 3 cm well-circumscribed mass, upper quadrant of left breast; thickened skin; diffuse increased breast density. Pathology: Hodgkin's lymphoma, nodular sclerotic type. *B,* The breast was enlarged, the nipple and areola were fixed, and there was slight discoloration of the skin of this breast.

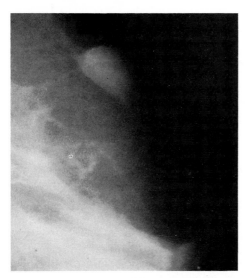

Figure 14–99. Systemic Hodgkin's disease with breast mass. A 69-year-old woman with known Hodgkin's disease and a clinically benign 0.5 × 1.5 cm breast mass. Mammography: 1.2 × 1.4 cm sharply defined mass considered medullary carcinoma. Excision biopsy: small discrete mass of Hodgkin's lymphoma.

The average age of the patient was 48.3 years, with the oldest being 80 and the youngest 24 years. This is a much older age than with the benign variety or with giant fibroadenoma, a good differential diagnostic point. A clinical mass was present in all cases except for one that was detected solely by mammography. No characteristic calcification was seen by x-ray except, on occasion, that of the fibroadenoma. All but one lesion occurred in dense glandular or coarsely nodular breasts. Treatment consisted of one radical, four modified radical, and two complete mastectomies, with one woman having tumorectomy only. No lymph node metastasis was demonstrated. Two women died of disease, one before 5 years and one 10 years following diagnosis.

At the M. D. Anderson Hospital and Tumor Institute, of 720 primary breast cancers, three malignant cystosarcoma phylloides

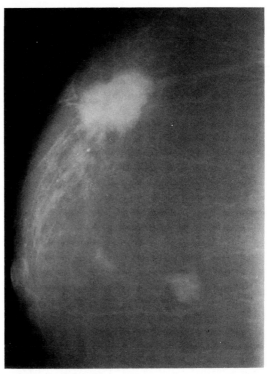

Figure 14–100. Primary breast carcinoma and leukemic metastases of the breast. A 78-year-old woman whose lymphatic leukemia was stable on chemotherapy; breast lump for one week; clinically cancer; question of leukemic metastasis. Mammography: 1.8 × 2.7 cm moderately invasive carcinoma containing stippled calcifications. Pathology (segmental resection): duct carcinoma with comedo and colloid pattern; small nodule of leukemia.

were diagnosed on the basis of recurrence. This 0.4 per cent incidence compared with that at Emory University. One case of the three did contain disease metastatic to the axillary lymph nodes.

Lymphoma

Primary lymphoma of the breast is also uncommon, occurring only four times in our series, for an incidence of 0.18 per cent of the total primary operable breast cancers. The ages of the women were 24, 29, 52, and 69

TABLE 14–29. Features of Breast Metastasis, Not Breast Cancer (Emory University)

Path. Type Cancers	Number	Patient Age (Years)				Detection				Axillary Lymph Nodes*			Tumor Path. Size (cm)				
		<40	40–50	51–60	60+	X P + −	X P + +	X P − +	X P − −	None	Low	All Levels	0	<1	1–2	2.1–5	>5
One	27	10	5	8	5	3	19	4	1	0	0	1*	†	3	4	6	2
Two	1	1	0	0	0	0	1	0	0	0	0	0*	0	0	1	0

X = x-ray; P = physical examination; + = positive; − = negative.
*27 not studied.
†13 no resection.

TABLE 14–30. Types of Breast Metastasis, Not Breast Cancer (Emory University)

Type Cancer	Number
Single Type	
Melanoma	3
Amelanotic melanoma	1
Anaplastic histiocytic lymphoma	1
Hodgkin's lymphoma	6
Squamous cell (neck)	1
Lymphocytic lymphosarcoma	4
Lytic bone lesion	1
Ovarian	1
Rhabdomyosarcoma (groin)	1
Lung	1
Bone marrow	1
Reticulum cell sarcoma	4
Alveolar soft tissue sarcoma (thigh)	1
Unclassified	1
Lymphosarcoma and soft tissue sarcoma	1

years. All presented with a breast nodule that was evident clinically and by x-ray. The masses were devoid of calcifications. One mass was less than 2 cm, two were 2 to 5 cm, and one was greater than 5 cm in diameter on gross pathology. Each occurred at a single site in the breast. One patient had a radical mastectomy, and three had tumorectomy with radiotherapy and/or chemotherapy. Lymph nodes were studied in two patients only, and both were positive at all levels. Systemic disease was not demonstrated at the time of diagnosis. Three of the patients died within five years, two with disease, and one died with disease six years after diagnosis.

Radiographically the masses were simply moderately circumscribed without identifying characteristics.

Metastatic Cancer to Breast from Distant Sites

M. D. Anderson Series

Only eight times in 728 cases of malignant breast lesions were the sites of the primary cancer other than the breast. These metastatic malignant masses included three melanomas (Fig. 14–97), two Hodgkin's disease (Figs. 14–98 and 14–99), alveolar rhabdomyosarcoma, one leukemia (Fig. 14–100), one lymphosarcoma, and one reticulum cell sarcoma. Usually, the metastatic nodule is mistaken for a circumscribed carcinoma of the breast. If the presence of widespread cancer is known and there are dense nodules in the breast, cancer metastatic to the breast should be suspected.

Emory University Series

During the study of 2209 primary operable breast cancers, 28 cases of breast metastasis from distant sites were encountered. One contained two types of cancer. Eight were bilateral, four simultaneous and four nonsimultaneous (Tables 14–29 and 14–30). This was an incidence of 1.2 per cent of all the 2,375 cancers included in the series, both primary and secondary, operable and inoperable. The oldest woman was 75 years, the youngest 19 years, with an average age of 45.1 years. Much of the data were incomplete, as 13 patients had only biopsy, 14 simple mastectomy, and one a whole-organ study. Most of the lesions were apparent either clinically or on x-ray. Thirteen were in fatty breasts or in fatty ductal hyperplasia, six in glandular breasts, and nine in coarsely nodular breasts.

There were no distinguishing radiographic features except for usually a circumscribed mass. Subject to five years' follow-up, 15 patients had died, 14 with systemic disease. Two were alive, and one had died by the ninth year of follow-up.

REFERENCES

Carstens PHB (1978): Tubular carcinoma of the breast. A study of frequency. Am J Clin Pathol 70:204.

Frable WJ, Kay S (1968): Carcinoma of the breast: histologic and clinical features of apocrine tumors. Cancer 21:756.

Hutter RVP, Foote FW, Farrow JH (1970): In situ lobular carcinoma of the female breast, 1939–1968. *In* Breast Cancer, Early and Late. Chicago, Year Book Medical Publishers, pp 219–220.

Male Breast Diseases

15

BACKGROUND

The occurrence of breast cancer in the male is so infrequent that oncologists see very few cases and thus place little emphasis on the disease. Even pathologic enlargement of the male breast is not common, may be confused with subcutaneous fatty deposition in the breast area, and usually regresses in a year or so. In a clinical setting, unless a male complains of a hard mass or enlargement of his breast so pronounced that he becomes self-conscious, little emphasis is placed on diseases of the male breast.

Embryologically the development of the male breast parallels that of the female until shortly after birth, when the maternal hormone effects (such as "witch's milk") disappear.

BENIGN

Normally the male breast radiographically produces a nipple shadow with varying amounts of fatty tissue beneath. At the most, histologically there are a few vestigial ducts.

There may be generalized enlargement of the male breast from increased deposition of fatty tissue that is associated with a mild degree of proliferation of the ducts.

Gynecomastia

Transient hypertrophy of the male breast is more common than is reported to the clinician. Normally the breast enlargement occurs at the time of puberty or at an advanced age. The two forms may be separated into pubertal and senile types, as only the hypertrophy at the older age must be differentiated from malignancy. Both forms are idiopathic without known relationship to endocrine disorders and do not differ significantly clinically, radiographically, or pathologically.

Pubertal

A significant number of males aged 12 to 16 or 18 years experience some degree of breast enlargement that usually disappears in three to six months. It may be only a 1 to 3 cm disk of tissue under the nipple, initially it may be unilateral, then bilateral, or it may be bilateral when first noted. In a limited number of these young males the enlargement is more marked and may persist as long as two to three years. These are the patients most often seen by the physician. Most of the gynecomastia per se is fibrous tissue with limited ductal elements, dense on x-ray against the background of fatty tissues.

Senile

The gynecomastia that occurs in men, usually after 50 years of age, is considered senile type. It too may be transient, unilateral, or bilateral.

Associated with Organic Disease

Breast enlargement in the male may be associated with developmental anomalies such as hypogonadism, frequently associated

289

with cryptorchidism and hypospadias, Klinefelter's syndrome, or Reifenstein's syndrome. Organic diseases also directly affect the developed testes as trauma, mumps orchitis, or neoplasms; indirectly their effect is through diseases of the adrenal cortex and thyroid gland as well as liver and chronic pulmonary diseases.

Hormones, Drug-Induced

Estrogens have regularly produced gynecomastia when used over long periods in treatment of carcinoma of the prostate. Even androgens have produced these changes in the male breast.

Digitalis causes gynecomastia and classically produces a distinct mammographic pattern when given over long periods (usually for heart disease): enlargement and proportions of the female breast, and fatty ductal hyperplasia frequently associated with typical calcifications. Experienced mammographers may have difficult recognizing mammograms of such breasts as being from a male patient.

Diagnosis

The most frequent complaint in the male breast is generalized enlargement or a palpable mass. This is usually gynecomastia and in the male results from increased deposition of adipose tissue that is associated with some degree of proliferating breast tissue (Fig. 15–1). As a result of this increased glandular tissue many of the usual benign processes occurring in the female breast occur in the male. Our present nomenclature for benign male breast lesions includes only gynecomastia with or without superimposed fibrocystic disease. Most of the increased size of the breast is due to the increased subcutaneous adipose tissue. The enlargement of the glandular tissue results either in a small rounded mass of glandular tissue just beneath the nipple, having primarily the appearance of the fibrous type of fibrocystic disease; or in a cystlike mass ranging from several millimeters up to 2 cm in size.

Also, from examples of male breast enlargement seen in Figure 15–1, the enlargement may be entirely due to fatty tissue or primarily due to fatty tissue with only remnants of the duct system just immediately beneath the nipple. The diagnosis of gynecomastia then becomes a relative one but should be reserved for the presence of a distinct rounded mass of tissue (Fig. 15–1B), an irregular deposit of fibroglandular tissue (Fig. 15–1C), or diffuse deposition of fibroglandular tissue (Fig. 15–1D). With mild to marked obesity in the male there is almost always increased deposition of fatty tissue in the breast area without evidence of gynecomastia.

Breast sonography in gynecomastia does not differ significantly from that of the normal female breast (Fig. 15–2). Gynecomastia with the fibrocystic disease that is usually associated with the female may be clearly noted in the more glandular male breast (Fig. 15–3). In these older men, particularly clinically, there arises the problem of differentiation of gynecomastia from carcinoma and, in the cases of gynecomastia in men with carcinoma of the prostate, the presence of metastatic prostatic carcinoma in the breast.

MALIGNANT

Incidence

The experience of a single individual with carcinoma of the male breast is extremely limited. Our experience of 87 male breast carcinomas at the M. D. Anderson Hospital and Tumor Institute over a 30-year period (1945 to 1975) was reviewed by Yap and Tashima (1979). My participation was during less than one third of that time. During that period there were 11,183 women with breast cancer, making the incidence of male breast cancer 0.77 per cent. Three men had bilateral carcinomas, with one man having them simultaneously.

Clinical Manifestations

The age range was 25 to 86 years, with the peak between the fifth and sixth decades. The presenting symptoms are listed in Table 15–1.

The delay in diagnosis ranged from one month to seven years. Gynecomastia was present in 14 per cent. Recorded masses ranged from 0.5 to 13 cm in diameter: 23 masses less than 2 cm, 38 masses 2 to 5 cm, and 14 masses over 5 cm in diameter. Out of the 46 cases of axillary lymph nodes available for study, in 16 cases the nodes were free of tumor. Without axillary lymph node metastasis there was a disease-free period of 97.8 months compared with 21 months when these nodes were involved with tumor.

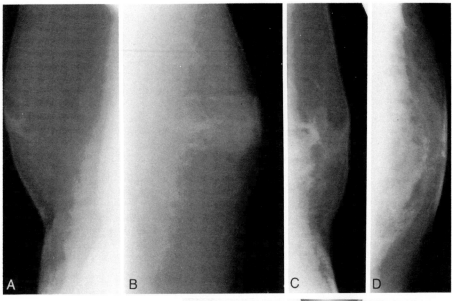

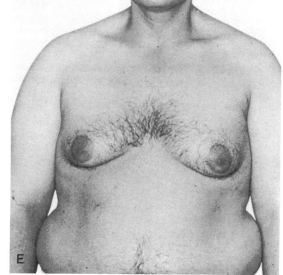

Figure 15–1. Enlargement of male breasts. *A,* Fatty deposition without increase in glandular tissue in a 63-year-old man. *B,* "Ball-like" or circumscribed gynecomastia in a 48-year-old man. *C,* Opposite breast in the 63-year-old man showing a less circumscribed gynecomastia. *D,* Generalized or diffuse glandular tissue in a 35-year-old man with gynecomastia. *E,* Twenty-one-year old male with bilateral gynecomastia.

In comparison with female breast cancer patients, the males were older and their carcinomas more centrally located, with greater involvement of the nipple. Spread and prognosis did not differ from the female patients in terms of tumor size and axillary lymph node status.

Diagnosis

Radiographic signs of carcinoma in the male breast, including calcification and nipple changes of Paget's disease, are identical to those in the female. Usually the lesions in the male breast are more advanced, so that the entire breast is involved and ulceration of the skin has occurred. The usual carcinoma of the male breast is readily recognized on the mammograms. A portion, however, tend to produce a well-circumscribed rounded central density very similar to gynecomastia

TABLE 15–1. Carcinoma of the Male Breast

Presenting Symptom	Per Cent
Painless mass	47
Mass, plus nipple retraction	22
Mass, plus nipple discharge	8
Mass, plus ulceration	9
Breast ulceration	9
Axillary mass	2
Painful mass	2

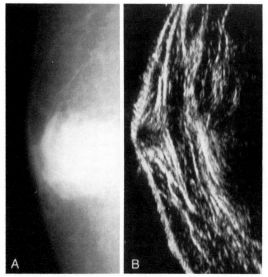

Figure 15–2. Unilateral gynecomastia. A 41-year-old man with a mass under the right nipple. The patient had been on digitalis for years. *A*, Mammography: 1.5 × 2 cm mass of fibroglandular tissue symmetrically located under the nipple, gynecomastia. Opposite breast: normal fatty tissue. *B*, Sonography: mostly subcutaneous fat but a central rounded area under the nipple, hypoechoic with varying types of echoes; benign. Pathology: gynecomastia.

(Figs. 15–4 and 15–5). The rounded density of gynecomastia is often associated with apparent diffuse skin thickening and may be diagnosed as carcinoma. This skin thickening is produced by the small breast having a greater arc of skin tangential to the x-ray beam, and in some males there is an actual overall increase in skin thickness compared with the female. Any one radiologist will have limited experience with male breast studies and must be extremely careful in his diagnosis by mammography.

Whole organ studies reveal other similarities of male breast carcinoma to female breast carcinoma (Figs. 15–6 to 15–8).

M. D. Anderson Experience

Our experience with male breast cancer at the M. D. Anderson Hospital and Tumor Institute was reviewed by Robinson and Montegue (1986). It concerned 39 men admitted for primary definitive treatment and 30 men for first treatment failure. The age ranged from 25 to 86 years with a median of 66 years. All patients had a mass or swelling, bloody nipple discharge, nipple retraction or ulceration, or an axillary or supraclavicular mass. One had a history of gynecomastia. Delays in diagnosis ranged from 2 to 24

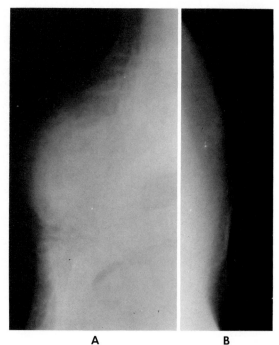

A   **B**

Figure 15–3. Gynecomastia. *A*, Cystic type. A 67-year-old man with carcinoma of the prostate; on estrogen therapy two and one-half years. Clinically: bilaterally enlarged breasts. Mammography 3.5 × 5 cm mass of fibroglandular tissue; gynecomastia. Pathology: gynecomastia with hyperplasia. *B*, A 69-year-old man with a clinical mass deep to the nipple. Mammography: gynecomastia with focal calcifications. Pathology: gynecomastia with fibrocystic disease. (The male breast frequently lacks the fatty contrast of the female breast.)

months: Those with a favorable stage averaged 10 months, while those with an unfavorable stage averaged 18 months.

Clinically the tumors ranged in size from 1.5 to 12 cm. There were no bilateral cancers. Twelve of 21 cases, six without and six with axillary lymph node metastases, had no evidence of disease 2 to 32 years following treatment. Radical mastectomy had generally been the treatment of choice, but more limited surgery with irradiation controlled the disease better with less disability. A 50 per cent ten-year survival was recorded for all these men with breast cancer, which compared favorably with the results in women with similar staged disease.

OBSERVATIONS

The spiculated mass of male breast carcinoma, usually with advanced secondary signs and all the characteristics of female breast carcinoma, including calcifications, is

Figure 15–4. A and B, Carcinoma of the male breast. A 59-year-old man with a breast lump for "several" months, no pain. Clinically: firm 2 × 3 cm mass with fixation of the nipple. Mammography: 1 × 1.5 cm fairly circumscribed mass attached to the right areolar skin, retraction of the nipple, probable thickening of the skin of the areola despite symmetric placement at the nipple; carcinoma. Pathology: infiltrating duct carcinoma, all 20 axillary lymph nodes free of tumor.

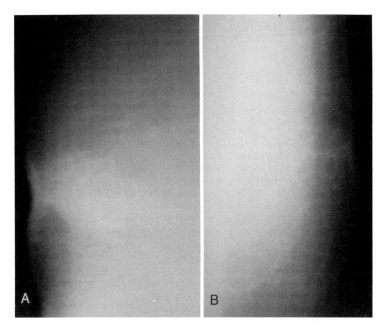

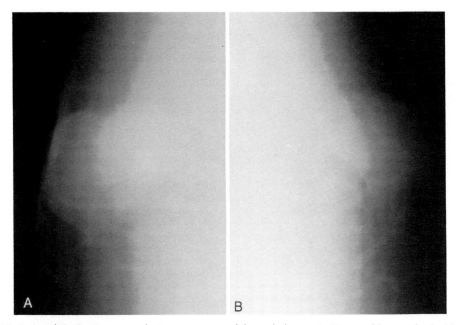

Figure 15–5. A and B, Carcinoma producing asymmetry of the male breast. A 57-year-old man who had been seeing his family physician for approximately one year for swellling of both breasts. Clinically: palpable tissue beneath both areolae, firmer on the right. Mammography: 1.5 × 2 cm rounded mass of tissue beneath each areola, more distinct on the right; a question of areolar skin flattening; masses symmetric in relation to the nipples. Gynecomastia on left, but asymmetry in breasts makes the right highly suspicious. Pathology: duct carcinoma of right breast; 18 axillary lymph nodes free of disease. The patient was free of disease four years later.

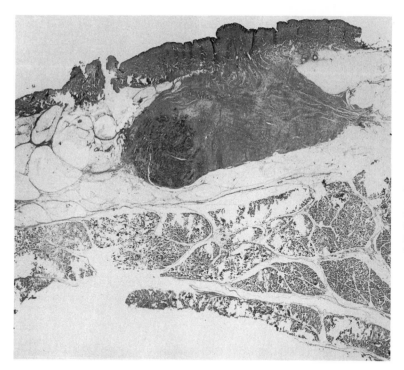

Figure   15–6.   Whole-organ mount of carcinoma in gynecomastia. The carcinoma of Figure 15–5 can be identified at the periphery of the rather bulky dense fibroglandular tissue of gynecomastia. The defect in the skin over the tumor was due to biopsy. Pathology: infiltrating duct carcinoma; all 24 axillary lymph nodes were free of tumor.

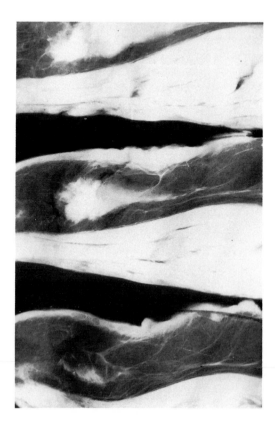

Figure 15–7. Slicer section of male breast carcinoma. A 58-year-old man presented with a breast mass of unknown duration. Clinically: bilateral gynecomastia with a poorly defined mass in the LOQ of the right breast. Mammography: bilateral gynecomastia measuring 2 × 2.5 cm in diameter, with a 1 cm irregular spiculated mass in its periphery LOQ right breast; carcinoma. The whole-organ slicer section of the radical mastectomy specimen, above, shows the carcinoma with that portion of the density toward the nipple gynecomastia.

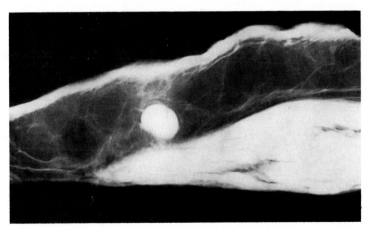

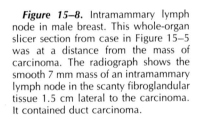

Figure 15–8. Intramammary lymph node in male breast. This whole-organ slicer section from case in Figure 15–5 was at a distance from the mass of carcinoma. The radiograph shows the smooth 7 mm mass of an intramammary lymph node in the scanty fibroglandular tissue 1.5 cm lateral to the carcinoma. It contained duct carcinoma.

not a diagnostic challenge to the average mammographer, and there has been little effort here to illustrate that. However, even to the most experienced mammographer the symmetric rounded ball of carcinomatous tissue beneath the areola can be confused with the dense fibrotic tissue of gynecomastia, similarly placed, with pseudothickening of the skin of the areola. Emphasis here has been directed to this lack of clear-cut distinction radiographically.

The persistent masses that clinically should tend to be transient, in men aged 40 to 60 years and older, should be viewed with considerable suspicion and do not require a full-blown clinical and radiographic diagnosis of carcinoma for investigation to be pursued.

Our Emory University experience has consisted of seven primary cases of male breast cancer during the period in which 2056 primary operable breast cancers were seen in females, for a rate of 0.35 per cent. Our data base contains only those cases having mammography prior to biopsy. In the M. D. Anderson series, nearly three fourths of male breast cancer patients had had a diagnostic work-up elsewhere prior to admission.

REFERENCES

Robison R, Montague E (1982): Treatment results in males with breast cancer. Cancer 49:403.
Yap HY, Tashima CK (1979): Male breast cancer: a natural history study. CA 44:748.

Ductal Epithelial Hyperplasia

16

BACKGROUND

Speculations on the relationship of benign breast processes to carcinoma have abounded. These implied histologic changes, usually proliferative, have been given a wide variety of designations, including chronic mastitis (Warren, 1940); benign lesions (Clagett et al., 1944); chronic cystic mastitis (Foote and Sterrart, 1945); cysts (Davis et al., 1964); large duct epithelial hyperplasia (Humphrey and Swerlow, 1968); ductal hyperplasia (Gallager and Martin, 1969); hyperplastic alveolar nodules (Wellings et al., 1975); and epitheliosis (Azzopardi, 1979).

In the 1950s our radiographic-pathologic study of breast calcifications led to the recognition of ductal hyperplasia by mammography. Once it was learned to avoid highly acid fixatives and stains to study these calcifications by light microscopy, it readily became apparent that denser flecks than glandular tissue on the mammograms were not all calcifications. On H & E preparations these were noted in areas of advanced ductal hyperplasia and were found to be produced

by ducts seen on-end packed with cells, analogous to a blood vessel seen on-end on a chest radiograph. This pattern was so often associated with breast carcinoma that for years we used ductal hyperplasia as a strong secondary sign of carcinoma (unpublished to avoid the appearance of the radiologist's practicing histopathology). Concurrently arose the hypothesis that carcinoma could well have its origin in this hyperplastic process.

Thus, very early in our experience with mammography we recognized the frequent association of ductal hyperplasia with carcinoma, its potential for masking a small carcinoma, its confusing fine calcifications, and its being a secondary sign of carcinoma (Egan, 1960).

Certain proliferative changes may be considered nonobligate precursors of malignancy. These histologic changes, which include the epithelial hyperplasias, papillomatosis, and atypias, have been reported to be associated with an increased risk of subsequent development of malignancy varying from 1.8 to 6 times the natural incidence of carcinoma (Fisher et al., 1975; Moskowitz et al., 1976; Page et al., 1978).

To us the term ductal (epithelial) hyperplasia seems most appropriate. It is purely the epithelial cells that are essential. The particular pattern of their arrangement is not contributory. "Papillomatosis" in this setting refers merely to piling up of the hyperplastic cells without true papillomata with fibrous stalks. "Atypia" indicates only a more bizarre appearance of these cells. Epitheliosis would be an acceptable synonym.

RADIOGRAPHIC, SONOGRAPHIC, AND SUBGROSS CORRELATION

Although the radiologist cannot predict precise histologic diagnoses, the mammographic appearance may suggest a dominant pattern of fibrocystic disease, especially proliferative epithelial processes. In a review of our work, Gallager could not break down which hyperplastic process (ductal hyperplasia, lobular hyperplasia) was more clearly related to carcinoma—in his term, was the "non-obligate precursor of cancer" (Gallager and Martin, 1969). Certainly, the radiologist should not be expected to compete with the pathologist in this decision.

Radiographically there are two forms of hyperplastic types of fibrocystic disease that may be recognized. Usually each is more commonly associated with the premenopausal type of breast, which has considerable fibroglandular tissues remaining. The breast is relatively firm and still retains moderate radiographic density. Both may be present to varying degrees in the same breast, but both are bilateral and have been described (Egan, 1964).

In ductal hyperplasia, rather prominent major ducts may be traced to a greater extent than normal into the breast. The ducts may be distinctly outlined in continuity into the third or even fourth arborization. They then become apparent as numerous ill-defined 2 to 3 mm densities that resemble snowflakes (Figs. 16–1 to 16–8). As a rule, these densities do not interfere appreciably with the radiographic study of the breast. At times, ductal hyperplasia is a useful secondary sign of carcinoma mammographically.

Lobular hyperplasia (adenosis) with numerous densities scattered throughout both breasts, often with one breast slightly more involved than the other, may be recognized. The densities are lobular or segmental in distribution. Some opacities are quite large and dense, obscure overlying trabeculae, and produce homogeneous areas. Their outlines mimic the irregular borders of certain cysts; other lesions with clear margins may suggest fibroadenomata. Some have almost straight edges as though restrained by the supporting ligaments (see Chapter 13). Less typically, the densities due to hyperplasia or adenosis may be sparse. Thus, it is difficult to differentiate ill-defined areas of conglomerate cyst formation or fat necrosis from areas of hyperplastic fibrosis.

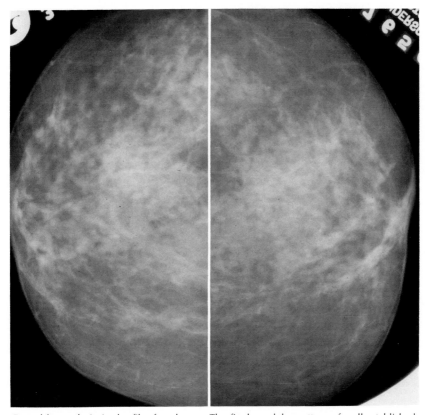

Figure 16–1. Ductal hyperplasia in the fibrofatty breast. The finely nodular pattern of well-established mammographic ductal epithelial hyperplasia in a 51-year-old premenopausal woman with histopathologic changes of ductal hyperplasia; a baseline study. The fatty content of the breasts makes the fluffy densities readily apparent.

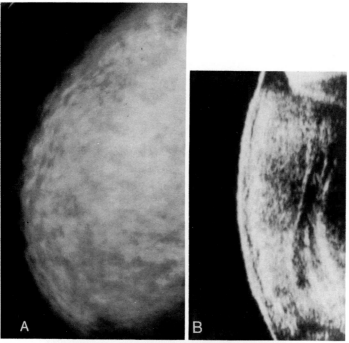

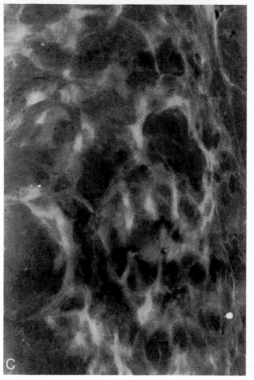

Figure 16–2. Ductal hyperplasia in a moderately dense breast. A 27-year-old woman with a questionable breast mass. *A,* Mammography: vague, fluffy, nodular densities outlined by a small amount of fatty tissue, a uniform appearance throughout both breasts. *B,* Sonography: diffuse, homogeneous high-level echoes with interspersed, evenly spaced, well-outlined fine anechoic (or low echoic) dotlike areas characteristic of ductal hyperplasia; scant subcutaneous adipose tissue. *C,* Slicer section: radiograph of 5 mm slicer section with poorly defined densities of ductal hyperplasia against the background of variously shaped globules of adipose tissue.

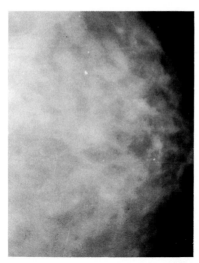

Figure 16–3. Denser ductal hyperplasia. A 34-year-old woman with a clinical nodule of the breast. Mammography: bilateral severe ductal hyperplasia in a radiographically dense breast. Pathology: fibrocystic disease, adenosis, papillomatosis, ductal epithelial hyperplasia.

Some areas of sclerosing adenosis (considered here as nonhyperplastic) may be microscopic in size or may exist in variably sized, ill-defined patchy densities on the mammogram; they may be diffuse, with or without coalescence of densities. Precise radiographic delineation of the specific density that will

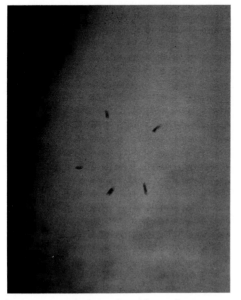

Figure 16–4. Very dense ductal hyperplasia. A 31-year-old woman with a paucity of generalized fatty infiltration of the breasts. An asymmetric density (wax markers) in this breast led to biopsy. Histopathologically well-established ductal hyperplasia was present.

be labeled sclerosing adenosis by the pathologist is not possible with any degree of certainty.

The radiologist may be overwhelmed by the multiplicity of densities in the breast on initial inspection of the mammograms; this need not cause confusion, as he can study each area and each nodule of each breast, initially and on follow-up studies, pinpointing areas of concern.

Thus, as the radiologist has difficulty identifying the less distinct form of lobular hyperplasia, it is less meaningful. However, ductal epithelial hyperplasia produces a useful, consistently recognizable, distinct form. The densities of ductal hyperplasia are associated with such histologic diagnoses as epithelial hyperplasia, papillomatosis, atypia, and even carcinoma in situ. Hyperplasia surrounded by periductal connective tissue contributes to the nodular densities. This mammographic appearance should not be confused with sclerosing adenosis, cysts, and fibroadenoma.

The recognition of ductal epithelial hyperplasia by sonography is not so consistently done as with mammography. There is usually an increased echoic activity associated with the hyperplastic areas of tissues. As those areas usually are small and diffuse, there is a homogeneous echo pattern throughout the breast. One area does not predominate unless there is significant coalescence of the hyperplastic cells to form pseudomasses. A fine diffuse black dot–like pattern is often clearly portrayed. The varying amounts of fat contribute to the level of echoes and their disorganization—the more fat, the more highly disorganized the echo pattern.

The subgross studies by radiography of 5 mm whole-organ breast slices correlates well with radiography of the intact breast and H & E light microscopy preparations. Such studies led to the realization that even in the ground-glass breast x-ray images of elderly women, glandular tissue often was still present. This prompted closer scrutiny of the high-resolution mammograms for faint shadows of ductal hyperplasia and the recognition of the very high risk pattern of "fatty ductal hyperplasia"—ductal hyperplasia in the physiologically older breasts.

Many facets of recognition and correlation of ductal epithelial hyperplasia are illustrated in Figures 16–2 to 16–8. The dense glandular breasts with a paucity of fat may prevent

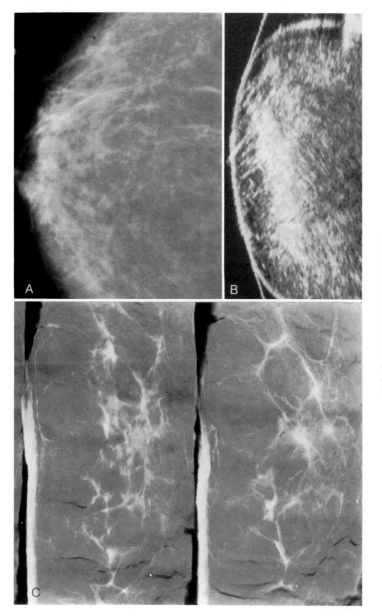

Figure 16–5. Ductal epithelial hyperplasia in a fatty breast. *A,* On the mammogram are typical diffuse patchy densities (snowflakes) with a coalescent area, e.g., small area superiorly, always of concern. This degree of fatty involution is termed fatty ductal hyperplasia. *B,* Sonography despite compression; high-level echoes, better organized and more uniform than in fatty or nodular breasts; interspersed small regular dark spots. *C,* Slicer section: small areas of fibroglandular tissue suspended in a background of almost complete fat, with a tendency to coalescence.

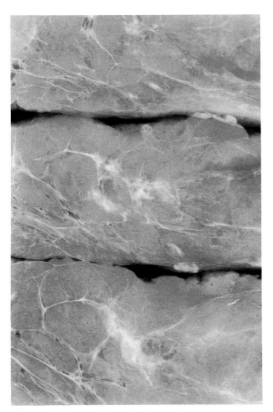

Figure 16–6. Small islands of ductal hyperplasia in fat. A 69-year-old woman studied for lobular carcinoma in one breast and duct plus intracystic papillary carcinoma in the other breast. In a large pendulous breast these small deposits could easily be overlooked, especially those in the top slicer, usually not seen on xeroradiography.

recognition of ductal epithelial hyperplasia (Figs. 16–3 and 16–4). Usually the underlying fine nodules can be seen with only a small amount of fat for contrast.

The epithelial hyperplasia pattern does occur frequently in the fatty, nearly atrophic breast, but the finely nodular pattern may be quite difficult to discern (Figs. 16–5 and 16–6). Recognition is very important, for in this physiologically older breast parenchyma, 14 per cent of our malignancies occurred in a pattern representing only 3.8 per cent of our study population. A markedly increased risk of cancer with ductal hyperplasia occurred after the age of 50 years, an age at which the fatty breast is more common and the radiologist is more apt to recognize the underlying hyperplastic pattern. Most definitions of mammographic parenchymal patterns (Wolfe, 1978) not only fail to include ductal hyperplasia per se but also do not recognize this very important physiologically older pattern of fatty ductal hyperplasia, in which we found a high rate of cancer biopsies (80 to 85 per cent).

The relatively high kvp used during xeroradiography of the breast tends to erase the contrast in the near-equal densities in fatty ductal hyperplasia of the thinly dispersed glandular tissues and the surrounding fatty involution. There are no sharply defined borders of the fluffy densities of ductal hyperplasia for the edge effect to be operative.

Figure 16–7. Whole-organ 5 mm slicer section from a breast containing a duct carcinoma with metastasis to an intramammary lymph node (rounded density above). On the mammogram fatty ductal hyperplasia could be identified but was difficult to reproduce photographically. A, This 14 kvp x-ray study clearly shows an area of ductal hyperplasia just above the lymph node. B, An H & E preparation of a slightly different area shows ductal hyperplasia between the India ink dots. Fatty infiltration predominates.

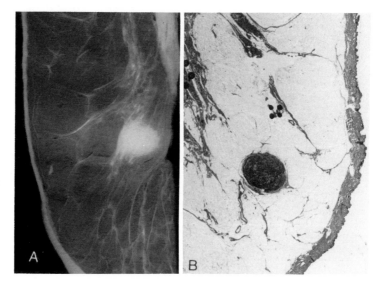

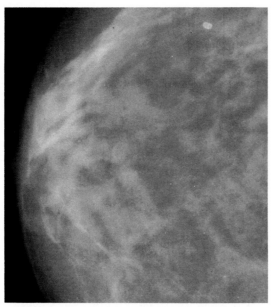

Figure 16–8. Ductal epithelial hyperplasia after prolonged use of digitalis. A 63-year old woman seen for checkup had been treated with digitalis for congestive heart failure for the past 15 years. This response of the breast to this steroid-like compound by some women is not unusual.

Recognition of fatty ductal hyperplasia by xeroradiography poses problems with this type of breast imaging.

HISTOLOGIC CORRELATION

Our whole-organ studies of intact, fatty breasts containing cancer demonstrate small islands of fibroglandular tissue scattered throughout the fatty tissue (Figs. 16–6 and 16–7). Multicentric sites of carcinoma, atypia, and epithelial hyperplasia are commonly found within these breasts. Other whole-organ studies have also shown areas of hyperplasia and malignancy both in the vicinity

of and remote from the main tumor mass (Gallager and Martin, 1969; Wellings et al., 1975). Fisher emphasized that mammary cancer is related to epithelial and not to stromal proliferation (Fisher et al., 1975). He found no correlation between histologic alterations and parenchymal patterns based on increasing density of the breast by stromal proliferation on mammography.

EMORY UNIVERSITY STUDIES

In our experience, proliferative ductal epithelial changes have had an association with breast carcinoma or were indeed preneoplastic. Systematically identifying these changes in the intact breast by mammography would help in selecting women at increased risk of developing clinical carcinoma. We reviewed our material to determine: (1) if proliferative breast diseases could be recognized in a consistent reproducible manner by mammography; (2) if there was a correlation between the radiographic and histologic findings; and finally (3) if there was any relation between this pattern and breast carcinoma.

Material and Patients

Long-Term Data

The prospective data (clinical, radiographic, histologic, and pathologic) were reviewed on 30,904 consecutive individual breast examinations. From these studies there were 3733 excisional biopsies with 3020 benign lesions and 713 primary operable breast cancers (Tables 16–1 and 16–2). These studies provided an overall relationship of ductal hyperplasia to carcinoma mammographically. At the initial interpretation of the mammograms the relative amounts of fatty, fibrous, and glandular tissues as well

TABLE 16–1. Total Mammograms, Breast Types, and Biopsies Associated with 713 Consecutive Breast Cancers

X-ray Breast Type	Number Mamm.	% Mamm.	Number Biopsies	Number CA	% Mammo CA	% Biopsies CA
Fatty (atrophic)	4004	13.0	400	112	2.80	28.0
Fatty DH	1160	3.7	144	103	8.88	72.0
DH	4388	14.2	564	205	4.16	36.2
Nodular	6088	19.7	940	103	1.69	11.0
Fibrofatty	12,968	42.0	1345	160	1.23	11.9
Glandular	2296	7.43	340	30	1.34	8.80
Total	30,904	100.00	3733	713	2.31	19.1

TABLE 16–2. Total Cases and Cases of Ductal Hyperplasia by Age Associated With 713 Cases of Primary Operable Cancers

Age (Years)	Total Cases						Cases With Ductal Hyperplasia					
	No. of Mamm.	% of Mamm.	No. of Biopsies	No. CA	% of CA	% Biopsy CA	No. of Mamm.	% of Mamm.	No. of Biopsies	No. of CA	% of CA	% Biopsy CA
21–30	3951	12.8	279	11	1.5	3.9	22	0.4	3	0	0	0
31–35	3029	9.8	274	23	3.2	8.4	142	2.6	12	0	0	0
36–40	4018	13.0	491	32	4.5	6.5	270	4.9	43	6	1.9	14
41–49	9364	30.3	1505	205	28.8	13.6	1531	28.0	262	51	16.7	19.5
50–59	5844	18.9	617	215	30.2	35.3	1875	33.8	175	80	25.9	45.7
60–69	3276	10.6	383	181	25.3	47.3	1458	26.3	193	154	50.0	79.8
≥70	1422	4.6	184	46	6.5	25.0	250	4.5	20	17	5.	85.0
Total	30,904	100.0	3733	713	100.0		5548	100.5	708	308	100.0	

as the glandular and ductal patterns were digitalized with 60 possible descriptive types of mammographic patterns in the complete print-out. From these, the ductal hyperplasia pattern was extracted. The pathologic reports on both benign and malignant diseases were available for reference and usually indicated whether or not hyperplastic activity was present in the breasts.

One-Year Data

The year 1977 was chosen for comparison with the 1963–1976 data as the first year in which noncancerous changes in the breast were routinely recorded by our pathologists in a detailed manner. During that year there were 1168 patient examinations, with 72 primary operable carcinomas and 180 benign biopsies. The mammograms on 208 patients studied that year who had prior mastectomy for carcinoma were reviewed, and particular attention was paid to the presence of fine nodules, distribution of glandular tissue, relative amounts of fatty involution, borderline calcification, and minimal distortion of architecture. These findings were correlated with any histologic descriptions of the prior mastectomy specimen, when available.

Findings

Long-Term Data

The long-term data revealed that 43.5 per cent of the patients with radiographic ductal hyperplasia who were biopsied had a malignancy. In contrast, 13.4 per cent of patients without an epithelial hyperplasia pattern who were biopsied had a malignancy (Table 16–1). This 3.2 times increased association of epithelial hyperplasia pattern with breast cancer appeared to be substantial. If the hyperplasia occurred in a breast with a fatty background, a subset we have labeled fatty

DH, the incidence of breast cancer was doubled (87 per cent).

One-Year Data

The radiographic pattern of ductal hyperplasia in the 1977 study showed a nearly twofold increased association with breast carcinoma when compared with a nodular breast pattern, approximately threefold when compared with a fibrofatty pattern, and fourfold when compared with a dense glandular pattern. Compared with all other breast types, the relative risk of ductal hyperplasia was 3.2 times (Table 16–3). The ductal hyperplasia pattern occurred in 19.2 per cent of patients, yet these patients harbored 44 per cent of the carcinomas. During a five-year follow-up, 16 of these patients developed breast cancer. Twelve of these were in breasts with the pattern of ductal epithelial hyperplasia on a fatty background, and four were in nodular, fibrofatty, or glandular breasts.

Additionally, 40.4 per cent of the 208 mastectomy patients had ductal hyperplasia. Also, the 1963–1976 data substantiated the increase in the 1977 data on the ductal hyperplasia with cancer. Multiple sites of breast cancer are also associated with ductal hyperplasia (Table 16–4). No other predictive mammographic risk pattern was observed in the many possible x-ray changes that had been computerized except the physiologically atrophic breast.

CLINICAL PROBLEMS

Clinically, the woman who has had one breast carcinoma is considered at increased risk for a second breast primary carcinoma for the rest of her life. Our data do not support this, particularly beyond a six-year interval. However, the increasing age with follow-up and the presence of severe ductal

TABLE 16–3. Total Mammograms, Studies Following a Mastectomy for Carcinoma, and Cancers Initially on Mammograms (1977 Study)

Breast Type	Total Mammograms in 1977 Study Population		Mastectomy Prior to 1977		Cancer Initially in 1977	
Fatty (atrophic)	72	6.2%	16	7.7%	0	0%
DH	224	19.2%	84	40.4%	32	44%
Nodular	248	21.2%	44	21.1%	20	28%
Fibrofatty, lobules	300	25.7%	28	13.5%	12	17%
Glandular	324	27.7%	36	17.3%	8	11%
Total	1168	100%	208	100%	72	100%

*Contains varying amounts of fat.

TABLE 16–4. Separate Pathologic Sites and Mammographic Parenchymal Patterns on 2056 Primary Operable Breast Carcinomas

Sites	Fatty	Glandular	Coarsely Nodular	Ductal Hyperplasia			Total
				Fatty	Fibronodular	Dense	
One	584	185	370	353	44	175	1719
Two	82	40	82	68	11	37	321
Three	9	3	2	1	0	1	16
Total	680	232	454	422	55	213	2056

hyperplasia most assuredly places such a women at increased risk (Fig. 16–9). In all woman with radiographic findings of ductal hyperplasia we recommend "yearly mammograms in addition to usual clinical follow-up examinations." Even without a previous history of breast carcinoma, this practice is rewarding (Fig. 16–10).

In the presence of ductal hyperplasia, any suspicious mammographic change is sufficient for biopsy. The finding of associated calcifications, which may even be widespread, is cause for localization, biopsy, and

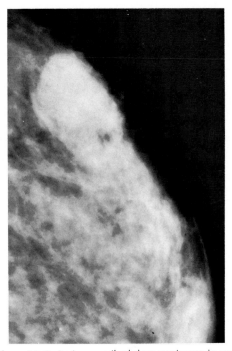

Figure 16–9. A circumscribed duct carcinoma in severe ductal epithelial hyperplasia. A 70-year-old woman who had a radical mastectomy 16 years before. Suspicious lump clinically. Mammography: 1.5 × 2 cm lobulated carcinoma, increased vasculature, stretching of the trabeculae, cluster of calcifications. Modified radical mastectomy for infiltrating duct carcinoma, intermediate grade, all 11 axillary lymph nodes free of tumor. The patient was living without disease three years later.

specimen radiography (Fig. 16–11) as is the faintest suggestion of asymmetric density or architectural change (Fig. 16–12). Such recommendations are based on astute observations of minute changes on high-resolution mammograms; they are not to be confused with the "aggressive" policy of recommending biopsy of every smudge on a xeroradiograph or a vague density on a mammogram. Obviously, many small carcinomas are overlooked in dense ductal hyperplasia; it is in this parenchymal pattern that the highest percentage of subsequent malignancies is detected. More careful evaluation of the initial mammogram may prevent this occurrence (Fig. 16–13).

The question of a prophylactic mastectomy for severe ductal hyperplasia is real at times (Fig. 16–14). In our experience, follow-up mammograms in less than one year are not the answer. A change sufficient for recognition usually requires a year or more; shorter interval studies tend to supply only a false sense of security. The woman often does not elect mastectomy unless a malignancy is present (Fig. 16–15).

Epithelial hyperplasia, papillomatosis, and atypia are histologic markers denoting patients who are at higher (3.2 times) than normal risk for the development of breast cancer. These high-risk markers may be reproducibly recognized on mammograms by a finely nodular parenchymal pattern. These changes can be recognized in all types of breasts but frequently are subtle in the fatty breasts, where they are often overlooked.

It is the combination of the physiologically older fatty breast and epithelial hyperplasia that constitutes the greatest increased risk of malignancy—over six times the risk without ductal hyperplasia. These mammographic changes must be recognized in all types of breasts but most importantly in the fatty breasts, in which they may be subtle and easily overlooked. The radiologist, surgeon, and pathologist must work as a team with

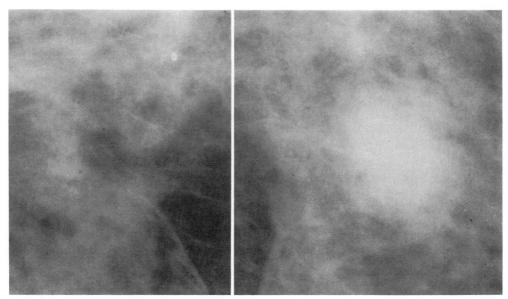

Figure 16–10. Dense ductal hyperplasia with carcinoma. A 50-year-old woman seen for a checkup on fibrocystic disease; bilateral aspirations three years before. Mammography: severe ductal hyperplasia bilaterally with a 1.4 × 1.5 cm moderately invasive carcinoma on the left. Pathology: duct carcinoma with moderate fibrosis; modified radical mastectomy; all 27 axillary lymph nodes free of tumor. The patient was alive and well 13 years later.

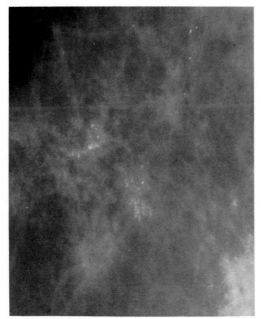

Figure 16–11. Comedocarcinoma on a background of severe ductal hyperplasia. A 64-year-old woman with lumpy breasts. Mammography: severe ductal hyperplasia with at least eight confluent densities containing stippled calcifications. These could be densities of ductal hyperplasia containing comedo-like calcifications or comedocarcinoma causing tissue response. Pathology: numerous foci of intraductal and infiltrative comedocarcinoma; marked ductal hyperplasia; modified radical mastectomy; all 21 axillary lymph nodes free of tumor. No evidence of disease four years later. Mirror-image biopsy of the opposite breast showed only marked ductal hyperplasia.

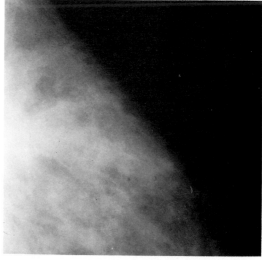

Figure 16–12. Carcinoma difficult to see in dense ductal epithelial hyperplasia. Mammography: fortunately the films revealed fine linear stranding from the density, partially seen here superiorly and toward the skin. A biopsy yielded a diagnosis of 1.2 × 1.2 × 1.5 cm duct carcinoma with fibrosis. One of 12 low axillary and 1 of 9 midaxillary lymph nodes were positive for metastatic carcinoma; modified radical mastectomy. The patient was free of disease seven years later.

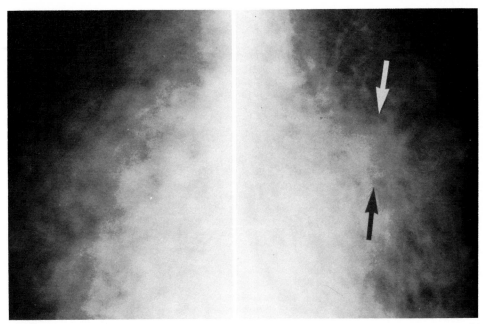

Figure 16–13. Large, moderatively invasive carcinoma overlooked in severe ductal hyperplasia. A 53-year-old woman with a breast lump for two weeks. Mother and maternal aunt had breast cancer. Clinically a 5 × 5 cm benign mass. Mammograms: The 2 × 2 cm spiculated carcinoma in the left breast was overlooked upon original review. Pathology: 2 × 2 × 2.2 cm duct carcinoma, severe ductal hyperplasia. Modified radical mastectomy with 0 to 14 nodes positive. Seven years later the patient was free of disease.

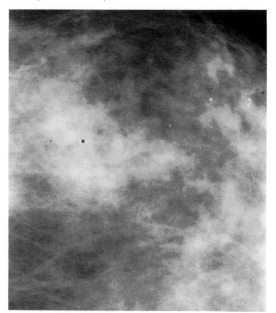

Figure 16–14. Multifocal intraductal carcinomas in ductal hyperplasia. A 67-year-old woman seen for a checkup. Clinically large breasts. Mammography: severe ductal hyperplasia with many areas of coalescence. The most prominent area was in the UOQ of the left breast; definite but less marked on the right. Biopsy revealed only intraductal carcinoma despite the suggestion of a mass. Mirror-image biopsy on the right showed severe ductal hyperplasia, no carcinoma. Left modified radical mastectomy: numerous diffuse deposits of intraductal carcinoma on a background of severe ductal hyperplasia and atypia; none of 18 nodes contained tumor. Three years later the patient was free of disease.

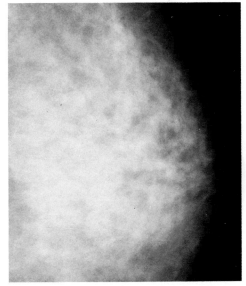

Figure 16–15. Ductal epithelial hyperplasia being followed by clinical examinations and radiography. A 62-year-old woman being followed for previous right mastectomy ten years earlier. Mammography: no interval change in ductal hyperplasia during annual studies. The alternative is prophylactic mastectomy, not desired by this patient.

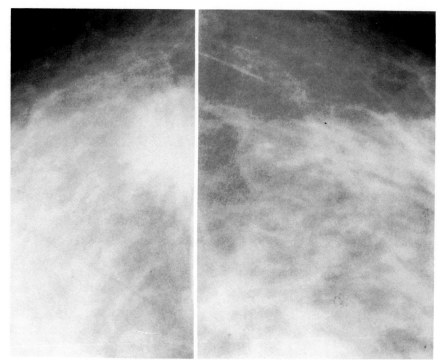

Figure 16–16. Combined types of duct carcinoma.

these breast changes in the formulation of criteria for biopsy, treatment planning, and recommendations for follow-up.

CASE HISTORY

Duct carcinoma in ductal epithelial hyperplasia. A 70-year-old woman had a red and itching left nipple "for a long time." Suspicious lump clinically. Mammography (Fig. 16–16, comparative CC views): 1.7 × 1.8 cm moderately invasive carcinoma. Sonography showed a hypoechoic, irregular mass with attenuation in the same area. Pathology: intraductal and ductal, intraductal and comedo carcinomas; modified radical mastectomy, nodes normal. Two years later the patient was free of disease.

This woman should have had a baseline mammogram years before, at least with the advent of

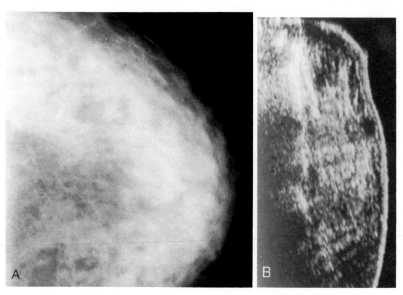

Figure 16–17. A and B, Initial study of ductal hyperplasia.

nipple changes. The ductal hyperplasia pattern would have dictated annual mammograms. This rather large carcinoma would have been detected much earlier.

CASE HISTORY

Carcinoma in severe ductal hyperplasia.

A 68-year-old woman with a 4 cm hard mass UIQ of the breast with skin dimpling. By history: 32 months previously there were clinically confusing changes, but a mammogram showed no dominant area. Present mammogram without comparative films (Fig. 16–17): ductal hyperplasia; in UIQ is a 2 × 3 cm irregular spiculated mass containing countless calcifications; bulges and thickens the overlying skin; moderately invasive and localized comedocarcinoma. Sonography: There was an irregular, hypoechoic mass attenuating the beam and causing disruption of the surrounding architecture. Pathology: infiltrating duct carcinoma with comedo elements; modified radical mastectomy: one node of Level I and one node of Level II of a total of 17 nodes positive for tumor. One year later the patient was free of disease.

This woman had a mammogram but was not put on an annual follow-up program. No doubt, some interval change or asymmetry would have been present prior to the carcinoma's reaching this large size and metastasizing.

CASE HISTORY

Whole-breast study of ductal hyperplasia.

A 48-year-old woman who had a right modified radical mastectomy for in situ carcinoma, judged lobular carcinoma in situ 20 years before. Upon review the diagnosis was concurred with. Recently the patient had mammography after a routine cyst aspiration. A cluster of calcifications not in a mass was localized; their removal was followed by specimen radiography. Only ductal hyperplasia and atypia were demonstrated histologically. But since several sites of in situ carcinoma had been demonstrated previously in the right breast, a left total mastectomy was performed at this visit.

A whole-organ study was carried out, and severe ductal hyperplasia was demonstrated (Fig. 16–18). Areas of atypia were seen, but no carcinoma was demonstrated in the left breast. The patient is alive and well nearly 20 years after the initial mastectomy. Radiographically this breast could have contained in situ, or even microinvasive, carcinoma.

Today lobular carcinoma in situ is followed clinically and by mammography without a mastectomy. Yet, having had one breast removed, this woman probably was relieved to have the second removed under these conditions.

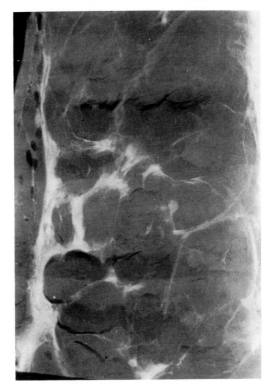

Figure 16–18. Follow-up of ductal hyperplasia.

OBSERVATIONS

Pathologists continue to speculate about the origin of breast carcinoma: that carcinoma arises de novo, from ductal and/or lobular hyperplasia, from atypical lobules, and in association with atypia and epithelial hyperplasia (Azzopardi, 1979).

Our data on ductal epithelial hyperplasia imply a strong relationship between this process and breast carcinoma. The data neither predict which women with ductal hyperplasia by x-ray will develop carcinoma (except for a higher risk in physiologically older breasts) nor which dense glandular breast will reveal a hyperplastic pattern by x-ray as fatty involution progresses. The progression from normal epithelium through hyperplasia, carcinoma in situ, and into invasive breast carcinoma has been suggested.

The recognition of ductal epithelial hyperplasia, papillomatosis, and atypia as nonobligate precursors of breast cancer resulted from the challenge to the radiologist to investigate less obvious x-ray changes and the response of the pathologist to study more thoroughly those poorly understood changes (Fig. 16–19).

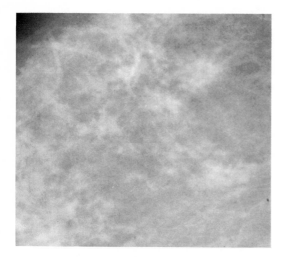

Figure 16–19. Ductal hyperplasia simulating fine breast calcification. A 62-year-old woman seen for routine baseline mammography. Clinically: soft normal breasts. Mammography: dense ductal hyperplasia with area of fatty ductal hyperplasia; confluent areas of the process highly suspicious with dense, tiny, almost calcific flecks that are more likely to be packed ducts than calcifications. Pathology: numerous discrete areas of intraductal carcinoma without invasion and with calcifications only 7 to 18 μ in size. (These were too small to be seen by x-ray.)

Figure 16–20. A 40-year-old woman with suspicious radiographic pattern of calcifications requiring localization and specimen radiography for study. The hyperplastic and atypical cells packing the lower duct would produce a similar density on the mammogram as the upper packed duct associated with periductal fibrosis and lymphocytosis. No area of infiltration was demonstrated in this breast.

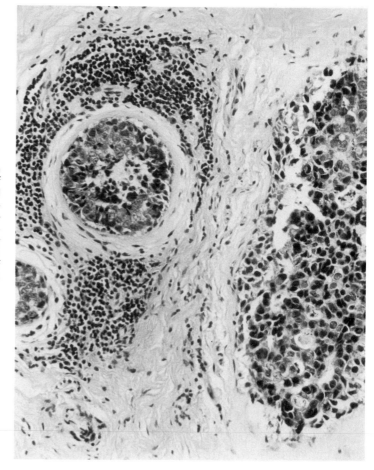

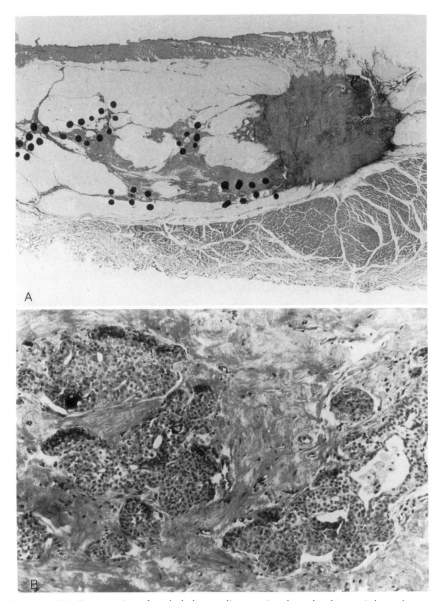

Figure 16–21. A, An H & E preparation of a whole-breast slicer section through a large scirrhous duct carcinoma. Near the mass is intraductal carcinoma (black dotted area), and at the extreme left is marked hyperplastic epithelial change. B, Intermediate changes that probably represent the transition of ductal hyperplasia into intraductal carcinoma and finally into highly invasive duct carcinoma.

Hyperplastic, atypical, and in situ carcinoma epithelial cells produce densities on the mammograms in two ways: (1) actual piling up of the cells within and packing of the lumen of the ducts; and (2) excitation by this process of periductal fibrosis (Fig. 16–20). The periductal fibrosis is more prominent the more atypical the epithelial cells.

Our hypothesis that ductal epithelial cells proceed into frank carcinoma is depicted in one slicer section that could be labeled the life history of breast carcinoma (Fig. 16–21) and one area of this evaluation as seen on light microscopy. Another hypothetical represention, with nuances of where irreversibility may occur, is depicted in Figure 16–22. Ductal epithelial hyperplasia occurs equally with comedo and duct carcinomas both intraductal and infiltrative (Fig. 16–19).

REFERENCES

Azzopardi JG (1979): Problems in Breast Pathology. Philadelphia, WB Saunders, p 113.

Black MM, Barclay TH, Cutler SJ, et al (1972): Association of atypical characteristics of benign breast lesions with subsequent risk of breast cancer. Cancer 29:338.

Clagett OT, Plimpton NC, Root GT (1944): Lesions of the breast. The relationship of benign lesions to carcinoma. Surgery 15:413.

Davis HH, Simons M, Davis JB (1964): Cystic disease of the breast. Relationship of carcinoma. Cancer 17:957.

Egan RL (1960): Experience with mammography in a tumor institution. Evaluation of 1,000 studies. Radiology 75:894.

Egan RL (1964): Mammography. Springfield, IL, Charles C Thomas, p 274.

Egan RL (1979): Estimated risk and occurrence of breast cancer in asymptomatic and minimally symptomatic patients. Cancer 43:871.

Fisher ER, Gregorio RM, Fisher B (1975): The pathology of invasive breast cancer. Cancer 36:1.

Foote FW, Stewart FW (1945): Comparative studies of cancerous versus non-cancerous breasts. I. Role of so-called chronic cystic mastitis in mammary carcinogenesis. Influence of certain hormones on human breast structure. Ann Surg 121:197.

Gallager HS, Martin JE (1969): Early phases in the development of breast cancer. Cancer 24:1170.

Humphrey LJ, Swerlow MA (1968): Large duct epithelial hyperplasia and carcinoma of the breast. Arch Surg 97:592.

Moskowitz M, Pemmaraju S, Fidler JA, et al (1976): On the diagnosis of minimal breast cancer in a screenee population. Cancer 37:2543.

Page DL, Vander Zwaag R, Rogers LW, et al (1978): Relation between component parts of fibrocystic disease complex and breast cancer. J Natl Cancer Inst 61:1055.

Warren S (1940): The relation of chronic mastitis to carcinoma of the breast. Surg Gynecol Obstet 71:257.

Wellings SR, Jensen HM, Marcum RG (1975): An atlas of subgross pathology of the human breast with special reference to possible precancerous lesions. J Natl Cancer Inst 55:231.

Wolfe JN (1978): Breast parenchymal patterns and the risk of breast cancer. Cancer Bull 30:36.

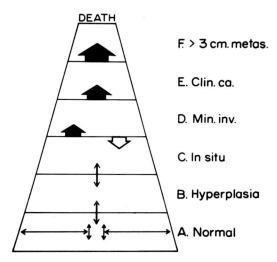

Figure 16–22. Hypothetical representation of progression from a large base of breasts with normal epithelial cells into and through a stage of benign hyperplasia. This could be considered a reversible process. From hyperplasia into in situ carcinoma there probably is a phase of reversibility, perhaps too subtle for light microscopic detection. Once in situ carcinoma is well established or in a microinvasive stage there may exist only a hypothetical reversibility. Formation of a mass, first on mammography, then clinically, signals a lethal process if uninterrupted.

Intramammary Lymph Nodes

17

BACKGROUND

With institution of clinical mammography, many unexplained changes in the breast appeared on the high-resolution studies. Some of these unfamiliar changes seen on the mammograms were resolved by comparing the mammograms with gross and microscopic studies in the surgical pathology laboratory. Small rounded shadows were frequently seen in breasts that were to be removed for cancer. In the 1950s, by directing the pathologist to these x-ray shadows in the breast previously ignored, lymph nodes were identified. Pathologists, surgeons, and anatomists were questioned about these nodes. None had heard of intramammary lymph nodes, but some were aware of deep pectoral nodes.

The evaluation of this new set of lymph nodes could perhaps elucidate the imprecise histologic staging of breast cancer, since approximately 25 per cent of Stage I lesions will actually be Stage II and a portion of Stage II cancers will have a lower mortality. Prognostic factors such as tumor size, status of the axillary lymph nodes, or histologic type of carcinoma are of value but have failed to select that group of women with localized disease and high mortality or those with regional disease and low mortality (Black and Kwon 1978; Fisher et al, 1978, 1980; Saigo and Rosen, 1980). No attention had been directed toward intramammary lymph nodes in prognosis. Since these disregarded nodes were rather common on mammograms, we examined our material to see if intramammary lymph nodes were of clinical or prognostic significance.

DEFINITION

To be intramammary the node had to be completely surrounded by fibroglandular tissue both on the radiograph of the 5 mm slicer section and on histopathologic preparations (Egan, 1970). This definition was mandatory, as at times it was difficult to differentiate intramammary lymph nodes high in the tail of the breast from low axillary lymph nodes. Also, the node in any part of the intact breast had to be clearly surrounded by fibroglandular tissue both on x-ray and later histologically. With rounded densities in the UOQ, or tail of the breast, labeling them intramammary lymph nodes is problematical unless careful histologic studies are done on the density and surrounding tissues (Fig. 17–1). The fibroglandular tissues may fall over the low axillary nodes, producing the appearance of being intraglandular. This was exemplified by Wolfe's (1977) illustration of 12 such nodes, which he called intramammary lymph nodes, none of which had histopathologic confirmation. In one other of his cases, histopathology was "heterotopic lymph nodes." This node probably would meet the criteria for an intramammary lymph node.

Another potential source of confusion is metastasis to the intramammary lymph node and replacement of all the lymphoid tissue of the node with carcinoma. Without recog-

313

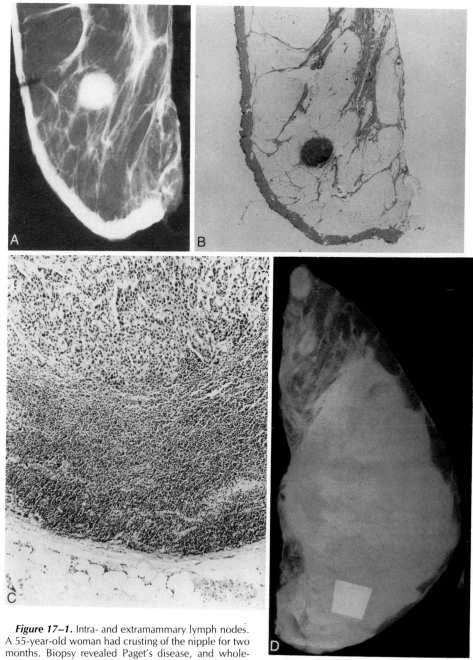

Figure 17–1. Intra- and extramammary lymph nodes. A 55-year-old woman had crusting of the nipple for two months. Biopsy revealed Paget's disease, and whole-organ studies showed the main mass of infiltrating duct carcinoma with comedo elements located centrally in the breast. There was one intramammary lymph node with metastatic carcinoma in the LOQ in slicer 19. The node was within fibroglandular tissue radiographically (*A*) and histologically (*B*). *C*, Photomicrograph of the node also shows surrounding fibroglandular tissue. *D*, A 39-year-old woman had bilateral subcutaneous mastectomies for atypical ductal hyperplasia. In contrast, the two low normal axillary lymph nodes are outside the dense breast tissue and are surrounded only by fat and fibrous tissue.

nizable residual lymphoid tissue this lesion would be indistinguishable from another tumor nodule. We did not encounter this problem in our series.

MATERIAL

The complete correlated clinical, radiographic, and pathologic studies on whole breasts done from May 1965 to September 1969 were reviewed. This report was confined to 158 breasts of 153 women and one man containing a primary operable carcinoma. Four were simultaneous bilateral primaries (eight breasts), three initial primaries, 13 second primaries, and the remainder unilateral primaries. Also, there were similar studies on 15 noncancerous breasts of 13 women: seven following previous mastectomy for carcinoma; four following bilateral mastectomy for fibrocystic disease; two for calcifications by x-ray; one for previous carcinoma, ipsilateral positive axillary lymph node; and one for cystosarcoma (by biopsy), borderline malignant. All cases were subject to 14 to 18 years' follow-up (Egan and McSweeney, 1983).

Intact breast specimens were used and consisted of the breasts and preparations described in the section on correlated clinical, radiographic, and pathologic whole-organ breast studies in Chapter 11.

RESULTS

Intramammary lymph nodes were demonstrated in 45 (28 per cent) of the breasts (Table 17–1). Fifteen breasts (10 per cent) with carcinoma contained a positive intramammary lymph node. The nodes ranged in

TABLE 17–1. Intramammary Lymph Nodes in 158 Whole-Breast Studies

Occurrence	Number of Breasts
One positive node	13
One negative node	23
Negative and positive	2
Many negative	7
No nodes	113

size from 3 mm to 15 mm, with the positive nodes 3 mm to 10 mm in size.

The positive intramammary lymph nodes occurred in all quadrants of the breasts: UOQ, 6; LOQ, 5; LIQ, 2; UIQ, 2; and central, 2 (Table 17–2). They occurred in the same quadrant as the reference carcinoma (primary abnormality) with at least one node in seven cases (Fig. 17–3) and in different quadrants in eight cases (Figs. 17–1 and 17–2). One breast contained nine nodes, with at least one node located in each of three quadrants; of these, two were positive and in the same quadrant as the carcinoma (Fig. 17–3). The positive nodes were associated with Stage I carcinoma in six cases, with two having a ten-year survival; and with Stage II in nine cases, with four having a ten-year survival (Table 17–3). Only two breasts contained a unicentric deposit of carcinoma of one histologic type, one Stage I with a 2 × 3 cm mass, and one Stage II with a 1.5 × 3 cm mass; both patients survived over ten years. The other 13 had multiple sites and/or multiple histologic types of carcinoma. The presence of positive intramammary lymph nodes per se had no demonstrable effect on prognosis in Stage II lesions but tended to indicate worsened prognosis in Stage I. Intramammary lymph node metastasis was associated with varied cell types of the primary carcinoma: five invasive duct; four duct with

TABLE 17–2. Location of Intramammary Nodes in 173 Breasts

	No. Breasts	No. Nodes	UOQ	UIQ	LOQ	LIQ	Central
Noncancer							
Single	3	3	2	0	0	1	0
>1 node	4	8	1	3	2	0	2
No nodes	8	0	0	0	0	0	0
Cancer							
Single node pos.	13	13	5	1	4	1	2
Single node neg.	23	23	8	3	7	2	3
>1 node pos.	2	7	3	1	2	1	0
>1 node neg.	7	18	7	3	6	1	1
No nodes	113	0	0	0	0	0	0

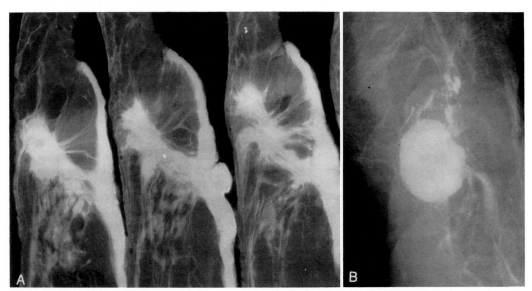

Figure 17–2. Intramammary lymph node with metastasis. A 75-year-old woman, gravida 2, para 1, 25 years post menopause; one maternal aunt with breast cancer. She had found a breast lump ten months before. Clinically and radiographically: moderately invasive carcinoma. Modified radical mastectomy. *A*, Infiltrating duct carcinoma, 1 × 2 × 2.5 cm, scirrhous type, UOQ, slices 13 to 18 (nipple 13 and 14) with 6 of 15 low axillary lymph nodes positive. *B*, A 6 mm intramammary lymph node, with metastasis, was in the LOQ, slice 31, of a total of 35 slices. The patient died five years later without evidence of breast cancer.

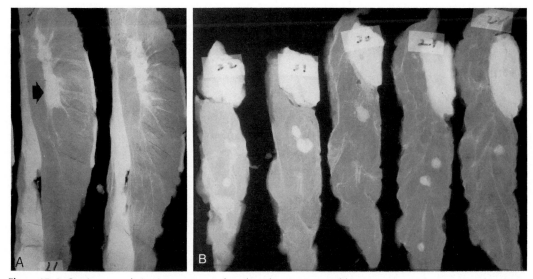

Figure 17–3. Carcinoma and nine intramammary lymph nodes. A 54-year-old woman, two years past natural menopause; no family history of breast cancer; lump in the breast for two months. Clinically and radiographically: highly invasive carcinoma. *A*, In slices 15 to 18 an infiltrating duct carcinoma UOQ (nipple in slice 13). *B*, Eight intramammary lymph nodes lateral to the tumor in slices 28 to 32 (four in LOQ and four in UOQ), two containing metastasis; the ninth node, normal, was in UOQ. Four years later the patient had a contralateral mastectomy for a primary duct carcinoma. Twelve years following the second mastectomy she had no evidence of disease.

TABLE 17–3. Ten-Year Survival With Positive, Negative, and Absent Intramammary (IM) Lymph Nodes in 158 Whole-Breast Studies With Positive Nodes Precedent Over Negative Nodes

	Positive IM Nodes	Per Cent	Negative IM Nodes	Per Cent	Absent IM Nodes	Per Cent
Stage I						
Survival	15*	79	2	33	62†	83
Nonsurvival	4	21	4	67	13	17
Stage II						
Survival	2	18	4	44	16	42
Nonsurvival	9	82	5	56	22	58
Total	30	19	15	9.5	113	72

*Includes three cases of intraductal carcinoma.
†Includes 13 cases of intraductal carcinoma.

scirrhous element; two duct with comedo element; one duct, tubular, and mucoid; one duct with Paget's disease; one Paget's disease and duct with scirrhous elements; and one mucoid.

The 15 noncancerous breasts had a similar incidence and distribution of intramammary lymph nodes as the cancerous breasts.

Metastatic deposits of carcinoma in the nodes did not tend to enlarge them compared with the nodes without carcinoma. Our observations have provided no connection of these intramammary lymph nodes with the usually accepted concept of lymphatic drainage of the breast toward the axillary or internal mammary lymph node–bearing areas.

For example, in Figure 17–1 drainage apparently was contrary, with a central carcinoma and a positive intramammary lymph node in the LOQ. A medial lesion could metastasize medially and inferiorly (Fig. 17–4), while metastasis followed the usual concept of drainage in Figure 17–5. About one half of the positive intramammary lymph nodes were in the same quadrant as the main tumor mass even when there were numerous nodes in several quadrants (Fig. 17–3).

IMAGING CHARACTERISTICS

Most of the intramammary lymph nodes were 5 mm or less in diameter and difficult

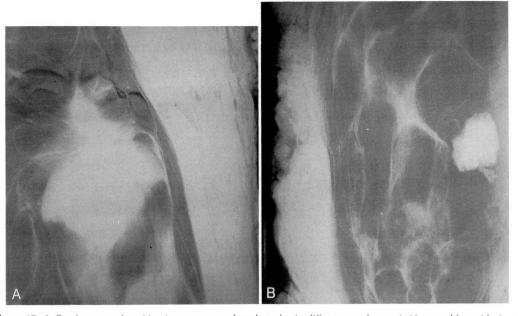

Figure 17–4. Carcinoma and positive intramammary lymph nodes in different quadrants. A 46-year-old gravida 2, para 2, no nursing; one maternal aunt with breast cancer; mass UIQ, present for several months. Study of the mastectomy specimen: *A,* Scirrhous carcinoma, 2.5 × 2 × 2 cm, UIQ from slices 6 to 11 (nipple slice 11). *B,* Intramammary lymph node slice 5, medial to and 4 cm inferior to the tumor, LIQ, with metastasis. Two low nodes of a total of 26 axillary nodes contained metastatic disease.

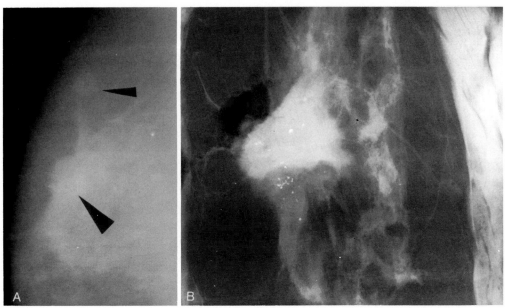

Figure 17–5. Intramammary node near carcinoma but free of tumor. A 48-year-old woman with a breast mass for one week. Previous panhysterectomy for endometriosis; no hormones, one child, not nursed. Clinically: 4 cm mass UOQ, one 2 × 3 cm axillary lymph node. *A,* Mammography: 1.7 cm moderately invasive carcinoma with uncountable calcifications (large arrowhead) and nearby intramammary lymph node (small arrowhead). *B,* 1.5 × 1.5 × 1.7 cm carcinoma in slices 13 and 14.

to define on mammography, especially when embedded in dense fibroglandular tissue. On the mammogram a discrete rounded or lobulated lesion in the glandular portion of the

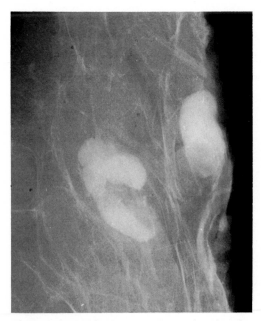

Figure 17–6. Two benign intramammary lymph nodes in a breast studied for carcinoma. The larger shows a large notch and is lobulated. The other is lobulated with a radiolucent area inferiorly, indicating fatty infiltration. Both are deep in the breast and surrounded by atrophic glandular tissue.

breast suggests the diagnosis of intramammary lymph node. The mass often will be considered a cyst, particularly in the proper age group. A small notch representing a hilum (Fig. 17–6) or a radiolucent center of fatty replacement (Fig. 17–5 and 17–7A) may indicate an intramammary lymph node on the mammogram. These fatty nodes are without metastasis, just as with axillary lymph nodes. Often positive nodes cannot be identified (Fig. 17–8). They can easily be confused with a small noncalcifying fibroadenoma (Fig. 17–9).

Breast sonography is not very rewarding with intramammary lymph nodes. The nodes are too small for visualization. If seen, they cannot be differentiated from other benign solid masses.

CLINICAL SIGNIFICANCE

If the pathologist is alerted and the breast is searched, histologic study may prove of prognostic value (Fig. 17–5). Otherwise, as in the past, they may not be properly studied. Now that the pathologists are more used to searching for these lesions, they may be an incidental finding (Fig. 17–8B). Being aware of the frequency of intramammary lymph nodes often does prevent confusion

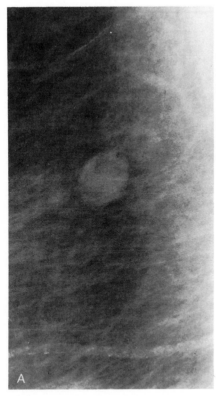

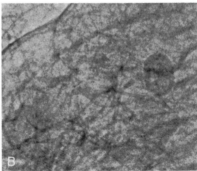

Figure 17–7. Two cases of normal intramammary lymph nodes. *A,* A 78-year-old woman with mastectomy for a 1.2 cm infiltrating duct carcinoma, UOQ right breast, with this node at the level of the nipple laterally. *B,* A 59-year-old woman also had mastectomy for RUQ duct carcinoma. This node (at 12 o'clock) was nonpalpable on histologic study; both were intramammary lymph nodes partially replaced with fat and with no metastasis. There were metastases in one low node in the patient shown in *A* and two low nodes in the patient shown in *B.*

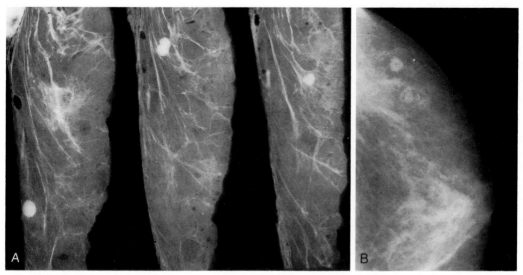

Figure 17–8. Positive and negative intramammary lymph nodes. *A,* A 54-year-old woman had a mastectomy for an infiltrating duct carcinoma in the UOQ right breast, Stage II, four lower axillary lymph nodes positive. The centralmost of the three intramammary lymph nodes on slices 22 to 24 LOQ contained metastatic deposits. *B,* An incidental finding in a left modified radical mastectomy for Stage I infiltrating duct carcinoma was this tumor-free intramammary lymph node lateral to the nipple.

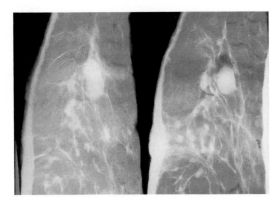

Figure 17–9. Fibroadenoma simulating intramammary lymph node. A 52-year-old woman had a modified radical mastectomy for a Stage I infiltrating duct carcinoma UOQ right breast. Radiographically this 7 × 10 mm smooth mass, approximately at 11 o'clock, was an intramammary lymph node. Actually it was a noncalcifying fibroadenoma. Note the ductal hyperplasia and dilated subareolar ducts.

(Fig. 17–10), as this node could have been labeled low axillary.

PROGNOSIS AND STAGING

The presence of intramammary lymph nodes with or without metastasis from a carcinoma in that breast often aids in assessing prognosis. Even with a 1.5 cm duct carcinoma with a scirrhous component, in the presence of normal intramammary lymph nodes a good prognosis exists (Fig. 17–11). Even though an intramammary lymph node contains metastatic deposits, prognosis is not necessarily affected with axillary lymph node metastasis already present in a Stage II tumor. (Fig. 17–12). Intramammary lymph nodes may be seen with multiple sites of carcinoma (Fig. 17–13).

There was a trend toward poorer prognosis in Stage I carcinomas with positive intramammary lymph nodes; these may represent some of the histologically Stage I carcinomas that are clinically Stage II. In Stage II, positive intramammary lymph nodes seemed to have no direct effect on prognosis (Table 17–3). They were more frequently associated with Stage II disease and perhaps merely represented advanced disease; their presence would indicate a greater likelihood of axillary metastatic disease. If these findings could be widely duplicated, intramammary lymph nodes could be of clinical importance. Conceivably, a Stage Ia—positive intramammary lymph node(s) but normal axillary nodes—could be defined and used.

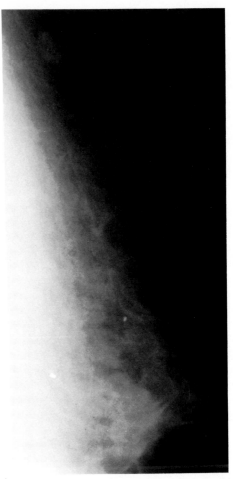

Figure 17–10. Duct carcinoma with negative intramammary lymph node. A 68-year-old woman with a breast mass that clinically was carcinoma. Mammography: severe ductal hyperplasia; 1 × 1.5 cm central moderately invasive carcinoma; intramammary lymph node with clear notch toward tail of breast. Pathology: duct carcinoma with productive fibrosis. Modified radical mastectomy, normal intramammary lymph node, 25 axillary lymph nodes free of tumor. The patient was alive and free of disease six years later.

CLINICAL APPLICATION

The practicality of applying this tedious, time-consuming, and expensive whole-breast study clinically can be questioned. A complete laboratory, two technologists, and one pathologist full-time, with five years of study and fewer than 200 breasts, plus a great deal of time on the part of the radiologist and surgeon, and much clerical assistance—this could be tolerated only under research conditions. However, during thorough routine breast studies, multiple histologic types of carcinoma are demonstrated. The knowledge

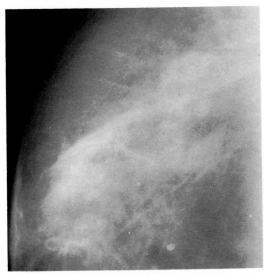

Figure 17–11. Poorly defined duct carcinoma with an intramammary lymph node. A 66-year-old woman being followed after left mastectomy three years before. Clinically: vague thickening UOQ. Initial mammography: vague density extending from subareolar area into UOQ, with stretching of the major subareolar ducts; a few scattered coarse and fine calcifications; straightening of two Cooper's ligaments above level of the nipple; rounded, partially hidden 6 mm mass; vague changes of carcinoma with possible intramammary lymph node. Pathology: intraductal and ductal carcinoma, two separate sites; a small intramammary lymph node with metastatic carcinoma. Modified radical mastectomy; 11 nodes Level I and 9 nodes Level II free of tumor. The patient was free of disease six years later.

that multiple sites of breast cancer are common and are of great significance in prognosis may stimulate more thorough breast studies. Lagios (1977) has shown good results with a much less extensive procedure in his radiographic-pathologic routine study of breast cancer, requiring only the added services of one technologist.

CASE HISTORY

Worsened prognosis with an intramammary lymph node.

A 56-year-old woman with a fullness of the right breast for three months; no family history of breast cancer; gravida 3, para 3; 18 months' nursing; five years postmenopausal. Clinically there was a subareolar thickening with a question of nipple flattening—suspicious enough to warrant biopsy. Mammography (Fig. 17–14). Pathology: 1.5 cm duct carcinoma, moderate fibrosis. Modified radical mastectomy; two intramammary lymph nodes with metastatic tumor; all 15 axillary lymph nodes free of disease. Death occurred 30 months later from disseminated breast carcinoma.

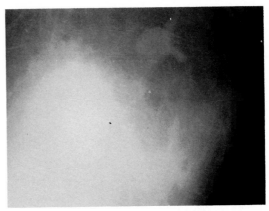

Figure 17–12. Positive intramammary lymph nodes in Stage II disease. A 54-year-old woman with a clinical carcinoma with palpable axillary lymph node extension. Mammography: highly invasive carcinoma UOQ with a discrete 1.2 cm mass nearby; suspected intramammary lymph node metastasis; density in axilla. Pathology: duct carcinoma with fibrosis. Radical mastectomy; 7 of 24 axillary lymph nodes positive at all levels, and one positive 1.1 cm intramammary lymph node. Distant metastases within three years.

With our present system of TNM staging this would be a $T_1N_0M_0$ (Stage I) lesion, clinically and histopathologically. However, a more precise staging indicating intramammary lymph node metastasis would have signaled a worsened prognosis.

CASE HISTORY

Intramammary lymph node with Stage II carcinoma.

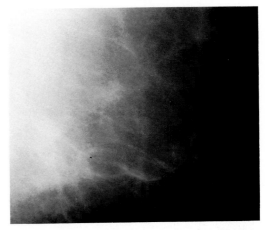

Figure 17–13. Two-duct carcinoma and positive intramammary lymph node. A 53-year-old woman with a clinically suspicious area. Mammography: 1.5 cm poorly defined carcinoma in lower breast; above and toward the nipple is a nearby 5 mm similar lesion, and farther above is a 4 mm discrete mass. There is associated adjacent skin flattening and increased vascularity. Pathology: two separate duct carcinomas and an intramammary lymph node with metastatic tumor. Modified radical mastectomy; all 19 axillary lymph nodes free of tumor. Nine years later the patient was free of disease.

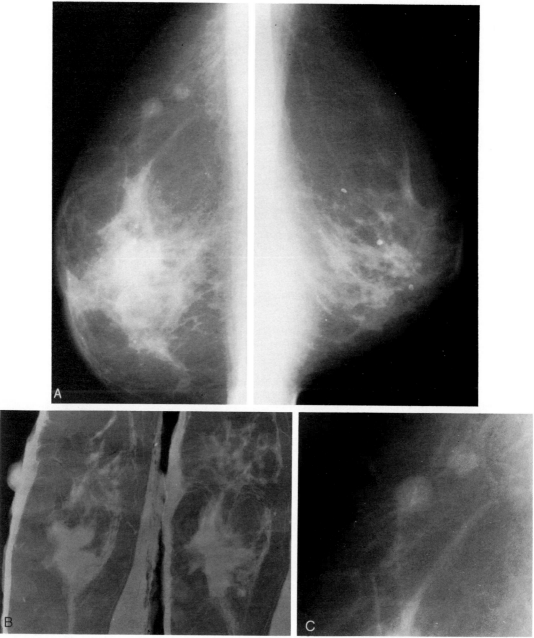

Figure 17–14. Case 1. Mammography: 1.5 × 1.8 cm ill-defined, moderately invasive, subareolar carcinoma with surrounding tissue reaction, stippled calcifications, areolar skin thickening, and increased vascularity; two intramammary lymph nodes probably positive. *B,* Slicer section through the carcinoma. *C,* Close-up of nodes.

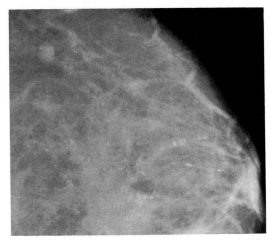

Figure 17–15. Case 2. Mammography: 2.2 × 2.5 cm moderately invasive duct carcinoma with calcifications of a comedo element, nipple and areola flattening, and increased vascularity; intramammary lymph node probably positive.

A 71-year-old woman, gravida 3, para 2, 20 years past menopause; one sister had breast cancer; nipple inverted all her life. Clinically: 4 cm central mass with nipple retraction. Mammography (Fig. 17–15). Pathology: 3 cm duct carcinoma with fibrotic component. Radical mastectomy; one intramammary, four low and maxillary of 24 axillary lymph nodes with metastases. Radiotherapy followed. Death from widespread breast carcinoma occurred 18 months later.

Despite more aggressive treatment, the clinical course was similar to that in the preceding case. The intramammary lymph node on mammography only suggested a more advanced carcinoma.

CASE HISTORY

Fibroadenoma simulating an intramammary lymph node.

A 42-year-old woman with a newly developed lung nodule; search for a primary site. Clinically the breasts were nodular but normal otherwise (Fig. 17–16). An intramammary lymph node could be part of a complex of carcinoma and metastasis. Sonography was suggested and demonstrated the solid nature of the process. After breast biopsy showed only fibroadenoma and fibrocystic disease, a primary bronchogenic carcinoma was demonstrated later at thoracotomy.

In this case the intramammary lymph node was misleading.

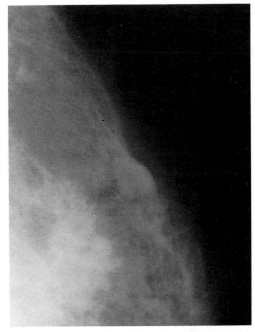

Figure 17–16. Case 3. Mammography: a lobulated smooth lesion bulging into the subcutaneous fat, a fibroadenoma; deep, a poorly defined area that could be fibrocystic disease with several small cysts.

REFERENCES

Black MM, Kwon CS (1978): *In* Gallager HS, Leis HP, Synderman RK, Urban JA (eds): Prognostic Factors in the Breast. St Louis, CV Mosby, p 297.

Egan RL (1970): Mammography and Breast Diseases. Baltimore, Williams & Wilkins, p 19, 70.

Fisher ER, Swamidoss S, Lee CH, et al (1978): Detection and significance of occult axillary node metastases in patients with invasive breast cancer. Cancer 42:2025.

Fisher ER, Redmond C, Fisher B (1980): Pathologic findings from the National Surgical Adjuvant Breast Project (Protocol No. 4). VI. Discriminants for five-year treatment failure. Cancer 46:908.

Hutter RVP (1980): The influence of pathologic factors on breast cancer management. Cancer 46:961.

Lagios, MD (1977): Multicentricity of breast carcinoma demonstrated by routine correlated serial subgross and radiographic examination. Cancer 40:1726.

Saigo PE, Rosen PP (1980): Prognostic factors in invasive mammary carcinomas 1.0 cm or less in diameter. Am J Clin Pathol 73:303.

Wolfe JN (1977): Xeroradiography: Uncalcified Breast Masses. Springfield, IL, Charles C Thomas, p 55.

Breast Masses

diagnosis, e.g., the circumscribed carcinoma that was not a benign mass; calcifications, not yet recognized by the pathologist, that were to lead to the huge area of in situ cancer; and ductal hyperplasia, which would lead to speculations of precancerous lesions.

The definition of a mammographic mass encompasses the specific localized density of elements found in the breast and also its distinction from other nonspecific, localized, less compact, and less well-outlined densities of coalescent tissues or altered architecture. In addition, a single area, the focal one, must be clearly delineated from amid numerous breast densities (Figs. 18–1 and 18–2). This delineation of a specific area requires a cautious judgment, as an immediate investigation is implied in the term "dominant mass," borrowed from the surgeon.

The mammographic classification of masses into solid and cystic is not as crucial as with sonography. Yet this distinction must

BACKGROUND

In the earliest mammograms, search was directed toward finding cancers, usually advanced and with secondary signs. Then followed efforts to establish the more obvious appearances of the normal breast in conjunction with benign and malignant patterns. Evolution of these patterns, established without any outside source of contradiction or competition, superficially flowed smoothly: (1) The vast, but consistently repetitive, parenchymal patterns of clinically "normal" breasts posed only fleeting problems; (2) the malignant characteristics fit those envisioned to be produced by infiltrative processes and were confirmed by daily comparisons with gross and microscopic pathology; and (3) the benign lesions, intermediate in the echelon, became relegated to less stimulating investigation and less vigorous study. These benign lesions, often mammographic dominant masses, were to pose startling challenges to

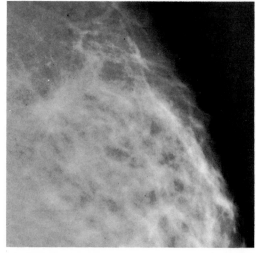

Figure 18–1. Moderately invasive small carcinoma mass. A 51-year-old woman seen for baseline mammogram for vague nodularity in the breasts. Mammography: 5 × 6 mm coarsely spiculated mass of carcinoma. Pathology: duct carcinoma Grade III with an infiltrating border. Modified radical mastectomy, 0 of 18 nodes positive. The patient was alive and well three years later.

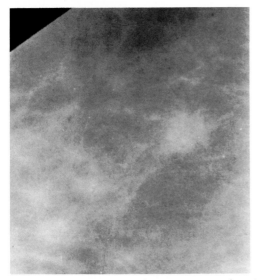

Figure 18–2. Small, moderately invasive mass of carcinoma. A 62-year-old woman with large breasts, clinically fatty. Mammography: 4 × 5 mm mass of carcinoma. Pathology: intraductal and duct carcinoma, Stage I (0 of 19 nodes positive); modified radical mastectomy; free of disease three years later.

masses. Nonhomogeneity, variation in overall density, and mixed borders of masses compound the problem. Yet a classification of mammographic masses can be derived that is greatly useful in establishing proper diagnoses (Table 18–1).

Additionally, masses must be related to patient age and whether their presence is single or multiple. Attempts to estimate prognosis based on the contour of the mass have been disappointing, except for the concept that the more fibrosis or scirrhous the element present, the worse the prognosis. Size of the mass clinically has strongly influenced the staging of breast cancer. Yet actual size, reliably measured only on mammograms or on gross pathology, lacks prognostic significance except in reference to the same histologic type of tumor. A medullary carcinoma with lymphoid stroma might reach a size of 2 cm before becoming apparent and still carry an excellent prognosis, whereas a 2 cm scirrhous duct carcinoma would have a grave prognosis.

be made in order for the clinician to aspirate the mass for diagnosis and treatment. Usually the clinical findings coupled with mammography suffice to proceed with needle aspiration of a mass. There is an advantage in classifying radiographic masses as calcified vs noncalcified. For maximal clinical usefulness, an attempt must be made to divide masses into benign and malignant ones.

The problems of overlapping benign and malignant characteristics of a mass, the borderline between an area of increased density and a true mass, and the separation of the dominant mass from surrounding densities prevent a concise classification of breast

MASS DENSITY

For recognition of the carcinomatous mass on the mammograms within the glandular tissue, there must be a definite increase in density of the carcinoma (Figs. 18–3 to 18–5). The highly cellular components of the masses are more tightly packed; reactive fibrosis develops in and about the tumor. There is often increased vascularity associated with the tumor as well as deposition of hemosiderin; furthermore, the actively growing cancer cells may have a higher affinity

TABLE 18–1. Radiographic Characteristics of Breast Masses

	Benign	Malignant
Relative density	Slight to marked increase	Always definite increase; denser than benign
Character of density	Homogeneous	Nonhomogeneous, densest at center
Shape	Round, oval; lobulated	Tentacled, ragged, spiculated, variable; spicules heavier toward nipple
Borders	Well-circumscribed, regular, and smooth; thin layer of surrounding fat	Poorly circumscribed, irregular, fuzzy, no halo
Surrounding tissues	Not invaded; displaced trabeculae pushed aside smoothly; no increased vascularity	Infiltrated; trabeculae retracted irregularly and thickened; increased vascularity
Calcifications	Coarse, isolated, few and countable; not punctate; more apt to have polarity; widely scattered; similar in density; may be in periphery of lesion	Numerous, punctate, uncountable; variable density; confined to a measurable area; less polarity, diffuse in lesion; more central
Relative size	Same size or smaller than clinical measurement	Larger than clinical measurement, often by a factor of 2 to 4

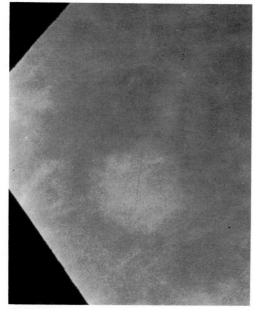

Figure 18–3. Faint mass of carcinoma. A 53-year-old woman with large breasts seen for checkup. Mammography: Routine views showed a very faint density in UOQ of the left breast. The area, radiographed using collimator made of a heavy copper pipe 1.5 inch inside diameter and 14 inches long, clearly demonstrates a 7 × 9 mm circumscribed carcinoma and a nearby intramammary lymph node. Pathology: medullary carcinoma with lymphoid stroma. Modified radical mastectomy; the intramammary and 21 axillary lymph nodes were free of tumor; the patient was alive and well 19 years later. Only with meticulous mammography is it possible to demonstrate clearly a medulllary carcinoma less than 1 cm in size.

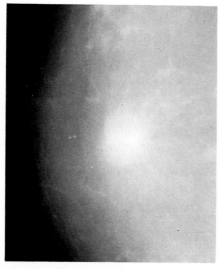

Figure 18–4. Dense mass of carcinoma with faint borders. A 50-year-old woman with a breast mass for three weeks that was clinically carcinoma. Mammography: homogeneously dense carcinoma with poorly defined borders. Pathology: duct carcinoma. Modified radical mastectomy; all 19 axillary lymph nodes free of tumor; the patient was alive and well five years later.

for minerals, with an actual increase in the calcium content in areas of necrosis.

The carcinoma is densest at its center owing to the more complete replacement of breast tissue by malignant cells. Some strands of the cells may extend outward from the central mass and be superimposed. The density of the mass decreases peripherally. At the extreme periphery the spiculated appearance is more frequently produced by retraction of the trabeculae toward the carcinoma rather than extension of the carcinoma (Fig. 18–1). As retraction progresses there is shortening of the ducts and retraction of the nipple toward the mass. Even in the densest portions of the glandular tissue, interspersed areas of radiolucent adipose tissue are usually present as well as some evidence of normal trabeculae and ductal structures. None of these can be seen through the dense portion of the mass of carcinoma—a good differential diagnostic point when an area of glandular tissue outlined by fat is noted.

MASS SIZE: CLINICAL VS RADIOGRAPHIC

When the size of the carcinomatous mass by palpation is significantly greater than that measured on the films, this becomes an important diagnostic point. The size of the mass by x-ray corresponds closely to that in the gross surgical specimen. The palpable mass may be two to four times the size measured on the mammograms (Figs. 18–6 and 18–7). The more infiltrative carcinomas, especially those associated with marked changes in the breast stroma peripheral to the lesion and thickening of the overlying skin, produce the greatest difference between the measurements from palpation and those from the mammograms.

MASS SHAPE AND BORDERS

An attempt to categorize the shape and borders of breast cancer masses by precise descriptive terms is near-impossible. Some of the lesions have consistently uniform growth patterns, but this is unusual. Most growth patterns are widely different and frequently reflect variations in cellular types. Figure 18–8 is representative of our whole-organ studies of breast cancer masses and illustrates problems in classification. Use of

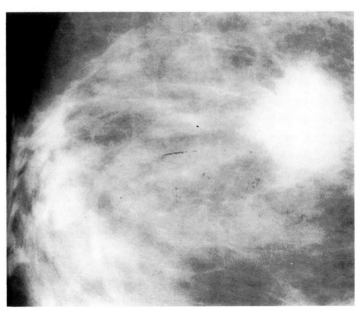

Figure 18–5. Moderately invasive mass of carcinoma causing retraction of the major ducts. A 75-year-old woman who had a breast mass for "months," clinically 3 × 5 cm cancer. Mammography: a 2.3 × 2.7 cm moderately invasive carcinoma with some portions of the periphery circumscribed but mostly spiculated, straightening the major ducts. Pathology: duct carcinoma with moderate fibrosis. Modified radical mastectomy, two of three Level I and none of seven Level II axillary lymph nodes positive. Free of disease two years later.

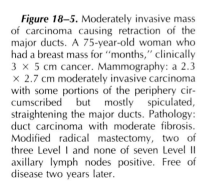

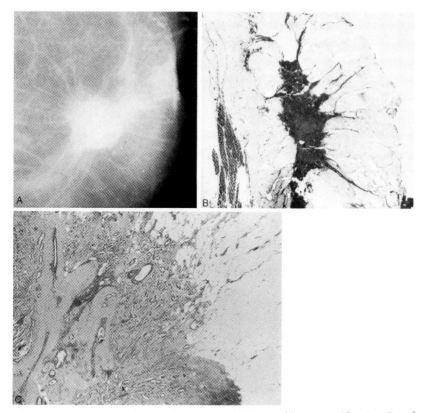

Figure 18–6. A to C, Markedly spiculated mass of carcinoma. A 66-year-old woman with a 6 × 7 cm breast mass with retracting nipple for three weeks. Clinically: 4 cm hard mass with nipple retraction; carcinoma. Mammography: 1.8 × 1.8 cm solid mass but highly infiltrative carcinoma with nipple inversion and areola retraction. Whole-organ slicer section showing the highly spiculated tumor mass with the fine strands being both infiltrating tumor cells and retractive elements. The photomicrograph illustrates the infiltrative processes but lacks the three-dimensional effect of the 5 mm thick radiographic specimen. Pathology: 2 × 1.8 × 1.6 cm duct carcinoma with marked fibrosis. Radical mastectomy, 6 of 28 Levels I and II axillary lymph nodes with metastases. Death from disseminated disease six years later.

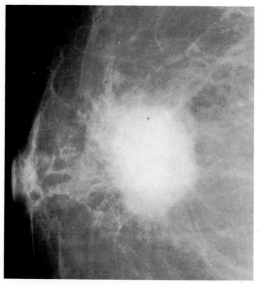

Figure 18–7. Large spiculated mass of carcinoma. A 64-year-old woman with a lump for two weeks, clinically 5 × 6 cm cancer, no mention of nipple retraction. Mammography: 2.2 × 2.9 cm dense spiculated mass of carcinoma, stippled calcifications; retractive phenomenon is more pronounced anteriorly with apparent fixation of the nipple. Pathology: duct and intraductal papillary carcinoma. Modified radical mastectomy; three of eight Level I and none of two Level II lymph nodes contained metastases (see Fig. 18–6). Alive without disease five years later.

a single cut (one plane) through the cancerous mass would obviate such problems. Yet, some remarks about the growth patterns of breast cancer are appropriate.

The irregular shape of the mass of carcinoma varies with the degree of invasion into the surrounding tissue and the degree of reactive fibrosis to this invasion. Two general contours result: highly invasive, represented by scirrhous carcinoma, which is irregular, tentacled, and spiculated; and circumscribed, which is smoother and in some areas has well-defined borders. Transition from one type to the other occurs; the two contours may exist in contiguous areas. The highly invasive carcinomas may have an ill-defined or faint central mass made up of a small central point of unusually long converging straightened trabeculae. One has the impression that there has been insufficient time for a real mass of cells to form. In contrast, a clearly circumscribed periphery of the carcinoma may suggest a benign lesion; it seems to be causing very limited reaction about it, so that the periphery must be searched carefully.

Serial sections through the masses of can-

cer reveal that three distinct contours of the margins actually can be categorized: (1) smoothly rounded, relatively small projections arising from the entire surface, pushing adjacent breast tissue aside with a hazy border on the mammograms (Fig. 18–9); (2) fine projections, 2 to 3 mm in length, appearing in the surrounding tissue as tiny peaks with a finely spiculated periphery to the solid mass on the mammograms (Figs. 18–6 and 18–7); and (3) coarse, irregular projections of varying lengths that represent ducts filled with tumor, thickened periductal connective tissues, and possibly tumor-laden periductal lymphatics that present as an irregular stellate mass with the periphery composed of coarse extensions into the surrounding breast tissue (Figs. 18–10 to 18–12). Most masses do not fit a distinct category throughout the periphery but are mixtures of borders (Figs. 18–13 and 18–14).

Highly Infiltrative Masses

In a highly infiltrative carcinoma (Fig. 18–6) the distorted trabeculae radiate peripherally from the mass. Trabeculae are very seldom seen traversing the carcinoma owing to the increased density of the tumor and distortion of the trabeculae when retracted toward the mass. Trabeculae may frequently be seen traversing a benign mass. Normal trabeculae may occasionally be seen traversing some portion of a more circumscribed carcinoma. The highly invasive carcinoma rarely exceeds 3 cm in diameter as measured on the mammograms. As this size is approached, diffuse changes of infiltration, reactive fibrosis, edema, and skin thickening cause progressive loss of delineation of its borders. As growth progresses, the primary site of the carcinoma may not be definitely demonstrated even with a more penetrating x-ray beam. In Table 18–2 are listed the more common infiltrative lesions.

The borders may not be clearly seen and evaluated (Fig. 18–15).

The glandular tissue of the breast lies between the two layers of superficial fascia. The trabeculae are anchored to the fascia posteriorly. A carcinoma causing shortening of the trabeculae and the ducts produces retractive signs evident peripherally in the breast, either at the attachment of the ducts to the nipple (Fig. 18–16) or in the skin overlying the mass.

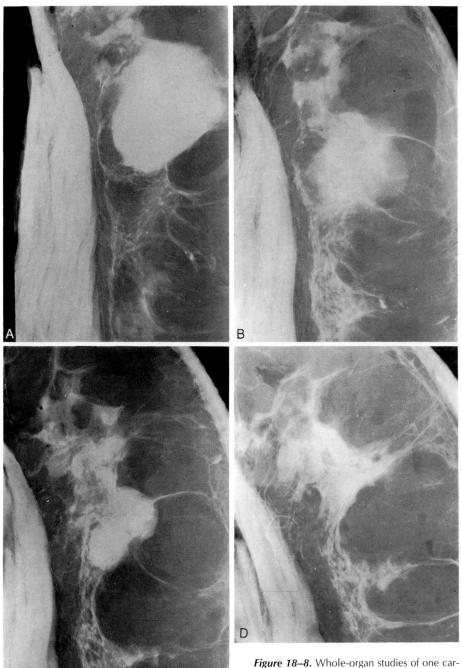

Figure 18–8. Whole-organ studies of one carcinomatous mass at 5 mm interval slices. A 57-year-old woman with a suspicious mass in the UIQ of the left breast. Mammography: 2 cm carcinoma with smooth and spiculated borders. Pathology: intraductal and duct adenocarcinoma UIQ. *A,* Slicer 4: 1.6 × 2.1 cm homogeneous, mostly smooth, bordered mass. Note marked ductal hyperplasia and intraductal carcinoma just below the lesion. *B,* Slicer 5: 1.3 × 1.5 cm coarsely spiculated mass. *C,* Slicer 6: 0.8 × 1.3 cm bilobed mass with calcifications. *D,* Slicer 7: 0.9 × 1.2 cm poorly defined nonhomogeneous mass with fine and coarse spiculations. Radical mastectomy; all 28 axillary lymph nodes free of tumor; 1 cm duct carcinoma LIQ of the same breast. The patient was living and well 17 years later.

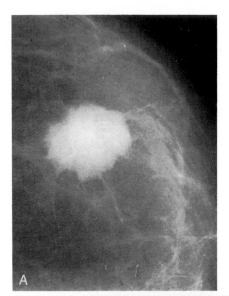

Figure 18–9. A, Circumscribed mass of carcinoma with nodular excrescences, silhouette sign. An 82-year-old woman with a clinical mass of carcinoma. Mammography: 1.8 × 2.3 carcinoma with smooth coarse nodular protuberances and several coarse spiculations; the vasculature was symmetric. These overlapping nodules produce double densities. B, Medullary carcinoma with lymphoid stroma demonstrating marked cellular anaplasia with a small number of lymphoid cells. The smooth margin against the fibrofatty tissue suggests a pseudocapsule. C, Medullary carcinoma with lymphoid stroma, with similar border showing marked lymphocytic reaction in the surrounding tissues. Pathology: duct carcinoma, with a cribriform pattern and productive fibrosis. Radiography suggests minimal fibrosis. Modified radical mastectomy; nodes free of disease; the patient was alive and well four years later.

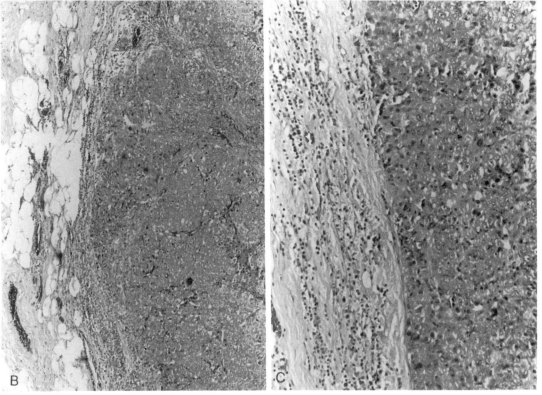

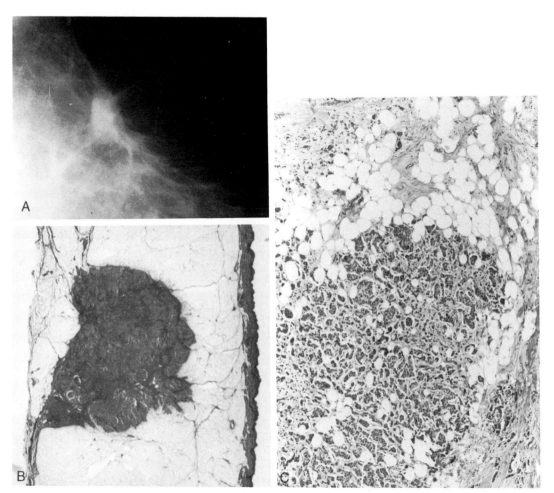

Figure 18–10. *A* to *C*, Coarsely spiculated mass of carcinoma. A 43-year-old woman with a soft movable 1 cm lump for two weeks. Mammography: 8 × 11 mm moderately invasive carcinoma. The whole-organ section shows a solid mass of tumor with varying sized nodular excrescenses in the periphery. The high-power photomicrograph shows one rather circumscribed peripheral nodule typical of this type of mass. Pathology: duct carcinoma Grade III with lymphocytic infiltration. Modified radical mastectomy; ten nodes Level I and ten nodes Level II free of tumor. The patient was alive and well three years later.

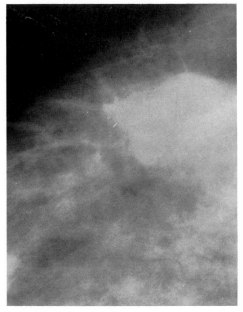

Figure 18–11. Moderately invasive mass of carcinoma. A 63-year-old woman with a mass that was clinically carcinoma. Mammography: homogeneously dense, coarsely spiculated mass stretching Cooper's ligaments into prominence. Pathology: duct carcinoma with mild productive fibrosis. Modified radical mastectomy; all 17 axillary lymph nodes free of tumor. The patient was alive and well nine years later.

TABLE 18–2. More Common Infiltrative Masses

Benign	Malignant
Abscess	Comedocarcinoma
Acute mastitis	Cystosarcoma phylloides
Adenosis (sclerosing)	Duct carcinoma
Fat necrosis	Intracystic papillary
Foreign body reaction	carcinoma
Hyalinizing fibroadenoma	Medullary carcinoma with
Organizing hematoma	lymphoid stroma
Scarring	Metastasis
With trauma	Most carcinomas
With inflammation	Sarcomas
Subareolar fibrosis	

Circumscribed Masses

The smoother portions of the borders of a circumscribed carcinoma may suggest a benign tumor (Figs. 18–8A and 18–17). The circumscribed carcinomas are most often mucin-producing, intracystic papillary, and medullary carcinomas. It is with such circumscribed lesions, those with areas of infiltration not too apparent, that secondary signs of carcinoma are searched for. Such changes include skin thickening, increased vascularity, and distal stromal changes, which make the diagnosis of carcinoma definite. Table

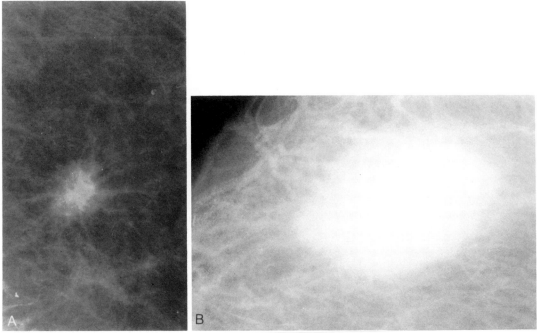

Figure 18–12. A, Coarsely spiculated carcinoma. A 67-year-old woman with pendulous breasts seen for baseline study. Mammography: 6 × 7 mm carcinoma. Modified radical mastectomy; all 21 axillary lymph nodes free of tumor. The patient was living and well nine years later. B, Circumscribed mass of carcinoma. A 67-year-old woman with a breast mass that clinically was carcinoma. Mammography: 3 × 5 cm circumscribed mass of carcinoma with radiating coarse spicules in portions of the periphery, marked increase in vascularity. Pathology: duct carcinoma with lymphocytosis. Modified radical mastectomy, all 19 axillary lymph nodes free of tumor. The patient was alive and well three years later.

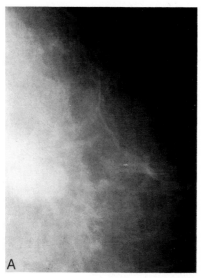
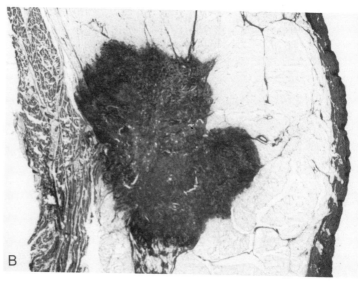

Figure 18–13. Mixed smooth and highly invasive borders of carcinoma. A 74-year-old woman with a breast lump for one month, clinically carcinoma. *A,* Mammography: a 1 × 1.8 cm well-circumscribed carcinoma with a contiguous 0.8 × 1.7 cm highly invasive portion superiorly. *B,* Whole-organ slicer photomicrograph showing portions of the periphery circumscribed and portions highly infiltrative. Pathology: duct carcinoma with productive fibrosis. Modified radical mastectomy; 0 of 18 axillary lymph nodes positive; no evidence of disease five years later.

18–3 lists the more common circumscribed masses.

Unusual Masses

Many times malignant masses produce unusual radiographic configurations, such as fanlike (Fig. 18–18) or nebular (Fig. 18–19).

A rather reliable differentiation between a solid mass of cancer and fibroglandular tissue is the absence of fat in the cancer. This is not always so, however (Fig. 18–20).

In first describing signs noted to be associated with cancer of the breast, the thought was to call attention to as many as possible so that they could be verified or refuted. To

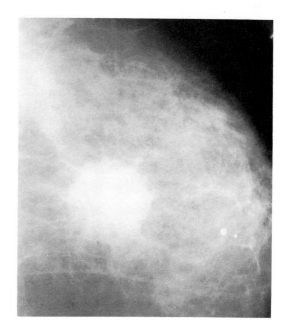

Figure 18–14. Partly smooth bordered mass of carcinoma. A 66-year-old woman with a breast lump that was clinically suspicious. Mammography: 2.3 × 2.4 cm mass containing stippled calcifications, with the anterior borders rather smooth and the posterior borders coarsely spiculated. Pathology: intraductal and duct carcinoma without a scirrhous element. Modified radical mastectomy, seven axillary lymph nodes free of metastasis; patient alive and well three years later.

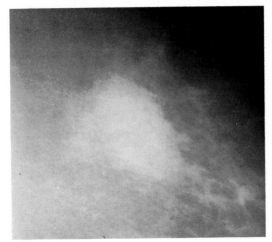

Figure 18–15. Poorly defined mass of duct carcinoma. Stage I infiltrating duct carcinoma, 1.5 × 2.8 cm, without fibrosis in a 62-year-old woman.

date, the silhouette sign has provoked little interest. It has proved reliable. The reason that multiple solid masses, such as fibroadenomata, do not cause this sign is not clear, unless it is related to the density of the lesion (Figs. 18–21 and 18–22.) No doubt, fat in the breast provides the necessary contrast in the breast, as air does in the lung; this sign usually is seen in fatty breasts.

Of 315 consecutive primary breast cancers, 237 revealed a mass on the mammograms. Of these cancers, 18 were smoothly rounded: five were cancer by x-ray, four were suspi-

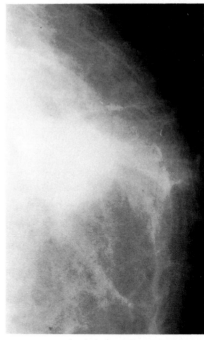

Figure 18–16. Moderately invasive mass of carcinoma. A 61-year-old woman with a breast lump for one week; nipple flattening; clinically carcinoma. Mammography: 1.7 × 2.1 cm carcinoma straightening trabeculae and stretching the major ducts into prominence. Pathology: duct carcinoma with a pattern of scirrhous type and an intraductal component; extensive lymphatic spread into distant quadrants. Modified radical mastectomy; 2 of 15 low axillary lymph nodes contained metastases. Free of disease two years later.

TABLE 18–3. More Common Circumscribed Masses

Benign	Malignant
Abscess	Carcinoid
Adenosis	Cystosarcoma phylloides
Cyst, galactocele	Intracystic papillary carci-
Cystosarcoma phylloides	noma
Fibroadenoma	Lymph node metastasis
Giant	Lymphoma—nodular
Hyalinized	Medullary carcinoma with
Adenolipoma	lymphoid stroma
Hemangioma	Mucinous carcinoma
Hematoma	Nonbreast metastasis
Intracystic papilloma	Sarcoma
Intraductal papilloma	
Gynecomastia	
Keloid	
Lymph node	
Lymphoma	
Neurofibroma	
Neurofibromatosis	
Nevus	
Nipple off-profile	
Prepubertal breast tissue	
Prosthesis	
Sebaceous cyst	

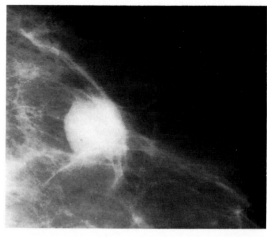

Figure 18–17. Benign mass with partly smooth and partly indistinct borders. A 61-year-old woman with a suspicious palpable lump. Mammography: a 1.5 × 1.5 cm mass with clear sharp borders posteriorly; the anterior borders are partially obscured by overlying trabeculae. The unusual findings are reversed: posterior clear and anterior indistinct. Pathology: intracystic papilloma.

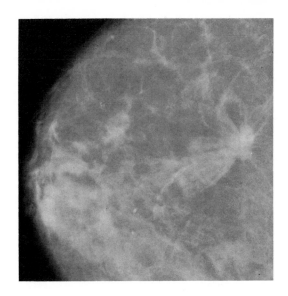

Figure 18–18. Highly infiltrative mass of carcinoma. A 58-year-old woman with nodular breast with a suspicious thickening on the left. Mammography: 6 mm nonhomogeneous mass with marked retractive phenomenon, causing fanning out of the trabeculae in all directions, especially anteriorly, on a background of severe ductal hyperplasia. Pathology: duct carcinoma, scirrhous type. Modified radical mastectomy; three of twelve Level I and two of eight Level II lymph nodes contained metastases. Patient died of widespread disease three and one-half years later.

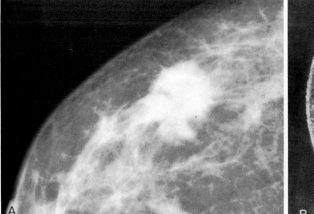
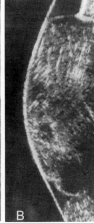

Figure 18–19. A and B, Duct carcinoma with a nebular configuration. A 61-year-old woman with a breast lump that is poorly evaluated clinically. Mammography: 2.1 × 2.1 cm infiltrative mass that appears to represent coalescence of at least four masses of carcinoma; background of fatty ductal hyperplasia. Sonography: irregular hypoechoic area, nonhomogeneous internal echoes, distorted surrounding breast architecture, mild attenuation on some scans. Pathology: duct carcinoma, ductal hyperplasia, atypia, papillomatosis. Modified radical mastectomy, five of twelve Level I and six of nine Level II axillary lymph nodes with metastases. The patient was free of disease after one-year follow-up.

Figure 18–20. Mass of carcinoma containing radiolucencies. A 53-year-old woman with clinically normal breasts seen for a checkup. Mammography: bilateral fatty ductal hyperplasia with an asymmetric dominant nodule. The 7 × 11 mm poorly outlined mass blends into the breast tissue in some areas, produces no retractive signs, and is honeycombed with small radiolucent areas. Increased vascularity makes it even more suspicious. Modified radical mastectomy; 17 axillary lymph nodes free of tumor; the patient was alive and well four years later.

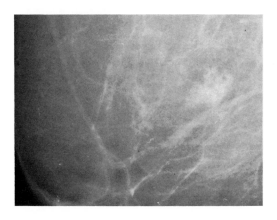

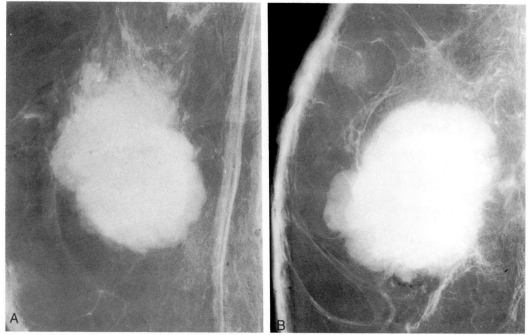

Figure 18–21. *A* and *B*, Silhouette sign of carcinoma. A 67-year-old woman with a suspicious breast mass that proved to be a 2.4 × 2.5 cm medullary carcinoma with lymphoid stroma. In the same breast were distant sites of duct carcinoma and an intraductal papillary carcinoma. The radiograph of the whole-organ slicer section of the modified radical mastectomy specimen illustrates the silhouette sign of carcinoma (all nodes were normal, no tumor after eight years). The first radiograph (*A*) is of slicer 21 and the second (*B*) of slicer 22, each 5 mm thick but contiguous. There is no intraductal component to medullary carcinoma with lymphoid stroma, but note the definite ductal epithelial activity above and below the mass in slicer 21 (that was confined to the area of mass). The calcifications were associated with the ductal hyperplasia.

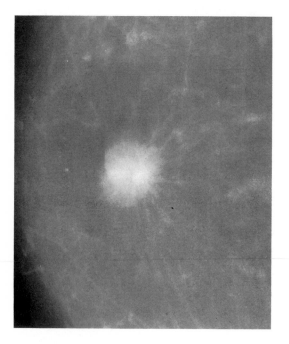

Figure 18–22. Silhouette sign. A 50-year-old woman with a suspicious breast lump for three months. Radiographically, this carcinoma, 9 × 15 mm, shows highly invasive spiculated areas in its borders as well as circumscribed areas and a silhouette sign that is found almost exclusively with carcinoma. Pathology: duct cell carcinoma with a scirrhous component; one low axillary node, of a total of 25 nodes at modified radical mastectomy, contained metastatic tumor. Patient living without disease three years later.

cious, and nine were labeled benign. Clinically they were: four cancer, three suspicious, and 11 benign or no dominant mass. The patient age range was 15 to 78 years, with eight under and ten over age 50 years.

Intermediate Masses

For classification purposes an intermediate, or combined, type of carcinomatous mass with varying degrees of both infiltrative and circumscribed borders may be included. Tumors may be more infiltrative in character or may have a more circumscribed appearance. Different histologic types of carcinoma can produce the same radiographic appearance. Metastatic deposits of breast carcinoma may exhibit entirely different growth patterns and histologic types. The radiologist must realize that he can often only suggest (on the basis of growth pattern), without assurance, the histologic type of carcinoma.

Mixed Type Masses

The coexistence of smooth and irregular margins in a single lesion may result from a number of possible causes. Three of them are: (1) the production of a cystic area in an infiltrative carcinoma; (2) a circumscribed carcinoma, such as an intracystic papillary carcinoma, showing marked invasion in one area of the periphery; and (3) a solid mass of well-circumscribed carcinoma growing in the periphery of a highly invasive tumor. These appearances are all manifestations of the ability of carcinomas of the breast to assume varied radiographic appearances rather than indications that infiltrative carcinoma is invading a nearby circumscribed lesion.

With fibroadenomata there frequently may be seen bosselated, smooth, wavy outlines or a notch. This must be differentiated from the demonstration of a double density, or silhouette sign, of the breast mass, which almost always indicates carcinoma. This is a function of the carcinoma's producing prolongations in different directions as opposed to the benign lesion's expanding more evenly from its center.

CALCIFYING MASSES

The density of calcification in a breast mass ranges from the large amorphous plaques to the faint, almost imperceptible, tiny flecks seen in ductal hyperplasia coalescing as a mass. Large breast masses, diffuse breast changes (inflammatory carcinoma), or blood-filled cysts may obscure calcifications. Less precise technical aspects, such as inadequate collimation or poor receptor systems, often prevent recognition of calcifications. Most of the various types of calcifications are illustrated in Chapter 27 as well as the differentiation, when possible, of benign and malignant calcifications in masses.

NONCALCIFYING MASSES

Differentiation of benign and malignant noncalcifying masses is more difficult without the frequently characteristic calcifications as an aid. Needle aspiration may be useful in establishing the presence of the benign cyst or the more ominous hemorrhagic cyst. In other lesions, some estimate of the nature of the mass may be reached by observation of the density, border, and number of masses as well as the surrounding breast tissue architecture and vascularity of the breast.

CYSTIC MASSES

The surgical tenet for years has been, "All dominant nodules of the breast must be removed and have microscopic examination." Concomitant with the growing use of mammography there was a trend toward aspiration of cysts: If the masses disappeared and the results of laboratory study were normal, this treatment sufficed. This policy seemed safer if mammography were used to study the remaining breast tissues. Multiple cysts caused problems, as the greater number increased the probability that one of them would not be completely aspirated. Once the decision to aspirate was made, it was necessary to follow with an open biopsy if the aspiration was not complete. This situation induced some surgeons to forego aspiration of any of the multiple cysts that was palpable. Nonpalpable ones demonstrated by mammography were less of a problem in treatment: They could be ignored.

Various forms of breast sonography were introduced to increase confidence in the management of breast cysts. The rounded mass on mammography was not always clearly differentiated from a solid mass.

NONCYSTIC MASSES

The noncystic benign mass most frequently encountered is the fibroadenoma. Typical calcifications may be sufficient for radiographic differentiation. Frequently multiple and bilateral, and often noncalcifying, masses in the young woman are not sufficient for differentiation if all breast masses are to be aspirated or surgically removed. Fear of radiation in the younger age group compounds the problem; sonography may be useful. It is helpful if the mass is related to patient age and multiplicity of lesions.

MASS NUMBER, PATIENT AGE, AND CANCER RISK

A reliable preoperative risk level for breast masses may be established based on the presence or absence of a single mass or multiple masses by x-ray and palpation. These findings are then related to the woman's age without regard to any x-ray or clinical characteristic of the individual breast mass or masses.

We, as well as other observers, have found that breast lumps are the most frequent complaint in breast diseases (Haagensen, 1986). The breast mass is the single most common indicator of breast cancer. All lumps are not biopsied; some of those not biopsied are benign and some are cancerous. As breast biopsy is a formidable procedure, any increased efficiency in selection of women for biopsy would be beneficial.

Among patients currently recommended for biopsy, no single clinical sign delineates minimal or maximal risk groups. Information such as age and status of menstruation in conjunction with physical findings provides some keys for assigning biopsy priorities, but these keys are insufficient for the establishment of a working biopsy hierarchy. When the decision to biopsy a breast is preceded by mammography, this diagnostic procedure enables the setting of strong priorities (Egan, 1972).

A partitioning of clinical mass findings by radiographic mass finding alone and then further refinement by age groups produce categorizations with a striking variation in the ratios of malignant to benign biopsies. These ratios suggest a provision for a meaningful guide to the assignment of biopsy priorities. Thus we proceeded to evaluate the nine combinations of simply no mass, single mass, and multiple masses by x-ray and clinical examination (Egan, 1975).

Emory University Subjects and Methods

To relate x-ray and clinical masses to breast biopsy priority we utilized, from Emory University Clinic, 17,288 consecutive studies on

TABLE 18–4. Various combinations of Dominant Breast Masses in 17,288 Clinical and X-ray Examinations on 6392 Patients

	Number of Breast Exams	Number of Biopsies	Number of Benign	Number of Malignant	Percentage of Breasts with Cancer	Percentage of Biopsies Cancerous
Type of Dominant Nodules						
clin. + +, x-ray + +	172	80	67	13	7.6	16.3
clin. +, x-ray + +	193	110	80	30	15.5	27.3
clin. −, x-ray + +	162	34	29	5	3.1	14.7
clin. + +, x-ray +	124	66	57	9	7.3	13.6
clin. +, x-ray +	1227	844	460	384	31.3	45.5
clin. −, x-ray +	522	117	76	41	7.9	35.0
clin. + +, x-ray −	389	97	95	2	0.5	2.1
clin. +, x-ray −	2198	886	746	140	6.4	15.8
clin. −, x-ray −	12,301	559	446	113	0.9	20.2
Total	17,288	2793	2056	737	4.3	26.4
Mass Categories						
clin. + +	685	243	219	24	3.5	9.9
clin. +	3618	1840	1286	554	15.3	30.1
clin. −	12985	710	551	159	1.2	22.4
x-ray + +	527	224	176	48	9.1	21.4
x-ray +	1873	1027	593	434	23.2	42.3
x-ray −	14,888	1542	1287	255	1.7	16.5
Total	17,288	2793	2056	737	4.3	26.4

+ = Solitary mass; + + = multiple masses; − = no mass.

6392 female patients that included history, physical examination, and mammography. These examinations resulted in 2793 biopsies, of which 2056 were benign (635 cyst aspirations, 320 fibroadenomas, and 1101 other benign lesions) and 737 were malignant by histopathologic study. There were 58 cancers demonstrated clinically or by mammography, usually in the opposite breast (not biopsied). These were omitted. The decision to biopsy a given breast was based on all available information obtained from the history, physical examination, and mammography and was not dependent solely on the presence or absence of the clinical mass. A clinical benign dominant nodule may have had a biopsy or been observed for up to six weeks prior to the decision to biopsy. Approximately four biopsies yielded one cancer.

The categories of no dominant mass, a single dominant mass, and multiple dominant masses determined by clinical examination were cross-tabulated with those same categories as determined by mammography. The frequency of biopsy and malignancies found is shown in Table 18–4. The choice of age intervals used in Tables 18–5 to 18–9 resulted from an examination of data from Table 18–4 in age groups, first in five-year intervals, then in one-year intervals, to find the age at any abrupt change of incidence of breast cancer.

Results

In the categories of clinical multiple masses, clinical solitary masses, and no mass clinically (Table 18–4) there were 24, 554, and 159 cancers, respectively. The cancer rate among clinical single masses was more than four times that of clinical multiple masses and 13 times that in breasts with no clinical mass.

The percentages of biopsies for cancer in column 6 of Table 18–4 reflect the biopsy selectivity and the overall rates. The 9.9, 22.4, and 30.1 per cent cancer in the "mass category" in this table of patients selected for biopsy indicates little variation. The clinical solitary mass and no clinical mass had similar rates of cancer per biopsy, while the clinical multiple mass rate was only one third of that rate.

When the clinical mass categories were considered with radiographic mass categories, a much wider variation in the rate of cancer per biopsy was seen. The rate varied from 2.1 per cent for clinical multiple masses and no mass on radiography to 45.5 per cent for solitary mass clinically and by x-ray.

TABLE 18–5. Various Combinations of Dominant Masses in 2405 Clinical and X-ray Examinations on Women Aged 0–32 Years

	Number of Breast Exams	Number of Biopsies	Number of Benign	Number of Malignant	Percentage of Breasts with Cancer	Percentage of Biopsies Cancerous
Type of Dominant Nodules						
clin. + +, x-ray + +	14	7	7	0	0	0
clin. +, x-ray + +	8	5	5	0	0	0
clin. −, x-ray + +	5	1	1	0	0	0
clin. + +, x-ray +	13	7	7	0	0	0
clin. +, x-ray +	151	93	88	5	3.3	5.4
clin. −, x-ray +	20	2	2	0	0	0
clin. + +, x-ray −	65	19	2	0	0	0
clin. +, x-ray −	429	180	174	6	1.4	3.3
clin. −, x-ray −	1700	54	49	5	0.3	9.3
Total	2405	368	352	16	0.7	4.3
Mass Categories						
clin. + +	92	33	33	0	0	0
clin. +	588	278	267	11	1.9	4.0
clin. −	1725	57	52	5	.3	8.8
x-ray + +	27	13	13	0	0	0
x-ray +	184	102	97	5	2.7	4.9
x-ray −	2194	253	242	11	.5	4.3
Total	2405	368	352	16	0.7	4.3
Percentage of total (Table 18–4)	13.9	13.2	17.1	2.2		

+ = Solitary mass; + + = multiple masses; − = no mass.

TABLE 18–6. Various Combinations of Dominant Breast Masses in 4317 Clinical and X-ray Examinations on Women Aged 0–38 Years

	Number of Breast Exams	Number of Biopsies	Number of Benign	Number of Malignant	Percentage of Breasts with Cancer	Percentage of Biopsies Cancerous
Type of Dominant Nodules						
clin. + +, x-ray + +	24	11	10	1	4.2	9.1
clin. +, x-ray + +	26	19	17	2	7.7	10.5
clin. −, x-ray + +	10	2	2	0	0	0
clin. + +, x-ray +	23	12	12	0	0	0
clin. +, x-ray +	242	148	133	15	6.2	10.1
clin. −, x-ray +	67	7	7	0	0	0
clin. + +, x-ray −	123	31	31	0	0	0
clin. +, x-ray −	724	301	289	12	1.7	4.0
clin. −, x-ray −	3078	116	106	10	0.3	8.6
Total	4317	647	607	40	0.9	6.2
Mass Categories						
clin. + +	170	54	53	1	0.6	1.9
clin. +	992	468	439	29	2.9	6.2
clin. −	3155	125	115	10	0.3	8.0
x-ray + +	60	32	29	3	5.0	9.4
x-ray +	332	167	152	15	4.5	9.0
x-ray −	3925	448	426	22	0.6	4.9
Total	4317	647	606	40	0.9	6.2
Percentage of total (Table 18–4)	25.0	23.2	29.5	5.4		

+ = Solitary mass; + + = multiple masses; − = no mass.

TABLE 18–7. Various Combinations of Dominant Breast Masses in 12,971 Clinical and X-ray Examinations on Women Over Age 38 Years

	Number of Breast Exams	Number of Biopsies	Number of Benign	Number of Malignant	Percentage of Breasts with Cancer	Percentage of Biopsies Cancerous
Type of Dominant Nodules						
clin. + +, x-ray + +	148	69	57	12	8.1	17.4
clin. +, x-ray + +	167	91	63	28	16.7	30.8
clin. −, x-ray + +	152	32	27	5	3.3	15.6
clin. + +, x-ray +	101	54	45	9	9.0	11.7
clin. +, x-ray +	985	696	327	369	37.5	53.0
clin. −, x-ray +	455	110	69	41	9.0	37.3
clin. + +, x-ray −	266	66	64	2	0.8	3.0
clin. +, x-ray −	1474	585	457	128	8.7	21.9
clin. −, x-ray, −	9223	443	340	103	1.1	23.3
Total	12,971	2146	1449	697	5.4	32.5
Mass Categories						
clin. + +	519	189	166	23	4.5	12.2
clin. +	2626	1372	847	525	20.0	38.3
clin. −	9830	585	426	149	1.5	25.5
x-ray + +	467	192	147	45	9.6	23.4
x-ray +	1541	860	441	419	27.2	48.7
x-ray −	10,963	1094	861	233	2.1	21.3
Total	12,971	2146	1449	697	5.4	32.5
Percentage of total (Table 18–4)	75.0	76.8	70.5	94.6		

+ = Solitary mass; + + = multiple masses; − = no mass.

TABLE 18–8. Various Combinations of Dominant Breast Masses in 10,870 Clinical and X-ray Examinations on Women Aged 39–62 Years

	Number of Breast Exams	Number of Biopsies	Number of Benign	Number of Malignant	Percentage of Breasts with Cancer	Percentage of Biopsies Cancerous
Type of Dominant Nodules						
clin. + +, x-ray + +	143	64	54	10	7.0	15.6
clin. +, x-ray + +	146	75	59	16	11.0	21.3
clin. −, x-ray + +	134	29	27	2	1.5	6.9
clin. + +, x-ray +	94	50	43	7	7.4	14.0
clin. +, x-ray +	772	526	295	231	30.0	43.9
clin. −, x-ray +	372	85	62	23	6.2	27.1
clin. + +, x-ray −	252	65	63	2	0.8	3.1
clin. +, x-ray −	1313	517	417	100	7.6	19.3
clin. −, x-ray −	7644	364	288	76	1.0	20.9
Total	10,870	1775	1308	467	4.3	26.3
Mass Categories						
clin. + +	489	179	160	19	3.9	10.6
clin. +	2231	1118	771	347	15.6	31.0
clin. −	8150	478	377	101	1.2	21.1
x-ray + +	423	168	140	28	6.6	16.7
x-ray +	1238	661	400	261	21.1	39.5
x-ray −	9209	946	768	178	1.9	18.8
Total	10,870	1775	1308	467	4.3	26.3
Percentage of total (Table 18–4)	62.9	63.6	63.6	63.4		

+ = Solitary mass; + + = multiple masses; − = no mass.

TABLE 18–9. Various Combinations of Dominant Breast Masses in 2101 Clinical and X-ray Examinations on Women Aged 63–100 Years

	Number of Breast Exams	Number of Biopsies	Number of Benign	Number of Malignant	Percentage of Breasts with Cancer	Percentage of Biopsies Cancerous
Type of Dominant Nodules						
clin. + +, x-ray + +	5	5	3	2	40.0	40.0
clin. +, x-ray + +	21	16	4	12	57.1	75.0
clin. −, x-ray + +	18	3	0	3	16.7	100.0
clin. + +, x-ray +	7	4	2	2	28.6	50.0
clin. +, x-ray +	213	170	32	138	64.8	81.2
clin. −, x-ray +	83	25	7	18	21.7	72.0
clin. + +, x-ray −	14	1	1	0	0	0
clin. +, x-ray −	161	68	40	28	17.4	41.2
clin. −, x-ray −	1579	79	52	27	1.7	34.2
Total	2101	371	141	230	10.9	62.0
Mass Categories						
clin. + +	26	10	6	4	15.4	40.0
clin. +	396	254	76	178	45.1	70.0
clin. −	1680	107	59	48	2.9	44.9
x-ray + +	44	24	7	17	38.6	70.8
x-ray +	303	199	41	158	52.1	79.4
x-ray −	1754	148	93	55	3.1	37.2
Total	2101	371	141	230	10.9	62.0
Percentage of total (Table 18–4)	12.2	13.3	6.9	31.2		

+ = Solitary mass; + + = multiple masses; − = no mass.

Breast examinations in the age group between 39 and 62 years (Table 18–8) accounted for 62.9 per cent of all examinations, 63.6 per cent of all biopsies, and 63.4 per cent of all malignancies. The 0 to 38 years group (Table 18–6) accounted for 25 per cent of all breast examinations, 23.2 per cent of all biopsies, and 5.4 per cent of all malignancies. In the 0 to 32 years group (Table 18–5) were 13.9 per cent of all breast examinations, 13.2 per cent of all biopsies, and only 2.2 per cent of all cancers. The 63 to 100 years group accounted for 12.2 per cent of all breast examinations, 13.3 per cent of all biopsies, and 31.2 per cent of all cancers.

In the 63 to 100 years group with a solitary mass clinically and by x-ray, only 213 breast examinations were done, or 1.2 per cent of the total examinations. Yet 138 cancers, 18.7 per cent of the total, were demonstrated out of 170 biopsies, which was only 6.1 per cent of the total number of biopsies. In this age group, 81.2 per cent of the biopsies were done for cancer.

Clinical Considerations

The incidence of cancer varied widely within the 0 to 38, 39 to 62, and 63 to 100 year groups. The number of biopsies in these groups ranged from 14 to 16 per cent of all breast examinations. Yet the rates of cancer per biopsy for these groups were 6.2, 26.3, and 62.0 per cent, respectively.

In each category each biopsy does not have an equal likelihood of yielding cancer; the surgeon is able to assign the relative risk of cancer to each biopsy. In addition to the ratio of cancer to biopsy for a category, assessment of radiographic and clinical factors of relative risk other than mass and age contributes to an increased priority scheme.

Beyond age 62, a high percentage of masses was associated with cancer; of 213 patients with a solitary mass clinically and on the mammogram, 138 of 170 biopsies were done for cancer, for a yield of 81.2 per cent. In the 43 patients in this category who were not biopsied, 12 cancers developed during a relatively short period of follow-up.

Of 389 patients with clinical multiple masses but no mass by x-ray, 97 biopsies produced two cancers, a 2 per cent yield. Of 180 patients under age 32 years biopsied for a clinical mass but no mass on mammography, there were six cancers, or 3.3 per cent.

With a single clinical and a single radiographic dominant mass, 1227 patients with 844 biopsies yielded 384 cancers, a 45.5 per cent biopsy rate of malignancy. Thus, 383 patients in this very high-risk category were not biopsied. Perhaps the effort extended in performing biopsy on the low-yield groups could have been applied to the patients in this nonbiopsy group to produce a substantial cancer yield. In the group of 151 patients 0 to 32 years old with a single clinical and radiographic mass, there were 93 biopsies with five cancers, one with calcification of cancer not associated with a mass, a 4.3 per cent yield.

Of 737 cancers by x-ray, 434 had a single mass; 48, multiple masses; 99, cancer type calcifications without a mass; and 156, no mass. Clinically, 534 cancers had a single mass; 23, multiple masses; and 159, no mass. At times there were radiographic or clinical signs, excluding calcifications and mass, that indicated the presence of breast cancer.

The surgically "dominant" mass in the breast may be defined as a lesion requiring an immediate histologic diagnosis (or cyst aspiration) or close observation for a short time to observe any change or lack of change on which to base the decision to biopsy. This surgical term is also used by the radiologist to indicate the presence of a definite mass in the breast.

Surgical investigation of all breast lumps without delay is an impossibility at present, for lack of facilities and personnel. At Emory University, where the number of operable lesions contains a uniquely high percentage (80 per cent) of Stage 0 or Stage I cancers, only 48 per cent of the clinical dominant masses were investigated surgically. At times it required reshuffling the operating room schedule to treat without delay a proven breast cancer.

Observations

The breast biopsy rate was the same for all age groups studied. The percentage of cancer per biopsy varied from 0 to 100 when the various combinations of mass (masses), no mass, and age were considered. Low priority (less than 5 per cent cancer) groups were as follows: in all age groups, no mass by mammography or clinically and no mass by x-ray and clinical multiple masses; for the 0 to 32 year group, all categories except single mass by radiography and clinically; and for the 0 to 38 year group, all categories except mass or masses both by mammography and clinically. Using this wide range in the ratios of cancer, priority for biopsy can be established for each group. The surgeon can use additional clinical assessment of relative risk to contribute to an increased priority scheme.

The placement of breast cancer patients into relative cancer risk groups could result in a more judicious use of the operating room, surgeon, and operating room personnel. Unavoidable waiting periods for elective, but often pressing, surgery in patients with breast disease cause patients to be lost to follow-up, create a false sense of security, and temper decisions to biopsy clinically dominant masses.

An objective appraisal of the likelihood of certain patients to have breast cancer will allow the establishment of priorities for operating room use. The same number of biopsies, or even more, could be done. The surgeon could schedule his desired limit of highly possible cancer patients one day and

a large number of likely benign biopsies on another date. This would prevent delays in treatment of breast cancer and avoid a large backlog of benign biopsies.

Proven cancer occurred 156 times without a clinical mass for biopsy (21 per cent) and in an additional 23 breasts (3 per cent) with multiple masses, causing concern over biopsy of the proper mass if biopsy were decided upon. This leaves little doubt, particularly since only one half of the clinical single dominant nodules were biopsied, of the necessity for mammography prior to every decision to biopsy the breast.

REFERENCES

Egan RL (1972): Mammography, 2nd ed. Springfield, IL, Charles C Thomas.
Egan RL (1975): Breast biopsy priority: Cancer versus benign preoperative masses. Cancer 35:612.
Haagensen CD (1986): Diseases of the Breast, 3rd ed. Philadelphia, W. B. Saunders Company.

19

Radiographic Skin Changes

BACKGROUND

Minute changes in the skin of the breast may be studied by mammography and sonography and often represent characteristics of breast disease processes. Localized or generalized, benign or malignant changes may result either from lesions indigenous to the breast or from systemic processes. Any lesion that develops from the skin or its accessory glands can occur in the breast. Systemic skin changes are reflected in the skin of the breast. Most changes in the skin of the breast noted on clinical examination, except for heat and color, are depicted on mammography, often before clinical recognition.

Most skin changes, if diffuse, occurring with breast cancer signal advanced disease and a poor prognosis. For this reason, proponents of high-contrast, short-latitude techniques of breast radiography discount the value of skin imaging. With xeroradiography of the breast, only advanced skin changes are recognized owing to the imprecise delineation of this structure. Yet frequently in our experience, subtle skin changes on the mammograms have been the red flag for recognition of serious disease processes. Even more subtle are similar changes of retraction and distortion of the superficial layer of the superficial fascia and the skin. Extremely slight skin changes are reflected on pendant whole-breast sonography.

SKIN LESIONS

These are of special interest because they may simulate lesions of the mammary glands. Malignant and benign skin and subcutaneous changes may be classified as local or diffuse and according to whether there is skin thickening, retraction, and edema.

Localized

Most of the localized lesions of the skin of the breast that produce changes on the mammogram are superficial and are readily recognized clinically. The technologist can usually suggest the nature of these lesions and alert the radiologist to their presence.

Benign

Most breast skin changes are self-limiting and result from trauma, poorly fitting brassieres and self-inflicted treatments, and irritating lotions, deodorants, and ointments. If such changes are long-standing, large areas of the skin of the breast may become involved.

Scars and Keloids. Many breast scars will go undetected on the mammograms or manifest only underlying alterations of the sub-

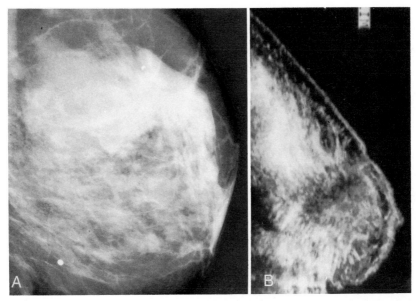

Figure 19–1. *A* and *B*, Skin scar after biopsy. A 66-year-old woman with a lump removed one year before; a thickening beneath the scar was rebiopsied six months later. Both benign. Mammography: distortion of parenchyma above level of nipple and disruption of the superficial fascia and subcutaneous tissues. Sonography: dimpling, distortion of the skin and underlying parenchyma.

cutaneous tissues or breast architecture (Figs. 19–1 and 19–2). There may be marked deformity of the breast following removal of large portions of the gland, especially in association with infection. The history is always desirable and helpful (see discussion of abscess in Chapter 13).

Scleroderma morphea may produce localized plaques in the skin of the breast (Fig. 19–3).

Nevi may be recognized on the skin of the breast (Fig. 19–4), especially when tangential to the x-ray beam. They may contain confusing flecks of calcification. A localized hema-

Figure 19–2. Biopsy complicated by infection. A 63-year-old woman, gravida 7, para 5, with a clinical breast mass for eight months. Original mammogram normal. Breast biopsy showed adipose tissue. A carcinoma clinically in the area of biopsy. Mammography: *A*, Four days post biopsy minimal skin changes UOQ. *B*, Seven weeks post rebiopsy, thickened, laminated skin in an area localized to the site of biopsy; an inflammatory process. Pathology: adipose tissue with foreign body granulomatous reaction and areas of organization. Ten months later the breast was normal clinically and by x-ray.

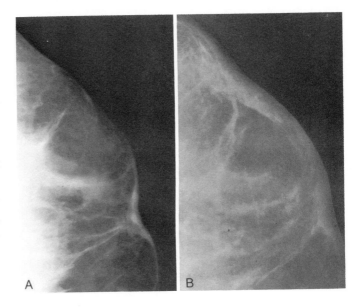

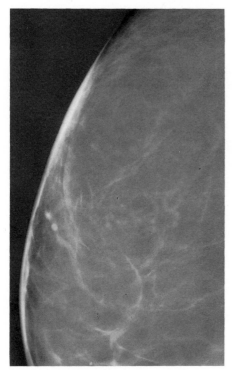

Figure 19–3. Scleroderma morphea. A 51-year-old white female with swelling of the breast for nine months and recent tenderness. Clinically: 4 × 6 cm area of hardened skin, mottled light pink hue, no underlying mass. Mammography: localized thickening of skin, minimal fibrosis beneath, no tumor, benign. Pathology: scleroderma morphea.

toma may be associated with the skin (Fig. 19–5).

Fibromata, sweat gland adenomata, mixed tumors of the sweat glands, and epidermal cysts are encountered (Figs. 19–6 to 19–8). In the periareolar area, apocrine glands may enlarge (Fig. 19–9); lesions may be localized to the nipple (Fig. 19–10 to 19–12).

Malignant

Melanoma, epithelioma, or breast carcinoma may be present as localized lesions of the breast skin (Fig. 19–13).

Generalized

Benign

Tuberculosis, granulomatous processes (Fig. 19–14), and von Recklinghausen's disease may produce diffuse skin lesions.

Malignant

An example of Hodgkin's disease has been illustrated (Chapter 14) to show generalized skin thickening of the breast.

SKIN RETRACTION

Localized

On the mammograms a small area of skin dimpling may be noted some distance from the carcinoma. With one end of the trabecula anchored at the chest wall and the other end inserted into the skin via Cooper's ligaments and the retinacula cutis, any shortening caused by fibrosis along the trabecular course is reflected in skin retraction. Tiny fibrotic strands may extend from the mass toward the skin (Fig. 19–15), but direct connection with the skin need not always be demonstrated on the mammograms. Often this early phase of skin retraction (Fig. 19–16), so graphic on the mammogram, cannot be appreciated by palpation or inspection even by an experienced observer under optimal lighting conditions.

Since it identifies the location of the un-

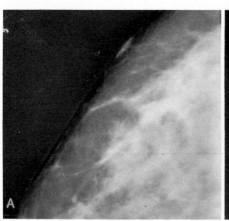

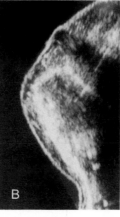

Figure 19–4. *A* and *B*, Nevus. A 55-year-old woman seen for routine checkup. Clinically: nodular breast with a nevus. Mammography showed only nodular breast and a nevus. Sonography: bulging of skin, marked attentuation by the nevus.

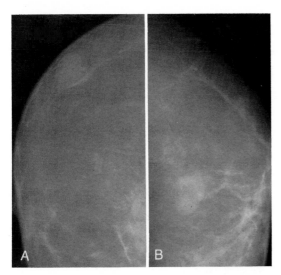

Figure 19–5. *A,* Hematoma that subsequently resorbed. A 53-year-old white female who bumped her breast seven days previously noted ecchymosis two days later. Clinically: no mass but disturbing ecchymosis. Mammography: 11 × 15 mm smooth lesion, from its location a sebaceous cyst (*B,* reversed image). Normal (done three weeks later; the ecchymosis had disappeared). Follow-up for three years; no clinical or radiographic abnormality.

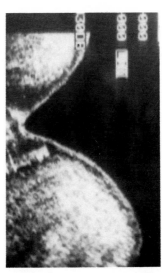

Figure 19–7. Epidermal cyst. A 40-year-old white female with a breast nodule present for one year. Clinically: 1.5 × 2 cm smooth mass fixed to the skin. Sonography: 1.5 cm anechoic smooth-margined mass, just below the skin medially in the breast, with increased through-transmission. Pathology: epidermal cyst.

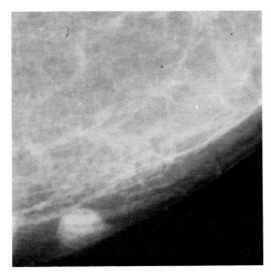

Figure 19–6. Epidermal cyst. A 45-year-old woman with a lump in the UIQ of the left breast for one year. Clinically: 1.5 cm firm mass under the skin. Mammography: 1 cm homogeneous benign lesion in the subcutaneous fat and attached to the skin, an epidermal cyst. Pathology: epidermal cyst.

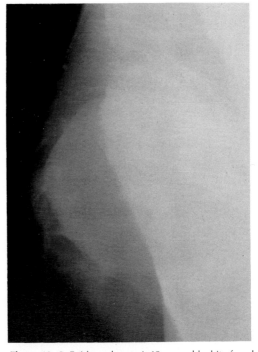

Figure 19–8. Epidermal cyst. A 48-year-old white female with a mass in the breast for an indeterminate number of years. Clinically: 10 × 5 cm hard, nodular, movable mass; no retraction or nodes. Mammography: 5 cm benign lesion, atypical fibroadenoma. Pathology: 4.5 × 4.2 × 4.0 cm cyst filled with white, amorphous, friable material; cyst wall 2 mm thick; epidermal cyst. (An unusually large cyst.)

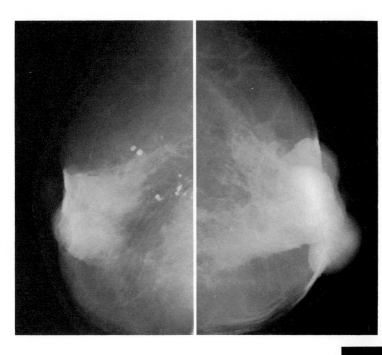

Figure 19–9. Bilateral apocrine gland hyperplasia and cyst formation. A 58-year-old white female with masses in both breasts for six months. Clinically: 4 × 4 cm carcinoma in left breast; 5 × 5.5 cm carcinoma in right breast; bilateral axillary metastases; Paget's disease of both nipples. Mammography: smoothly margined densities, subareolar in location; thickening and deformity of the overlying skin; bilateral carcinomas. Pathology: bilateral apocrine gland hyperplasia with numerous cysts ranging from 10 mm to 45 mm in size.

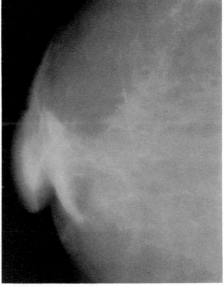

Figure 19–10. Granuloma of the nipple area. A 67-year-old black female. Clinically: subareolar mass. Mammography: subareolar dense abscess with localized skin and nipple thickening. Pathology: granuloma of the nipple area suggestive of tuberculosis.

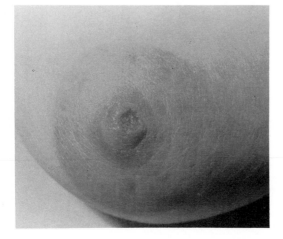

Figure 19–11. Keratosis of the nipple. A 41-year-old woman with a keratotic plaque on the left nipple for several years. Removal of the keratotic material revealed a moist clean surface.

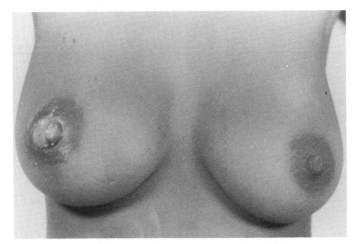

Figure 19–12. Chancre of the skin of the breast in a 26-year-old woman who presented with an open lesion of the skin of the areola and side of the nipple. Darkfield studies established the etiology as syphilis.

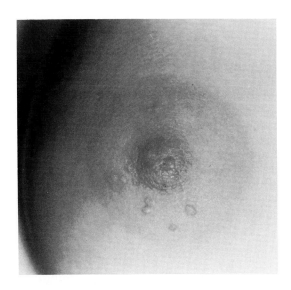

Figure 19–13. Breast carcinoma with satellite skin nodules. A 52-year-old woman with a large central clinical breast carcinoma and matted axillary lymph nodes. Pathology: biopsy of the breast mass and a skin nodule, both carcinoma. Despite radiotherapy, distant metastases occurred within six months.

Figure 19–14. Mastitis with duct stagnation. A 67-year-old woman with a serous nipple discharge, fullness under the areola, and itching of the skin of the areola. Clinically: fullness under the areola without a true mass; numerous small skin nodules. Pathology: marked duct ectasia; all the changes were thought to be related to reaction to the debris within the major ducts.

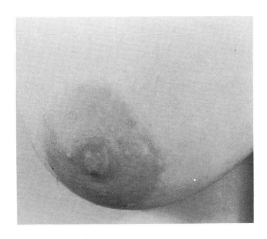

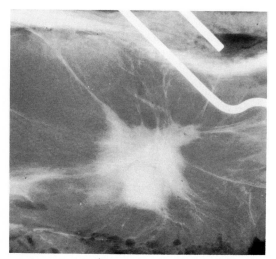

Figure 19–15. Cooper's ligament stretched into prominence. A 58-year-old woman with a suspicious lump clinically and a 1 × 1.1 cm moderately invasive carcinoma. The whole-organ slicer section clearly shows the Cooper's ligament retracted into prominence. Pathology: scirrhous duct carcinoma; modified radical mastectomy; 22 nodes normal; the patient was alive and well 14 years later.

derlying mass, the retraction sign is of obvious importance clinically—a most important sign in the diagnosis of carcinoma. For a definite clinical diagnosis of carcinoma, demonstration of skin retraction by signs of plateau formation, dimpling, or deformity of the breast is usually mandatory. Radiograph-

ically skin retraction is also a reliable diagnostic sign (Figs. 19–17 to 19–21). Although two mammograms of the breast are obtained at right angles, the entire skin of the breast is not shown in profile. Evidence of skin retraction and/or thickening in an area not in profile may be identified by a bandlike density similar to a wrinkle in the skin of the breast. The skin overlying a lesion may be studied more thoroughly with additional views that show it in profile (Fig. 19–22).

Generalized

Sonographic studies of the pendant breast in the water bath readily demonstrate minimal skin retraction. At times the breast wrinkles badly or takes on a wavy contour (Fig. 19–23).

SKIN THICKENING

Localized

Benign

A limited area of skin thickening is usually associated with the localized area of skin retraction, which appears on the mammograms to be overlying the carcinoma. This skin thickening is also evident radiographically before it is recognized clinically. With such limited skin retraction, it may be diffi-

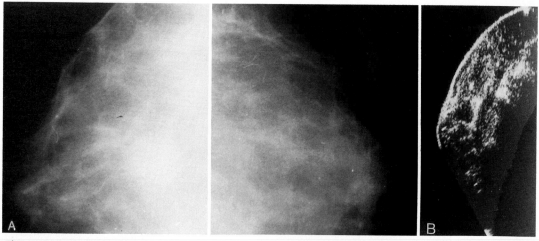

Figure 19–16. Retraction of superficial layer of fascia. A 45-year-old woman with a breast lump for three to five months. Clinically a mass of carcinoma. *A,* Mammography: marked asymmetry of the superficial layer of superficial fascia in the upper portion of the right breast. Fine strands of straightened trabeculae can be seen extending from the 1.2 × 1.5 cm moderately invasive central carcinoma to the fascia. Straightened subareolar ducts are beginning to fix and retract the nipple. *B,* Breast sonography shows that the retractive changes are primarily anterior to the mass and extend to flatten and retract the overlying skin. Pathology: Stage I duct carcinoma with elements of fibrosis.

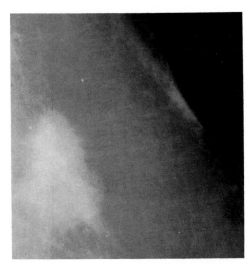

Figure 19–17. Small area of skin retraction remote from carcinoma. A 74-year-old woman with a breast lump for one month; clinically suspicious but without skin changes. Mammography: 1.4 × 1.9 cm moderately invasive carcinoma containing stippled calcifications, causing straightening of Cooper's ligaments, and producing a small overlying area of skin retraction. Pathology: duct carcinoma with desmoplasia. Modified radical mastectomy; all 21 axillary lymph nodes free of tumor. The patient was free of disease four years later.

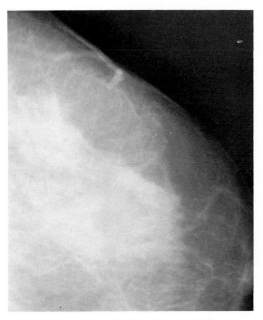

Figure 19–19. Very early skin change with breast carcinoma not appreciated clinically even with optimal lighting and careful examination. The poorly defined mass is readily diagnosed as carcinoma after noting the prominent ducts leading to it, the increased vasculature, and skin changes.

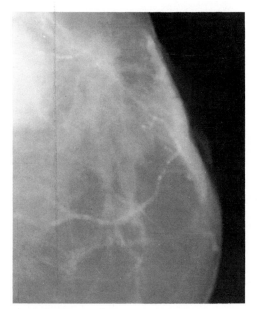

Figure 19–18. Carcinoma producing local skin retraction at some distance from the tumor. A 63-year-old woman with "pulling" in her breast. Clinically: 3.5 × 4.5 cm hard lesion with skin dimpling with certain maneuvers of physical examination. Mammography: 1.8 × 2.9 cm coarsely spiculated carcinoma, stretching Cooper's ligaments to retract a distant area of skin. Pathology: duct carcinoma, scirrhous type. Modified radical mastectomy; 3 of 18 axillary lymph nodes with neoplasm. The patient was alive and well two years later.

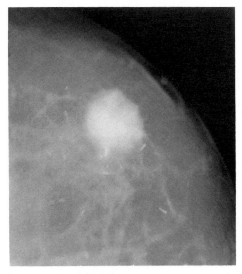

Figure 19–20. Moderately invasive carcinoma producing local skin retraction that can be recognized even though not in profile. The patient, a 54-year-old woman, had noted a breast lump five months before but skin dimpling only recently. Clinically, a 2.5 × 3.5 cm mass was felt with skin retraction in certain positions. On the mammograms and gross sectioning, the carcinoma was 1.5 × 1.7 cm.

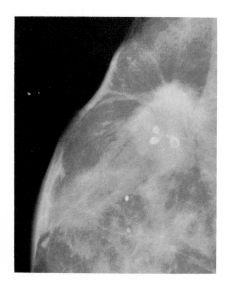

Figure 19–21. Localized skin retraction and thickening with a superficial breast carcinoma. A 64-year-old woman with a breast mass and early skin dimpling. Mammography: moderately invasive 1.7 × 2 cm carcinoma; straightening of Cooper's ligament with adjacent skin retraction and thickening; radiographically operable. Pathology: duct carcinoma with fibrosis; radical mastectomy; 3 lower of a total of 27 axillary lymph nodes with metastasis. The patient died six years later without evidence of breast carcinoma (complications of a stroke).

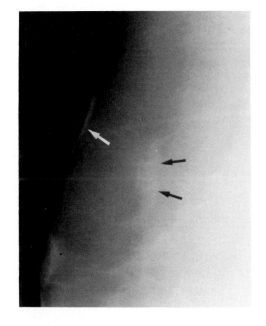

Figure 19–22. Special spot view in mediolateral position. The breast is rotated so that the skin adjacent to a carcinomatous mass (black arrows) is tangential to the x-ray beam. The skin changes (white arrow) were not apparent on routine views. There was a question of skin retraction clinically; the carcinoma was readily palpable.

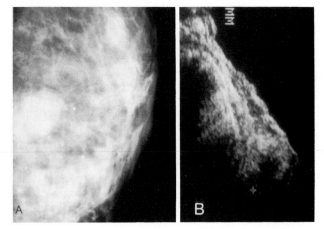

Figure 19–23. Wavy contour of the skin from carcinoma. A 75-year-old woman with a clinically suspicious mass. *A,* Mammography: circumscribed carcinoma with indistinct periphery and several areas of coalescent fibroglandular tissue. *B,* Sonography: two contiguous hypoechoic areas with nonhomogeneous internal echoes; retraction of the skin in an undulating fashion. Pathology: duct carcinoma with anastomosing sheets of cells, necrosis, two separate foci of intraductal carcinoma. Modified radical mastectomy, all 19 axillary lymph nodes free of tumor. The patient was alive and well 30 months later.

cult to be certain whether the skin is actually thickened or only distorted by the retraction. Early local skin changes about the areola usually are not appreciated clinically.

Localized, minimal skin thickening and occasionally some degree of retraction occur following biopsy of a benign lesion. Unless complicated by infection, the mammogram reverts to normal in 10 to 14 days. Marked deformity of the breast, clinically evident after massive biopsies, is not associated with thickened skin or with retraction of the skin involved with carcinoma. Mammoplasties involving removal of much of the breast tissue produce no unusual changes in the remaining skin. Usually no evidence of the previous surgery is reflected on the mammograms. Occasionally, however, infolding of the skin over a massive biopsy site produces an appearance of minimal skin thickening or retraction. Keloid formation should be obvious on the mammograms.

Trauma (biopsy, needle aspiration, heat, bruise) may be the cause of localized skin thickening of the breast (Fig. 19–24).

Mondor's disease is difficult to demonstrate on mammography, as the affected vein is retracted and becomes difficult to image.

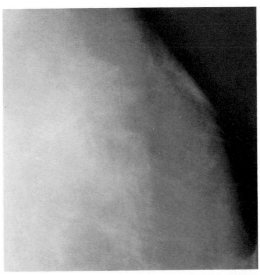

Figure 19–25. Poorly defined carcinoma producing thickening of the adjacent skin. A 52-year-old woman was aware of a breast mass for six months. Slight flattening of the skin is produced.

Brassiere syndrome merely produces increased inframammary skin thickening unless other areas of the breast are chronically irritated.

Fat necrosis, so frequently seen in the subcutaneous area, may be associated with

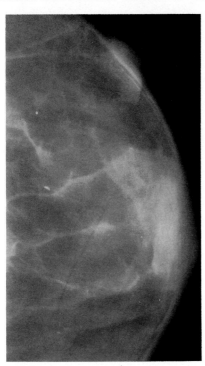

Figure 19–24. Second-degree burn. A 66-year-old white female with subareolar inflammatory changes and axillary lymph node enlargement. Application of a hot water bottle to the breast resulted in a second-degree burn; note blister on the skin.

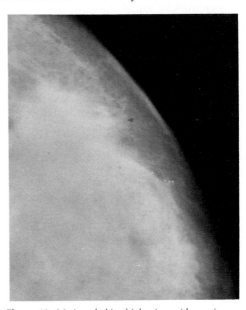

Figure 19–26. Local skin thickening with carcinoma. A 44-year-old woman whose gynecologist observed a breast lump for one year. Clinically: highly suspicious mass. Mammography: 2.5 cm highly invasive carcinoma with thickening of the overlying skin. Pathology: duct carcinoma with scirrhous elements. Modified radical mastectomy; two of three tail of breast lymph nodes with metastasis, none of 12 axillary lymph nodes with metastasis. Two years later after a course of chemotherapy the patient was living and well.

skin thickening. A hematoma also may be located in the subcutaneous area and produce skin thickening.

Malignant

Primary breast carcinoma produces skin thickening without retraction or with flattening only (Figs. 19–25 to 19–28).

Generalized

Benign

Cardiac decompensation (Fig. 19–29) or similar generalized anasarca can produce massive diffuse skin thickening. A greater effect may be apparent in the breast that remains more pendant than its mate.

When severe, thyroid disease, manifested by myxedema, can have the appearance of the breast shown in Figure 19–30.

Diffuse hemorrhage into the breast may cause increased density of the breast and diffuse skin thickening (Fig. 19–31).

Acute bacterial infections, as well as chronic forms such as breast abscess, produce generalized skin thickening.

Lactation mastitis may be severe enough to cause thickening of the skin of the entire breast.

Granulomatous processes such as sarcoidosis or tuberculosis (Fig. 19–32) produce generalized skin thickening.

The skin of the breast may be normally unusually thick, or there may simply be no explanation for this mammographic finding (Fig. 19–33), or there may be idiopathic breast hypertrophy (Fig. 19–34).

Rapid weight loss, such as with carcinoma of the esophagus or anorexia nervosa, can be accompanied with diffuse skin thickening (Fig. 19–35).

Of course, no series of breast cases would be complete without an example of the breast caught in the wringer (Fig. 19–36).

Malignant

Diffuse skin thickening with primary breast cancer may progress from a localized to a generalized extent (Figs. 19–37 and 19–38), be associated with skin thickening of another etiology (Fig. 19–39), or begin in a diffuse fashion from a deep carcinoma (Figs. 19–40 and 19–41). Even early diffuse skin thickening with carcinoma indicates a poor prognosis (Figs. 19–42 and 19–43).

Progressive thickening of the skin, with

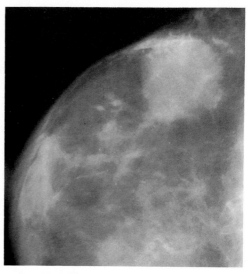

Figure 19–27. Well-defined carcinoma producing flattening and thickening of skin adjacent to the mass. This 52-year-old woman was aware of a lump in her breast for over six months.

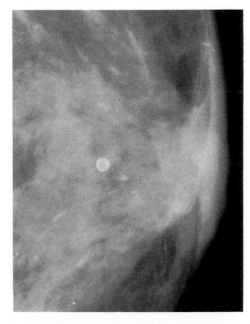

Figure 19–28. Thickened periareolar skin with Paget's disease of the breast. A 59-year-old woman with nipple, then areolar, then breast skin changes "for years" that progressed despite ointments, salves, soaks, and other home remedies. A central lump found one day before. Mammography: Coarse calcifications of secretory disease interspersed with fine calcifications of comedocarcinoma; vague central density with thickened skin of the areola. Pathology: intraductal carcinoma and comedocarcinoma with scirrhous elements. Modified radical mastectomy; 5 of 19 Level I and II lymph nodes with metastases. Death occurred 25 months later with disseminated carcinoma.

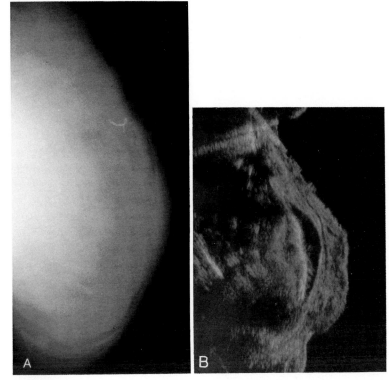

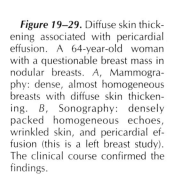

Figure 19–29. Diffuse skin thickening associated with pericardial effusion. A 64-year-old woman with a questionable breast mass in nodular breasts. *A,* Mammography: dense, almost homogeneous breasts with diffuse skin thickening. *B,* Sonography: densely packed homogeneous echoes, wrinkled skin, and pericardial effusion (this is a left breast study). The clinical course confirmed the findings.

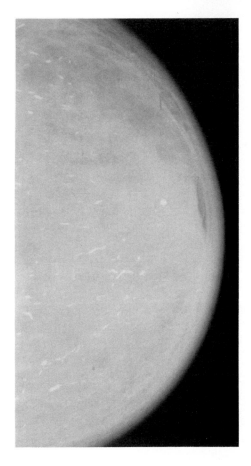

Figure 19–30. Diffuse skin thickening associated with generalized myxedema. A 71-year-old woman studied as part of a routine work-up for persistent thyroid disease. Edema and diffuse skin thickening were equal bilaterally.

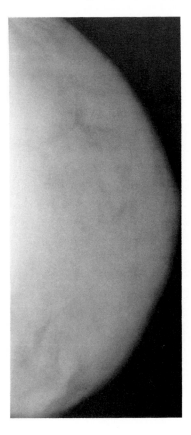

Figure 19–31. Diffuse breast hemorrhage. Hemorrhage occurred in a 38-year-old woman following a biopsy nine days previously for fibrocystic disease. Clinically a large mass was felt, but upon biopsy there were only changes of fibrocystic disease and marked hemosiderin deposits in the glandular tissue. Mammography shows diffuse increased density in the breast.

Figure 19–32. Diffuse tuberculosis of the breast. A 67-year-old white female with enlarging breast for an indefinite period. Clinically: diffuse enlargement and turgidity of the breast, skin edema, and carcinoma. Mammography: diffuse density throughout the breast without demonstrable mass but with diffuse skin thickening and carcinoma. Pathology: tuberculosis of the breast.

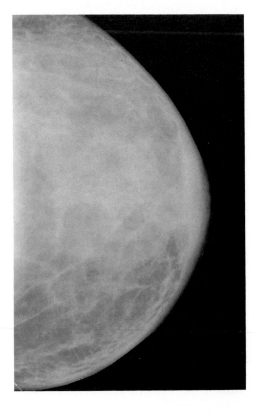

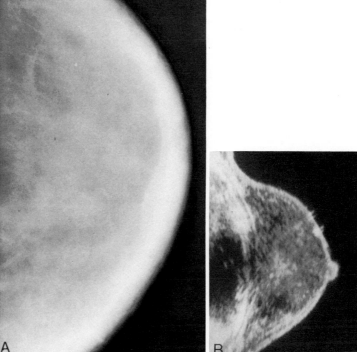

Figure 19–33. *A*, and *B*, Idiopathic diffuse skin thickening. A 31-year-old woman with nodular breasts. No pregnancies, no known systemic disease. Mammography: fibroplasia with marked diffuse skin thickening, etiology unknown. Pathology: fibrocystic disease of the breast.

A

B

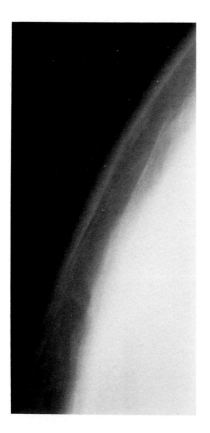

Figure 19–34. Idiopathic breast hypertrophy with skin thickening. A 39-year-old woman with enlarging breasts for several months. Heaviness and a dull ache were her major complaints. Histologically the skin and breast tissue appear normal. Hormonal readjustments usually arrest or produce regression of the process.

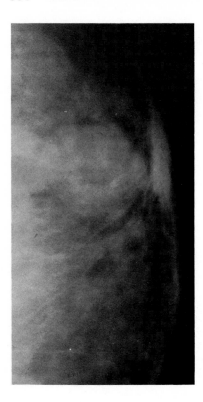

Figure 19–35. Diffuse skin thickening with a breast mass. A 73-year-old woman with a firm left subareolar mass. Mammography: 2 × 2 cm subareolar mass, slightly lobulated, outlined by fat. The mass appears benign but is associated with diffuse skin thickening. There has been a recent 80 lb weight loss due to a number of gastrointestinal problems, and the skin of the opposite breast was similarly increased in thickness. Biopsy revealed a sclerosing fibroadenoma.

Figure 19–36. Breast caught in wringer. A 54-year-old black female who presented with osteolytic metastases and a history of having caught her breast in a washing machine wringer several months previously. Clinically: carcinoma of the breast. Mammography: localized, slightly laminated, thickened skin, without underlying mass; benign.

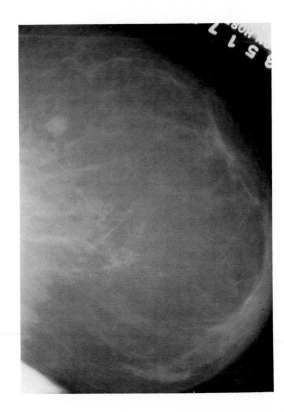

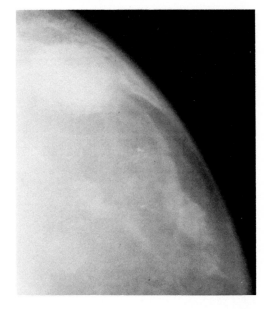

Figure 19–37. Local skin thickening extending into diffuse thickening. A 64-year-old woman with a breast mass for months, heaviness in her breast for one week. Mammography: 1.8 × 2.4 cm moderately invasive carcinoma just beneath an area of quite thickened skin that involves the skin of the entire breast; inoperable. Pathology (needle biopsy): duct carcinoma.

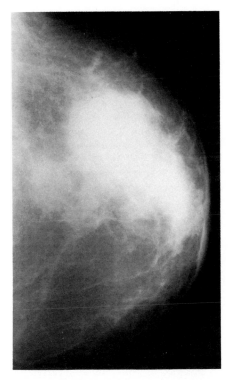

Figure 19–38. Very early diffuse skin thickening with medullary carcinoma with lymphoid stroma. A 59-year-old woman with a breast mass that had doubled in size during the past month. Mammography: 2.8 × 3 cm circumscribed carcinoma with skin thickening 4 cm superiorly and 6 cm inferiorly to the nipple and increased vascularity. Pathology: medullary carcinoma with lymphoid stroma. Modified radical mastectomy; all 19 axillary lymph nodes free of tumor. The patient was alive and well four years later. This case radiographically is borderline operable, but an area of the breast skin anterior to the inframammary skin crease is normal in thickness. See Figure 19–42 regarding prognosis. (At times minimal skin thickening does not reproduce well from screen-film studies.)

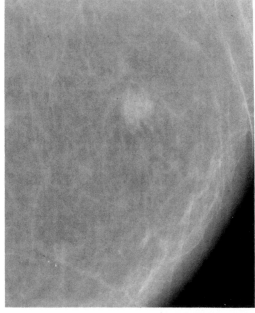

Figure 19–39. Nonpalpable duct carcinoma. A 55-year-old woman seen for a general physical examination prior to coronary triple bypass surgery; bilateral breast pain. Mammography: 9 mm moderately invasive carcinoma. Note massively thickened skin (present bilaterally) due to cardiac problems. Pathology (lumpectomy): duct carcinoma, sclerosing type, Grade III. Two years later there was no apparent breast problem.

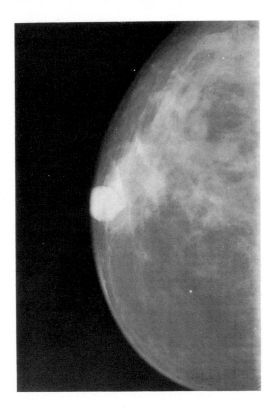

Figure 19–40. Subareolar carcinoma and skin thickening. A 69-year-old woman who lost more than 100 lb in the past year; general checkup; fatty breasts. Mammography: 8 × 9 mm spiculated subareolar carcinoma with diffuse skin thickening. Pathology: Stage I duct carcinoma. The patient was alive and gaining weight 18 months later.

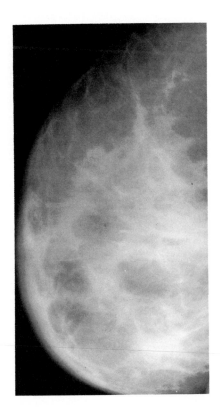

Figure 19–41. Progression of the process of diffuse skin thickening associated with breast carcinoma. The thickening extends toward the inframammary crease, then into the skin of the portion of the superior breast, with the skin of the tail of the breast being the last to thicken. The diffuse density in the breast almost obscures the faint calcification in the mass, poorly reproduced.

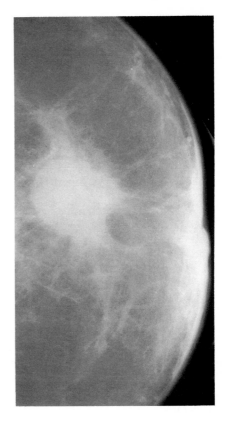

Figure 19–42. Early diffuse skin thickening with poor prognosis. A 66-year-old woman with a breast lump for "months" that measured 4 × 5 cm clinically and was located in the 10 o'clock position. Mammography: 2.8 × 3 cm moderately invasive carcinoma with increased vascularity and early diffuse skin thickening. Pathology: duct carcinoma with desmoplasia. Modified radical mastectomy; 4 (low) of 22 axillary lymph nodes with metastases. Distant metastases two years later. (See Figure 19–38 regarding prognosis.)

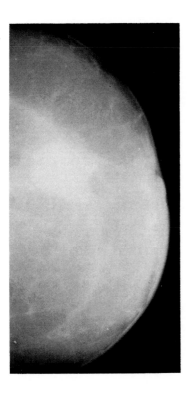

Figure 19–43. Borderline early diffuse skin thickening with carcinoma. A 77-year-old woman with a clinically palpable left breast mass but otherwise normal breasts. Mammography: large, fatty breasts containing a 2.5 × 3 cm moderately invasive carcinoma producing fixation of the nipple, increased breast density partially obscuring the mass, and increased skin thickening. Pathology: duct carcinoma with intraductal elements. Modified radical mastectomy; 1 of 12 axillary lymph nodes contained metastatic deposits. This definite skin change compared with the right breast probably is an extremely early phase of diffuse skin thickening. (There was normal skin near the inframammary crease.) It's always better to err in the direction of operability to assure the maximum therapy for the breast cancer patient. This patient was living and well three years later.

involvement of a large area of the skin overlying a carcinoma, occurs as the clinical finding of plateau formation, dimpling, or retraction becomes more obvious. With very deep-seated lesions, skin thickening may be evident at a distance from the area overlying the carcinoma during the development of these findings prior to local skin changes. The initial area of this distal skin involvement seen on the mammograms is just below the areola in the dependent portions of the breast. This location suggests a relationship between the increased vascularity of the breast and possible interference with drainage through the engorged veins. Larger portions of the skin of the breast become evenly and diffusely thickened. This early skin involvement is devoid of the *peau d'orange* effect, and the skin remains soft and pliable. Skin thickening of this type, 8 to 10 mm, is

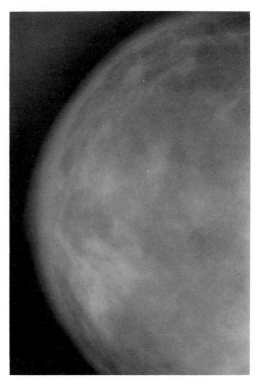

Figure 19–45. Massive thickening of skin of entire breast. Diffuse carcinoma of the entire breast is present, obscuring almost all structures. The widened strands in the subcutaneous fat are markedly dilated lymphatics. Clinically this skin was thickened and firm but of normal temperature.

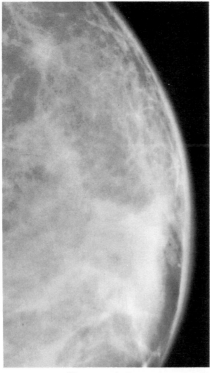

Figure 19–44. Infiltration of dermis by comedocarcinoma. A 53-year-old woman with tenderness and thickening of the breast for two weeks. Clinically: question of a subareolar carcinoma; no palpable skin changes. Mammography: comedo type calcification, several coalescent areas producing small masses and a carcinoma approximately 2.5 cm in the subareolar area; diffuse skin thickening. Pathology: intraductal carcinoma and comedocarcinoma. Modified radical mastectomy; at least four sites of carcinoma, with the largest being 2.5 cm subareolar in location; infiltration of the dermis; all 19 nodes free of tumor. The patient was alive and well two years later.

often not evident clinically but is obvious on the mammogram.

With carcinoma, the skin of the entire breast and that overlying the axilla may be diffusely thickened to more than 1 cm, with the nipple and areola densely thickened and fixed. These changes may be associated with inflammatory carcinoma, with or without involvement of the dermal lymphatics. Marked diffuse skin thickening has not been found in benign inflammatory disease, in radiation reaction, after axillary dissection with or without radiation therapy, or after axillary perfusion. Some milder degree of skin thickening may be present with these conditions as well as with massive involvement of axillary lymph nodes by lymphoma, squamous carcinoma of the hand, or melanoma.

Early diffuse skin thickening, associated with inoperable breast carcinoma, has been observed to increase during radiation therapy but later regresses. This thickening is assumed to be a natural progression of the disease, temporarily unchecked by therapy,

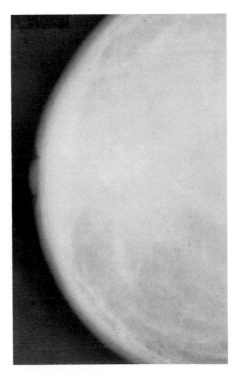

Figure 19–46. Diffuse skin thickening of breast in presence of clinical inflammatory carcinoma. This diagnosis cannot be made from the mammograms, which do not depict heat, pain, or color. Mammographically the lesion is the same as in Figure 19–47, noninflammatory carcinoma with skin thickening.

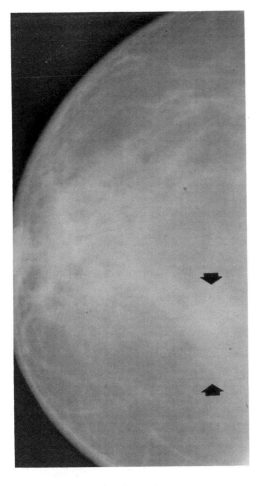

Figure 19–47. Diffuse thickening of skin of entire breast has occurred. The primary mass can still be seen (between arrowheads), although almost obscured. The quality of such mammograms is poor owing to the required increase in kvp, for penetration. Skin this thick often is soft, pliable, and clinically normal.

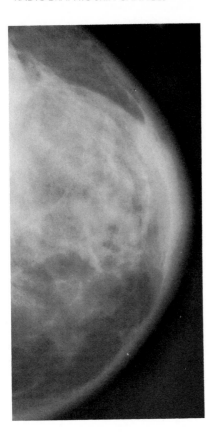

Figure 19—48. Marked diffuse thickening of the skin of breast associated with inflammatory carcinoma. The primary mass of cancer is obscured; the quality of the mammogram is poor owing to the increased thickness and density of the tissues. The patient, a 58-year-old woman, had rapid onset of swelling, pain, redness, and increased heat in the breast.

for most breasts without initial skin thickening that are irradiated show no, or only minimal, skin thickening during therapy.

Diffuse skin thickening is produced by increase in dermal collagen and actual increase in amount of tissue, rather than by edema (Fig. 19–44). This possibly is a reactive phenomenon to altered lymph flow. Actual infiltration of the dermis can occur. Small rounded densities beneath the skin represent lymphatics dilated with fluid and/or tumor cells (Fig. 19–46); if noted alone, this may have the same prognostic significance as diffuse skin thickening.

It is re-emphasized here (see Chapter 26) that inflammatory carcinoma is not a radiographic diagnosis, and only diffuse skin thickening can be noted. The degree of that thickening can be estimated, but inflammatory carcinoma cannot be differentiated from noninflammatory carcinoma (Figs. 19–45 to 19–48).

Subareolar Cancers

20

BACKGROUND

Normal anatomic and variants of normal anatomic structures as well as benign and malignant lesions in the subareolar area characteristically pose special problems in imaging and interpretation. There is much overlapping of benign and malignant diagnosis in this region. In almost all breasts subareolar changes are present and are frequently asymmetric. This perhaps is the most difficult part of the breast to evaluate clinically. For maximum assessment of changes in the breast, the pathologist who receives material for study from this area must be alerted to its source. This is such an important consideration that the term "subareolar fibrosis" was coined to distinguish subareolar changes from similar intramammary changes.

Both benign and malignant subareolar changes may or may not be associated with a palpable mass or fullness, nipple changes or fixation, retraction or eczema, a wide range of types of nipple discharge, stretching or dilatation of the major ducts, and calcifications. All are associated with diagnostic problems, and all occur in many combinations.

Most of the usual endogenous and exogenous breast lesions occur in the subareolar area and are not unlike lesions elsewhere in the breast. Features of the more perplexing subareolar lesions of the breast will be classified, illustrated, and emphasized in an effort to reach the differential diagnosis of cancer.

ASSOCIATED WITH MASS

The ever-present major subareolar ducts with varying degrees of periductal reaction and fibrosis can produce either a pseudomass or a thickening or can mask, both clinically and radiographically, a discrete mass in the area. Typical mammographic lesions, such as the benign fibroadenoma (Fig. 20–1) or the

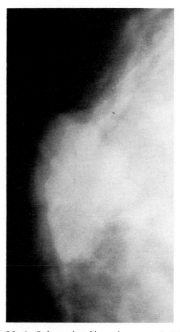

Figure 20–1. Subareolar fibroadenoma. A 26-year old woman, gravida 2, para 2, nursing, with a breast lump. Clinically: nodular breasts with a 2 × 2.5 cm lobulated freely movable mass beneath the right nipple. Mammography: 1.5 × 2.5 cm subareolar fibroadenoma and a similar 6 × 9 mm lesion below the level of the nipple. Pathology: fibroadenomata.

365

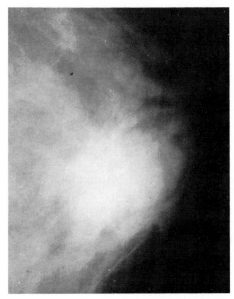

Figure 20–2. Circumscribed subareolar carcinoma. A 62-year-old woman with a breast lump for one month. Clinically: periareolar mass with nipple discharge. Mammography: 1.2 × 2 cm well-circumscribed mass anteriorly with indistinct borders posteriorly—considered carcinoma. Pathology: duct carcinoma, axillary lymph nodes free of tumor. The patient was free of disease four years later.

circumscribed carcinoma (Fig. 20–2), may be distinguished, although with more difficulty and less confidence, in the subareolar area. Asymmetry may not be sufficient for the histologic diagnosis, and secondary signs are useful (Fig. 20–3). A confident differentiation may not be possible (Fig. 20–4). Despite previous surgical procedures on the breast in

Figure 20–4, biopsy was mandatory to establish the etiology of such marked asymmetric changes, which were not explained radiographically. In Figure 20–5 the most pronounced asymmetry is the glandular portion of the two breasts, yet the most significant area was the immediate subareolar site with the highly suspicious density. The thickened areolar skin and borderline increased vascularity heightened concern. The symmetric placement of the carcinoma in relation to the nipple is more suggestive of subareolar fibrosis. The asymmetric placement of the lesion in relation to the nipple (Fig. 20–6) is more common with carcinoma. The diffuse increase in density of the right breast also supports the conclusion of malignancy rather than a benign process such as inflammation, but this is not absolute. Similarly, the areolar skin changes favor malignancy but can be produced by an inflammatory process. Many subareolar carcinomas are highly invasive, with poor prognosis despite a relatively small size and minimal clinical findings as in this case.

Subareolar fibrosis is usually bilateral and often very symmetric as in Figure 20–7. The radiologist was not overly concerned by this common appearance; even after being apprised of the bleeding left nipple, he could delineate no definite area of greater concern. The small carcinoma in this breast was completely masked radiographically. On routine mammograms a carcinoma may be so nearly masked that additional complementary stud-

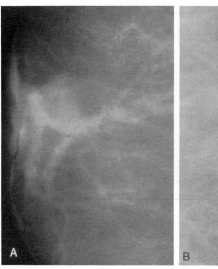
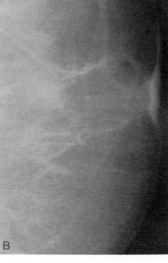

Figure 20–3. A and B, Clinically occult subareolar carcinoma. A 62-year-old woman who had a biopsy of an axillary lymph node, pathologically a poorly differentiated malignancy. Clinically: normal breasts. Mammography: 1.3 × 1.5 cm circumscribed subareolar carcinoma with increased vascularity. Pathology: duct carcinoma. Radical mastectomy; axillary lymph node metastases all levels. Distant metastases within a year.

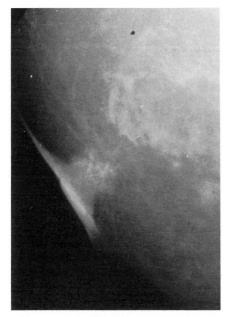

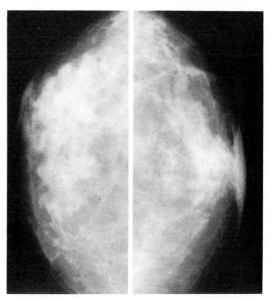

Figure 20–4. Small subareolar carcinoma. A 50-year-old woman with a lump under left areola. Prior surgery: 1957, right and left reduction mammoplasty; 1967, cyst removed from the right breast; 1974, cyst removed from the right breast. Mammography: asymmetric changes under the right nipple; carcinoma vs subareolar fibrosis. Pathology: duct carcinoma. Modified radical mastectomy (followed by chemotherapy); one low node of a total of 29 axillary lymph nodes contained tumor. Three years later, no evidence of disease.

Figure 20–5. Asymmetry of subareolar areas. A 66-year-old woman with a breast mass for three weeks. Clinically: a 3 cm subareolar suspicious mass. Mammography: different-appearing breasts. Right: prominent major subareolar ducts, marked ductal hyperplasia anterior third of the breast. Left: less tissue anterior third of breast, thickened areola with underlying triangular density, inflammation vs tumor. Pathology: (left) 2.5 cm main mass of tumor, intraductal and scirrhous duct carcinoma; satellite nodules in three quadrants; infiltration of the dermis UIQ and LOQ. Modified radical mastectomy; all ten nodes level I and four nodes Level II free of tumor. The patient was alive without disease five years later.

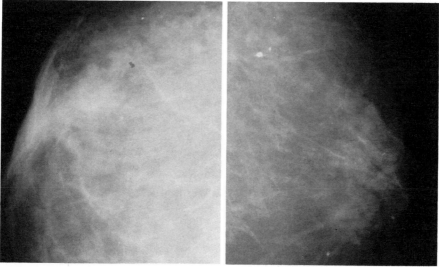

Figure 20–6. Diffuse central carcinoma. A 59-year-old woman with a "drawing" of her right nipple. Clinically: firmer, fuller subareolar area on right. Mammography: 1.4 cm spiculated carcinoma in the immediate subareolar area with diffuse density throughout the central portion of the right breast. Pathology: duct carcinoma with scirrhous element, multifocal. Modified radical mastectomy, 6 of 19 low axillary and midaxillary lymph nodes with metastases. Death from disseminated disease 42 months later.

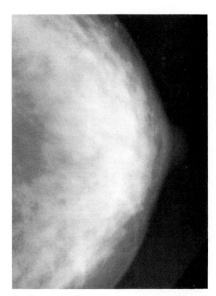

Figure 20–7. Small carcinoma masked by subareolar fibrosis. A 53-year-old woman with a bleeding nipple. Bilateral dilated ducts and subareolar fibrosis by mammography. Upon resection a small papillary carcinoma with microinvasion was demonstrated; nodes negative; patient alive and well three years later. (The opposite breast had the same x-ray appearance.)

ies are necessary (Fig. 20–8). Clinical suspicion and sonography aided greatly in this case.

ASSOCIATED WITH NIPPLE CHANGES

Various nonspecific nipple changes occur in many malignant processes in the breast and must be differentiated from similar lesions with a benign etiology. The more common nipple changes producing concern include fixation and/or retraction, intradermal changes, and discharge.

ASSOCIATED WITH FIXATION AND/OR RETRACTION

The nipple may be fixed in position and fail to become erect upon stimulation; this is often associated with at least a mild degree of retraction (Fig. 20–9). Search for an underlying carcinoma is imperative. Congenital nipple retraction by patient history (often unreliable) can still be associated with breast cancer. The retractive process may progress to complete inversion of the nipple (Fig. 20–10). Carcinoma producing retraction of the nipple may be located at varying depths in the breast (Figs. 20–4 and 20–10).

Most of the nipple changes illustrated thus far are readily seen when associated with shortening of the major ducts by fibrosis and scarring related to the carcinoma. Often, carcinomas contiguous with the base of the nipple and surrounding areolar skin are highly infiltrative and actually invade the nipple and areolar skin, producing such marked fixation of these structures that retraction is limited (Fig. 20–11). The nipple may appear bulbous. These advanced nipple and areolar changes usually imply poor prognosis, whereas simple nipple retraction has no more significance than retraction of the skin adjacent to a carcinoma elsewhere in the breast. In contrast to skin invasion and fixation, the highly infiltrative carcinoma may produce marked retraction without actual skin invasion (Fig. 20–12) and still have a less guarded prognosis.

ASSOCIATED WITH INTRADERMAL CHANGES

Various stages of scaling, crusting, eczema, weeping, and ulceration of the nipple may be associated with an underlying breast cancer. Long-term nipple discharge may be an irritant to the skin of the summit of the nipple. Prolonged nipple retraction may predispose to uncleanliness, collection of detritus, infection, and skin changes. The single most significant lesion of the skin of the nipple is Paget's disease of the breast. Biopsy of the involved nipple skin will verify the presence of a breast carcinoma, and mammography will outline its nature and extent (Fig. 20–13). Clinically, other dermal changes may simulate Paget's disease (Fig. 20–14).

ASSOCIATED WITH DISCHARGE

Nipple discharge may be intermittent or continuous, tinged with numerous colors, vary widely in consistency, and be a barely perceptible oozing or a copious flow. Of concern to the patient and her physician is the often elusive etiology, its significance, and the necessity to correct it. Cytology, x-ray contrast studies of the ducts, and mammography may be helpful. Localization of the offending area and surgical removal, if

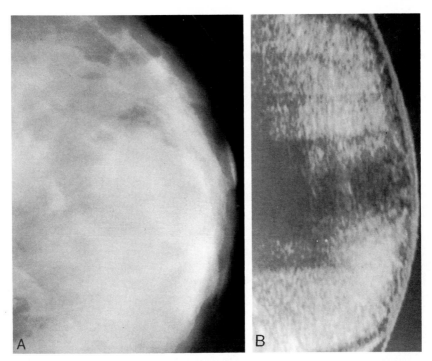

Figure 20–8. Poorly defined subareolar carcinoma. A 68-year-old woman with a clinically suspicious subareolar mass. *A*, Mammography: poorly defined mass, approximately 4 cm, subareolar carcinoma. *B*, Sonography: hypoechoic irregular mass with nonhomogeneous internal echoes, attenuation of the beam. Pathology: duct carcinoma. Modified radical mastectomy, all 22 axillary lymph nodes free of tumor. Patient was alive without disease 35 months later.

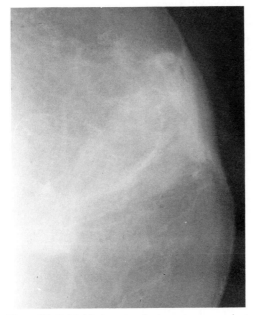

Figure 20–9. Highly invasive duct carcinoma producing marked retraction. The shortening of many of the major subareolar ducts toward the nipple is producing early areolar retraction and minimal or no nipple retraction. Correct positioning is important in evaluation of nipple retraction.

correction and/or diagnosis is required, is the optimal approach.

Some authors (Leis et al., 1985) claim knowledge of association of every type of nipple discharge with breast cancer. In our experience the highest risk of cancer has been in the presence of a sanguineous or serosanguineous discharge from a single duct. The bleeding nipple most commonly indicates an intraductal papilloma. Green, black, white, and serous discharges may be from breasts harboring a cancer, but the discharge is usually related to some form of fibrocystic disease, such as duct ectasia or subareolar fibrosis (Figs. 20–7 and 20–15).

ASSOCIATED WITH MAJOR DUCT CHANGES

The major ducts are involved in all subareolar changes of both benign and malignant breast diseases. Their involvement per se, except for harboring intraductal lesions such as papillomata or intraductal carcinomas, is manifested by stretching or dilatation. Any

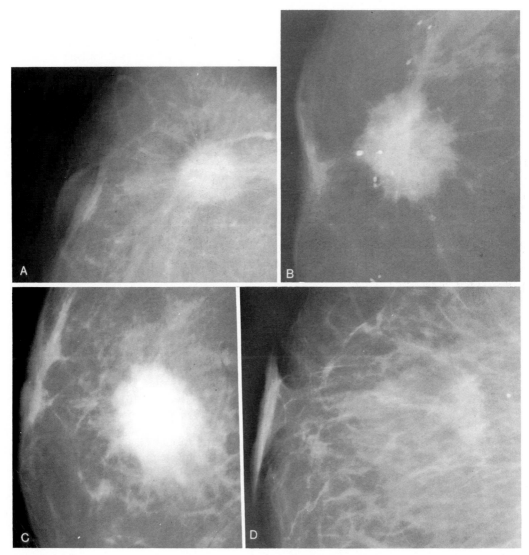

Figure 20–10. *A,* Complete inversion of the nipple produced by a highly invasive duct carcinoma. The major ducts are barely visible despite marked nipple retraction. This 72-year-old woman with noticed gradual retraction of the nipple for several months. *B–D,* Three other duct carcinomas at different depths in the breast producing nipple retraction. The size of these subareolar carcinomas is not particularly related to the degree of retraction.

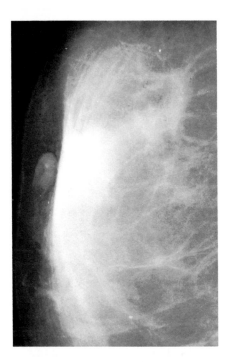

Figure 20–11. Highly invasive subareolar carcinoma. An 80-year-old woman with firmness and dimpling of the areola. Mammography: 1.8 × 2 cm moderately circumscribed carcinoma in the immediate subareolar area producing marked subareolar reaction; thickening and flattening of the areola with fixation of the nipple. Slightly above and deeper in the breast is an irregular separate 1.2 × 2.2 cm mass suggestive of comedocarcinoma. Pathology: one duct carcinoma with fibrosis invading the skin and a separate comedocarcinoma with fibrosis. Modified radical mastectomy; 4 of 19 axillary lymph nodes contained metastases. Three years later, widespread metastases.

Figure 20–12. Highly invasive subareolar carcinoma. A 70-year-old woman with a lump and "drawing in" of her nipple for an indefinite time; clinically cancer. Mammography: 8 × 12 mm highly invasive carcinoma, stippled calcifications, nipple retraction. Pathology: duct carcinoma with productive fibrosis. Modified radical mastectomy; 1 low of a total of 18 axillary lymph nodes contained metastatic deposits. The patient was free of disease four years later.

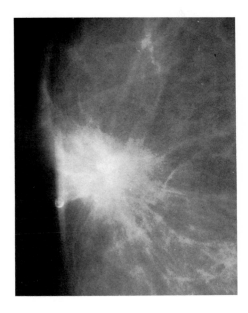

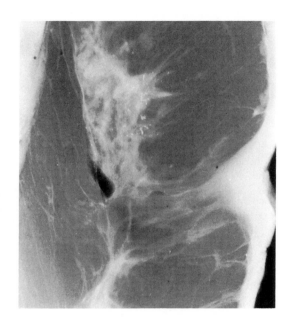

Figure 20–13. Paget's disease. A 68-year-old woman with mild nipple retraction, otherwise normal breasts clinically. Mammography: (not shown) 9 × 13 mm area of stippled calcifications of comedocarcinoma type and increased density just above the level of the nipple; a few flecks of calcification along the major ducts suggest Paget's disease of the fixed nipple. Whole-organ slicer radiograph: the mass is some distance from the major subareolar ducts, yet marked straightening of the ducts and nipple retraction is present. Pathology: intraductal and ductal carcinoma, intraductal carcinoma and comedocarcinoma, Paget's disease of the nipple. Modified radical mastectomy; 21 axillary lymph nodes free of tumor. Patient was alive and free of disease 12 years later.

Figure 20–14. Nonspecific subareolar lesion. A 31-year-old woman with scaling and crusting of the nipple, diffuse hardness about the areola; clinically Paget's disease. Mammography: asymmetric diffuse nonspecific changes in the subareolar area; carcinoma vs subareolar fibrosis. Pathology: intense nonspecific chronic inflammatory cell reaction, pseudoepitheliomatous hyperplasia and focal ulceration; no malignancy.

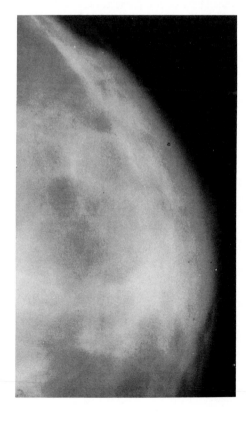

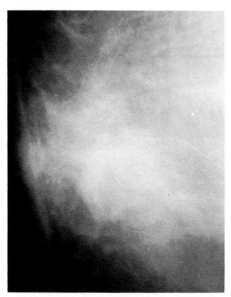

Figure 20–15. Subareolar fibrosis vs carcinoma. A 42-year-old woman with nipple discharge, fullness and heaviness under the areola, poor response to hot soaks. Nonspecific clinical findings. Mammography: masslike density with nonspecific secondary changes; favor carcinoma over subareolar fibrosis or abscess. Pathology: diffuse subareolar chronic inflammatory reaction, probably related to a chronic abscess; no carcinoma (compare Fig. 20–22).

straightening of the normal curvilinear course of the ducts is abnormal. Some degree of dilatation of the major ducts is always present. Both may occur simultaneously (Fig. 20–16). A tortuous, beaded, wormy appear-

ance of the dilated ducts is clearly seen when there is minimal periductal fibrosis (Fig. 20–17). The dilatation may be localized in some ducts (Fig. 20–18). Simple cysts are merely local dilatations of the ducts, but the local dilatation of a major subareolar duct may have a different etiology. The lesion in Figure 20–19 was a local collection of grumous material from the ruptured major duct that had been walled-off as a discrete lesion.

ASSOCIATED WITH SUBAREOLAR FIBROSIS

One of the most difficult mammographic exercises is the differentiation of subareolar carcinoma and fibrosis. The frequency and importance of this benign entity mammographically deserves greater emphasis. At times the best appraisal may end with a 50-50 chance of carcinoma. A subareolar carcinoma may be unilateral, bilateral, or in an area of subareolar fibrosis (Fig. 20–20). Clinical information and complementary studies usually produce further confusion (Fig. 20–21). If a dominant area in the subareolar density is demonstrated by mammography, this must be viewed with great concern and localized for surgical removal and histopathologic studies (Fig. 20–22).

Early subareolar carcinomas are amenable to treatment and good prognosis, just like

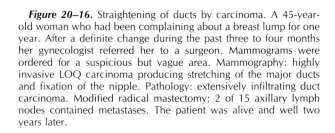

Figure 20–16. Straightening of ducts by carcinoma. A 45-year-old woman who had been complaining about a breast lump for one year. After a definite change during the past three to four months her gynecologist referred her to a surgeon. Mammograms were ordered for a suspicious but vague area. Mammography: highly invasive LOQ carcinoma producing stretching of the major ducts and fixation of the nipple. Pathology: extensively infiltrating duct carcinoma. Modified radical mastectomy; 2 of 15 axillary lymph nodes contained metastases. The patient was alive and well two years later.

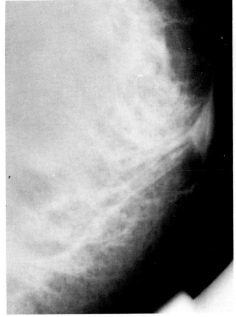

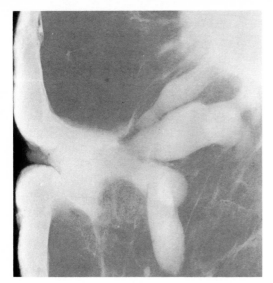

Figure 20–17. Duct ectasia. A 57-year-old woman (professor's wife) with a breast lump known only to her for over two years. Clinically an advanced cancer with palpable lymphadenopathy. There were satellite nodules around the primary focus of a scirrhous carcinoma and distant sites of duct carcinoma, also desmoplastic. The radiograph of the whole-organ slicer section of the radical mastectomy shows the individual dilated major duct without periductal reaction. Axillary lymph nodes at all levels contained metastases. Death occurred from widespread metastases two and one-half years later.

Figure 20–18. Duct ectasia. A 64-year-old woman studied for a Stage I duct carcinoma of the breast. The whole-organ slicer radiograph shows two ducts bluntly dilated with a third one longer (no carcinoma in this section). Clinically this area was difficult to evaluate.

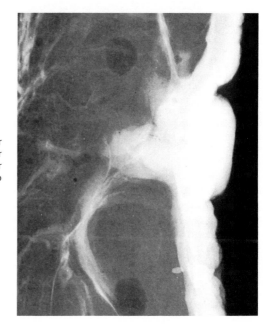

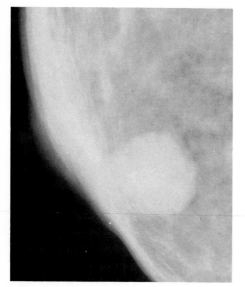

Figure 20–19. Ruptured ectatic duct. A 58-year-old woman with pain under her nipple for several weeks. Clinically: thickening under areola. Mammography: sebaceous cyst vs dilated duct. The pain subsided with conservative treatment, but the lesion was removed for verification of a benign etiology.

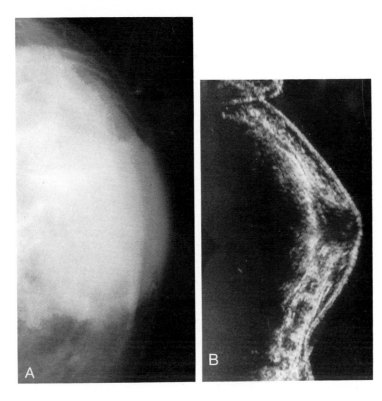

Figure 20–20. A 63-year-old woman with a clinical subareolar fibrosis. *A,* Mammography: 1.5 cm scirrhous carcinoma containing calcifications in lower border of dense subareolar fibrosis. Note fold of retracted skin. *B,* Sonography: Irregular area of marked subareolar attenuation consistent with fibrosis. Pathology: 7 × 9 mm invasive duct carcinoma with marked desmoplasia, subareolar fibrosis. The small carcinoma could not be separated from fibrosis on sonography and its size was poorly judged by x-ray. Modified radical mastectomy; 1 of 24 axillary lymph nodes contained tumor. The patient was alive and well 29 months later.

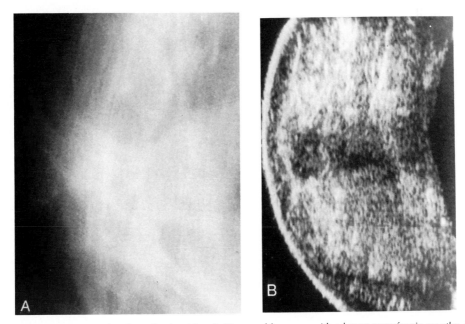

Figure 20–21. Sonography with subareolar densities. A 63-year-old woman with a breast mass for six months. Clinically: a 2 cm subareolar carcinoma. Mammography: poorly outlined density in the subareolar area that is more likely to be subareolar fibrosis than carcinoma. Sonography: intense alteration of the sonar beam; large irregular area of distortion and attenuation. Significance not clear. Pathology: chronic inflammatory changes.

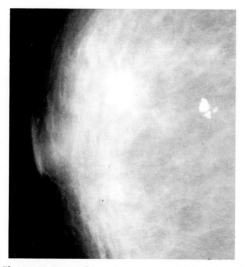

Figure 20–22. Inflammatory vs neoplastic subareolar changes. A 73-year-old woman studied for large clinically fatty breasts. Mammography: fatty ductal hyperplasia with increased density and a 5 mm mass in the right subareolar area; carcinoma is favored over inflammatory etiology. Pathology: 5 mm duct carcinoma, duct ectasia, papillomatosis. Modified radical mastectomy; all 19 axillary lymph nodes free of tumor. The patient was alive and well two years later (compare Fig. 20–15).

carcinomas in other portions of the breast. "Central" breast carcinomas have historically been associated with a poor prognosis owing to the greater likelihood of internal mammary lymph node metastases (compared with upper outer quadrant lesions). This possibility can be largely reduced by a vigorous diagnostic approach.

ASSOCIATED WITH CALCIFICATIONS

The differential diagnosis of calcifications in the subareolar area is similar to that of subareolar fibrosis. Most of the benign calcifications result from intraductal detritus, but with advanced changes of plasma cell mastitis the calcifications are also beyond the ducts as a result of chemical or foreign body reaction. The uncountable fine calcifications of malignant processes within the ducts usually pose no problem. As always, it is the intermediate or borderline types that present uncertainties. Again, those of a suspicious nature must be localized, removed, and studied by light microscopy.

CASE HISTORY

Subareolar carcinoma presents problems in a young woman.

Mrs. G. B. is a 30-year-old woman and mother of three children; all pregnancies and deliveries were normal, the last occurring at age 27 years. She nursed the last two children for six months each. She had noted intermittent nodules in her breast described as "milk ducts" by her obstetrician-gynecologist. She noted a persistent one, different to her, just under the lower edge of the left areola. She was not sure how long it had been there, but for one whole year she had called her physician's attention to it. During this period of observation he assured her, "fibrocystic disease, don't worry." When she called his attention to the nipple retracting, he referred her to a surgeon. Mammography was obtained (Fig. 20–23).

This case illustrates the disasters that befall many young women who are unfortunate enough to harbor an elusive subareolar cancer, the severity of subareolar cancer before it attracts the attention of a physician, and the resultant poor prognosis once the lesion has invaded the nipple and areola.

CASE HISTORY

Bloody nipple discharge leads to detection of breast cancer.

Mrs. G. T. presented with a history of a bloody nipple discharge for one month. She was a 74-year-old woman with no family history of breast cancer. The bleeding started spontaneously, was intermit-

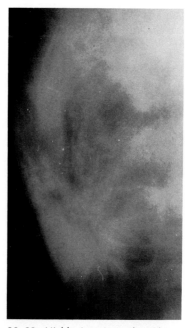

Figure 20–23. Highly invasive subareolar carcinoma. Clinically: suspicious mass with nipple retraction. Mammography: highly invasive 9 × 11 mm carcinoma extending into the skin of the areola. Sonography confirmed the presence of cancer. Pathology: scirrhous duct carcinoma. Radical mastectomy; lymph node metastases at all levels. Despite chemotherapy, distant metastases appeared within two years.

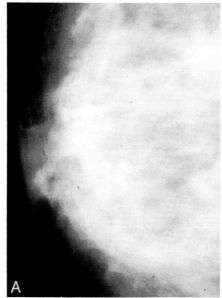
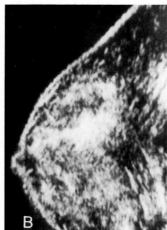

Figure 20–24. Bleeding papilloma and nearby carcinoma. Clinically a single-duct bloody discharge. A, Mammography: density and distorted architecture above the nipple; moderate subareolar fibrosis. b, Sonography: single dilated major duct. Resection: intraductal papilloma; nearby 6 mm duct carcinoma. Modified radical mastectomy; no additional tumor; all 21 axillary lymph nodes free of tumor. The patient was free of disease five years later.

tent, and could be initiated by pressing the tissues below the nipple between her thumb and forefinger. It was staining her brassieres and bedclothes. Clinically this was a single-duct bloody nipple discharge. Mammography and sonography were obtained (Fig. 20–24).

It has been our experience that often bloody nipple discharge is of a benign nature. However, we welcome it as a means of obtaining mammograms on women in the breast cancer age range.

OBSERVATIONS

Wrestling with this subareolar problem for 30 years has produced no easy solutions. The only prudent approach is the use of high-quality mammograms bolstered with a strong suspicion of pathology and keen observation.

The team approach, with close cooperative efforts, will minimize delays and errors. The clinician may be alerted to the presence of inflammation or to its absence. The radiologist may recognize cancer calcifications or the growth pattern of a malignant mass. In the final evaluation the pathologist can be productive only when he is apprised of the whole clinical picture.

Nipple discharge is an important clinical entity (Leis et al., 1985), being the chief complaint of 7.4 per cent of 7588 patients undergoing breast surgery. Most nipple discharges are due to benign disorders. But of 503 patients with watery, serous, serosanguineous, and sanguineous discharges, 13.3 per cent had cancer, 7.2 per cent had precancerous lesions, and 11.9 per cent had mild to moderate atypical changes. The surgeon looks to the radiologist for as much help as possible with these discharges, since surgical exploration is mandatory even if there is no palpable mass or any abnormal cytologic change.

REFERENCE

Leis HP Jr, Cammarata A, LaRaja RD (1985): Nipple discharge: Significance and treatment. Breast, Diseases of the Breast (April–June)11:6.

Peripheral Breast Carcinoma

21

BACKGROUND

The extent of the mammary tissues on the chest wall is highly variable. In most women it is confined to the eminent portion of the breast. In others it may extend across the midline at the sternum, to the clavicle or into the axilla above, into the inframammary crease below, and beyond the posterior axillary line laterally. No simple single mammographic projection includes all these anatomic areas, and, in fact, some areas cannot be projected onto the mammogram. Fortunately, when the breast extends beyond the usual boundaries, it is in a thin sheet and is readily palpable except when high into the axilla. The bandlike, irregularly compressed tissues at the inframammary crease interfere with palpation. Aberrant breast tissue or supernumerary breasts pose additional problems.

One of the first radiologists to be instructed in mammography noted that his first lesson was to study carefully all edges of the mammogram. These "edges" may show only a single straightened trabecula, a suggestion of a rim of a mass, or some density of altered architecture. These are red flags indicating the necessity to proceed with supplementary views.

Thus, breast cancers in the extreme periph-eral portions of the breast present such special problems in imaging, diagnosis, evaluation, and treatment that particular attention to these lesions is mandatory. Fortunately, breast cancers in such locations are unusual, as there is a paucity of breast tissue to harbor the lesion. The experience of any one oncologic surgeon is limited; the pattern of spread of the disease is inconsistent. At treatment planning sessions I have been impressed with the great concern of the surgeon about the difficulty of en bloc resection, complete removal, and primary closure. Thus, the frequent unavoidable morbidity and the high mortality rate make these peripheral cancers a challenge to the team of diagnostic radiologist, oncologic surgeon, therapeutic radiologist, and chemotherapist.

CHEST WALL

The mediolateral and oblique mammographic views were so designed that the central x-ray beam traversed the retromammary space at the chest wall to project the maximum breast tissue onto the receptor. Inclusion of a part of the chest wall assured study of the base of the breast. Even this arrangement did not project all of the base of the breast beyond the convex rib cage. With the introduction of rigid cassettes for screen-film receptors and xeroradiography it became impossible to include the chest wall while maintaining a short object-receptor distance. Angulation, special compression, and tugging on the breast often were required (Fig. 21–1). Sometimes surprises may be in store if the deep portion of the breast is studied. In this breast in an attempt to image a partially seen large carcinoma (Fig. 21–2), two more separate lesions were demonstrated.

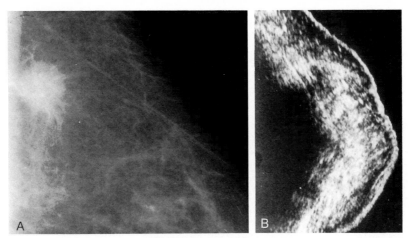

Figure 21–1. Deep carcinoma requiring special positioning maneuver and spot view to demonstrate. A 72-year-old woman seen for baseline study for follow-up of right mastectomy in 1963. Clinically: normal breast without evidence of recurrent disease. *A,* Mammography: Routine views showed a suggestion of stranding high supposedly at the chest wall. Pulling the breast, angulation of the beam and spot views demonstrated a 9 × 10 mm moderately invasive carcinoma, a second primary lesion. *B,* Sonography: irregular hypoechoic area, on pectoral muscles, attenuation, distant skin flattening. Pathology: duct carcinoma, Grade III. Modified radical mastectomy; 0 of 11 nodes positive. The patient was alive and well three years after second primary.

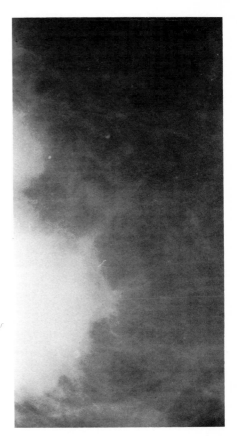

Figure 21–2. Three separate carcinomas. A 54-year-old woman with a lump. Clinically: breast mass with axillary metastases. Mammography: large fatty breasts, at least three separate foci of carcinoma (all against chest wall) measuring 4 × 3 cm, 1.3 × 1.5 cm, and approximately 5 mm (calcifications) in size; increased vascularity. The largest is coarsely spiculated and more invasive. Pathology: duct and comedo carcinoma. Radical mastectomy; at least five sites of infiltrative duct and comedo carcinomas with widespread foci of intraductal and intraductal comedo carcinoma; 8 of 27 axillary lymph nodes of all levels with tumor. Distant metastases appeared before completion of radiotherapy.

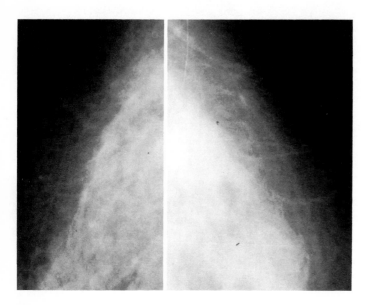

Figure 21–3. Deep, high chest wall carcinoma. A 67-year-old woman with a breast lump for less than seven days; mother and mother's sister had breast cancer. Mammography: 1.3 × 1.8 cm moderately invasive carcinoma deep in the UIQ of the left breast; increased vascularity. Pathology: duct carcinoma with fibrosis. Modified radical mastectomy; all 14 axillary lymph nodes free of tumor. The patient was alive and well six years later.

Figure 21–4. Carcinoma high in medial quadrant of the breast. This 63-year-old old woman presented with this near-ulcerating lesion of the left breast. It had been considered a "boil not related to the breast" by her family physician and treated with hot soaks for an indefinite time. Clinically: fixed lesion, bilobed, axillary lymph nodes producing bulging of the axilla. Mammography (not shown): some overall increase in density of the left breast; mass only vaguely suspected; poorly projected. Pathology (incision biopsy): duct cell carcinoma. Widespread metastases before completion of radiotherapy.

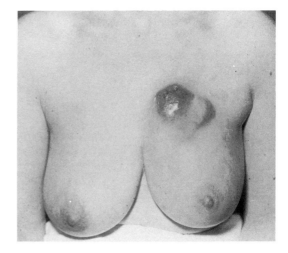

HIGH DEEP

A variation of the chest wall carcinoma is a similarly deep one high in the upper quadrant of the breast (Fig. 21–3). These lesions may be so deep that they are not easily detected by the woman herself. Despite the aggressive nature of the illustrated tumor, its excitation of distant glandular response, its increased vascularity, and its proximity to the axillary lymph nodes, it was still a Stage I lesion histologically. The high, deep carcinoma in the inner quadrant is one of the most difficult to project onto the film (Fig. 21–4).

TAIL OF THE BREAST

Often the axilla is more easily studied than the chest wall, as there may be considerable fat in the axilla and the receptor can readily be placed behind the lesion (Fig. 21–5). But

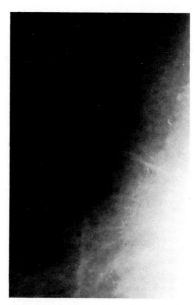

Figure 21–6. Carcinoma high and deep in the tail of the breast. A 54-year-old woman with a suspicious breast mass for three weeks. Mammography: approximately 1.4 cm highly invasive spiculated carcinoma. Routine views were not sufficient, but a special spot view (above), was required for demonstration; the technologist could feel the mass. Pathology: duct carcinoma with fibrosis. Modified radical mastectomy, 2 low of 19 axillary lymph nodes contained metastases; five years later no evidence of disease.

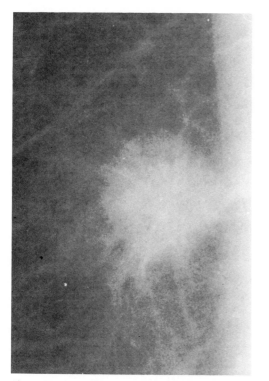

Figure 21–5. Small cancer high in the tail of the breast. A 52-year-old woman with a clinically suspicious mass high in a pendulous breast. Routine mammography was unrewarding. Spot-view radiograph of the area: This is an enlargement of a portion of a coned-down spot view demonstrating a 1 cm spiculated lesion near the chest wall. Fibroglandular tissue extends even deeper. This acrobatic accomplishment required tube angulation, rotation of the patient, and vigorous pulling of the breast from the chest wall. Some deep lesions defy demonstration with screen-film receptors.

the lesion may also be deep in the axilla and only the anterior portion of the tumor studied (Fig. 21–6). A vigorous technologist (on a stoic patient) may visualize a carcinoma in the tail of the breast on the craniocaudad projection (Fig. 21–7). By properly positioning the patient the axilla can readily be studied by sonography (Fig. 21–8).

INFRAMAMMARY CREASE

The weight of a pendulous breast, irritation from a brassiere, and poor ventilation produce poorly assessed palpable changes at the inframammary crease. On mammography there is actual thickening of a 1 cm band of skin in this area as well as disorganization of the supporting structures (Fig. 21–9). Radiography of this portion of the breast may be difficult (Fig. 21–10). One of the important considerations in treatment of a carcinoma in this area is complete resection of the tumor and the possibility that skin grafting will be required. In both cases (Figs. 21–11 and 21–12), it is clearly seen that the tumors are readily resectable. In Figure 21–13 there is

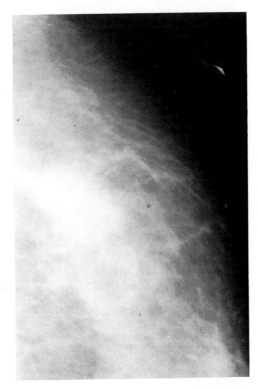

Figure 21–7. Exaggerated craniocaudad view to show tail of breast lesion. This nonpalpable 7 × 8 mm lesion in a 54-year-old woman seen for baseline studies required localization for removal. Maximal rotation of the patient, posterior compression, and pulling of the breast forward was necesary for this coned-down spot view of the lesion. Such "heroics" are often necessary to bring Stage 0 or Stage I breast carcinoma to treatment. This is especially true for high leisons; their tendency to early metastasis to the axillary lymph nodes demands earlier detection.

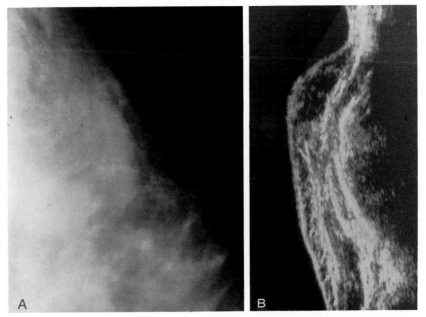

Figure 21–8. Carcinoma in the tail of the breast. A 39-year-old woman with a mass in the tail of the breast, by needle biopsy infiltrating duct carcinoma. A, Mammography: 3 × 3.3 cm moderately invasive carcioma high in the tail of the breast. B, Sonography: irregular, poorly demarcated tumor with jagged borders, nonhomogeneous internal echoes, resting on the pectoral muscles with bulging of the skin. Despite the needle biopsy one week before the examination it was decided that the process was truly an inflammatory (inoperable) carcinoma. Following radiation and chemotherapy, distant metastases occurred within a year after diagnosis.

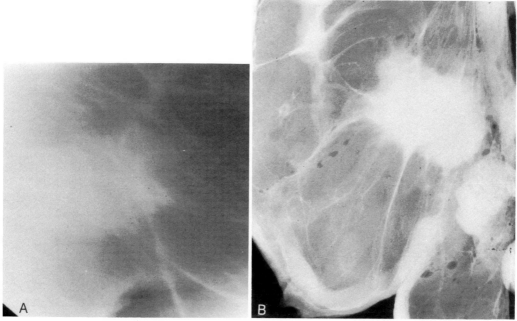

Figure 21–9. Carcinoma at the inframammary crease. A 72-year-old woman with a suspicious breast mass at the inframammary crease. The spot mammogram shows the lesion to be resectable even though the margins of the tumor extend almost to the pectoral muscle. *A*, On spot-view mammogram, a 1 × 1.6 cm coarsely spiculated mass. *B*, Whole-organ slicer section. Pathology: duct carcinoma, scirrhous type. Radical mastectomy; 4 low of 22 axillary lymph nodes contained tumor and three separate sites of duct carcinoma were present. Death from widespread disease eight months later.

Figure 21–10. Carcinoma at the inframammary crease. A 63-year-old woman with a small breast lump UOQ. Clinically: Changes at 6 o'clock position are highly suspicious. Mammography: 1.5 × 2 cm highly invasive carcinoma at the inframammary crease with stippled calcification and increased vascularity. The large sagging breast made examination difficult owing to overlapping of structures, but the chest wall and inferior breast skin are judged to be of normal thickness; operable. Pathology: duct carcinoma with productive fibrosis. Modified radical mastectomy; 4 of 21 low and midaxillary lymph nodes contained tumor. Liver metastases within six months.

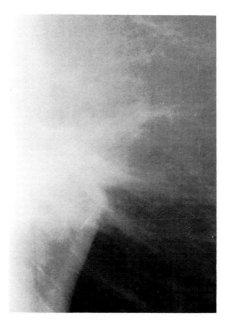

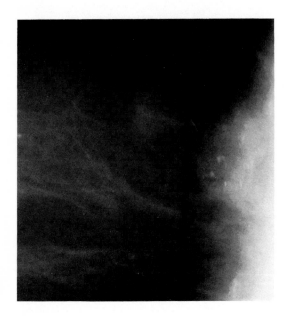

Figure 21–11. Carcinoma at the inframammary crease. A 69-year-old woman with a suspicious mass at the 6 o'clock position. Mammography: 1.5 cm highly invasive carcinoma containing calcifications at the inframammary crease and an 8 mm moderately invasive carcinoma anterior to this tumor. Pathology: 2 cm and 1 cm infiltrating duct carcinomas, scirrhous type. Modified radical mastectomy; 2 low of 19 axillary lymph nodes with metastases. Death two years later with disease.

Figure 21–12. Circumscribed carcinoma at the inframammary crease. A 54-year-old woman had problems with her brassiere inferiorly. Clinically: a carcinoma. Mammogrpahy: well-localized 2.7 × 3.6 cm carcinoma; the retromammary space and overlying skin clear of tumor (usual skin thickening at the chest wall). Modified radical mastectomy was uneventful for this medullary carcinoma with lymphoid stroma without axillary metastases. The patient was free of disease five years later.

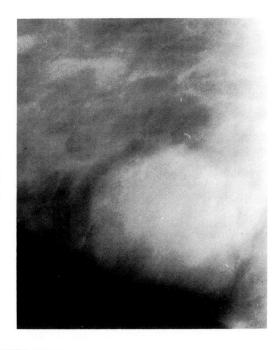

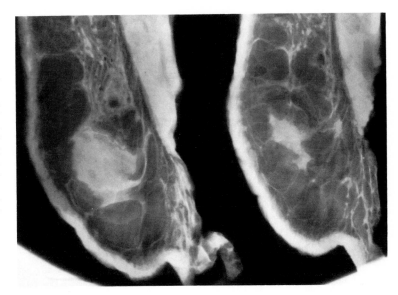

Figure 21–13. Carcinoma at the inframammary crease. A 55-year-old woman with a breast mass that was clearly resectable on mammography and the whole-organ slicer radiography. Despite a radical mastectomy and all axillary lymph nodes being free of metastases, she died 18 months later from widespread metastases. Pathology: 1.3 × 1.5 cm duct carcinoma with mild desmoplasia; all 22 axillary lymph nodes free of tumor.

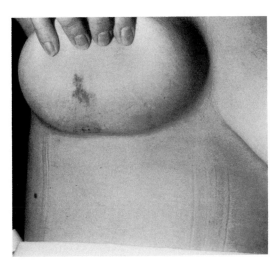

Figure 21–14. Large clinically obvious carcinoma, infraclavicular in location. A 67-year-old woman with a slowly growing breast "sore" for six months or a year. Clinically the lesion was near ulceration and was not fixed to the chest wall. Mammography was not attempted owing to the difficulty in projecting it onto the receptor. Axillary lymph node metastasis was producing the fullness in the axilla. This duct carcinoma was not resectable at surgery; internal mammary lymph node metastasis was suspected. Despite radiotherapy of the chest wall and regional node-bearing areas after the radical mastectomy, she died of disease two years later. Small lesions in this area must be detected clinically and usually are, with breast tissue being easily palpable. Mammography in the extreme periphery of the breast is most difficult.

another relatively small carcinoma at the inframammary crease, radiographically even more readily resectable.

OBSERVATIONS

Radiologists recognized the problems of projecting deep-seated breast lesions against the chest wall onto the film, even when pliable nonscreen systems snugly followed the contour of the chest wall on the mediolateral view. With the advent of rigid cassettes for xeroradiography and screen-film receptors, the problem became greater, and led to reports in the literature. The oblique, or Cleopatra, view was resurrected, along with more tugging on the breast, in an attempt to offset this deficiency. The problem remains.

Prognosis of cancers in most of the locations described is poor. This relates to (1) advanced stage of disease when detected, (2) lack of experience in treating the lesions, (3) inconsistent spread of the malignancy, and (4) surgical problems of en bloc resection and primary closure (Fig. 21–14).

In our experience with carcinoma at the inframammary crease we have seen no long-term survival with duct carcinoma regardless of the size, the stage, or the apparent radiologic resectability of the carcinoma. We have presented one case of medullary carcinoma with lymphoid stroma in this location that had an improved prognosis. No reports for comparison have been encountered in the literature.

Intracystic Papillary Carcinoma

22

BACKGROUND

With the advent of mammography and the ability to recognize intracystic papillary lesions of the breast, it has become helpful to specify a distinct clinical entity, intracystic papillary carcinoma. The diagnosis and treatment planning then can be individualized for the woman with this unusual neoplasm. Papillary lesions of the breast include epithelial hyperplasia, single and multiple intraductal papillomata, intracystic papilloma, intracystic carcinoma, and papillary carcinoma. Of these lesions, the intracystic papillary ones are the least uniformly categorized and treated.

As recorded by Geschickter (1945), "carcinomatous intracystic growths" were of considerable interest to Velpeau (1856), Bryand (1887), Selling (1898), Hart (1927), and Ewing (1935). Both the solid and the cystic forms of papillary growths were usually regarded as Grade I cancer by these workers. Geschickter (1945) exemplified the confusion and lack of

confidence in differential diagnosis when he treated 110 benign intracystic papillomata by excision (with six recurrences), 46 additional ones with simple mastectomy, and 47 with radical mastectomy. In 197 intracystic growths considered malignant he used similar diverse treatments, with 36 recurrences. In the benign lesions the average age was 55 years, and 48 per cent had nipple discharge. The malignant variety had 19 per cent nipple discharge and occurred equally in each decade from age 30 to age 70 years.

Intracystic papillary carcinomas have also been combined with all types of papillary carcinomas with disregard for the predominantly cystic characteristic of the papillary intracystic lesions. Haagensen (1986), in his series of 1420 breast cancers, noted that 18 of 130 papillary carcinomas were intracystic. With 30 of the papillary carcinomas there was blood-tinged discharge. Of 64 patients with these papillary carcinomas who were subject to ten-year follow-up, 47 had a radical mastectomy, 5 had simple mastectomy, and 12 had local excision; there were 10 recurrences. The women with papillary carcinomas had 70 per cent ten-year survival.

Review of our cases of intracystic papillary carcinomas, many studied in detail with long-term follow-up, enables a better understanding of these uncommon tumors. Given their tendency to multiplicity and bilaterality and the difficulty in differentiating benign and malignant forms histologically on frozen section, any aid in diagnosis and treatment planning should be explored.

INCIDENCE

At Emory University, of 2209 primary operable breast cancers with up to 20 years' follow-up having clinical, radiographic, and pathologic studies, 19 were intracystic papillary lesions (Table 22–1). This was only 0.9

TABLE 22–1. Intracystic Papillary Lesions With Clinical Features, Histology, Treatment, and Follow-up

Case No.	Age (Years)	Family History	Use of Hormones	Complaint	Length of Complaint	Size of Lesion	Stage	Treatment	Years Follow-up	Status	Comments
1	55	none	none	mass	5 weeks	2 × 3 cm	1	simple mast.	16	living, N.E.D.	multiple foci
2	59	"	"	"	6 months	5 × 9 cm	2	"	2	dead, disease	single focus
3	66	"	"	"	3 weeks	1.5 cm; 2.5 cm	1	rad. mast.	12	living, N.E.D.	multiple foci
4	67	"	"	"	3 months	2.5 cm; 2.5 cm; 2 cm	2	"	5	dead, N.E.D.	" "
5	75	2 sisters	"	"	6 months	1 to 5 cm	1	mod. rad. mast.	4	dead, disease	" "
6	75	none	men. 1 year	"	12 months	1.5 × 1.7 cm	0	" " "	11	living, N.E.D.	simult. primaries, opposite duct cell
7	79	1 sister	men. 6 months	"	5 weeks	2.5 × 3 cm	0	" " "	8	dead, N.E.D.	single focus
8	45	1 aunt	men. 3 months	"	3 weeks	1.2 × 1 cm	1	" " "	1	living, N.E.D.	
9	60	1 aunt	none	"	4 weeks	0.6 × 0.8 cm	0	aspiration, excision; later mod. rad. mast.	1	living, N.E.D.	multiple foci
10	60	"	"	"	1 year	1; 3 × 4 cm	0	rad. mast.	11	living, N.E.D.	also 1 cm scirrhous cancer
11	71	2 sisters	men. 1 year	"	3 weeks	2 × 2 cm	bn.	excision	3	"	no malignant cells
12	74	none	none	"	1 year	0.5 cm; 1.5 × 2 cm	1	rad. mast.	0	no follow-up	2 separate, invasive
13	77	"	"	"	2½ years	1.2 cm; 1.5 cm; 2 cm	1	rad. mast.	10	living, N.E.D.	multiple foci
14	78	"	"	"	4 days	3 × 4 cm	0	simple mast.	3	dead, N.E.D.	single focus,
15	78	"	"	"	3 months	4 × 5 cm; 2 cm	0,1	mod. rad. mast.	2	living, N.E.D.	2 areas lobular in situ
16	83	"	"	"	3 years	1 to 4 cm	0	aspiration, observation	3	living, disease	multiple foci, bilateral
17	83	1 sister	"	"	15 years	12 × 13 cm	bn.	aspiration, simple mast.	2 mo.	living, N.E.D.	no malignant cells
18	85	none	"	"	5 years	5.5 × 7 cm	bn.	aspiration, observation	5	living, disease	no malignant cells
19	91	"	"	"	5 days	2 × 2 cm	0	biopsy	1	living, N.E.D.	single lesion

Men. = menopausal; mod. = modified; rad. = radical; bn. = benign.
Cases 1–6 had whole-organ studies; staged on basis of axillary lymph nodes.

per cent of the total cancers. Four of these had correlated clinical-radiographic-pathologic whole-organ studies, subject to 14 to 18 years' follow-up.

CLINICAL FEATURES

The age range was 45 to 84 years (median age 62.4 years); gross size of the intracystic papillary carcinomas by x-ray was 1 to 13 cm in diameter; and knowledge of the presence of a mass in each case ranged from 5 days to 15 years. None had nipple discharge. Two thirds of the lesions were multiple; one was centrally located (filling the whole breast); and the others were in the upper outer quadrant or diffusely located in the breast. One woman had bilateral simultaneous multiple foci, and one lesion occurred as a simultaneous primary lesion opposite a duct carcinoma. Ten tumors occurred in fatty breasts, four with ductal hyperplasia, one in a glandular breast, and four in coarsely nodular breasts.

RADIOGRAPHIC FEATURES

On mammography the noninfiltrating intracystic papillary lesions present as well-circumscribed round, oval, bilobed, or lobulated dense masses, usually in physiologically older breasts (Figs. 22–1 and 22–2). Once an area of infiltration about the periphery is apparent on the mammogram, the lesion appears as a duct carcinoma (Fig. 22–2 D–F). Prognosis is closely related to invasiveness and stage of disease (Figs. 22–3 and 22–4). Sonography produces a complex mass (Fig. 22–5).

Even though microscopically the malignant cells are confined to the inner border of the hemorrhagic cyst, the irregular changes external to the cyst wall in the nearby tissue will indicate to the radiologist the likelihood of carcinoma (Figs. 22–1B and 22–3). Apparently this is a tissue reaction to the presence of carcinoma within the cyst, less marked than with an actual invasion that produces a spiculated mass outside the cyst, often with punctate calcifications (Fig. 22–2C). The periphery of the cyst is easily studied, as the lesion often occurs against a background of fatty tissue in older women.

Myriad extremely fine calcifications (Fig. 22–2A) in the cancerous mass are typical but are obscured on the mammogram by the dense blood in the cyst. Upon invasion, the usual various-sized, coarser type of calcifications of an infiltrating duct carcinoma are

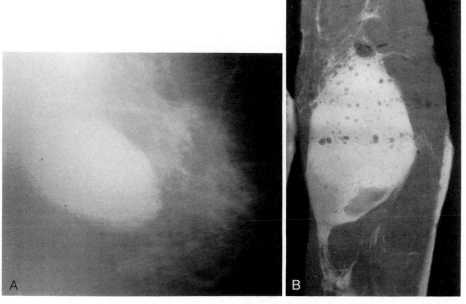

Figure 22–1. A 79-year-old woman with breast mass for "five weeks," 38 years post menopause; one sister and one aunt with breast cancer. Clinically a 5 × 10 cm cyst, probably benign. On x-ray (A) and slicer section (B) a 2.5 × 3 cm intracystic papillary carcinoma. Histologically a single focus of intracystic papillary carcinoma, noninvasive. Modified radical mastectomy; 19 lymph nodes negative. The patient lived without disease for over eight years before dying of a stroke (Case 7, Table 22–1.) Dark areas are air pockets in thawing blood.

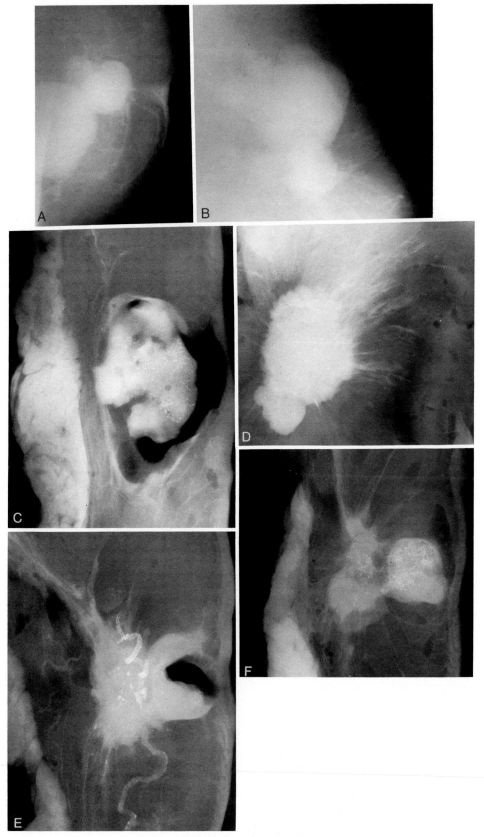

Figure 22–2 See legend on opposite page

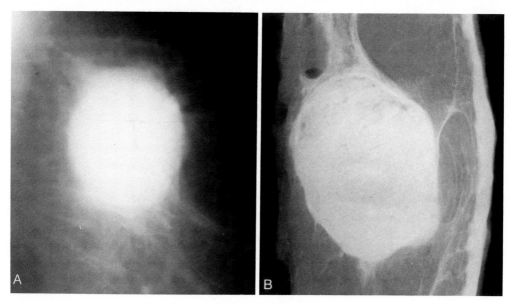

Figure 22–3. One intracystic papillary carcinoma as part of bilateral simultaneous carcinomas. A 75-year-old woman with mass in left breast for 12 months. No family history of breast cancer, five children, nursed 50 months, menopausal hormones. Mammograms (*A*) and slicer radiograph (*B*) showed a well-circumscribed mass, left breast, most likely an intracystic papillary carcinoma (based on density and protuberance); 1.6 cm moderately invasive primary carcinoma on right (not shown). Pathology: bilateral primary tumors: intracystic papillary carcinoma with peripheral infiltration in left breast and intraductal and invasive duct carcinoma in right breast. No axillary lymph node metastasis. Bilateral modified radical mastectomy; the patient is living without disease for over 11 years. The slicer section is through the intracystic papillary lesion while still partially frozen; nearby fluid in small cysts has melted. (Case 6, Table 22–1.)

produced (Fig. 22–2*C*). Histologically the infiltrative lesion (Fig. 22–2*B*) could be distinguished as an infiltrating duct carcinoma without any elements of an intracystic papillary carcinoma. A nearby focus of intraductal carcinoma was also noted in this case.

PATHOLOGY

Histologically the benign intracystic papillary lesion is characterized by a well-developed fibrovascular stroma in its fronds, whereas the stroma associated with an intracystic papillary carcinoma is scantier and is often absent in some areas (Fig. 22–6). As in other papillary lesions of the breast, the most reliable histologic criterion for distinguishing intracystic papillary carcinoma from papilloma is the demonstration of two cell types,

epithelial and myoepithelial, in the benign lesions.

Needle aspiration of the intracystic lesions reveals blood, but cytologic examination of the aspirate does not provide a reliable differentiation, as the epithelium aspirated may be scanty and not cytologically diagnostic of malignancy.

Histopathologic evaluation may often be complicated by a large volume of tissue available for study. Much of this tissue may be necrotic, with only small areas showing diagnostic features of malignancy. Since a limited part of the periphery can be studied microscopically, care may be required in sampling the proper tissue. Mammography and radiography of the specimen may be helpful in pinpointing the most productive area. These lesions can recur if not completely removed, and a second biopsy may be ne-

Figure 22–2. Multiple and varied intracystic papillary carcinomas. A 75-year-old woman with a mass in her right breast for six months. Clinically: 5 × 8 cm firm mass. Two sisters with breast cancer. *A* and *B*, Typical appearance on x-ray. *C*, Slicer section with noninvasive intracystic papillary carcinoma: thick-walled cyst; irregular projections into the cyst; blood thawed and leaked out, leaving myriad fine calcifications. *D*, Similar lesion in same breast with very highly infiltrative element with the x-ray appearance of duct (scirrhous) carcinoma. *E*, Note different types of calcifications in another lesion near the skin showing fine calcifications in the cyst but coarser ones in the infiltrative area. *F*, Two areas of intracystic lesions producing an invasive mass. Modified radical mastectomy; three nodes negative; the patient died after four years with extensive disease. (Case 5, Table 22–1.)

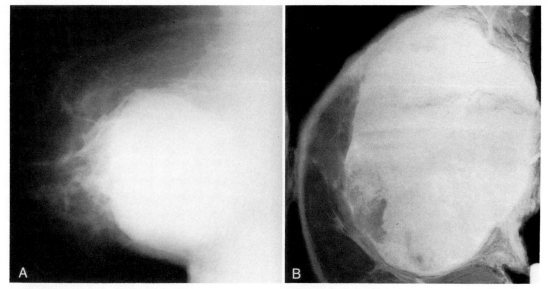

Figure 22–4. Advanced intracystic papillary carcinoma. A 59-year-old woman, mass in breast for six months; 22 years past surgical menopause; six children, nursed over 90 months. Clinically: a 10 cm circumscribed carcinoma. Mammograms: 5 × 9 cm intracystic papillary carcinoma, borders not sharp; local skin thickening; marked increase in vascularity; invasive. Slicer section: large circumscribed carcinoma. Pathology: intracystic papillary carcinoma with few areas of focal infiltration, most borders smooth. As large positive axillary nodes had already been demonstrated, the elected treatment was simple mastectomy plus postoperative irradiation. The patient died with disease in two years. (See Fig. 22–3 for comparative changes of a confined and infiltrative lesion.) (Case 2.)

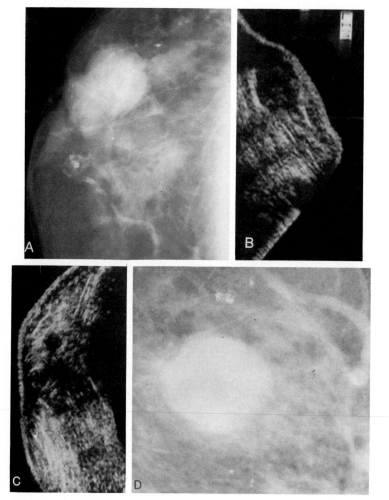

Figure 22–5. Bilateral intracystic papillary carcinomas. A 77-year-old woman with a large, firm right breast mass and onset of leg edema. Mammography: 3.5 × 4.5 cm on right (D) and 2 cm on left (A) dense masses suggesting intracystic papillary carcinomas. Sonography: rather well-demarcated, yet not sharp, borders; nonhomogeneous internal echoes; increased through-transmission (sonograms reversed for mirror image with mammogram). Pathology: intracystic papillary carcinomas, bilateral. Patient is living without disease despite intermittent cardiac decompensation.

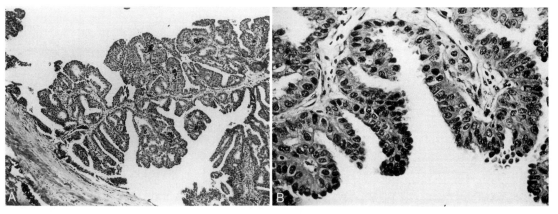

Figure 22–6. Intracystic papillary carcinoma. The delicate fibrovascular stroma is covered by a typical epithelium of one cell type. The absence of myoepithelium is essential for diagnosis. *A,* × 200, *B,* × 500.

cessitated by regrowth or, just as plausible, the appearance of an undetected carcinoma at the site of the previous excision. Since lesions are frequently multiple, with some of these small and poorly recognized, the cause of residual carcinoma on rebiopsy may be one of these smaller lesions having grown. With this surgical-histologic approach, wide excision is indicated so that the entire lesion and its periphery may be studied using a permanent histologic preparation.

RADIOGRAPHIC COURSE

Development

Intracystic papillary carcinoma begins as a papillary growth into the lumen of a duct or lobule, usually at a distance from the nipple. As it enlarges it blocks the duct with formation of a cyst. The intracystic papillary lesion is friable and bleeds easily, enlarging the cyst while the wall becomes progressively thicker. During this noninvasive stage nothing more than a discrete mass is evident on the mammograms. Such a mass is homogeneous. As it reaches 2 cm in diameter, enough hemosiderin has been concentrated from repeated hemorrhages that the cyst is characteristically very dense, unlike a cyst of fibrocystic disease, a fibroadenoma, or even a medullary carcinoma (Fig. 22–1). The lesions may be bilateral and usually are multicentric (Table 22–1). The characteristic fine, numerous calcifications are rarely seen by x-ray of the intact breast through dense blood in the cyst (Fig. 22–2A).

Differential Diagnosis

Intracystic Papilloma

The intracystic papilloma has a fibrovascular stalk, is most frequently located in a major subareolar duct (Figs. 22–7 and 22–8), infrequently produces a palpable mass, but produces a bloody discharge that may be diagnostic cytologically. Sonography does not differentiate the two lesions (Fig. 22–9). The historical controversy that is centered on the relationship of intraductal papilloma to carcinoma has been presented by Haagensen (1986). Available evidence supports his contention that these papillomata begin as benign lesions and remain so. This is especially true in reports after 1950, in which more careful clinical and pathologic descriptions permit a clearer classification. Excision suffices in treating the bleeding intracystic papilloma. The intracystic papillary carcinomas are usually located deeper in the breast and lack free communication with excretory ducts, but the papilloma may also be so located (Fig. 22–10).

Other Breast Cancers

The radiographic differentiation of intracystic papillary lesions is largely from circumscribed carcinomas (Figs. 22–11 and 22–12). The medullary carcinomas occur in younger women with more fibroglandular tissue; the mucin-producing carcinomas are less dense but occur in older women and stand out sharply against a fatty background; hemorrhage into a duct carcinoma to produce a cystic appearance in a portion of the periphery is rare. Pneumocystography can aid in

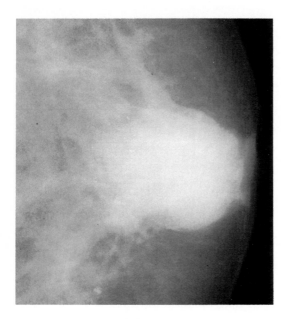

Figure 22–7. Intracystic papilloma. A 64-year-old woman with intermittent bloody nipple discharge. Clinically: dark bloody nipple discharge could be expressed from a single duct; poorly circumscribed subareolar mass, most likely carcinoma. Mammography: 2.5 × 3 cm circumscribed homogeneously dense mass attached to the nipple; location suggests papilloma vs dilated duct. Pathology: intracystic papilloma.

Figure 22–8. Intracystic papilloma. A 72-year-old woman with a 4 × 5 cm mass for six months; occasional bloody nipple discharge. Mammograms showed a very dense 4 × 4.5 cm homogeneous rounded lesion, smooth anteriorly but indistinct borders posteriorly; radiographically an intracystic papillary carcinoma. Note the proximity to the nipple. Pathology (excision biopsy): intracystic papilloma without evidence of carcinoma. The patient died eight years later without evidence of disease.

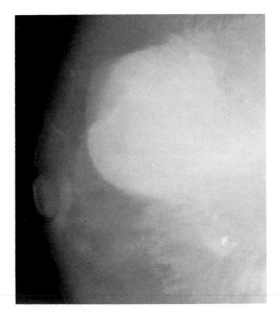

Figure 22–9. Intracystic papilloma. A 61-year-old woman with a breast lump and slight nipple inversion. *A,* Mammography: 1.5 × 1.8 cm circumscribed homogeneously dense mass, either intracystic papillary carcinoma or circumscribed carcinoma on a background of epithelial hyperplasia. *B,* Sonography: demarcated complex mass. Pathology (biopsy): benign papillary cystic lesion; rule out carcinoma. Mastectomy: region of mass, intraductal papillomata (probably one is the 5 mm lesion toward the nipple), epithelial hyperplasia, adenosis, microscopic cysts; UOQ, fibrosis, epithelial hyperplasia, adenosis; focal hyalinizing and calcified fibroadenoma, fibrocystic disease. No recurrence after two years.

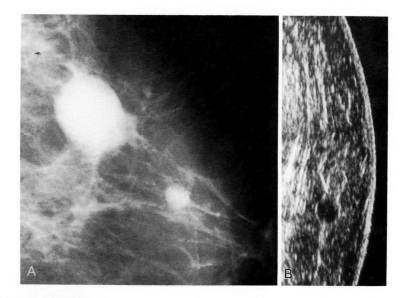

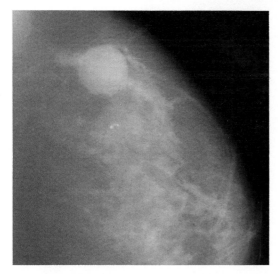

Figure 22–10. Intracystic papilloma at a distance from the nipple. A 71-year-old woman with a mass aspirated for bloody fluid; no malignant cells. Two sisters had breast cancer. Mammography: dense circumscribed mass (patient in the age group of intracystic papillary carcinoma). Pathology (excision biopsy): intracystic papilloma without evidence of malignancy. Patient last seen five years later for cerebrovascular accident; no breast pathology.

Figure 22–11. A 69-year-old woman with a breast mass for several months. Clinically: a firm mass with nipple retraction. Mammograms: a 5 × 7 cm and a 2.5 × 2 cm circumscribed mass, quite dense; probably intracystic papillary carcinoma. Modified radical mastectomy; 22 lymph nodes negative. Pathology: mucin-producing carcinoma. There are no distinguishing differential radiographic features; this is an unusually dense mucin-producing carcinoma.

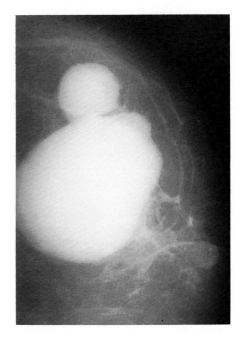

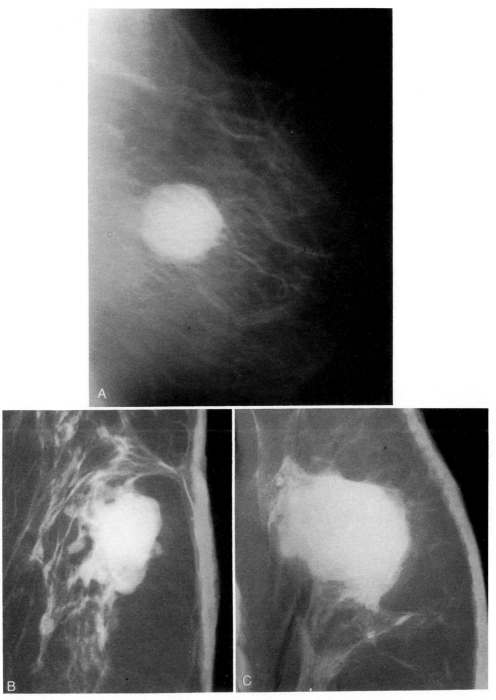

Figure 22–12. A 63-year-old woman, mass in breast for seven days, 25 years post surgical menopause. Clinically: 4 cm firm mass. *A–C,* Mammogram and radiographs of two slicer sections: 1.5 × 2.5 cm smooth-margined mass but overlying skin changes; circumscribed carcinoma. Pathology: medullary carcinoma; 19 axillary lymph nodes negative. Patient was living without disease 14 years. This mass is not nearly so dense as the intracystic lesions but has smooth borders in some areas.

establishing the presence of an intracystic lesion but not its benign or malignant character.

CLINICAL COURSE

Multiplicity

The occurrence of multiple intracystic papillary carcinomas in one breast is common (Fig. 22–13). In fact, local recurrence after excision of one malignant tumor may well represent the growth of a new mass to recognizable size. In Figure 22–2 there were at least seven distinct separate carcinomas identified on the whole-breast study. Even then, some of these masses may have been the coalescence of more than one separate primary lesion.

Bilaterality

The indolent growth of the intracystic papillary carcinoma in one breast may provide the opportunity for the frequent appearance of a similar lesion in the opposite breast. Bilaterality was a common occurrence (five cases) in our series and has been illustrated in a number of the cases included (Table 22–1).

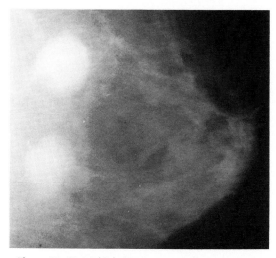

Figure 22–13. Multiple intracystic papillary carcinomas. A 79-year-old woman with a palpable mass in the UOQ of the breast. The opposite breast had been removed one and one-half years before for a Stage I duct carcinoma. Mammography: A 1.5 cm circumscribed homogeneously dense mass corresponding to the one palpable in the UOQ and a similar 1.2 cm lesion LIQ, nonpalpable. Pathology: intracystic papillary carcinomas. Modified radical mastectomy; all 19 axillary lymph nodes free of tumor. The patient died 11 years later free of breast carcinoma.

Occurrence With Other Cancers

Three of the five intracystic papillary carcinomas occurring as a single histologic type of cancer were infiltrating (Table 22–2), with two being noninfiltrating. Twelve of the lesions occurred with duct carcinoma, one with lobular carcinoma, and one with duct and lobular carcinoma. With a slow-growing tumor in the older woman, it is not surprising that intracystic papillary carcinoma occurs with other cancers in the same breast (Figs. 22–14 and 22–15) as well as in other cases demonstrated (Table 22–1). All these tumors having whole-organ studies were associated with foci of duct carcinoma in the same breast. One woman (not included in Table 22–2), three years after treatment for the first primary operable intracystic papillary carcinoma, returned with an inflammatory carcinoma of the opposite breast. It had a typical x-ray appearance of intracystic papillary carcinoma and an infiltrating carcinoma by needle biopsy. We have seen Paget's disease of the nipple and an intracystic papillary carcinoma in the same breast.

Treatment

Ten patients had radical mastectomy, five had modified radical mastectomy, three had total mastectomy, and one had a biopsy only. Study of permanent preparations of generous amounts of tissue does not always lead to the proper histologic diagnosis. Recurrence with histologically benign lesions and similar treatment for both benign and malignant types emphasize this difficulty.

In 5- to 14-year follow-up from the files of the Armed Forces Institute of Pathology, based on histologic characteristics and to a great extent on the clinical course, 4 of 17 malignant and 5 of 35 benign intracystic papillary lesions were misclassified (Kraus and Neubecker, 1962). After review of 48 intracystic carcinomas of all types at the Mayo Clinic from 1920 to 1954, Gatchell et al. (1958) concluded that these lesions were "more a gross than microscopic entity." In Haagensen's (1986) 14 papillary carcinomas subject to ten-year follow-up and treated with less than complete mastectomy, there were ten recurrences.

This potpourri of data emphasize (1) the tenuousness of histologic diagnosis historically—even today, permanent sections rather than frozen sections are generally required for diagnosis of papillary lesions; (2) the

TABLE 22–2. Features of Intracystic Papillary Carcinoma

Path. Type Cancers	Number	Patient Age (Years)				Detection				Axillary Lymph Nodes			Path. Tumor Size (cm)					Path. Sites			Survival: Alive/Dead (Years)			
		<40	40–50	51–60	60+	XP +–	XP ++	XP –+	XP ––	None	Low	All Levels	0	<1	1–2	2.1–5	>5	1	2–5	6+	<5	5–9	10–19	20+
One	5	0	1	2	2	1	3	0	1	5	0	0	0	1	2	2	0	3	2	0	2/0	0/0	2/0	1/0
Two	13	0	3	2	8	0	9	3	1	9	1	3	0	0	4	6	3	3	10	0	5/3	2/1	1/1	0/0
Three	1	0	0	0	1	0	1	0	0	1	0	0	0	0	0	1	0	0	0	1	0/1	0/0	0/0	0/0
Total	19	0	4	4	11	1	13	3	2	15	1	3	0	1	6	9	3	6	12	1	7/4	2/1	3/1	1/0

X = x-ray; P = physical examination; + = positive; – = negative.

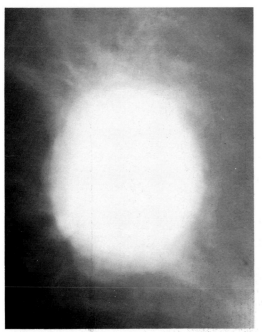

Figure 22–14. A 66-year-old woman with a breast mass for two to three weeks. Clinically: 3 × 4 cm hard mass UOQ. A 2 cm high UOQ duct carcinoma with a medullary component; just faintly seen a 1.2 × 1.7 cm intracystic papillary carcinoma near the nipple, clinically unsuspected. No axillary lymph node metastasis. (Case 3.)

practicality of clinically considering all intracystic lesions as malignant; and (3) the need for complete mastectomy if surgery is performed.

The length and the extent of breast surgery must be considered in the elderly patient. Diagnosis by needle aspiration may be unreliable. A frozen-section study adds time to the surgical procedure, often is unrewarding, and may necessitate a second operation (Case 9). Since these lesions are often multiple (Cases 3–5, 9, 12, 13, and 16, the ones not studied may be malignant. Circumscribed carcinomas in older women that may be confusing radiographically may also require conservative treatment; the question could be resolved by needle aspiration to demonstrate the blood-filled cyst. Total mastectomy, with examination of the lower axilla and extension of the surgery if indicated, is adequate treatment for well-circumscribed intracystic papillary lesions (Case 17) but not clearly invasive lesions (Case 2). Recurrence after a complete mastectomy for one of the circumscribed lesions has not been recorded.

A few cases are presented to represent the various treatment regimens utilized in our series over the past 20 years: simple mastectomy (Fig. 22–16), modified radical mastectomy (Fig. 22–17), observation with reliance

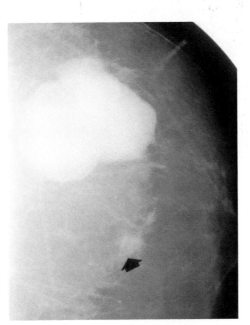

Figure 22–15. Intracystic papillary carcinomas and one duct carcinoma. This 60-year-old woman presented with a cystic lump in the breast. Clinically: a dominant nodule that would be biopsied. Mammograms: one 2 cm, one 3 cm, and one 3.5 cm intracystic papillary carcinoma, and one 6 mm infiltrative duct carcinoma (arrowhead). Pathology: same, with smallest lesion being infiltrating duct carcinoma.

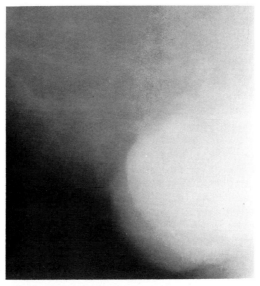

Figure 22–16. Single intracystic papillary carcinoma. A 78-year-old woman with a breast mass of unknown duration bulging the skin; leg edema. Mammography: 5.5 × 5.5 cm homogeneous discrete mass, probably an intracystic papillary carcinoma. Needle aspiration; dark blood; insufficient cells for diagnosis. Simple mastectomy; intracystic papillary carcinoma completely within its capsule. The patient is still living four years later.

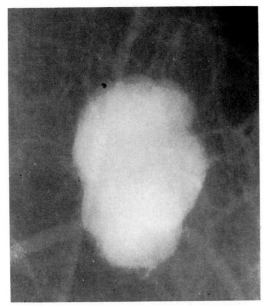

Figure 22–17. Intracystic papillary carcinoma. A 60-year-old woman with a palpable mass present for at least three months. Mammography: homogeneously dense, circumscribed, bosselated 2.6 × 3.7 cm mass. The silhouette, even though faint, suggests malignancy; the absence of the fine protuberances or the mulberry effect of medullary carcinoma, and lobulation leads to the most likely diagnosis of intracystic papillary carcinoma. Pathologic examination confirmed this diagnosis. Foci of intraductal carcinoma were identified. All 18 axillary lymph nodes were free of tumor after modified radical mastectomy.

on cytology (Fig. 22–18), and observation (Fig. 22–19).

Prognosis

In the five cases of intracystic papillary carcinoma as the only histologic type of carcinoma there were no deaths, with three women subject to more than ten years of follow-up and one to 20-year follow-up. There were four women alive and four dead at five years, and one alive and five dead at ten years, when a second histologic type of cancer was present. The woman with the additional duct and lobular carcinomas died prior to five years. The five- and ten-year survival rates were 58 per cent and 40 per cent, respectively. Only four cases had axillary lymph node metastases, three at all levels, all in the women having two histologic types of carcinoma present.

CASE HISTORY

The patient was an 83-year-old spinster who had had a gradually enlarging left breast mass for well

over ten years. It had not bothered her. She went to her primary-care physician owing to recent weight loss. Menarche was at 12; she was 33 years post natural menopause; one sister has breast cancer; and the patient had received no hormonal therapy.

On clinical examination there was marked scoliosis, resulting in the right rib cage being located near the right iliac crest. The right breast was atrophic, whereas the left measured 15 cm in size and contained a large bosselated cystic mass. The skin over the larger and more lateral portion of the mass was dark, dry, and thinned to almost "cracking." The two more central lobulations appeared to communicate with the one large lesion (Fig. 22–20).

Radiographically the right breast was fatty, with several plaques of old fibroadenoma type calcifications measuring up to 8 mm in size. The left breast was almost filled with a smoothly lobulated, very dense mass measuring 12 × 13 × 14 cm. A small amount of normal fibrofatty tissue was recognized in the tail of the breast and above the inframammary crease. No secondary signs of malignancy or evidence of invasiveness were demonstrated (Fig. 22–21). The diagnosis was intracystic papillary carcinoma with areas of calcifying necrotic material; the tumor was noninvasive and operable.

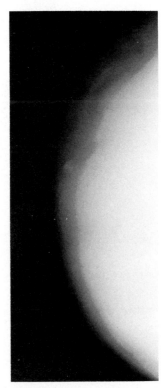

Figure 22–18. Intracystic papillary lesion, borderline malignancy. An 85-year-old woman with a mass filling most of the breast, present five to nine years. Mammography: lobulated homogeneous mass pushing aside fibroglandular tissue; intracystic papillary carcinoma. Pathology (aspiration): old blood and sufficient cells to suggest papilloma. At last follow-up 11 years later, the patient was alive without spread of disease.

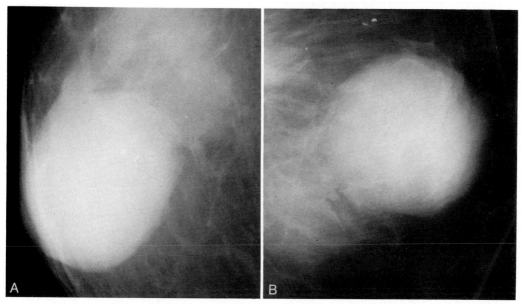

Figure 22–19. Bilateral intracystic papillary carcinoma (ICPC) being followed by mammography. An 83-year-old woman with bilateral breast masses for over eight years. Seven years prior to these mammograms the initial radiographic study showed similar but smaller lesions. Needle aspiration of dark blood and tissue fragments confirmed the mammographic diagnosis of ICPC. An average of two follow-up studies per year showed slow increase in size of the masses: on the right (A) 3 × 3.5 cm, and on the left (B) 3.5 × 4 cm. At the time of this last mammogram there was no evidence of infiltrative disease. These central lesions may well be benign, of only academic interest.

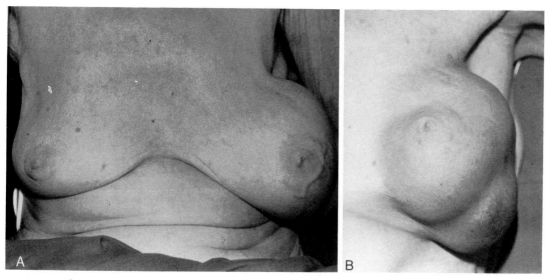

Figure 22–20. Appearance of the breasts: Frontal (A) and oblique (B) views of the left breast.

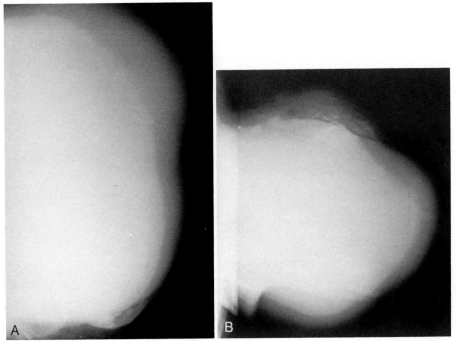

Figure 22–21. Mammograms. Craniocaudad (*A*) and mediolateral (*B*) views showing the breast almost completely filled with a smooth, lobulated, very dense mass.

A needle aspiration yielded 275 ml of dark bloody liquid, reducing the mass by 50 per cent. Cytologic study showed atypical cells but was not diagnostic of carcinoma. One week later a complete mastectomy was performed, with excision of several low axillary lymph nodes. Radiography of the specimen better demonstrated the mass (Fig. 22–22A). Upon sectioning, dark blood was seen to be under great pressure. The sliced specimen (Fig. 22–22B and C) demonstrated the circumscribed cyst containing projections of tumor from its wall. The patient had tolerated the procedure well and was living and well one year later. The final histopathologic diagnosis was intracystic papilloma. The benign designation was based on the presence of abundant fibrovascular stroma covered by two distinct cell types, epithelial and myoepithelial (Fig. 22–23).

OBSERVATIONS

Treatment of intracystic papillary carcinomas must be individualized in elderly women, who may be poor surgical risks or have short life expectancies. The circumscribed cyst on x-ray will not have produced metastasis, and many of these carcinomas will never, or very slowly, become invasive. Our treatment is based on x-ray appearance, clinical judgment, and, when necessary, needle aspiration to establish the presence of a cyst that contains blood. It consists of close follow-up with mammography and clinical examination or complete mastectomy without biopsy. With progression of reaction about the lesion as seen by x-ray or evidence of invasiveness, mastectomy may become imperative.

In selected patients who are poor surgical risks and have a noninvasive lesion on x-ray, surgery could carry a greater risk than periodic follow-up (Cases 16–18).

Despite the more advanced age of these patients, prognosis is good, barring the presence of other histologic types of carcinoma, especially duct carcinoma.

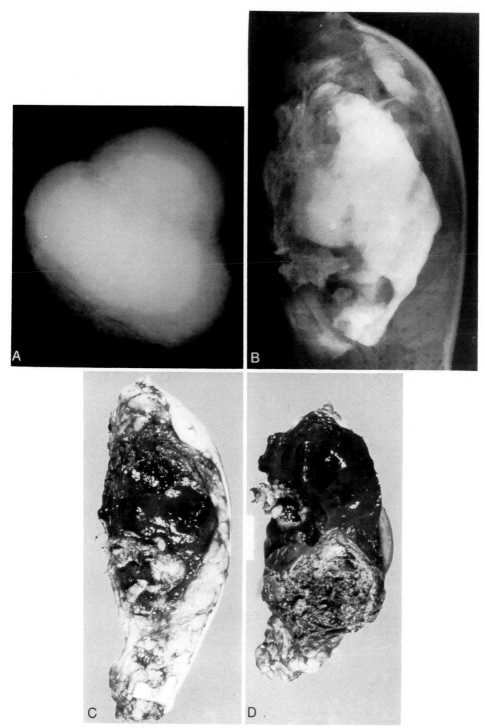

Figure 22–22. A, Radiograph of the simple mastectomy specimen better demonstrating the trilobed appearance of the large tumor mass. B, Radiograph of the midplane of the breast corresponding to the mediolateral mammogram. Numerous nodules of tumor project into the once blood-filled cyst wall. Centrally there are nonspecific calcifications, coarser than the ones associated with intracystic papillary carcinoma. C and D, Photographs of the hemorrhagic lesion.

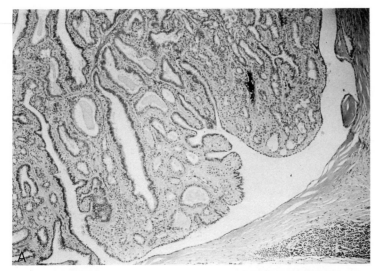

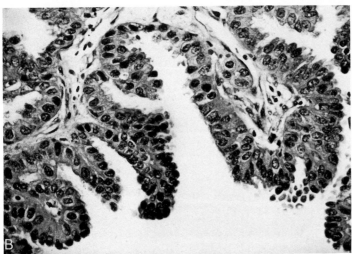

Figure 22–23. *A,* Intracystic papilloma. The presence of abundant fibrovascular stroma and two epithelial cell types distinguishes this tumor from malignant papillary neoplasms (× 20). *B,* The histologic appearance.

REFERENCES

Egan RL (1976): Mammography, 2nd ed. Springfield, IL, Charles C Thomas, p 135.

Egan RL (1970): Mammography and Diseases of the Breast. Baltimore, Williams & Wilkins, pp 19, 70.

Egan RL (1964): Mammography. Springfield, IL, Charles C Thomas, p 141.

Gatchell FG, Dockerty MB, Clagett OT (1958): Intracystic carcinoma of the breast. Surg Gynecol Obstet 106:347.

Geschickter CF (1945): Diseases of the Breast, 2nd ed. Philadelphia, JB Lippincott, p 511.

Haagensen CD (1986): Diseases of the Breast, 3rd ed. Philadelphia, WB Saunders, p 250.

Kraus FT, Neubecker RD (1962): The differential diagnosis of papillary tumors of the breast. Cancer 15:444.

Tabár L, Péntek Z (1976): Pneumocystography of benign and malignant intracystic growths of the female breast. Acta Radiol [Diagn] 17(6):829.

Medullary Carcinoma With Lymphoid Stroma

23

BACKGROUND

Certain malignant masses in the breast are rather well delineated by palpation, by x-ray, and by sonography. These include primarily intracystic papillary, mucoid, medullary, some duct, and papillary carcinomas, and sarcomas. On both radiographic and histologic examination all these masses show varying elements of invasiveness into the surrounding tissues and elicit some degree of response from these tissues.

One special type was called medullary by Moore and Foote (1949) owing to its characteristic circumscribed nature, its softness, and its hemorrhagic appearance. Richardson (1956) accepted this tumor as a pathologic entity. McDivitt et al. (1968) applied somewhat varying diagnostic criteria than strictly medullary carcinoma. Haagensen (1986) considered "circumscribed" carcinoma its proper name because of this striking clinical feature. Ridolfi et al. (1977) reviewed 192 breast carcinomas and reclassified 57 as medullary, 79 as atypical medullary, and 56 as nonmedullary (with some features of medullary) carcinomas. We much prefer the more specific term "medullary carcinoma with lymphoid stroma" to the less specific descriptive term "medullary" or "circumscribed," which can apply to many other breast masses.

The incidence of medullary carcinoma, where reported, ranged from 4.3 to 7 per cent. Ten-year survival rates ranged from 68 per cent (McDivitt et al., 1968) to 84 per cent (Ridolfi et al., 1977). Death, when it occurred, was usually within five years of diagnosis. Bilaterality of breast carcinoma occurred in 10 of 57 of the patients of Ridolfi et al. (1977): The opposite breast lesion was usually duct carcinoma, which preceded the medullary carcinoma by 8.8 years. The size of medullary carcinomas was 3.4 cm compared with 3.1 cm for duct carcinomas (McDivitt et al., 1968); the lesions of both types were of equal size (2.9 cm) in the studies of Ridolfi et al. (1977). Twenty-one per cent of the patients with typical medullary carcinoma had axillary lymph node metastasis compared with 42 per cent of those with duct carcinomas (Ridolfi et al., 1977).

Azzopardi (1979) concluded that for a diagnosis of typical medullary carcinoma there must be (1) at least 75 per cent syncytial growth pattern; (2) completely circumscribed pattern; (3) substantial mononuclear stromal infiltrate; (4) a very small in situ component, or none; (5) large neoplastic cells; and (6) exclusion, if a reasonable doubt exists, of the diagnosis of "medullary carcinoma with lymphoid stroma." Our 68 cases of medullary carcinoma with lymphoid stroma fulfill these criteria.

INCIDENCE AND AGE

The overall incidence of medullary carcinoma with lymphoid stroma varies according to age group in each series of patients. In our breast cancers it is 3.3 per cent, our

405

patient population tending to be younger. This lesion can occur from the early 20s to the late 70s with a mean age of about 50 years. The youngest patient in our series having medullary carcinoma with lymphoid stroma was 27 years of age, and the oldest patient was 83 years (average 51.2 years).

DIAGNOSIS

Physical Examination

On palpation the medullary carcinoma with lymphoid stroma may be so well delineated and so much softer than the usual duct carcinoma that a benign tumor could be suspected. The skin overlying the mass may even bulge. On occasion the skin may have a pinkish hue, a clue that central hemorrhage and necrosis has occurred within the tumor. Needle aspiration of this large tumor may yield the diagnosis of malignancy.

Radiographic Examination

The medullary carcinoma varies in the degree of infiltration and the appearance of its borders. Usually it is a circumscribed carcinoma with sufficient evidence of invasion about the entire periphery for a diagnosis of carcinoma (Figs. 23–1 and 23–2). The many minute projections from the surface overshadow each other on the radiograph so that each is blurred, resulting in a strictly indistinct border (Fig. 23–3). The mass with these small excrescences may be likened to a mulberry viewed from above (Fig. 23–4). These tumors frequently have a hemorrhagic and necrotic center (Fig. 23–5). The less usual pattern of medullary carcinoma with lymphoid stroma is a highly infiltrative pattern on the mammogram (seen progressively in Figs. 23–6 to 23–8). This tumor has a density similar to that of other carcinomatous masses. It can usually be differentiated from a fibroadenoma, a lesion that, when large,

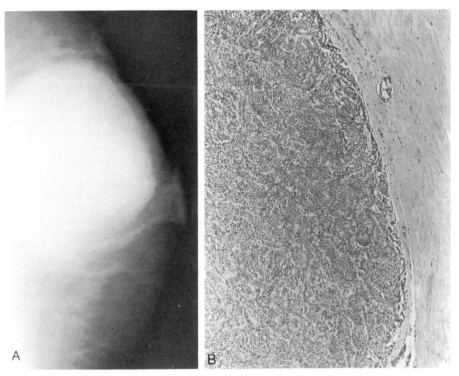

Figure 23–1. Medullary carcinoma with lymphoid stroma. A 60-year-old woman with an enlarging breast. A 6 cm mass with questionable skin fixation was present clinically. *A,* On mammography the 5.5 × 6 cm carcinoma was well circumscribed, bulging the skin. Pathology: medullary carcinoma with lymphoid stroma. *B,* Characteristic rounded periphery. Cells grow in solid sheets without duct formation. Lymphoid stroma is diffuse throughout the mass. A pseudocapsule is apparent. Modified radical mastectomy; axillary lymph nodes free of tumor. The patient was living and well six years later.

Figure 23–2. Medullary carcinoma with lymphoid stroma, thought to be a cyst clinically. A 43-year-old woman with a breast mass for 12 to 14 months, clinically a 2 cm cyst. *A,* Mammography finally was obtained and a 2 cm circumscribed carcinoma was noted on a background of ductal hyperplasia. *B,* Sonography confirmed the presence of a malignant mass: hypoechoic area, irregular jagged borders, nonhomogeneous internal echoes, and increased through-transmission. All suggested a medullary carcinoma in a woman in this age group. Pathology: 2 cm medullary carcinoma with lymphoid stroma; all nodes free of tumor; modified radical mastectomy. The patient was alive and well three years later.

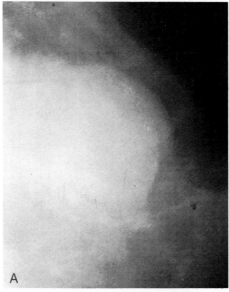
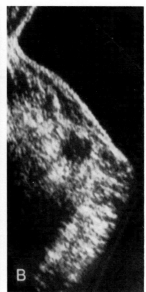

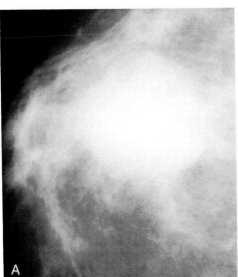
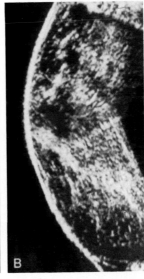

Figure 23–3. Less distinct borders of medullary carcinoma with lymphoid stroma. A 52-year-old woman with a breast mass for three months; mother had breast cancer. Clinically: 4 × 5 cm hard mass. *A,* Mammography: 3 × 3.5 cm partially circumscribed medullary carcinoma. *B,* Sonography: slightly irregular hypoechoic mass, nonhomogeneous internal echoes, surrounding architecture distorted. Pathology: 3 × 3.5 × 3.5 cm medullary carcinoma with lymphoid stroma. Modified radical mastectomy; all 19 nodes free of tumor; patient alive and well three years later.

Figure 23–4. Medullary carcinoma with lymphoid stroma containing a central fibrotic area. This 58-year-old woman, surgical menopause age 37 years, had noted a breast lump for two and one-half months. Clinically: a 2.5 cm circumscribed carcinoma. The bosselated 2.5 × 3 cm homogeneous carcinoma had areas of both smooth and indistinct borders suggestive of medullary carcinoma; background of severe ductal hyperplasia. Pathology: 2.5 cm medullary carcinoma with lymphoid stroma; hyalinized fibrotic center. After modified radical mastectomy all 19 axillary lymph nodes were free of tumor. Twelve years later the patient was free of disease.

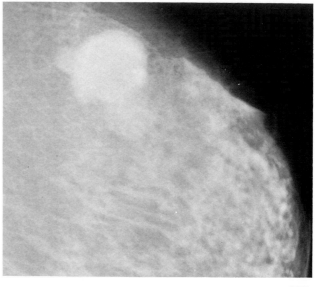

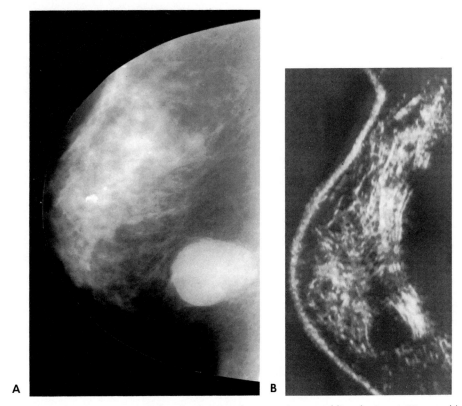

A   **B**

Figure 23–5. Medullary carcinoma with lymphoid stroma demonstrating central liquefaction. A 56-year-old woman with a breast lump for one week, clinically a 2.5 cm mass. *A*, Mammography: 2.5 × 3 cm circumscribed carcinoma, intracystic papillary vs medullary carcinoma; age favors the latter. *B*, Sonography: well-demarcated mass with low-level internal echoes and increased through-transmission, which suggest a cyst with internal debris such as an intracystic papillary carcinoma. Pathology: medullary carcinoma with lymphoid stroma with a large area of central necrosis. Modified radical mastectomy; all 18 axillary lymph nodes free of tumor. Eighteen months later the patient was free of disease.

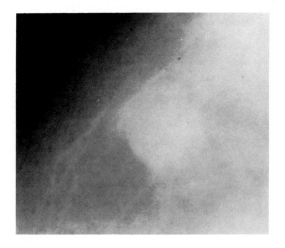

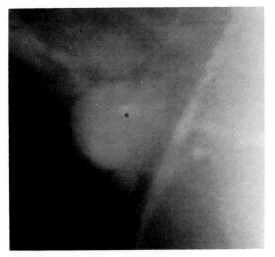

Figure 23–6. Medullary carcinoma with lymphoid stroma and axillary lymph node metastases. A 39-year-old woman with a 2 × 3 cm firm mass UOQ of her breast. Mammography: 1.8 × 2 cm moderately invasive, but slightly circumscribed, carcinoma in the tail of the breast. Pathology: medullary carcinoma with lymphoid stroma. After a modified radical mastectomy two of nine nodes were positive at Level I and nine nodes were free of disease Level II. Five years later the patient was free of disease.

Figure 23–7. Medullary carcinoma with massive axillary lymph node metastases. A 54-year-old woman with a breast lump for "several months." Clinically: 3 × 4 cm hard mass UOQ with large axillary lymph nodes, questionably matted. Mammography: 2 × 2.2 cm circumscribed carcinoma (lower density) with large low axillary lymph nodes. Pathology: medullary carcinoma with lymphoid stroma. Radical mastectomy; 12 of 24 lymph nodes positive, all levels. Death from widespread disease three years later.

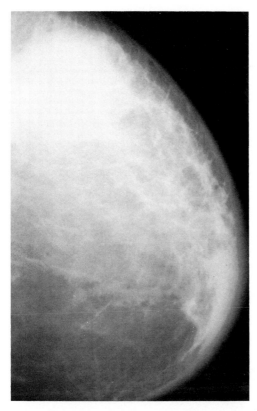

Figure 23–8. Highly infiltrative and diffuse medullary carcinoma with lymphoid stroma. This 55-year-old woman admitted knowing that there was something wrong with her breast for over two years. This lesion was inoperable; there were massive axillary nodes both on x-ray and clinically.

Sonographic Examination

On breast sonography a rather well-demarcated solid mass is evident. The borders may be so smooth that differentiation from a fibroadenoma is not clear-cut. However, the internal echoes and increased through-transmission may be quite different from that of a fibroadenoma. Mammography may be helpful in the diagnosis. As calcification may still be absent or minimal in a fibroadenoma at this age, calcification will not be an aid in differential diagnosis by sonography.

Most of the lesions that we studied by ultrasound were fairly well demarcated (at times almost as smooth as a fibroadenoma but definitely invasive on x-ray), bulged the skin, and had increased disruption of the surrounding architecture. An increased anterior border has been noted. Most of the lesions had at least a slightly irregular border with minimally potentiated posterior border and increased through-transmission. The internal echoes were not as homogeneous, with more variation in size than those in the fibroadenoma; the fibroadenoma had a greater tendency to gross lobulation or bosselation.

The homogeneity of the cellular structure of the medullary carcinoma, without dramatic reflective interfaces unless there has been necrosis and scarring, provides an almost liquid-like path to the ultrasound beam. As a result, there may be rather markedly increased through-transmission. The internal scarring, even to a slight degree, produces areas of high-level echoes on the background of the usual more homogeneous echo pattern. Central liquefaction can produce a complex mass on sonography.

Pathologic Study

Histologically the tumor is made up of closely packed, structureless, uniform cells. Varying numbers of lymphocytes are found within the tumor, hence the term "medullary carcinoma with lymphoid stroma." A similar tumor without lymphoid stroma must be differentiated. The invasive edge of this tumor varies in aggressiveness.

In parts of the periphery a zone of surrounding lymphocytic infiltration along with a thin band of encircling fibrotic reaction may give an impression of a pseudocapsule. In larger tumors with marked central necrosis, hemorrhage, and liquefaction with only a thin rim of tumor remaining, the lesion

also may be quite dense. Unlike the more highly infiltrative carcinomas, medullary carcinoma with lymphoid stroma has more nearly the same size by palpation as on the mammogram or on gross pathology.

Radiographically suspicious calcifications are not an integral part of medullary carcinoma with lymphoid stroma but were found in 15 breasts harboring this type of carcinoma—12 times associated with a mass and 3 times without a mass. Careful search then was required to dissociate these flecks from the mass of medullary carcinoma with lymphoid stroma per se. This tumor was associated with the more glandular and dense breast parenchymal pattern 34 times—9 times in glandular breasts, 8 times in denser ductal hyperplasia, and 17 times in dense, coarsely nodular breasts. Yet it was associated just as frequently with the fatty type parenchyma—fatty breasts 25 times and with fatty ductal hyperplasia 9 times.

grossly will be confused with intracystic papillary carcinoma.

The tumor is made up of strands or masses of usually monotonous closely packed cells without a fibrous matrix. The cells are large and highly anaplastic, have large and hyperchromatic nuclei, and vary in size and shape. Multinucleated bizarre giant cells, degeneration within the tumor, and squamous cell metaplasia are typical changes of medullary carcinoma with lymphoid stroma. We did not demonstrate a true intraductal phase of this carcinoma. Six whole-organ studies demonstrated only three breasts with a single histologic type of this tumor.

Variations of breast carcinomas that include a medullary pattern without lymphocytic infiltration and circumscribed duct carcinoma with marked lymphocytosis are only suggestive patterns that do not fit into the true category of medullary carcinoma with lymphoid stroma. Such lesions have been included with infiltrating duct carcinoma.

CLINICAL MANIFESTATIONS

The medullary carcinoma with lymphoid stroma is associated with premenopausal or menopausal age, is rather well circumscribed, and carries a better prognosis than most invasive duct carcinomas. The average duration of symptoms with medullary carcinoma with lymphoid stroma is somewhat longer than with duct carcinoma. There are fewer dramatic changes in the early phase of the growth period with medullary carcinoma with lymphoid stroma, since this is a softer lesion in the more glandular breast of younger women. There are fewer secondary signs, such as skin dimpling or nipple retraction, as with infiltrating duct carcinoma. If discovered at a small size, this lesion might be considered a fibroadenoma or even a tense cyst. The greatest diameter of the tumor in our series at diagnosis was approximately twice that of duct carcinoma.

Only eight lesions were less than 1 cm in size; 23 were less than 2 cm; 37 were greater than 2 cm; and three were larger than 5 cm, with an average diameter of 2.2 cm. Most of the lesions (45) were apparent on x-ray and physical examination, with an equal number being found either by x-ray or by physical examination only. Seven tumors occurred under observation following at least one normal mammogram and physical examination.

Multiplicity

Multiple medullary carcinomas with lymphoid stroma do occur in the same breast (Fig. 23–9). In such cases they are near-equal in size, are located in different quadrants of the breast, and are considered simultaneous primary carcinomas. In our 14 such cases this produced no discernible difference in the clinical course of the patient.

Bilaterality

Bilateral simultaneous primary medullary carcinomas with lymphoid stroma also occur (Fig. 23–10). Both tumors have the appearance of a primary lesion so that there is little necessity to speculate that one could be a contralateral metastatic deposit. To us the latter occurrence is quite infrequent, as it did not occur in our series. The second primary

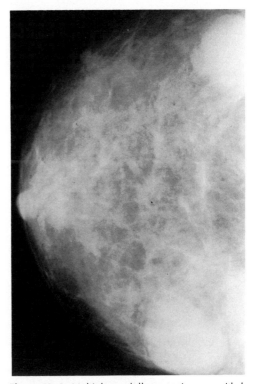

Figure 23–9. Multiple medullary carcinomas with lymphoid stroma in the same breast. A 43-year-old woman with a mass in UOQ of the right breast for three months. Clinically: suspicious masses in UOQ and UIQ of the right breast. Mammography: 3.5 × 4 cm UIQ and 2.5 × 3 cm UOQ circumscribed lobulated masses that suggest medullary carcinoma even though this is an unusual occurrence. Pathology: two medullary carcinomas with lymphoid stroma, both with central fibrosis. All 18 lymph nodes free of disease; modified radical mastectomy. The patient was free of disease six years later.

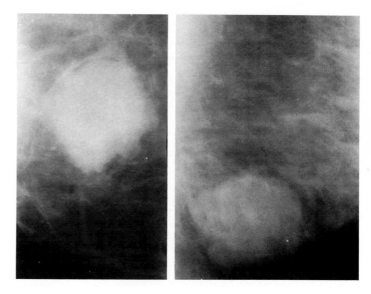

Figure 23–10. Bilateral primary medullary carcinomas with lymphoid stroma. A 45-year-old woman with a mass in the LOQ of each breast. Clinically: bilateral breast masses, 4 cm on the right and 3 cm on the left. Mammography: 3 × 3.5 cm lobulated, circumscribed mass right and 3 cm circumscribed mass left LOQ each breast. Pathology: bilateral primary medullary carcinoma with lymphoid stroma. All lymph nodes free of tumor after bilateral modified radical mastectomies. The patient was alive and free of disease four years later.

is more frequently a duct carcinoma. Bilateral primary carcinomas did occur nine times (all nonsimultaneous).

Occurrence With Other Cancers

Medullary carcinomas with lymphoid stroma occur with other distinct histologic types of carcinoma in the same area of the same breast (Fig. 23–11) or in different quadrants of the same breast (Fig. 23–12).

Fourteen of the 68 patients had two or more distinct deposits of medullary carcinoma with lymphoid stroma in the same breast; seven in the 48 breasts containing only one histologic type of tumor (Table 23–1). In 17 breasts there was one additional histologic type of tumor, 16 having duct and one having mucinous carcinoma. In three cases two other types of carcinoma were present, two with duct and lobular and one with duct and mucinous.

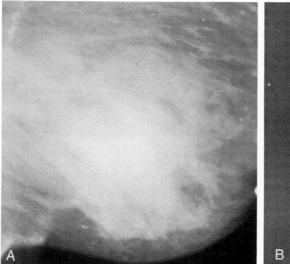
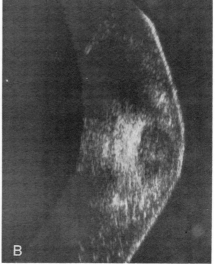

Figure 23–11. Medullary carcinoma with lymphoid stroma surrounded by comedocarcinoma. A 77-year-old woman with a clinical mass filling most of the lower half of the breast. *A,* Mammograms: 2.5 × 3 cm homogeneous circumscribed mass surrounded by calcification of comedocarcinoma with density and architectural distortion associated with the large area of calcification. *B,* Sonography: well-demarcated mass containing many nonhomogeneous internal echoes, increased through-transmission, surrounded by architectural reaction. Pathology: medullary carcinoma with lymphoid stroma surrounded by comedocarcinoma. Two distinct histologic types of carcinoma in the same breast.

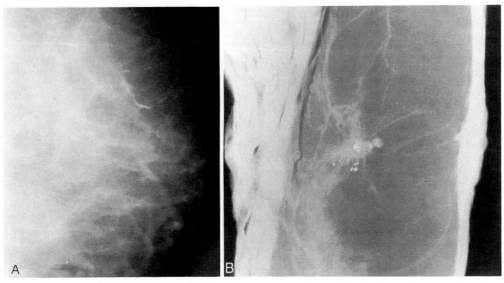

Figure 23–12. Medullary carcinoma with lymphoid stroma in one quadrant of the breast, with a comedocarcinoma in another quadrant. A 42-year-old woman with a breast lump for four days. *A,* Mammography: 4 cm circumscribed carcinoma at the 6 o'clock position; calcification pattern UOQ right breast. *B,* Whole-organ slicer radiograph for better demonstration of the calcification. Pathology: medullary carcinoma with lymphoid stroma and an intraductal comedocarcinoma. All 16 nodes free of disease. The patient was living and well 14 years later.

Miscellaneous

Medullary carcinoma with lymphoid stroma may have atypical features (Fig. 23–13). This tumor may have an aggressive radiographic appearance but still have a guarded prognosis (Fig. 23–14). Medullary carcinomas with lymphoid stroma in peripheral areas of the breast are difficult to image (Fig. 23–15).

Seldom is a nonpalpable medullary carcinoma with lymphoid stroma of less than 1 cm detected in the dense nodular breasts of the younger woman usually harboring this tumor. However, it can occur in the older woman with fatty breasts (Fig. 23–16).

The pathologist must make the final decision as to which of these circumscribed carcinomas are medullary carcinomas with lymphoid stroma (Fig. 23–17). Sonography in this case (Fig. 23–17) would have raised a question of that diagnosis.

TREATMENT

In the Emory University series of medullary carcinomas with lymphoid stroma, 32 of the carcinomas were treated by radical mas-

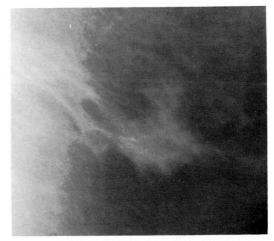

Figure 23–13. Medullary carcinoma with lymphoid stroma having atypical features histologically. A 60-year-old woman with a lump in the tail of the left breast. Clinically this mass was benign, but enlarged axillary lymph nodes were palpable. Mammography: 1 × 2 cm moderately invasive carcinoma with extension superiorly and posteriorly. Pathology: typical pattern of medullary carcinoma with lymphoid stroma associated with unusual histologic features: expansile borders, small foci of tumor peripherally interprted as satellitosis, and a 1 cm adjacent similar tumor. Modified radical mastectomy: three of four nodes positive at Level I, and 7 of 14 nodes positive at Level II. Six years later death from metastases occurred. Without circumscription this could not be included with the typical medullary carcinoma with lymphoid stroma.

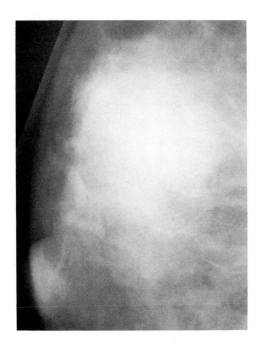

Figure 23–14. Medullary carcinoma with lymphoid stroma; aggressive radiologically but with guarded prognosis. A 47-year-old woman has been watching a breast mass grow over the past five months. Mammography: only partly circumscribed but mostly invasive 2.4 × 3 cm mass with spiculations, increased vascularity, and borderline early diffuse skin thickening. Pathology: medullary carcinoma with lymphoid stroma. Modified radical mastectomy: all 21 axillary lymph nodes free of tumor. The patient was free of disease four years later. This lesion histologically was circumscribed.

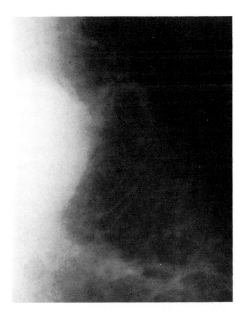

Figure 23–15. Tail of breast medullary carcinoma with lymphoid stroma. A 52-year-old woman with a 3 cm breast mass UOQ. Mammograms: 2.5 × 3 cm circumscribed carcinoma consistent with medullary type in this age group. Pathology: medullary carcinoma with lymphoid stroma; modified radical mastectomy; 1 low node of a total of 19 axillary lymph nodes with metastatic tumor. The patient was alive and free of disease seven years later.

Figure 23–16. Nonpalpable medullary carcinoma with lymphoid stroma. A 77-year-old woman studied for large fatty breasts. Mammography: 9 × 10 mm circumscribed carcinoma. Pathology: medullary carcinoma with lymphoid stroma. Modified radical mastectomy; all 20 axillary lymph nodes free of tumor. The patient was living and well 13 years later. (Smallest of this type tumor in our series.)

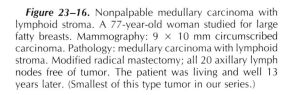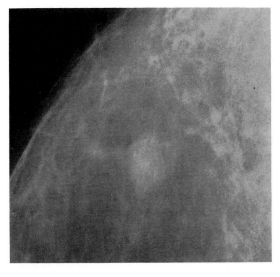

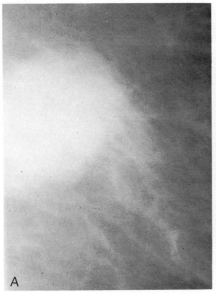
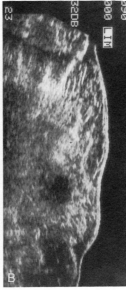

Figure 23–17. Circumscribed duct vs medullary carcinoma with lymphoid stroma. A 49-year-old woman with a breast mass for three months; mother had breast cancer. *A,* Mammography: 2.6 × 2.6 cm circumscribed carcinoma. *B,* Sonography: well-demarcated hypoechoic mass; non-homogeneous high-level internal echoes; suggestion of attenuation of the beam. Pathology: duct carcinoma associated with lymphocytosis. Modified radical mastectomy; 2 low of 19 axillary lymph nodes with metastases. The patient was alive and free of disease 18 months later.

tectomy, 30 by modified radical mastectomy, three by total mastectomy, and the remaining three by tumor excision and radiotherapy.

The frequency and level of axillary metastasis are noted in Table 23–1. In the 48 patients with a single histologic type tumor, axillary lymph node metastases were present in only seven cases higher than Level I.

PROGNOSIS

Despite the increased size of the mass of pure medullary carcinoma with lymphoid stroma in our series, after five years the survival rate was 76 per cent; at ten years it was 61 per cent. All the deaths in the series were from breast cancer, and all of these were within five years of treatment. With additional histologic types of carcinoma in the breast, two deaths did occur after five years, both from cancer (Table 23–2).

Three patients had been treated with radiation owing to age and poor surgical risk.

CASE HISTORY

Medullary carcinoma with lymphoid stroma can be a real clinical problem in the young woman with dense nodular breasts (Fig. 23–18).

This 34-year-old woman, gravida 4, para 4, had had an uncomplicated delivery four months before. She had nursed for one month, during which time she repeatedly complained to her physician about a fullness in the upper part of her right breast. During nursing he attributed the nodularities to "milk ducts." Following cessation of nursing he attributed the changes to fibrocystic disease.

An x-ray technician friend suggested she ask her doctor for a mammogram. The study showed a classic 2 cm circumscribed carcinoma against the background of young dense fibroglandular tissue without secondary changes. Surgical consultation was followed by an open biopsy and diagnosis of medullary carcinoma with lymphoid stroma. This,

TABLE 23–1. Features of Medullary Carcinoma With Lymphoid Stroma

Path. Type Cancers	Number	Patient Age (Years)				Detection				Axillary Lymph Nodes*			Tumor Path. Size (cm)					Path. Sites		
		<40	40–50	51–60	60+	X P + −	X P + +	X P − +	X P − −	None	Low	All Levels	0	<1	1–2	2.1–5	>5	1	2–5	6+
One	48	15	15	10	8	3	34	5	6	3	8	7	0	6	16	24	2	41	7	0
Two	17	1	4	6	6	4	10	2	1	11	2	3	0	2	6	8	1	11	6	0
Three	3	0	1	0	2	1	1	1	0	1	0	2	0	0	1	2	0	2	1	0
Total	68	16	20	16	16	8	45	8	7	43	10	12	0	8	23	34	3	54	14	0

X = x-ray; P = physical examination; + = positive; − = negative.
*Three cases not studied.

TABLE 23–2. Follow-up of 68 Medullary Carcinomas With Lymphoid Stroma Alone or Associated With One or Two Other Histologic Types of Carcinoma

	One Type		Two Types		Three Types		Total	
	No.	% Alive	No.	% Alive	No.	% Alive	No.	% Alive
Patients treated ≥ 5 yrs ago	22		7		3		32	
Alive	22	100	5	71	2	66	29	91
Dead, breast cancer	0*		2†		1		3	
Dead, not breast cancer	0		0		0		0	
Patients treated ≥ 10 yrs ago	10		4		1		15	
Alive	10	100	3	75	0	0	13	87
Dead, breast cancer	0		1		1		2	
Dead, not breast cancer	0		0		0		0	
Patients treated ≥ 20 yrs ago	1		0		0		1	
Alive	1	100	0		0		1	100
Dead, breast cancer	0		0		0		0	
Dead, not breast cancer	0		0		0		0	

*Seven died of breast cancer within five years of treatment.
†Four died of breast cancer within five years of treatment.

in turn, was followed by a modified radical mastectomy, showing all 19 axillary lymph nodes free of tumor. Five years later the woman was alive without evidence of disease.

CASE HISTORY

Medullary carcinoma with lymphoid stroma deep in the breast.

This 47-year-old woman reportedly practiced

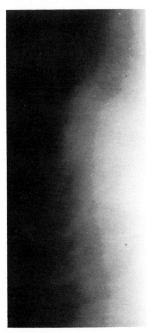

Figure 23–18. Medullary carcinoma with lymphoid stroma as a problem in the young.

breast self-examination after a baseline mammogram three years previously. She had felt a thickening, or difference, in the breast five months earlier and what she termed a lump two months later. This did not seem to change for a month or so but then became more alarming to her.

Clinically the patient had rather firm pendulous breasts with a definite hard deep-seated mass. No other clinical signs were present. A mammogram was followed by sonography (Fig. 23–19).

Such a homogeneous, circumscribed carcinoma without calcification in this age group is highly suggestive of the diagnosis. The only secondary sign of malignancy was increased vascularity. A 3 cm duct carcinoma probably would be producing diffuse disease in the breast, perhaps even inflammatory changes.

Pathologically this proved to be a medullary carcinoma with lymphoid stroma. Examination of the modified radical mastectomy specimen showed no other site of carcinoma; all 19 axillary lymph nodes were free of tumor. The patient was alive and free of disease three and a half years later.

OBSERVATIONS

Three out of nine of our medullary carcinomas having whole-organ studies were associated with a separate smaller deposit of invasive duct carcinoma in the same breast. Necrosis and liquefaction within the mass of tumor was fairly common, and the overlying skin on occasion was reddened as a reaction.

Better prognosis is anticipated if a strict histopathologic diagnosis is established. This is in spite of the frequent occurrence of medullary carcinoma with lymphoid stroma in

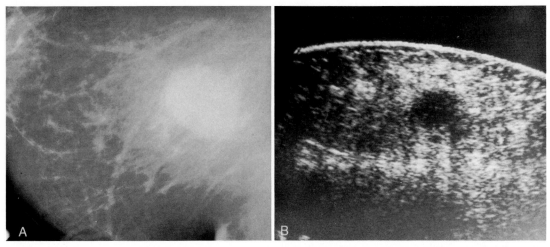

Figure 23–19. *A*, Mammography: 3 cm homogeneous mass with indistinct borders; slightly lobulated; increased vascularity. *B*, Sonography: irregular solid mass; fairly well demarcated; nonhomogeneous internal echoes; no attenuation; increased reflectivity surrounding the mass.

the denser breasts of younger women; the procrastination in exploration of the breast in young women; discovery of the tumor at a larger size; multiplicity; and bilaterality of the disease.

No true intraductal component of medullary carcinoma with lymphoid stroma was encountered even though whole-organ studies were done on six breasts with this carcinoma; the lesions were multiple in 14 instances, and bilaterality did occur.

Metastasis, death, or complications of this carcinoma usually occur within five years, more often three years; prognosis beyond that period of follow-up is extremely good.

REFERENCES

Azzopardi JG (1979): Problems in Breast Pathology. Philadelphia, WB Saunders, p 286.

Haagensen CD (1986): Diseases of the Breast. 3rd ed. Philadelphia, WB Saunders, p 790.

McDivitt RW, Stewart FW, Berg JW (1968): Tumors of the Breast. Atlas of Tumor Pathology, Washington, DC, Armed Forces Institute of Pathology. Second Series, Fascicle 2.

Moore OS Jr, Foote FW Jr (1949): The relatively favorable prognosis of medullary carcinoma of the breast. Cancer 2:635.

Richardson WW (1956): Medullary carcinoma of the breast. Br J Cancer 10:415.

Ridolfi RL, Rosen PP, Port A, Kinne D, Mike V (1977): Medullary carcinoma of the breast. A clinicopathologic study with 10-year follow-up. Cancer 40:1365.

Mucinous Carcinoma

BACKGROUND

Mucinous carcinoma of the breast is considered a rather indolent, slow-growing tumor with better prognosis than the average breast carcinoma. Beyond this generalization, specific reports of nodal metastasis and prognosis vary, even in more recent series. For example, Azzopardi (1979) cites variations in the incidence of axillary lymph node metastasis ranging from 36 per cent down to 4 per cent with the suggestion, "This difference needs explaining." Such variations suggest parallel radical vs conservative treatment regimens. There was the obvious difference between pure mucinous carcinomas with a 10 per cent mortality and mixed mucinous carcinomas with a 29 per cent mortality.

In our series an additional factor may well contribute to the poorer prognosis with pure mucinous carcinomas, namely, multiplicity of histologic types of carcinomas in the same breast. Two of 18 mucinous carcinomas (11 per cent) occurring in the breast without additional histopathologic types of carcinoma had only low-node metastasis, with no woman dying of her disease. However, 20 of 47 patients with additional carcinomas (43 per cent) had node metastasis, with 13 (28

per cent) having positive nodes at all three levels.

DEFINITION

Special mucin stains will demonstrate some mucin in almost all breast carcinomas. The term "mucin-producing carcinoma" is reserved for those lesions that have abundant mucin, with clumps or nests of carcinoma cells floating in pools of mucin. This tumor is usually classified as a circumscribed carcinoma. Numerous synonyms include gelatinous carcinoma, colloid carcinoma, and mucoid or mucin-producing carcinoma. The term relating to mucin is much preferred; some authors decry the terms "gelatinous" and "colloid."

We feel that there should be separation into typical, or pure, mucinous carcinomas in sharp distinction from the impure types of duct carcinomas with varying amounts of mucin.

INCIDENCE AND AGE

The incidence of mucinous carcinoma averages approximately 2 per cent in most series (Veronesi and Gennari, 1960; McDivitt et al., 1968). The incidence in our series of 3.2 per cent was similar, but slightly higher. Haagensen (1986) reported an incidence of slightly over 4 per cent of this type of carcinoma.

CLINICAL FEATURES

The reported age for this tumor ranges from 54 years (McDivitt et al., 1968) to 68.6 years (Silverberg et al., 1971). Our average age, 62.5 years, falls between these two reports. The youngest patient was 23 years and the oldest 81 years of age.

Clinically, this uncommon tumor is often soft and poorly defined (although at times clearly delineated), and lacks most of the

TABLE 24–1. Features of Mucinous Carcinoma

Path. Type Cancers	Num-ber	Patient Age (Years)				Detection				Axillary Lymph Nodes			Path. Tumor Size (cm)					Path. Sites		
		<40	40–50	51–60	60+	X P +–	X P ++	X P –+	X P ––	None	Low	All Levels	0	<1	1–2	2.1–5	>5	1	2–5	6+
One	18	1	2	6	9	1	17	0	0	16	2	0	0	1	6	10	1	16	2	0
Two	43	2	2	11	28	11	27	4	1	24	7	12	0	10	17	11	5	31	12	0
Three	4	2	0	2	0	0	3	0	1	2	0	2	0	0	2	1	1	3	0	1
Total	65	5	4	19	37	12	47	4	2	42	9	14	0	11	25	22	7	50	14	1

X = x-ray; P = physical examination; + = positive; – = negative.

usual definite signs of retraction. Usually, if palpable, it is in an area of thickening or fullness of undetermined origin. It may be too soft to be palpable. At times a bulky tumor will bulge the skin. McDivitt et al. (1968) reported an average size of 3.8 cm. Of our tumors, 36 per cent were less than 2 cm in greatest diameter, 11 were under 1 cm, and only 7 were greater than 5 cm in diameter (Table 24–1).

Over three quarters of the mucinous carcinomas occurred in fatty breasts or in those with fatty ductal hyperplasia; 38 per cent were associated with ductal hyperplasia; and only 22 per cent were in glandular or nodular breasts. Most of these carcinomas were ob-vious both clinically and by x-ray, with only one single mass not being detected by physical examination.

RADIOGRAPHIC FEATURES

Radiographically, the mucin-producing carcinomas may lack many of the criteria of carcinoma. They are perhaps the least dense of all carcinomas, often no denser than a cyst (Fig. 24–1). However, the peripheral evidence, such as trabecular distortion and retraction, is usually more marked in some areas than the fibrotic portion of advanced fibrocystic disease, which produces the ill-

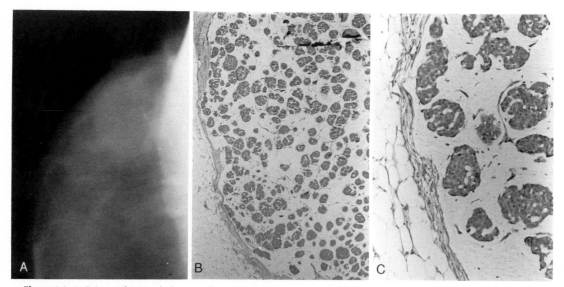

Figure 24–1. Faint, soft, rounded mass of mucinous carcinoma. A 64-year-old woman with a questionable nodule in the opposite breast. Clinically: "in spite of the mammograms, a normal breast." *A*, Mammography: 2.5 cm circumscribed carcinoma. Pathology: mucin-producing carcinoma. *B*, This type of invasive duct carcinoma has an expansile rounded periphery. Malignant epithelial cells appear to float within a mucinous background. *C*, Upon magnification mucin may be identified within the clumps of cells. Modified radical mastectomy; all 21 axillary lymph nodes free of tumor. The patient was alive and well 12 years later.

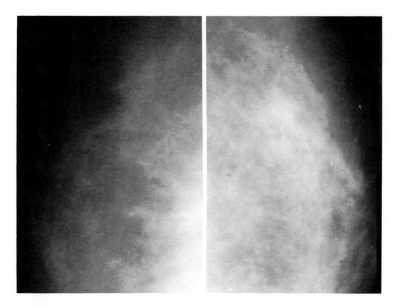

Figure 24–2. Poorly defined mucinous carcinoma. A 56-year-old woman with a suspicious thickening UOQ left breast. Mammography: severe ductal hyperplasia, more pronounced on left. Against this background are two asymmetric poorly defined areas, each approximately 1 cm in diameter. Pathology: mucinous carcinoma 3 × 4 × 4 cm. Modified radical mastectomy; five nodes at Level I and nine nodes at Level II free of tumor. The patient was alive and well seven years later.

defined borders of a cyst (Fig. 24–2). Careful study will reveal definite trabecular distortion or a tail about some portion of the mass. A rounded, circumscribed, fairly dense mass against fatty tissue (Fig. 24–3), or less dense against fibroglandular tissue (Fig. 24–4), may be present. A faint, rounded type of calcification may be present in the lesion. Secondary signs, such as minimal skin changes or increased vascularity, may lead to the diagnosis of malignant disease. Although mucin-producing carcinomas are not commonly found in the breast, great care must be taken to evaluate subtle changes that may indicate their presence. As there is frequently an absence of firmness and retraction, the mucin-producing carcinomas may be overlooked clinically. The radiologist may also be confused by this tumor. Mucinous carcinomas may be multiple (Figs. 24–5 and 24–6).

The mass of mucinous carcinoma may present an irregular contour without significant retractive phenomenon (Fig. 24–5, the superior mass). At times the mass may appear infiltrated by fat (Fig. 24–5, both masses; Fig. 24–6, the anterior mass). An unusual type of round, dense, coarse, scattered calcification frequently occurs in the area of the carcinoma but not specifically within the mass or elsewhere in either breast (Fig. 24–6).

The absence of significant clinical changes with mucinous carcinoma suggests that this type is a slow-growing carcinoma, as large lesions may be nonpalpable (Fig. 24–1) or even occult (Fig. 24–5). Our infrequent whole-organ study on this carcinoma did demonstrate a multiplicity of sites (Fig. 24–

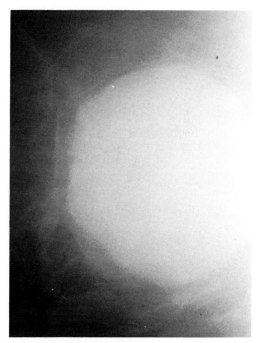

Figure 24–3. Circumscribed carcinoma, mucinous type. A 74-year-old woman who for an indefinite period had a breast lump that was clinically suspicious. Mammography: 5.7 × 5.8 cm circumscribed homogeneously dense carcinoma, most likely intracystic papillary in a woman in this age group. Pathology: mucinous carcinoma, extending deeply to within 1 cm of the fascia. Modified radical mastectomy; 12 Level I and 11 Level II nodes free of metastasis. The patient was free of disease five years later.

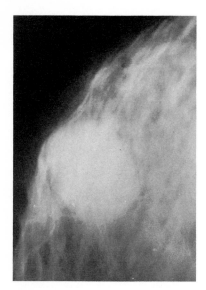

Figure 24–4. Mucinous carcinoma. A 69-year-old woman with a breast lump for one month; palpable LIQ. Mammography: 2.3 × 2.7 cm circumscribed carcinoma bulging the superficial layer of superficial fascia. Pathology: mucinous carcinoma, Grade III. Modified radical mastectomy; all 27 axillary nodes without tumor. The patient was free of disease four years later.

Figure 24–5. Irregularly shaped mucinous carcinoma. A 69-year-old woman with a diagnosis of mucin-producing carcinoma from an excised axillary lymph node. Clinically: normal breast. Mammography: 2 cm and 2.5 × 3 cm carcinomas with faint calcifications, intervening infiltration. Pathologically: two separate nodules of mucinous carcinoma of the breast. Radical mastectomy; all 25 axillary lymph nodes in the specimen free of tumor. When last seen two years later, the patient was free of disease.

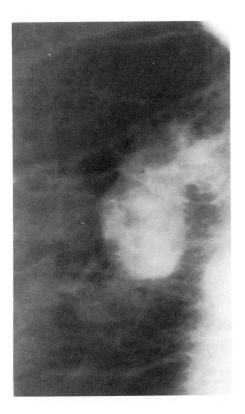

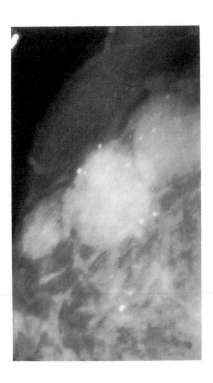

Figure 24–6. Calcifications with mucinous carcinoma. A 58-year-old woman with a lump in her breast for four years. Clinically: possible cancer. Mammography: 1.5, 2.5, and 3 cm carcinomas with minimal invasion but with typical round coarse calcifications of mucinous carcinoma. Pathology: three separate sites of mucin-producing carcinoma. Modified radical mastectomy; 22 axillary lymph nodes without metastasis. The patient was alive without disease eight years later.

Figure 24–7. A 59-year-old woman, seven years post menopause, nulliparous; no family history of breast cancer; partial amputation of the breast 22 years previously for fibrosarcoma; now firm nodule LIQ. *A,* A 6 × 10 mm mucinous carcinoma LIQ, slices 7 and 8; intramammary lymph node slice 4, LIQ; no metastasis (*B*). There were multiple small sites of mucinous carcinoma scattered throughout the breast. A 1.8 cm axillary lymph node noted on the mammogram was free of tumor. She had a modified radical mastectomy and was free of disease 13 years later.

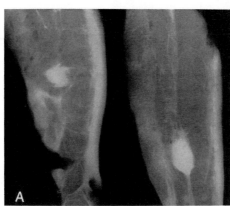
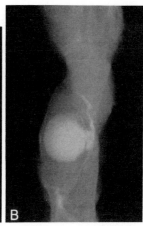

7). Hemorrhage into one of these carcinomas apparently is infrequent (Fig. 24–8).

Many of these carcinomas have progressed to a definite suspicious mass clinically (Figs. 24–9 and 24–10). Even so, these lesions still have good prognosis. In both cases (Figs. 24–9 and 24–10), after modified radical mastectomy, all axillary lymph nodes were free of tumor. The women were alive without disease 13 and 11 years, respectively, following surgery. Infrequent atypical calcifications may be seen in mucinous carcinomas (Fig. 24–11). Sonography has been helpful in this ill-defined carcinoma (Fig. 24–12).

PATHOLOGY

Grossly, the mucinous carcinoma is well delineated, almost encapsulated, and of jelly-like consistency. Its homogeneous appear-

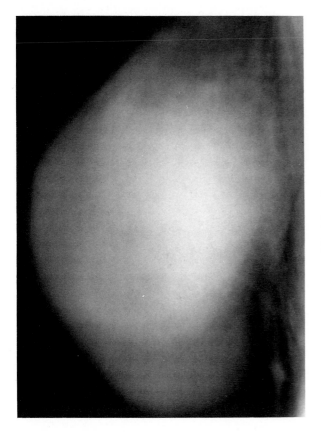

Figure 24–8. Hemorrhage into a mucinous carcinoma. A 51-year-old woman with a breast lump for over one year. Clinically: cystic mass. Mammography: invasive cystosarcoma phylloides or intracystic papillary carcinoma, 7 × 10 cm. Pathology: 10 cm cystic mass filled with old dark blood, on one wall of which was a mucin-producing carcinoma. Stage I lesion. The patient was free of disease 12 years later.

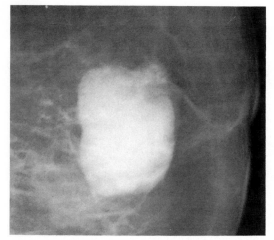

Figure 24–9. Mucinous carcinoma. Well-circumscribed mucinous carcinoma in a 67-year-old woman with a vague mass in the central portion of the breast. Mammograms: 3 × 4 cm discrete mass; only part of periphery indistinct; circumscribed carcinoma. Pathology: 3 × 4 cm mucin-producing carcinoma of the breast.

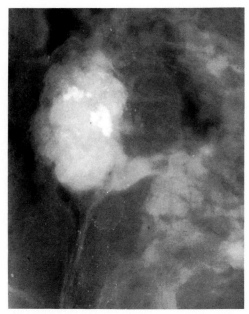

Figure 24–11. Whole-organ slicer of mucinous carcinoma. The lobulated mass is not highly invasive but contains fine and coarse calcifications.

ance clearly sets it off from the surrounding breast tissues. The contents are so friable that good frozen sections may be made only with some difficulty.

The pathologist must be able to distinguish pure from mixed carcinomas. The greater the ductal element of the carcinoma, the poorer the prognosis. The individual cells tend to form scattered acini from which lakes of mucinous material are secreted; these isolated clumps of cells appear to float on pools

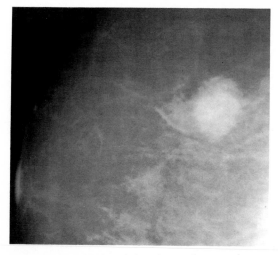

Figure 24–10. Moderately invasive mucinous carcinoma. Patient was a 75-year-old nulliparous woman. Clinically: moderately firm, fixed 2.5 × 3 cm carcinoma. Mammograms: moderately invasive carcinoma, 1.5 × 2 cm. Pathology: 2 cm mucin-producing carcinoma.

of this mucus. The intraductal component is infrequent, being clearly demonstrated as the only histologic type of malignancy in three of 18 of our mucinous carcinomas. Some areas of these in situ lesions also may secrete copious amounts of mucinous material.

CLINICAL COURSE

Even though the carcinomas per se are histologically pure mucinous carcinomas, it is important to make the clinical distinction of the single type of carcinoma vs multiple histologic types present in the same breast.

Multiplicity

In approximately 10 per cent of mucinous carcinomas, there were multiple sites of this tumor. In the 18 cases in which there was a single histologic type, three had an intraductal component of mucinous carcinoma. In 40 cases the mucinous carcinoma was associated with duct carcinoma, in one case with lobular carcinoma, in one case with medullary carcinoma with lymphoid stroma, and in one case with tubular carcinoma. In two cases there was both duct and lobular carcinoma; in two cases duct carcinoma and medullary carcinoma with lymphoid stroma were also present.

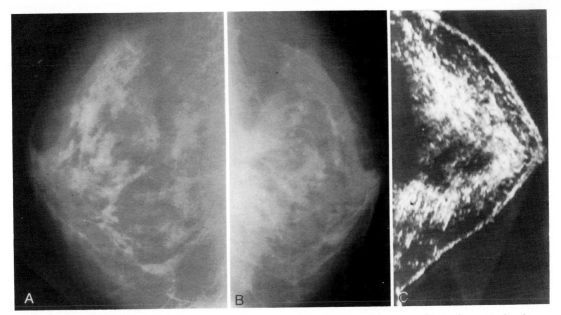

Figure 24–12. Sonography useful with a mucinous carcinoma. A 58-year-old woman felt a change in her breast. Clinically: thickening UOQ left breast. Mammography: ductal hyperplasia in left breast (reversed for comparison) on previous mammogram (*A*), then with a definite interval change in mid–left breast on mammogram 13 months later (*B*). *C*, Sonography (second study): hypoechoic area, jagged borders, nonhomogeneous internal echoes, shadowing; carcinoma. Pathology: mucin-producing carcinoma with an area of lobular carcinoma. Modified radical mastectomy; all 19 axillary lymph nodes free of tumor; the patient was alive and well four years later. This increase in tissue at this age is ominous, but the confirmation of the concern by sonography is welcome.

Bilaterality

Mucinous carcinoma can occur bilaterally. Bilateral primary carcinomas were present 11 times in our series; all were nonsimultaneous and in most cases the opposite breast contained a different type of carcinoma. In two of these cases, however, both primary mucinous carcinomas were of a single histologic type.

Treatment

Primary treatment consisted of radical mastectomy in 19 cases, modified radical mastectomy in 40 cases, total mastectomy in 2 cases and biopsy with tumorectomy in 4 cases. Whole-organ studies were available in seven cases; one of these thorough studies failed to demonstrate an additional carcinoma in that breast.

Prognosis

The prognosis is better for the lesion that meets stringent microscopic criteria for delineation of the typical mucinous carcinoma. In these pure cases in our series, even with rather large tumors, axillary lymph nodes were free of tumor in all but two cases (both having only low-node involvement) and no distant metastatic disease occurred. From Table 24–2, the two breast cancer deaths in patients having only mucinous carcinomas were in women with nonsimultaneous primary carcinomas with infiltrating duct carcinomas as the second lesion. Two women with nonsimultaneous bilteral mucinous carcinomas were free of disease five and seven years, respectively, after treatment of the second primary carcinoma.

CASE HISTORY

Large mucinous carcinoma. This 58-year-old woman had noted a right breast lump for at least seven months. She was gravida 3, para 3, and had nursed for a total of six months; her mother had a breast cancer. Clinically the 5 × 6 cm mass was firm, was freely movable, and in certain positions caused a bulging of the skin. The etiology was uncertain. Mammograms and sonograms were obtained (Fig. 24–13).

Pathology: Mucinous carcinoma. Modified radical mastectomy; all 21 axillary lymph nodes free of tumor. The patient was living without evidence of disease 32 months later.

TABLE 24–2. Follow-up of 66 Cases of Mucinous Carcinoma Alone or Associated With One or Two Other Histologic Types of Cancer

	One Type		Two Types		Three Types		Total	
	No.	% Alive	No.	% Alive	No.	% Alive	No.	% Alive
Patients treated ≥ 5 years ago	10		17		1		28	
Alive	9	90	14	82	1	100	24	86
Dead, breast cancer	1*		3†		0‡		4	
Dead, not breast cancer	0		0		0		0	
Patients treated ≥ 10 years ago	2		8		1		11	
Alive	1	50	5	63	0	100	6	55
Dead, breast cancer	1*		3		0		4	
Dead, not breast cancer	0		0		0		0	
Patients treated ≥ 20 years ago	0		2		0		2	
Alive	0	0	1	50	0	0	1	50
Dead, breast cancer	0		1		0		1	
Dead, not breast cancer	0		0		0		0	

*Nonsimultaneous bilateral with infiltrating duct carcinoma.
†Nine died of breast cancer within five years of treatment; one other cause.
‡One died of breast cancer within five years of treatment.

OBSERVATIONS

The more rigid the criteria for pure mucinous carcinoma, the better the prognosis for the lesion that fulfills them. The death rate or the axillary lymph node metastasis from these tumors is very low even when they have a multiple presence in the same breast. This is despite larger than average masses. The greater the element of duct carcinoma, the more the lesion becomes clinically like duct carcinoma.

The association of even the pure mucinous carcinoma with other histologic types of tumor, especially duct carcinoma, whether in the same breast or in the opposite breast, portends a marked increase in axillary lymph node metastasis (43 per cent, and to all nodal levels 29 per cent) and a similar reduction in survival.

Conservative treatment is possible with the single histologic type of pure mucinous carcinoma, but more aggressive treatment is necessary in the presence of infiltrative ductal elements and axillary lymph node metastasis.

Radiographically, the differential diagnoses are the usual rather well-circumscribed noncalcifying carcinomas. In the older woman this is most frequently intracystic papillary carcinoma. In younger women

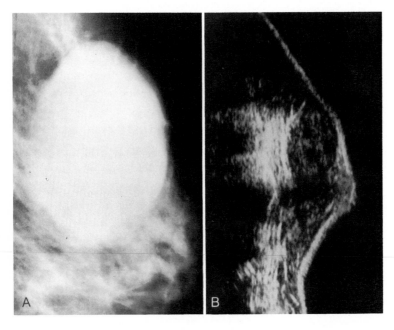

Figure 24–13. *A,* Mammography: There was a slightly lobulated, dense 4.2 × 5.5 cm mass with smooth borders anterolaterally; indistinct anterior border. Differential diagnosis: fibroadenoma, cystosarcoma phylloides, or circumscribed malignancy such as medullary carcinoma. *B,* Ultrasound: Fairly well-demarcated (except for lateral borders) hypoechoic mass; slightly lobulated borders; enhanced posterior borders; increased through-transmission. The internal echoes were so diffuse and nonhomogeneous that they appeared as nearby breast tissue. The lesion bulged the skin; there was no disrupted architecture.

medullary carcinoma with lymphoid stroma is more common. In all age groups sarcomas must be considered.

REFERENCES

Azzopardi JG (1979): Problems in Breast Pathology. Philadelphia, WB Saunders, p 296.

Haagensen CD (1986): Diseases of the Breast, 3rd ed. Philadelphia, WB Saunders, p 798.

McDivitt RW, Stewart FW, Berg JW (1968): Tumors of the Breast. Atlas of Tumor Pathology, Second series, Fascicle 2. Washington, DC, Armed Forces Institute of Pathology.

Norris HJ, Taylor HB (1965): Prognosis of mucinous (gelatinous) carcinoma of the breast. Cancer 18:879.

Silverberg SG, Kay S, Chitale AR, Levitt SH (1971): Colloid carcinoma of the breast. Am J Clin Pathol 55:355.

Veronesi U, Gennari L (1960): Il carcinoma gelatinoso della mammella. Tumori 46:119.

Paget's Disease of the Breast

25

BACKGROUND

Velpeau (1856) described the eczematous nipple lesion that we now recognize as part of Paget's syndrome of the breast. He did not realize that such lesions were associated with a mammary carcinoma. Paget (1874) again described similar nipple changes that resisted all local and general treatment. He did recognize subsequent discovery of a cancer "beneath or not far from the diseased skin." He noted, "For the sequence of cancer after the chronic skin disease is so frequent that it may be suspected of being a consequence and must be always feared."

As late as 1956 there was controversy regarding the etiology of Paget's disease of the breast. Haagensen (1956) devoted equal space to each of two hypotheses for the origin

of Paget's disease: (1) a lesion arising on the summit of the nipple that infiltrates the mammary tissues below; and (2) a lesion arising in the glandular breast tissue with extension into the epidermis of the nipple.

This confusion lessened with the advent of mammography, when the radiographic examination of the breast with Paget's disease of the nipple always, in our experience, demonstrated an intramammary cancer. At times mammography demonstrated a lesion in the breast with calcification extending toward the summit of the nipple, leading to discovery of clinically unsuspected Paget's syndrome of the breast.

Two such cases, first studied in 1956, that led to the clinical realization of the true nature of Paget's carcinoma of the breast are presented in Figures 25–1 and 25–2. With the first case the clinicians were not convinced that a central carcinoma was present despite nipple changes of Paget's disease and a mammographic carcinoma. Shortly thereafter, however, with the second case I was able to get the whole breast for the first conclusive study of the nature of Paget's disease of the breast. In those days, breasts were frozen in dry ice and cut into slices 1 cm thick on the machinist's band saw. Hence, metallic chips do show in the radiographs of the specimens.

This constant association of Paget cells of the nipple with an underlying duct cell carcinoma, however, does not provide the precise origin of the pagetoid cells. Azzopardi (1979) gleaned the following four hypotheses from the literature of the genesis of Paget cells in the epidermis: (1) altered melanocytes, (2) a form of squamous carcinoma, (3) adenocarcinoma cells, and (4) in situ origin in the epidermis. Even though the third view of tumor cell migration has the widest support, he ended by saying, "But the evidence remains inconclusive."

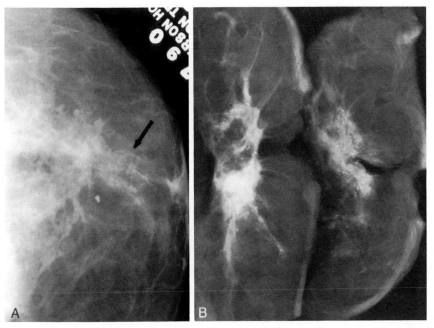

Figure 25–1. Paget's disease of the breast. A 59-year-old woman with nipple discharge accompanied by erosion; no palpable mass. *A*, Mammography showed a calcification pattern of carcinoma with only a faint surrounding density; intraductal carcinoma. Pathologically: intraductal carcinoma with Paget's disease of the nipple; 0 of 24 axillary lymph nodes positive. *B*, Slicer section after incision biopsy, better delineating the calcification following the course of the ducts.

INCIDENCE AND AGE DISTRIBUTION

Our series at Emory University included 40 women and one man with Paget's disease of the breast. This disease constituted 2.0 per cent of the total number of primary operable breast carcinomas. This incidence may actually be higher because unnoticed or subclinical pagetoid changes of the nipple are frequently overlooked for lack of thorough histopathologic study of the nipple.

The age of patients with Paget's carcinoma of the breast is not significantly different from the age of the usual breast cancer patient. The average age of our patients was 57.3 years, with the oldest being 77 and the youngest 31 years.

CLINICAL FEATURES

Changes of the nipple may be slight, with only an itching or burning sensation. Discoloration, thickening, and roughening of the epidermis follow. Scaling progresses into erosion with weeping and intermittent crusting. This indolent process responds partially and temporarily to creams and ointments but is always progressive. A saucer-like ulceration or a transverse crevice in the nipple may result and, when cleaned, has a reddish, granulomatous appearance. Spotting on the brassiere is caused by leakage of serum mixed with a small amount of old blood without true nipple discharge. The entire nipple becomes involved, with flattening taking place. The erosion eventually extends to the areola and in time may cover a great portion of the skin of the breast. Destruction, crusting with scarring, and retraction obliterate the normal configuration of the nipple and areola.

A clinical staging of Paget's carcinoma of the breast is pertinent to the understanding of the natural history of the disease, the treatment planning, and the prognosis.

Nonspecific Nipple Complaints

In the early stages of invasion of the nipple epidermis the patient complains of itching and a burning sensation and possibly a nipple discharge (Fig. 25–3). A true nipple discharge can be produced by Paget cells within the major subareolar ducts and lactiferous sinuses prior to changes in the nipple epidermis. Visual examination usually is nor-

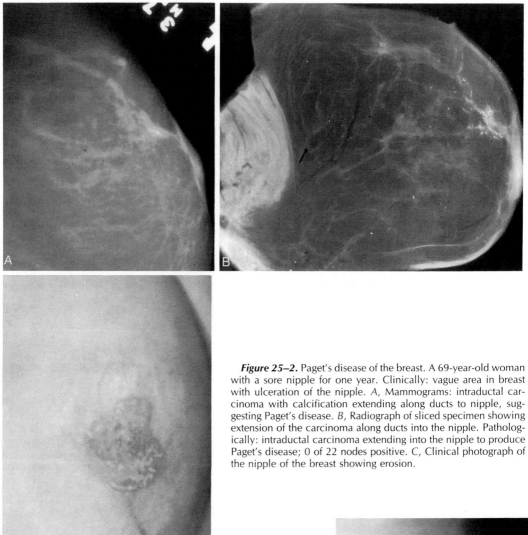

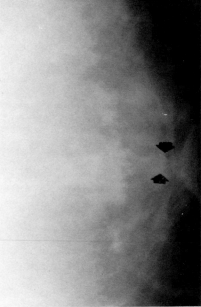

Figure 25–2. Paget's disease of the breast. A 69-year-old woman with a sore nipple for one year. Clinically: vague area in breast with ulceration of the nipple. *A,* Mammograms: intraductal carcinoma with calcification extending along ducts to nipple, suggesting Paget's disease. *B,* Radiograph of sliced specimen showing extension of the carcinoma along ducts into the nipple. Pathologically: intraductal carcinoma extending into the nipple to produce Paget's disease; 0 of 22 nodes positive. *C,* Clinical photograph of the nipple of the breast showing erosion.

Figure 25–3. Clinically unrecognized Paget's of the nipple. A 50-year-old woman had noted itching and burning of the nipple for months with recent progressive retraction. Clinically only mild nipple retraction was apparent. Mammography revealed a 3 × 4 cm spiculated subareolar carcinoma; fixed nipple. Pathologically: infiltrating duct carcinoma with Paget's disease of the nipple; axillary lymph nodes were free of metastasis.

mal. Mammography shows the mammary carcinoma, which is often still intraductal. Histopathologically, at this stage the Paget cells occur singly, usually in the basal portion of the epidermis. These are readily recognized as large cells with very prominent, irregular, hyperchromatic nuclei against a clear, slightly granular cytoplasm. Mitoses may be noted. Nipple biopsy confirms the diagnosis, and the patient is treated as for any intraductal or microinvasive duct carcinoma. Prognosis is very good.

Reddening and Eczema of the Nipple

With slightly more infiltration of the epidermis by small clumps of Paget cells, the nipple may take on a blush to bright red color. It appears smoother than its mate (Fig. 25–4). Further infiltration may produce an eczema. Microscopically the cornified layer of the epidermis remains intact, but underneath there is widespread infiltration both with Paget's cells and with lymphocytes. As no tumor is palpable, the prognosis remains good.

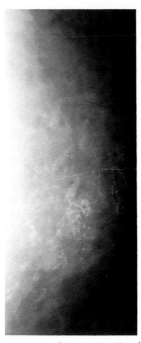

Figure 25–4. Paget's disease associated with diffuse calcifications of breast carcinoma. A 57-year-old woman had a smooth reddened itching nipple with intermittent discharge for three months. No mass was palpable. The diagnosis was primarily intraductal comedocarcinoma with limited microinvasion; lymph nodes were free of disease.

Erosion of the Nipple

The progression to erosion of the nipple is insidious. Spotting on the brassiere may lead to discovery of a crusted area on the nipple. When cleaned, a small, reddened, moist area is seen. This may respond temporarily to ointments and cleaning but invariably recurs and enlarges (Fig. 25–5). A crevice or an irregularly placed ulceration in the nipple may be produced, exuding a serous blood-tinged discharge from a reddened granulomatous area. Paget cells may be found throughout the epidermis of the nipple, but in the area of erosion the epidermis is replaced by Paget cells. Prognosis is worsened but remains good despite the long-term history of the presence of breast carcinoma.

Nipple Changes and Breast Tumor

The entire surface of the nipple may become eroded. The changes in the skin may extend onto the areola and beyond into the skin of the breast, erasing the areolar landmark (Fig. 25–6). The longer the course of pagetoid changes in the nipple, areola, and skin of the breast, the greater the likelihood of a mass being palpable clinically (Fig. 25–7). With a palpable primary breast carcinoma the probability of axillary lymph node metastasis is greatly increased. Treatment and prognosis then become similar to those for other Stage II breast carcinomas.

Breast Tumor, No Nipple Changes

The more aggressive infiltrating carcinomas may produce a breast mass in advance of nipple changes. The nipple changes will be present only microscopically (Fig. 25–8). The treatment and prognosis then become similar to those for any other similar infiltrating breast carcinoma. A nodular breast may mask the tumor (Fig. 25–9). Sonography may be positive (Fig. 25–10).

Nine times Paget's disease occurred in fatty breasts, 13 times with fatty ductal hyperplasia, four times with dense ductal hyperplasia, and five times in glandular or coarsely nodular breasts. Eleven cases without a mass and three with a mass were found by x-ray alone. All the cases had x-ray features of carcinoma; one developed under observation. Eleven of the cases without a mass by x-ray had some clinical abnormality and some palpable abnormality upon gross pathology.

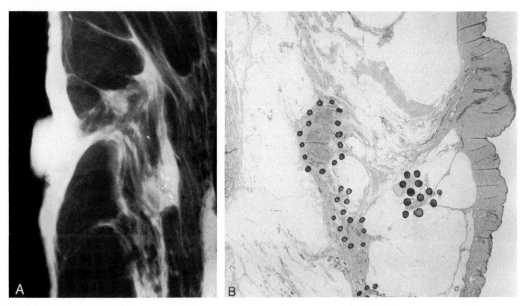

Figure 25–5. Paget's disease in a 67-year-old woman with tenderness of the nipple for six months. Minimal nipple erosion was noted only after mammograms revealed a nonpalpable central breast cancer. *A,* Whole-organ slicer sections through the area of calcification and pseudomass. *B,* H&E stains of section, carcinoma outlined by black dots. Pathologically: intraductal carcinoma and comedocarcinoma: 18 axillary nodes free of tumor.

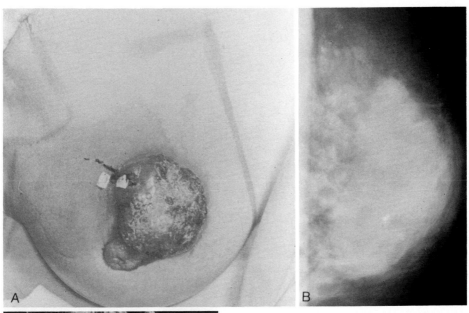

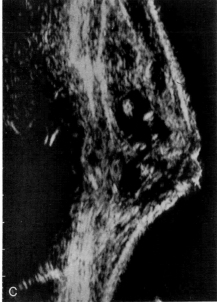

Figure 25–6. Extensive Paget's disease of nipple and areola. A 52-year-old woman with a breast mass enlarging for over one year. Nipple and areolar changes "for years." *A,* Clinically: whole breast a mass. Involvement of the nipple and areola with pagetoid skin changes. *B,* Mammography: Central carcinoma extending to a thickened areola; calcifications to the base of the nipple; retracted nipple; widespread skin changes. *C,* Sonography: In the central area of the breast is an irregular mass with nonhomogeneous internal echoes, architectural changes, irregular skin about nipple. Pathologically: 4 × 6.5 cm comedocarcinoma and infiltrating duct carcinoma with scirrhous element; Paget's disease. There were six low and midaxillary lymph nodes with metastasis.

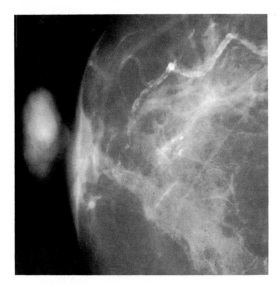

Figure 25–7. Paget's disease of the nipple. A 58-year-old woman with a swollen nipple for four months; no palpable mass. Mammograms: 1 × 1.5 cm area of stippled calcifications beneath a bulbous nipple. Pathologically: intraductal and microinvasive duct carcinoma with Paget's disease of the nipple. Axillary lymph nodes free of metastasis.

Figure 25–8. Large duct carcinoma and Paget's disease. A 55-year-old woman with a left breast mass for an unknown period. Clinically: carcinoma (no nipple changes noted). Mammography: 2.8 × 4.2 cm dense, moderately invasive carcinoma on a background of fatty ductal hyperplasia. Pathology: duct carcinoma. Modified radical mastectomy: none of 25 axillary lymph nodes with metastasis; Paget's disease of the nipple. The patient was alive and well three years later.

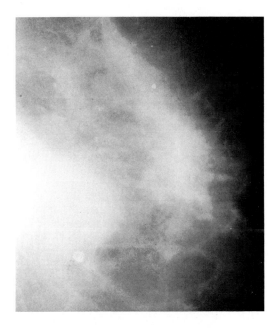

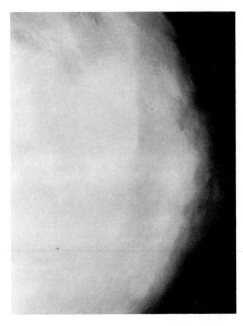

Figure 25–9. Early Paget's disease in a dense young breast. A 46-year-old woman with a history of recent intermittent right nipple discharge. Clinically the breasts were firm and nodular. Mammography: diffusely scattered areas of clustered punctate calcifications in the breast, suggesting comedocarcinoma. They are seen in the subareolar area but not in the nipple. Pathology: widespread comedo intraductal carcinoma with three sites of invasive tumor, one being beneath the nipple; Paget's disease. Modified radical mastectomy; 2 of 29 axillary lymph nodes with metastatic tumor. Three years later there was no evidence of disease.

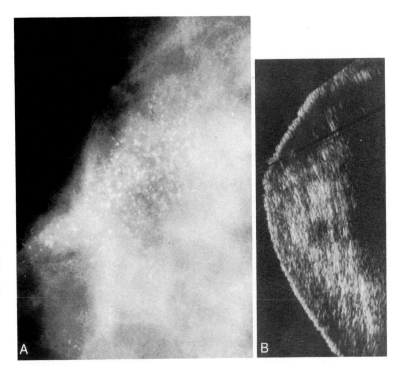

Figure 25–10. Comedocarcinoma with Paget's disease. A 46-year-old woman with a breast mass growing for three months. Clinically: suspicious thickening UIQ and redness of the nipple. *A,* Mammography: 1.5 × 3 cm area of calcification without mass typical of comedocarcinoma, extending into the nipple, suggesting the presence of Paget's disease. *B,* Sonography: slightly irregular hypoechoic area with moderate shadowing. Pathology: intraductal and comedocarcinoma, Paget's disease of the nipple. Modified radical mastectomy; all 20 axillary lymph nodes free of tumor; fibrocystic disease consisting of adenosis, papillomatosis, epitheliosis, fibrosis, and microcysts. The patient was alive and well three years later.

Of the 17 cases with a radiographic mass, 14 had a palpable abnormality and 13 of these had an abnormality on gross pathology. In 26 cases the lesions were 0 to 2 cm in size, with three being more than 5 cm in greatest diameter.

RADIOGRAPHIC CHANGES

The usual lesion of the breast producing these changes in the nipple is an intraductal carcinoma limited primarily to the ducts, with little tendency for invasion of surrounding tissues. This lack of invasion into the glandular tissue and the absence of a mass may lead to clinical confusion as to the etiology of the nipple changes. In 75 per cent of our cases of Paget's disease of the breast, the primary lesion was not palpable, even though its extent was usually outlined graphically on the mammogram by typical stippled calcifications. Almost any histologic type of carcinoma of the breast can produce Paget's disease. The radiographic appearance of the mammary cancer will depend to a degree on the histologic type.

The radiographic diagnosis of Paget's carcinoma is apparent only if there is demonstrable nipple erosion or if fine calcifications can be traced from the deeper carcinoma along a major duct into the nipple. Occasionally the nipple is bulbous.

HISTOLOGIC CHANGES

The carcinoma in the breast grows along the lumen of a major duct into the nipple. Large vacuolated pagetoid cells are found in the epidermis of the nipple and epithelium of the major ducts. In our series, although only 25 per cent of the carcinomas were palpable, in all instances the underlying malignancy was demonstrable by mammography. Axillary lymph nodes are seldom involved until the carcinoma of the breast becomes palpable, at which time the incidence of positive axillary lymph nodes increases sharply.

CLINICAL COURSE

Mass vs No Mass

Paget's disease of the breast may be much better appreciated if the syndrome is reduced simply to the absence or presence of a mass of breast carcinoma. This relates particularly to diagnosis, size of tumor, metastatic spread, and prognosis.

With the use of mammography (Tables 25–1 and 25–2), more cases were detected by mammography alone and all cases were detected by x-ray. Of the patients without a mass by x-ray only three had low axillary lymph node metastasis, but when a mass was present, nearly one half had metastasis to all three levels of axillary lymph nodes. Obviously, the size of the mass recorded by gross pathology was also much greater when a mass was present by x-ray. Usually the size of the mass on gross pathology when no mass was demonstrated by x-ray indicated the extent or area of involvement rather than a discrete mass size.

Multiplicity

In 13 cases there were two to five distinct sites of carcinoma in the breast associated with Paget's disease, often distant from the central one under the nipple that was considered the source of the nipple changes. In five breasts there were more than six separate sites of tumor. These less aggressive tumors, especially those without a mass, were often microscopically invasive only. In only one case was a purely intraductal carcinoma, without demonstrable invasion, the only histologic type of tumor found. In the other 22 cases without mass the intraductal component was associated with infiltrating duct carcinoma.

In three breasts, in addition to a duct carcinoma, there was an instance of mucoid carcinoma, lobular carcinoma, and papillary carcinoma.

Bilaterality

Seven patients had bilateral Paget's disease of the breast—all nonsimultaneous and opposite Paget's disease without a mass, each also being without a mass. These lesions contained an abundance of nonaggressive intraductal components frequently associated with comedo type intraductal carcinoma, which, in turn, is often present as bilateral breast carcinoma. These slowly evolving carcinomas perhaps differ from those that produce a mass in Paget's disease, in which there were no bilateral carcinomas in this series.

Treatment

In Paget's disease of the breast without a mass the treatment was radical mastectomy

eight times (four of these had whole-organ studies), modified radical mastectomy twelves times, and complete mastectomy four times. In those patients with an x-ray mass, radical mastectomy was the treatment in ten, modified radical mastectomy in six, and complete mastectomy in one.

Prognosis

Without a mass, the crude five-year survival was 87 per cent, and ten-year survival was 78 per cent. With a mass, the five-year survival was 40 per cent, and there was no ten-year survivor.

CASE HISTORY

A 55-year-old white housewife presented with a two-month history of crusting of her left nipple associated with scanty discharge (Fig. 25–11A). There had been some diffuse tenderness, a sensation of burning, and enlargement of the breast accompanying these nipple changes. The patient was ten years beyond a natural menopause. One sister and one niece had breast cancer.

Clinically the left breast was larger than the right: A 2 mm area of erosion of the nipple was covered by a crust. No masses, lymphadenopathy, or other abnormality was found in either breast.

Mammography disclosed two clusters of calcification in the deep central portion of the left breast (Fig. 25–11B). These were stippled calcifications of carcinoma and could be traced along the ducts well into the nipple; a radiographic diagnosis of Paget's carcinoma was suggested. (Fibroglandular tissue, without a mass, appears very dense on this 0.5 cm sliced section.)

A biopsy of the central portion of the lesion of the left nipple was obtained, and subsequent study revealed typical pagetoid changes (Fig. 25–11C). One week later a left radical mastectomy was performed. The clinical course was uneventful, and the patient has remained without breast problems for the past ten years. She has been followed with yearly mammograms. Of incidental interest is that she had developed a squamous cell carcinoma of the wrist.

The mastectomy specimen was frozen overnight and cut into 27 sagittal sections 5 mm thick. On gross examination of the subareolar area there were dilated ducts or cysts measuring about 1 mm across and filled with yellow-white opaque material. Nineteen axillary lymph nodes removed from the specimen were found free of tumor.

In Figure 25–11C the carcinomatous tissue can be seen following the ducts to the summit of the nipple, showing the small defect from the biopsy. Figure 25–11D–G shows the typical appearance of most of the carcinoma. The tumor was confined to the ducts for the most part, but microinvasion was observed in other sections. This was classified as a comedo

TABLE 25–1. Features of Paget's Disease of the Breast Without Mass

Path. Type Cancers	Num- ber	Patient Age (Years)				Detection				Axillary Lymph Nodes			Path. Tumor Size (cm)					Path. Sites			Survival: Alive/Dead (Years)			
		<40	40–50	51–60	60+	X P +–	X P ++	X P –+	X P ––	None	Low	All Levels	0	<1	1–2	2.1–5	>5	1	2–5	6+	<5	5–9	10–19	20+
One	23	2	7	9	5	15	7	0	1	20	3	0	14	2	2	4	1	14	6	3	14/3	0/2	3/1	0/0
Two	1	0	0	1	0	0	1	0	0	1	0	0	0	1	0	0	0	0	1	0	0/0	0/0	1/0	0/0
Total	24	2	7	10	5	15	8	0	1	21	3	0	14	3	2	4	1	14	7	3	14/3	0/2	4/1	0/0

X = x-ray; P = physical examination; + = positive; – = negative.

TABLE 25–2. Features of Paget's Disease of the Breast With a Mass

Path. Type Cancers	Num- ber	Patient Age (Years)				Detection				Axillary Lymph Nodes			Path. Tumor Size (cm)					Path. Sites			Survival: Alive/Dead (Years)			
		<40	40–50	51–60	60+	X P +–	X P ++	X P –+	X P ––	None	Low	All Levels	0	<1	1–2	2.1–5	>5	1	2–5	6+	<5	5–9	10–19	20+
One	15	0	5	4	6	3	12	0	0	6	1	8	4	0	3	7	1	10	4	1	7/6	1/1	0/0	0/0
Two	2	0	1	0	1	0	2	0	0	1	1	0	0	0	1	1	0	0	2	0	1/1	0/0	0/0	0/0
Total	17	0	6	4	7	3	14	0	0	7	2	8	4	0	4	8	1	10	6	1	8/7	1/1	0/0	0/0

X = x-ray; P = physical examination; + = positive; – = negative.

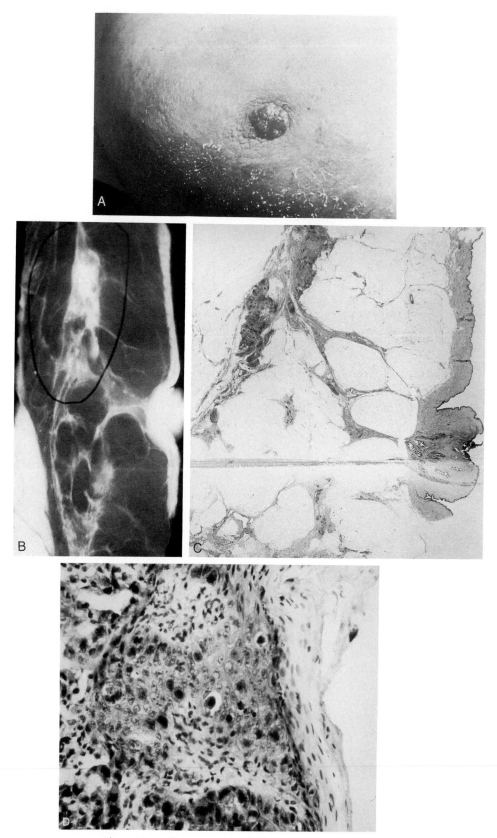

Figure 25–11 *Illustration and legend continued on opposite page*

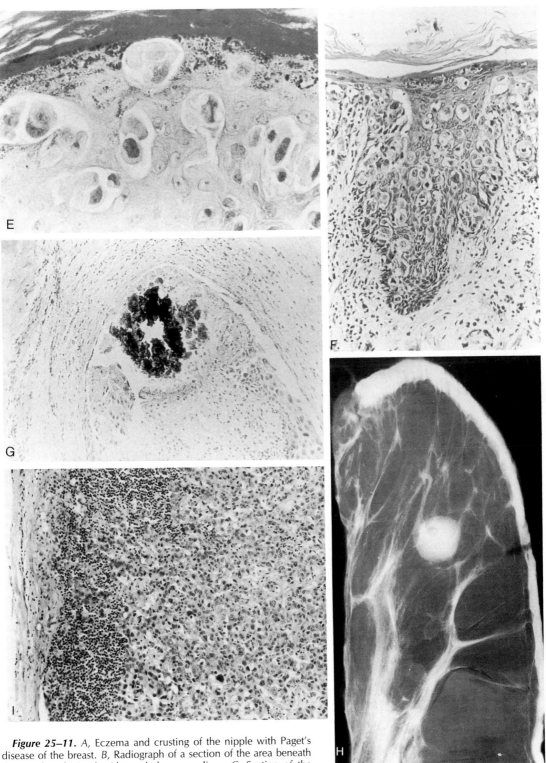

Figure 25–11. *A,* Eczema and crusting of the nipple with Paget's disease of the breast. *B,* Radiograph of a section of the area beneath the nipple, obtained with a whole-organ slicer. *C,* Section of the nipple showing crusting, and whole-slicer section through central carcinoma (dark area) and nipple. *D,* Large vacuolated Paget's cells within the epidermis. *E,* Higher power of Paget's cells. *F,* Extension deep into dermis. *G,* Low power of one of the ducts showing intraductal debris associated with comedocarcinoma with von Kossa stain of the comedocarcinoma. *H,* Intramammary lymph node LOQ containing metastasis. *I,* Microscopic section of lymph node containing tumor.

type carcinoma. There were pagetoid cells within the breast. Figure 25–11G is a modified von Kossa stain of an area of the comedo type carcinoma with the calcifications staining black. An intramammary lymph node was present (Fig. 25–11H and I).

Paget's carcinoma of the breast is a syndrome of carcinoma within the breast with secondary changes in the epithelium of the nipple. The carcinoma is usually located centrally in the breast, is intraductal or minimally invasive, and can be of almost any morphologic type of breast cancer.

OBSERVATIONS

Confusion as to the etiology of the nipple changes is understandable. Such changes have been mistaken for Bowen's disease of the skin. The usual lesion of the breast that produces pagetoid changes of the nipple is an intraductal or mildly aggressive ductal carcinoma with little or no invasion to produce a palpable mass. These carcinomas could easily be overlooked by the pathologist on gross sectioning just as any other intraductal carcinoma without specimen radiography might be overlooked.

This absence of a palpable carcinoma in the mastectomy specimen in 40 per cent of Gallager's cases (1985) led him to conclude that Paget's disease of the nipple could be invasive or noninvasive and, as in the vulva, was a "peculiar form of carcinoma that arises from the skin derived from the epithelium of the primitive milk ridge." In only one fourth of our patients was the primary lesion palpable in the intact breast, even though it was clearly outlined on the mammograms in all instances. Specimen radiography may be necessary to demonstrate the true nature of Paget's syndrome of the breast.

Paget's carcinoma of the breast need not be considered the result of a bizarre carcinoma; it simply results from a central breast carcinoma. Growth along the nonobstructing ducts indicates the presence of a less aggressive carcinoma that will produce clinical signs in a later period of growth. Clinicians may not recognize a central carcinoma of the breast as a true etiologic agent for Paget's carcinoma of the nipple. Histologic evidence

of Paget's carcinoma of the nipple can be considered a definite sign of carcinoma of the breast, thereby making frozen-section prior to mastectomy unnecessary.

Paget's carcinoma convincingly supports our long-held belief that breast cancer is a lengthy, indolent disease. The deep cancer must precede nipple changes, and the nipple changes progress over many years prior to metastases of the cancer beyond the breast. Such cancers are readily detectable by mammography years before they become life-threatening. In our experience, high-resolution mammography has never failed to demonstrate the smallest Paget's carcinoma.

Paget's disease of the breast has been associated with almost every known histologic type of breast carcinoma. This includes medullary, mucinous, and noninvasive intracystic papillary carcinoma. Even when it has been difficult or impossible to demonstrate additional histologic types of carcinoma in a particular breast, it is still most likely that the Paget's changes of the nipple have resulted from some form of duct or intraductal carcinoma: (1) Often intraductal carcinomas are associated with circumscribed carcinomas; and (2) a widespread intraductal component of circumscribed carcinomas is most unlikely. Any pagetoid changes of the nipple other than through the collecting duct system extending into the nipple is always pseudo-Paget's disease.

REFERENCES

Azzopardi JG (1979): Problems in Breast Pathology. Philadelphia, WB Saunders, p 258.

Gallager HS (1985): Malignant breast diseases: pathology. In Harper P (ed): Ultrasound Mammography. Baltimore, University Park Press, p 97.

Haagensen CD (1956): Disease of the Breast. Philadelphia, WB Saunders.

Paget Sir J (1874): On disease of the mammary areola preceding cancer of the mammary gland. St Barth Hosp Rep 10:86.

Velpeau A (1856). A Treatise on the Diseases of the Breast and Mammary Region. Translation from the French by Mitchell Henry. London, Sydenham Society.

Inflammatory Carcinoma

26

BACKGROUND

The poor prognosis of carcinoma of the breast associated with inflammatory signs in the overlying skin has been recognized for many years. Bell in 1811 referred to "the unpropitious beginning" of a breast tumor when the overlying skin was of purple color and was accompanied by shooting pains. Isolated case reports (Klotz, 1869; Volkmann, 1875; Rodman, 1909) appeared in the literature from time to time, and the condition was referred to by a variety of names: mastitis carcinomatous gravidarum and lactatum, acute carcinoma, acute brawny cancer, carcinoma mastoides, acute medullary carcinoma, acute mammary carcinoma, acute encephaloid cancer, inflamed cancer, and acute scirrhous carcinoma, among others (Lee and Tannenbaum, 1924).

All observers agreed that the inflammatory signs associated with carcinoma of the breast were of ominous prognostic significance; the condition remained ill defined until it was established as a clinical entity by the classic work of Lee and Tannenbaum in 1924. Since that time, several large series (Meyer et al.,

1948; Barber et al., 1961; Haagensen, 1986; Robbins et al., 1974) have been reported. Controversy still exists as to the best approach for improved treatment of this lethal disease.

Although inflammatory carcinoma is not a common manifestation of carcinoma of the breast, it is so striking that the clinician is quite impressed and recalls vividly the poor prognosis associated with clinical signs of inflammation. By the same token, the clinical manifestations are so unusual that they are often misinterpreted by the physician who is first consulted. The lack of recognition of this phase of breast carcinoma results in long delays in establishing the existence of a true nonbacterial process.

Thickened skin of the breast not associated with inflammatory changes is less striking; in fact, it is often overlooked by the examiner. The pathologist also frequently fails to recognize skin thickening, which may be improperly attributed to obliquity of the microscopic section or retraction of the biopsy specimen. Likewise, there may be failure to appreciate the significance of thickening if no tumor cells are recognized in the skin or dermal lymphatics. Histopathologic study of the skin of the entire breast is not routinely done. Skin thickening of the breast is so graphically recorded on the mammograms as a radiographic diagnostic aid that its explicit relationship to prognosis is invaluable.

In our experience, diffuse skin thickening of the breast not associated with signs of inflammation is just as important a sign of lethality as clinically inflammatory cancer.

The diagnoses of all reported cases of inflammatory carcinomas of the breast have not been based on rigid criteria. We have adopted Lee's definition that inflammatory carcinoma of the breast is "of rapid growth, the overlying skin becoming edematous, red to purplish in color, dimpled, brawny and having elevated edges after the manner of erysipelas." He suggested that at least 25 per cent of the skin of the breast must be affected.

439

Rapid growth is implied clinically, but radiographically the natural history of inflammatory carcinoma is not unlike that of other infiltrating duct carcinomas. The diagnosis of inflammatory cancer remains a clinical one, with radiologic and pathologic confirmatory studies.

Taylor and Meltzer (1938) indicated two clinical varieties of inflammatory carcinoma: (1) primary, in which the inflammatory signs simultaneously accompanied the clinical evidence of cancer arising in a previously normal breast; and (2) secondary, in which the inflammatory signs appear in a breast harboring a cancer for a long time, usually after prior biopsy and/or treatment either in the original site or in the opposite breast. Our consideration of inflammatory breast carcinoma completely excludes all cases of the secondary variety. The presence of a mass is usually known, particularly by mammography, prior to the primary inflammatory phase.

STUDY SERIES

Two series of patients with inflammatory carcinoma of the breast in which the author was involved were reviewed, compared, and contrasted.

One was from M.D. Anderson Hospital and Tumor Institute (MDAH) and consisted of 2145 cases of carcinoma of the breast during the ten-year period from September 1, 1952 to August 31, 1961. On 127 cases there were clinical annotations of redness, infection, and/or edema on the charts. All cases in which signs were considered to be due to local changes of necrosis of the skin, fungation, or inflammatory reaction surrounding a biopsy site were discarded. Inflammatory changes in the chest wall, operative site, or the remaining breast following treatment for a noninflammatory cancer also were excluded. The cases in which definitive treatment was not performed at that institution were excluded as well. The study then was composed of 31 inflammatory carcino-mas in 30 women. The diagnosis was confirmed histologically in each instance.

The second study comprised all patients with a diagnosis of inflammatory breast carcinoma who were seen and treated at Emory University Cinic during the 20-year period from 1960 to 1980. Among 3261 consecutive cases of all recorded breast cancer, 79 were considered to be primary inflammatory carcinoma. A total of 146 secondary inflammatory carcinomas was excluded. Again, any secondary signs of inflammation had caused exclusion of patients. In all cases the diagnosis was confirmed histologically except for ten cases that were confirmed by clinical course and x-ray changes alone.

INCIDENCE AND AGE

The reported incidence of inflammatory carcinoma varies with each institution. It is usually less than 1 per cent of the total breast cancers in a general hospital but may be as great as 2 to 4 per cent in an oncologic hospital. Our experience with primary inflammatory carcinoma has ranged from 1.4 to 2.4 per cent of total cancers. It constitutes 1.4 per cent (Lee and Tannenbaum, 1924), 1.5 per cent (Haagensen, 1971), 1.7 per cent (Barber et al., 1961) and 4 per cent (Taylor and Meltzer, 1938) of all breast cancers.

The women in our series ranged in age from 27 to 83 years with an average of 51.4 years—not unlike the age range for all breast cancers.

CLINICAL MANIFESTATIONS

A specific breast lump is not the usual first manifestation of inflammatory carcinoma (Table 26–1). Instead, the woman notices tenderness or pain, overall firmness, enlargement or heaviness of the breast, a pinkish or dusky appearance to the skin of the breast, or an occasional brawniness of the skin. She may volunteer the information that changes appeared suddenly and advanced rapidly be-

TABLE 26–1. Presenting Symptoms in Patients With Primary Inflammatory Carcinoma of the Breast

	Mean Age (Years)	Mass	Diffuse Enlargement	Pain	Heaviness	Not Recorded	Average Duration	Range Duration
MDAH	48.1	50.0%	26.7%	16.7%	3.3%	3.3%	5 mo	1 wk–16 mo
Emory	52.7	36.7	21.5	27.8	6.3	7.7	3.6 mo	1 wk–31 mo

TABLE 26–2. Reasons for Delay in Treatment of Inflammatory Carcinoma

	Poor Medical Advice	Ignorance	Patient Neglect	Economic Reasons	Fear	Not Stated
MDAH	34.6%	23.1%	23.1%	7.7%	3.3%	8.2%
Emory	27.8*	15.2	31.6	1.3	20.3	3.8

*In two cases, mammography was considered normal initially.

fore she consulted a physician. The duration of symptoms may be a few days to more than a year (Table 26–2). A few of our patients admitted delays from 6 months to 2.5 years. Over one fourth of the women had been treated for infection for periods ranging from a few days to several months.

Inflammatory carcinoma typically occurred in large breasts, usually associated with marked generalized obesity. Large, pendulous breasts were specifically noted in most patients. With the average breast carcinoma, retractive signs were frequently present. In contrast, inflammatory carcinoma produced generalized and global enlargement of the involved breast without contracture or local retraction. Only in very few instances did the breast fail to show concomitant enlargement with the malignant inflammatory process.

Two of the most distinctive features of inflammatory carcinoma of the breast are redness and edema of the skin, not especially related to the tumor (Table 26–3). Both signs may be present to satisfy the definition of inflammatory carcinoma. The reddened area may vary in hue between deep red and purple, and its periphery is sharply demarcated (erysipeloid). Skin edema often is readily apparent as *peau d'orange*.

Despite the bulk of the tumor and the frequency of cutaneous satellite metastases, the skin usually remains intact. The lesions begin so deep in the large breasts that there is involvement of most of the breast at the earliest discovery.

Although increased heat was noted in over one half of our cases, it is likely that this subjective finding would have been much more frequent with keener observation and more complete notation of the physical findings.

Patients with inflammatory carcinoma of the breast are very susceptible to the development of carcinoma in the other breast. Meyer et al. (1948) reported bilateral involvement in 13 per cent of patients in their series. Rogers and Fitts (1956) reported an incidence of 30 per cent, while Barber et al. (1961) gave an incidence of 26 per cent. The high incidence of bilateral involvement has also been stressed by other investigators (Taylor and Meltzer, 1938). Thirty per cent of the patients in our MDAH series developed bilateral disease, with bilateral simultaneous lesions in one patient. In the Emory University series, bilateral simultaneous inflammatory carcinomas occurred in three patients, with the opposite breast subsequently being involved in 28 per cent of the cases. All these figures are considerably in excess of the 6 to 8 per cent of carcinoma of the breast in general reported by Meyer et al. (1948).

The exact reasons for the frequency of inflammatory carcinoma are not clear. In our experience, however, diffuse or multicentric carcinoma in one breast tends to be accompanied by carcinoma in the opposite breast, both primary and metastatic. Also, a very large number of inflammatory carcinomas have spread beyond the confines of the breast upon initial presentation of the patient. Spread to the opposite breast then could simply be another manifestation of disseminated disease, just as supraclavicular lymph node metastasis is.

It has been suggested, notably by Schumann (1911), that a causal relationship exists between pregnancy and inflammatory carcinoma of the breast. However, the findings of other investigators (Lee and Tannenbaum, 1924; Meyer et al., 1948; Rogers and Fitts, 1956; Barber et al., 1961) indicate that the development of inflammatory carcinoma is

TABLE 26–3. Clinical Involvement of Skin and Axilla in Inflammatory Carcinoma

	Area Skin Involved						Axillary Lymph Nodes
	100%	*50–100%*	*50%*	*25–50%*	*25%*	*Not Recorded*	
MDAH	20.0%	56.6%	16.7%	3.3%	3.3%	—	100.0%
Emory	16.4	63.3	3.8	6.3	—	10.2	87.3

not influenced by pregnancy. The latter view is supported by findings in our MDAH series, in which only one patient of the 30, or 3.3 per cent of the group, developed cancer during pregnancy or in the immediate postpartum period.

All patients were married or had been married. Five patients had never achieved pregnancy. One patient was pregnant when first seen. Two of the remaining 24 women who gave a history of pregnancy recounted an interval of 15 and 36 months, respectively, between the end of the pregnancy and the development of signs of cancer. In the remaining 22 patients, at least 48 months elapsed between the end of pregnancy and the onset of the clinical diagnosis of inflammatory carcinoma of the breast.

DIAGNOSIS

The average physician encounters inflammatory carcinoma uncommonly. Thus, initially he may be inclined to consider other disease entities, such as (1) true acute bacterial infection, such as abscess; (2) duct ectasia and chronic subareolar abscess; (3) inflamed cyst; (4) necrosis with a medullary carcinoma; (5) carcinoma *en cuirasse;* or (6) skin involvement by advanced carcinoma.

Physical Examination

Upon clinical examination the areola is usually normal in position and outline. However, some degree of retraction, flattening, or inversion of the nipple is present in about one half the patients. Crusting of the nipple, erosion, or discharge from the nipple may be elicited in over 10 per cent of cases. The discharge may be bloody. Twenty-five to 100 per cent of the skin may be involved (Table 26–3).

Clinically, the homolateral axillary lymph nodes are involved in almost all cases (Table 26–3). The lymph nodes are discrete and movable 50 per cent of the time but are matted or fixed to surrounding tissue or overlying skin in one third of the patients. Their status is not always recorded. The homolateral supraclavicular lymph nodes may be involved at the time of the initial examination in at least 50 per cent of the cases.

Fixation of the carcinoma to the underlying pectoral muscle is frequently present. Such fixation is judged by restriction of movability of the tumor on the actively contracting muscle.

Dermal lymphatic engorgement may be advanced at least six weeks before signs of inflammatory carcinoma appear. The presence of clinically recognized dermal lymphatic engorgement with tumor cells does not indicate that inflammatory carcinoma will develop. The clinical finding of engorged dermal lymphatics alerts the clinician to the poor prognosis.

Many of the patients will develop carcinoma in the opposite breast, mostly primary carcinomas of a noninflammatory nature. The patients may present with a double primary inflammatory carcinoma, with a simultaneous primary inflammatory and a noninflammatory carcinoma, or with metastases from the breast involved with inflammatory carcinoma. The axillary lymph nodes on the side of the second breast lesion are often involved. It is difficult to determine which breast may be the source.

In our two series the right breast was involved in 59 cases and the left breast in 54 (four cases were bilateral simultaneous inflammatory carcinomas).

Radiographic Examination

The mammograms do not record heat or color. The radiologist can neither diagnose inflammatory carcinoma of the breast nor differentiate diffuse skin thickening due to inflammatory carcinoma from that due to noninflammatory carcinoma of the breast. His observations should be purely objective.

Mammograms were obtained on 43 per cent of our patients. Generalized skin thickening was present in all cases, although in some it was mild. In 82 per cent of the women there was generalized increased density of the affected breast, and in one third a mass was seen through the increased density. However, in the others the mass was obscured by a further increase in density. In two patients the overall increase in breast density was apparent only after careful comparison with the opposite breast in retrospect. Other nonspecific radiographic signs of vascular engorgement, increase in size of the breast, and axillary adenopathy aided in suggesting the diagnosis.

Mammograms of breasts with diffuse thickening of the skin associated with carcinoma often are of poor quality. This results not only from the increased thickness and density of the overlying skin but also from the associated diffuse carcinoma within the breast. The mammograms, however, can always be of sufficiently good quality to record the skin thickening.

There are three usual types of skin thickening projected on the mammograms that are associated with breast carcinoma: (1) localized skin thickening adjacent to the mass; (2) localized skin thickening inferior to the areola and at a distance from the carcinoma; and (3) diffuse skin thickening of the entire breast. Each type may be evident radiographically before it is apparent clinically. No differentiation between inflammatory and noninflammatory carcinoma of the breast is attempted by mammography.

Lymphatic channel engorgement with carcinoma is recorded on the mammograms as massive by dilated lymphatics streaking toward the nipple through the subcutaneous fat as a result of malignant cells spreading along the lymphatic channels and suspensory ligaments.

The sequence of events leading to diffuse thickening of the skin may be reconstructed by study of many mammograms made at various stages of tumor growth (Fig. 26–1). Both noninflammatory and inflammatory carcinoma of the breast have identical patterns of growth radiographically (Fig. 26–2). The inflammatory type of carcinoma can be differentiated clinically only by the final erysipeloid appearance of the skin. The original lesion in both types is an invasive carcinoma located deep in the glandular substance of a pendulous breast that is difficult to examine clinically. The growth pattern of the carcinoma apparently produces fewer clinical signs of retraction, and a less distinct mass may be noted on physical examination. Marked dilatation of the subcutaneous veins is evident on the mammograms.

It can be postulated that there is interference with vascular drainage of the breast resulting from the increased mass of densely packed carcinoma cells and breast tissue and from actual invasion of the subcutaneous tissues by carcinoma. There may be similar interference with the lymphatic drainage, as large axillary nodes have already been formed. Local skin retraction and thickening is seldom seen with this type of lesion. By the time the primary lesion is 2 to 3 cm in size on the mammograms, there is the beginning of thickening of the skin inferior to the areola. At this stage an overall increase in density of the breast is noted. Progression to diffuse infiltration of the entire breast tissue by carcinoma is rapid (Fig. 26–3).

The production of diffuse skin thickening occurs simultaneously. Radiographic study at this more advanced stage seldom reveals a distinct mass; a needle biopsy of almost any portion of the breast usually results in a histopathologic diagnosis of carcinoma. In the early stage of diffuse skin thickening, the carcinoma may be palpable. The mass often feels three to four times its actual size, as the palpating fingers include the skin thickening and the fibrotic reaction about the mass as part of the carcinoma. As more extensive involvement of the breast and skin takes place, no distinct mass is palpable (Fig. 26–4). There is a period when the primary carcinoma is no longer palpable but is still seen on the mammogram (Fig. 26–5). Inflammatory carcinoma may mimic metastatic disease clinically (Fig. 26–6).

Sonographic Examination

Breast sonography adds little information. Thickening of the skin is poorly appreciated by sonography. Usually, by the time of the examination the cancer is so advanced that most of the breast shows only evidence of increased density and distortion of the echoes throughout the breast. On occasion, before changes are so advanced, the mass will be detected but usually only when it is still apparent on the mammograms.

PATHOLOGIC STUDIES

The primary tumor mass is a large, highly invasive duct carcinoma with marked desmoplasia when observed radiographically. The primary mass is not always studied histologically. Study of an area of spread of the tumor within the breast or the skin may be used as the confirmatory diagnosis. For example, only one third of our diagnoses were established by open biopsy. Aspiration biopsy of the breast and/or skin or skin ellipses from representative areas of redness and edema usually furnished the diagnosis.

Microscopically, a wide variety of carcinomas produce inflammatory carcinomas: infiltrating duct combined with intraductal; scirrhous; large cell; small cell; and even circumscribed carcinomas. Most are classified

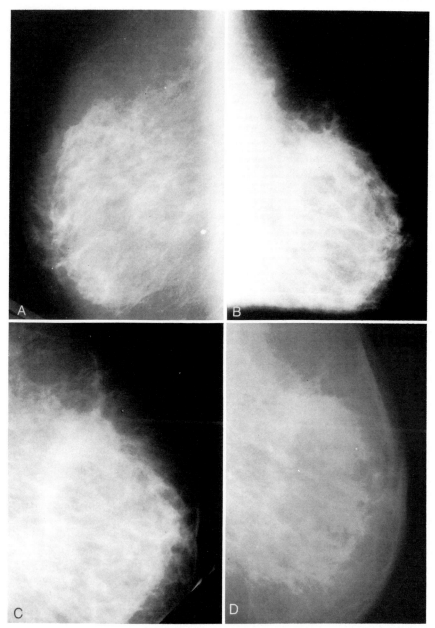

Figure 26–1. Rapid development of an inflammatory lesion. A 61-year-old woman seen for routine checkup for nodular breasts. Mammography: on original bilateral studies (*A* and *B*), severe diffuse ductal hyperplasia in pendulous breasts; increased density on the left with a 1.8 × 2 cm moderately invasive carcinoma UOQ. Three months later, physical examination "benign," with the radiographic carcinoma (*C*) measuring 2 × 2.4 cm in size. Two months later all signs of inflammation present (by history for less than seven days) radiographically (*D*); diffusely thickened skin with localized retraction, edema, and increased density throughout the breast. Pathology (biopsy): duct carcinoma with fibrosis, extensive intravascular and lymphatic spread with carcinoma in the dermal lymphatics. Death occurred from disseminated disease 11 months following diagnosis.

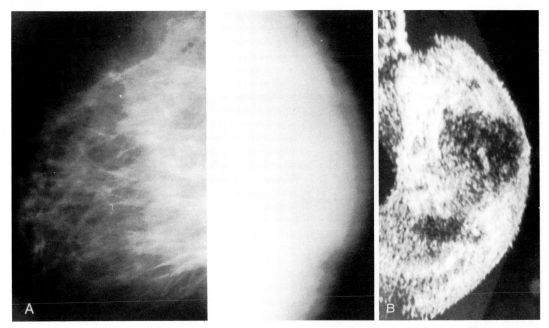

Figure 26–2. Inoperable, noninflammatory breast carcinoma. A 52-year-old woman with a hard, swollen, tender left breast for three days. *A*, Mammography: almost homogeneously dense left breast with an indistinct central mass approximately 3.5 × 5 cm in size. These diffuse changes indicate inoperability. *B*, Sonography: diffuse high-level echoes with evidence of fatty tissue; large irregular bilobed hypoechoic 5 × 8 cm mass with nonhomogeneous high-level internal echoes; 41 decibels were required for this study. Pathology (needle biospy): duct carcinoma; disseminated disease and death in 18 months.

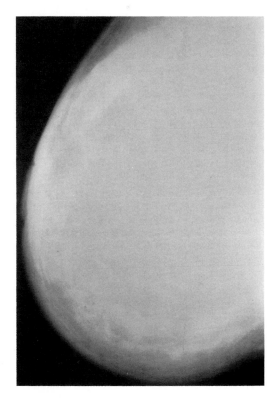

Figure 26–3. Advanced inflammatory breast carcinoma. A 66-year-old woman with pain, swelling, hardness, and redness of the breast for months. Mammography: diffuse density, massive skin swelling, and edema of the breast obscuring all internal structures. Dilatation of subcutaneous lymphatics is apparent superiorly. Pathology (biopsy only): primary duct breast carcinoma. Distant metastases were already present.

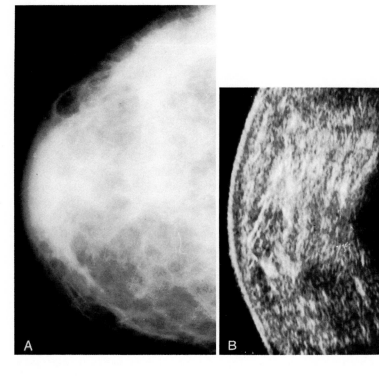

Figure 26–4. Inflammatory carcinoma. A 39-year-old woman with heaviness, pain, enlargement, and firmness in the right breast gradually increasing; recently the skin about the areola became discolored. Clinically: large vague area of increased induration in UOQ; all signs of inflammatory carcinoma. A, Mammography: 3 × 4.5 cm highly invasive carcinoma containing fine stippled calcification extending to the nipple, suggesting associated Paget's disease; diffuse skin thickening; diffuse edema; inoperable breast carcinoma. B, Sonography: high-level distorted echoes through the breast, most marked laterally with an irregular hypoechoic area; question of skin thickening beyond compression band. Pathology: duct carcinoma. Widespread metastases six months later.

Figure 26–5. Occult inflammatory carcinoma. An 80-year-old woman with an axillary lump with pain, swelling, and redness of the breast. Clinically: axillary mass; no breast mass but inflammatory process. Mammography: 1.5 × 2.5 cm poorly defined central carcinoma, diffuse breast edema, diffuse skin thickening; inoperable breast carcinoma. Pathology: duct carcinoma in biopsy of an axillary lymph node (no other surgery). The patient died 20 months later with widespread disease. The diffuse breast edema and skin thickening could be the result of matted axillary lymph nodes.

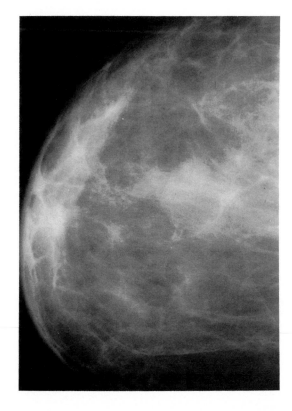

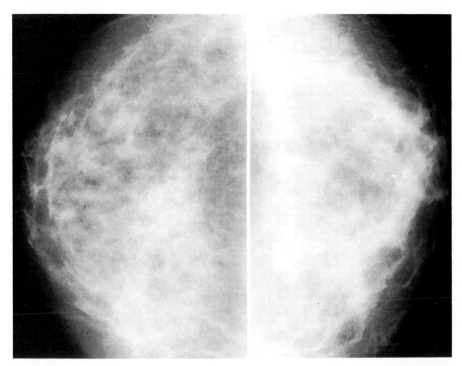

Figure 26–6. Inflammatory carcinoma. A 61-year-old woman with an inoperable lung cancer for two years and a clinically inflammatory lesion of the left breast. Mammography: severe ductal hyperplasia, poorly defined 2 cm mass upper quadrant of the left breast, diffuse densities in the breast, early diffuse skin thickening; inoperable primary breast carcinoma rather than a lung metastasis. Pathology: intraductal comedo, comedo and duct carcinoma with productive fibrosis. The patient died of lung cancer (three years after that diagnosis) one year later.

as undifferentiated, with a few classified as moderately differentiated or well differentiated. Only a few lesions show marked lymphocytosis suggestive of a reaction to the "inflammatory process."

There is no histologic explanation of why some breasts react with signs of inflammation to the presence of carcinoma cells within the breast or the skin. With advanced signs, the subdermal lymphatics usually contain emboli of carcinoma cells. However, such emboli are also found in diffuse skin thickening associated with noninflammatory breast carcinoma. My postulation is that there is an allergic biologic effect, with the skin reacting to the presence of the carcinoma cells in one case but not reacting to them in an inflammatory way in another case. This phenomenon would be analogous to an outbreak of hives after eating shellfish in one person but not in another.

In the Emory University study, on 18 patients there were available skin biopsy slides and blocks in addition to incisional or aspiration breast biopsy (Table 26–4). Nine had been interpreted as negative for skin involvement. In none could involvement of the skin by carcinoma be demonstrated, even upon many deeper cuts. Generous skin ellipses of areas of redness and edema were studied.

TABLE 26–4. Skin Involvement Histologically With Carcinoma and Survival in 18 Patients (Emory University)

Skin Involvement	No. of Patients	Status	Average Survival (Months)
None	5	Dead	33
Dermal lymphatics	5	Living	4, 4, 6, 8, and 24
Dermal lymphatics	4	Dead	41
Dermal lymphatics and infiltration of dermis	4	Dead	20

All showed dermal edema, focal perivascular lymphocytes, dilated dermal lymphatics, and small blood vessels but no demonstrable lymphatic metastasis. Each of these patients had had a mass from 2 to 30 months. The remaining nine cases fulfilled the histologic criteria of inflammatory carcinoma in the skin: plugging of the lymphatics of the upper dermis by carcinoma cells alone or associated with infiltrating carcinoma in the deeper dermis. It appears that there is no specific histologic skin lesion consistently associated with clinical inflammatory carcinoma.

TREATMENT

The methods of initial therapy are shown in Tables 26–5 to 26–7. The miscellaneous treatment groups included hypophysectomy; oophorectomy; estrogens alone; oophorectomy and male hormones; combinations of x-ray, hormones, and chemotherapy; and x-ray with surgery and/or chemotherapy and hormones.

The results of treatment of inflammatory carcinoma of the breast are disappointing. In most cases, spread beyond the breast has occurred when the patient is first seen. Palliation then must be the aim, and radiation therapy has proved the best means of accomplishing that, at least locally.

Treves (1952) reviewed his experience and collected reports on 262 cases of inflammatory carcinoma for which the treatment had been radical mastectomy. Only four patients survived five years, and there was no long-term survivor. Treves appealed to surgeons to stop treating this disease with radical mastectomy. However, Rogers and Fitts (1956) and Barber et al. (1961) continued to advocate radical mastectomy. In their combined series of 60 patients, only six lived five years; again, there was no long-term survivor. Most other surgeons have reported no five-year survi-

vors following radical mastectomy (Byrd and Stephenson, 1960; Richards and Lewison, 1961; Donegan, 1967). In 33 patients treated by supervoltage irradiation, Wang and Griscom (1964) reported an average survival time of 26.3 months (Table 26–6).

Surgery in our series was reserved for reducing the increased bulk of breast tissue caused by the generalized enlargement from the inflammatory carcinoma. In this way, radiation therapy of an already large breast could be rendered technically adequate.

PROGNOSIS

Nine of our patients having supervoltage radiation for definitive therapy have survival beyond five years. One was a 19-year survivor (personal case). The choice between radical surgery and nonoperative measures in the treatment of this disease was often readily solved, as in 77 per cent of the patients the disease was beyond the scope of surgical resection when first seen. The treatment and results of treatment in the seven patients whose disease could possibly be considered within the scope of surgical resection are shown in Table 26–7. This table fails to indicate the present choice of treatment: protracted irradiation to the breast and regional lymph nodes following the least possible surgical interference.

In two thirds of cases the development of metastases, other than in the axillary and supraclavicular lymph nodal areas, appeared within 12 months of the time the patient was first seen. In some patients, metastases were recognized for the first time as late as two years following radiation therapy. The most frequent sites of metastases were the skeleton and the intrathoracic contents (lungs, pleura, and mediastinal contents). Each of these areas was involved in almost all the patients who had metastases. The peritoneum and

TABLE 26–5. Treatment of Inflammatory Breast Carcinoma and Length of Survival After Treatment Began (MDAH and Emory University)

Initial Treatment	No. of Patients	Average Free Interval (Months)	Average Local Control (Months)	Average Survival (Months)
X-ray only	46	8	12	24
X-ray and hormones	26	8	11	23
X-ray and mastectomy	8	8	24	30
Miscellaneous	27	8	12	23
None	2	0	2	6

TABLE 26–6. Reported Results of Treatment of Inflammatory Carcinoma

Reporter	No. of Patients	Primary Method of Treatment	Duration of Survival (Months)	Year of Report
Barber et al.	53	Radical mastectomy	25.0	1961
Byrd and Stephenson	19	Various	16.0	1960
Donegan	38	Various	18.5	1967
Droulias et al.	69	Various	21.5	1976
Egan	107	Various	24.0	1987
Haagensen	87	Various	19.0	1971
Lee and Tannenbaum	28	Radical mastectomy	2.4	1924
Richards and Lewison	19	Various	20.0	1961
Taylor and Meltzer	25	Radical mastectomy	21.3	1938
Wang and Griscom	33	Ortho- and supervoltage	26.3	1964

intraperitoneal structures were involved in one half of the patients with known metastases. Other sites were the ovaries and retroperitoneal and cervical lymph nodes.

Reactivation of the primary tumor following irradiation occurred in one third of the patients: In almost all of them the reactivation took place within 12 months of treatment, in two, it occurred 2 years following treatment.

INFLAMMATORY VS NONINFLAMMATORY DIFFUSE SKIN THICKENING

The diffuse skin thickening seen by x-ray that is produced by breast cancer has the same appearance whether the cancer is clinically inflammatory or noninflammatory. There are almost identical radiographic findings in these two variants of breast carcinomas, one inflammatory and the other noninflammatory (Fig. 26–7 and 26–8).

Thickening of the skin of the breast produced by both inflammatory and noninflammatory carcinoma was evaluated in contemporary cases. The less advanced diffuse skin thickening of a noninflammatory carcinoma produces no significant difference on the mammograms from the early skin changes of inflammatory carcinoma.

Frequently, in order to indicate the degree of skin involvement, the term "inflammatory or near-inflammatory carcinoma" was used in reporting the mammograms. On several occasions carcinomas were so reported; the clinicians emphatically pointed out that no evidence of inflammation was present but later agreed that inflammatory carcinoma developed as "predicted from the mammograms." There are no radiographic criteria for predicting which breast with thickened skin will develop clinical inflammatory signs.

Twelve patients with inflammatory carcinomas having admission mammograms were reviewed, with only the degree of minimal and maximal skin thickening being noted. Consecutive cases with mammograms of breasts with skin thickening associated with noninflammatory carcinoma, also without

TABLE 26–7. Results of Treatment of Seven Patients (MDAH) Possibly Within Scope of Surgical Resection

Treatment	Free Interval (Months)	Local Control (Months)	Survival (Months)
Radical mastectomy and postoperative irradiation	2	6	6
Radiation and simple mastectomy for large breast	3	6	8
Radiation	12	12	24
Radiation	4	6	10
Radiation and simple mastectomy for large breast	8	14	28
Radiation	97	97	97*
Radiation	72	72	72*

*Died, no evidence of disease.

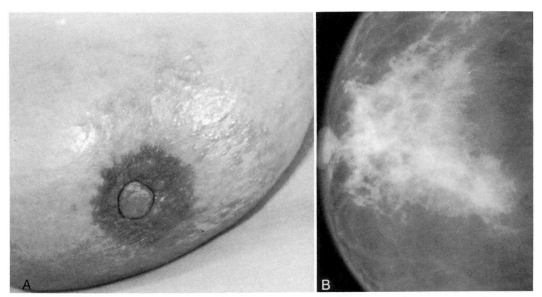

Figure 26–7. Inflammatory carcinoma with mass of carcinoma visible. A 73-year-old woman with pain and hardness of the left breast for several weeks. *A*, Clinically: inflammatory signs, no dominant mass palpable engorgement of dermal lymphatics. *B*, Mammography: visible 1.8 × 2.6 cm moderately invasive carcinoma despite diffuse breast density and edema with skin thickening. Pathology (needle biopsy): duct carcinoma. Death from disseminated disease occurred 20 months later.

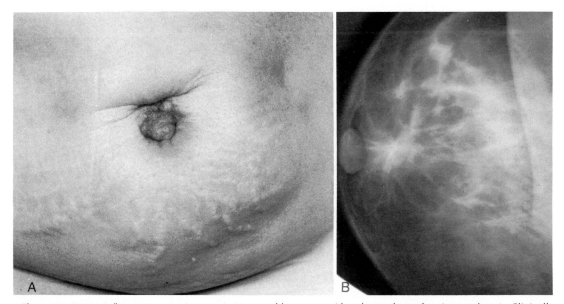

Figure 26–8. Noninflammatory carcinoma. A 65-year-old woman with a breast lump for six months. *A*, Clinically: diffuse disease, retracted nipple and skin, engorged lymphatics, no evidence of inflammation. *B*, Mammography: central and subareolar highly invasive carcinoma, diffuse skin thickening; inoperable. Pathology: needle biopsy, duct carcinoma, carcinoma in the skin. Death eight months later with no evidence of inflammatory disease.

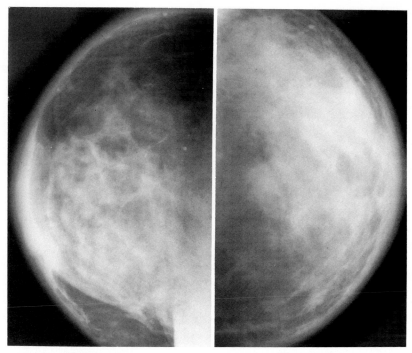

Figure 26–9   Figure 26–10

Figure 26–9. Inflammatory cancer. A 40-year-old woman with a breast mass, inflammatory changes, engorged dermal lymphatics. Mammography: diffuse carcinoma, massive skin changes. Needle biopsy: carcinoma of the breast. Death ensued eight months later. (Compare Figure 26–10.)

Figure 26–10. Noninflammatory cancer. A 57-year-old woman with a breast lump for ten years, slowly growing. Clinically: diffuse hard breast, engorged lymphatics. Mammography: diffuse carcinoma, marked skin thickening. Needle biopsy: carcinoma of the breast. Death occurred 14 months later. (Compare Figure 26–9.)

TABLE 26–8. On the Basis of Diffuse Skin Thickening on the Mammograms, 12 Matched Cases of Inflammatory and Noninflammatory Carcinoma of the Breast (MDAH)

Skin Thickness (mm)		Inflammatory Carcinoma		Noninflammatory Carcinoma	
Min.	Max.	Treatment	Survival (Months)	Treatment	Survival (Months)
2	4	Baclesse	82 (liv.)	Simple mastectomy, postoperative irradiation	14 (exp.)
3	5	Baclesse, gold grain implant	12 (exp.)	Simple mastectomy, postoperative irradiation	7 (exp.)
2	7	Oophorectomy, Baclesse	13 (exp.)	Oophorectomy, adrenalectomy, systemic	35 (exp.)
2	7	Baclesse, oophorectomy, systemic	9 (exp.)	Radical mastectomy, postoperative irradiation	3 (exp.)
1.5	5	Baclesse	12 (exp.)	Cortisone	3 (exp.)
1.5	3	Palliative irradiation, oophorectomy	5 (exp.)	Simple mastectomy, postoperative irradiation	23 (exp.)
1.5	4	Simple mastectomy, oophorectomy, systemic	22 (exp.)	Radical mastectomy, postoperative irradiation	63 (liv.)
1	6	None	4 (lost)	Radical mastectomy, systemic	62 (leukemia; lost)
1.5	5	Baclesse, oophorectomy	8 (exp.)	Radical mastectomy, systemic	14 (exp.)
1.5	2.5	CO-60 curative dose, systemic	14 (liv.)	Baclesse, radium implant, systemic	53 (exp.)
1.5	3	Baclesse, gold grain implant	13 (liv.)	Simple mastectomy, systemic	17 (exp.)
2	12	Palliative irradiation, oophorectomy, systemic	8 (exp.)	Radical mastectomy	11 (exp.)

previous treatment or biopsy and without ulceration or fungation, were reviewed and matched with the 12 inflammatory carcinomas on the basis of minimal and maximal skin thickening. Examples of matched pairs are shown in Figures 26–7 to 26–10.

Table 26–8 indicates the degree of skin thickening, the treatment, and the survival of the patients with matched cases of inflammatory and noninflammatory carcinomas of the breast. Diffusely thickened skin indicates an equally poor prognosis for both types of carcinoma. The ominous inflammatory type of carcinoma often receives more conservative treatment. The poor results with surgery in noninflammatory carcinoma of the breast, despite tolerance doses of irradiation postoperatively, suggest that mammography would be an invaluable aid in treatment planning. Diffuse skin thickening, even though not appreciated clinically, carries the same poor prognosis as clinical inflammatory carcinoma.

CASE HISTORY

The mammograms (Fig. 26–11) revealed diffuse skin thickening in the clinically normal breast of a 57-year-old patient being observed routinely following previous radical mastectomy. Biopsy of the skin was carried out on the basis of the mammograms, and normal skin was found on histolopathologic study. Two months later a massive tumor grew out through the biopsy site. Biopsy of this material showed carcinoma of the breast, indicating that carcinoma cells may lie in the thickened skin unsuspected by the clinician and unrecognized by the pathologist. As the mammograms show skin thickening far beyond that appreciated clinically and as cancer cells apparently can be present in clinically normal skin, one wonders whether the incision for surgical amputation of the breast at times may be through carcinoma.

OBSERVATIONS

Radiographically, a highly infiltrative carcinoma seldom exceeds 2 or 3 cm in diameter before the entire breast becomes diffusely dense and the skin becomes diffusely thickened. Skin thickening, either local or diffuse, is a frequent and highly suggestive x-ray sign of carcinoma. To the radiologist, any carcinoma with diffuse skin involvement could be inflammatory in type. The clinician's inability

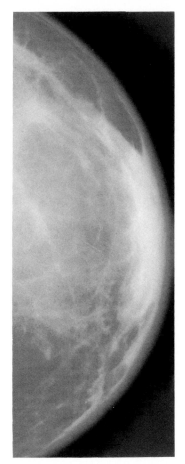

Figure 26–11. Mammogram that shows marked skin thickening due to carcinoma, yet the skin is still soft, pliable, and normal clinically.

to palpate the malignant mass in a breast diffusely involved by inflammatory carcinoma, or to appreciate diffuse thickening of the skin, leads him to suspect some special type of carcinoma.

The redness and heat are more apparent and as such are more impressive. The opinion of some surgeons that in inflammatory carcinoma of the breast the skin may become almost twice as thick as normal indicates the general clinical appreciation of skin thickening. One inflammatory carcinoma had skin 18 times normal thickness. Some cases without redness and heat have had skin 20 to 30 times normal thickness. From a purely objective standpoint, the radiologist has no reason to consider inflammatory carcinoma of the breast as other than a manifestation, through skin thickening, of an advanced stage of the cancer.

The reason for signs of inflammation associated with breast carcinoma in some individuals is not clear, and endless hypotheses have been proposed. The explanation perhaps is simple: Some women's skin reacts to allergenic substances by the production of generalized hives; some women's skin reacts locally to breast cancer by signs of inflammation.

REFERENCES

Barber KW Jr, Dockerty MB, Clagett OT (1961): Inflammatory carcinoma of the breast. Surg Gynecol Obstet 112:406.

Bell C (1816): A system of operative surgery. Harford, Hale and Hosmer 2:136.

Byrd BF Jr, Stephenson SE Jr (1960): Management of inflammatory breast cancer. South M J 53:945.

Donegan WL (1967): In Spratt JS Jr, Donegan WL (eds): Cancer of the Breast. Philadelphia, WB Saunders, p 167.

Droulias CA, Sewell CA, McSweeney MB, Powell RW (1976): Inflammatory carcinoma of the breast. Ann Surg 184:217.

Haagensen CD (1986): Diseases of the Breast, 3rd ed. Philadelphia, WB Saunders, p 808.

Klotz HH (1869): Uber Mastitis carcinomatosis grandarum et lactatum. Halle.

Lee BJ, Tannenbaum NE (1924): Inflammatory carcinoma of the breast. Surg Gynecol Obstet 39:580.

Meyer AC, Dockerty MD, Harrington SW (1948): Inflammatory carcinoma of the breast. Surg Gynecol Obstet 87:417.

Richards GJ Jr, Lewison EF (1961): Inflammatory carcinoma of the breast. Surg Gynecol Obstet 113:729.

Robbins GF, Shah J, Rosen P, Chu F, Taylor J (1974): Inflammatory carcinoma of the breast. Surg Clin North Am 54:(4), 801.

Rodman WL (1909): Acute carcinoma of the breast. Ann Surg, p 69.

Rogers CS, Fitts WT Jr (1956): Inflammatory carcinoma of the breast. Surgery 39:367.

Schumann E (1911): A study of carcinoma mastoides. Ann Surg 54:69.

Taylor GW, Meltzer A (1938): "Inflammatory carcinoma" of the breast. Am J Cancer 33:33.

Treves N (1952): The inoperability of inflammatory carcinoma of the breast. Surg Gynecol Obstet 109:240.

Wang CC, Griscom NT (1964): Inflammatory carcinoma of the breast; results following orthovoltage and supervoltage radiation therapy. Clin Radiol 15:168.

Volkmann R (1875): Beitraege zur Chirurgie. Leipzig, p 319.

27

Breast Calcifications

BACKGROUND

Calcifications displayed radiographically are intriguing in any part of the body. This applies particularly to the breast. Intramammary calcifications have provided confusion to the mammographer, appeal to the surgeon to explore less specific mammographic changes in the breast, incentive to the pathologist to associate benign breast changes with carcinoma, and a vehicle for establishing the team approach to detect, diagnose, and treat breast cancer. The readily recognized calcific particles in the breast even furnish a link between the inexact art of clinical mammography both with the abstract concepts of biostatisticians who analyze data of the complexities of breast diseases and with scientists who extract unbiased digitalized information from the mammogram.

Radiographic calcifications are seen in over one half of the cancers of the intact breast and in over three fourths of the cancers of sectioned breasts by correlated radiographic-histologic whole-organ studies. Calcifications can be demonstrated by light microscopy in almost all duct carcinomas. Typical calcifications within the cancerous mass add little to the x-ray diagnosis, as the mass itself is usually characteristic. Yet with subtle changes, such as altered architecture and asymmetry, the contribution of even a few calcifications is immeasurable.

History

In a review of Salomon's illustrations published in 1913, calcifications could be recognized in his radiographs of the breast specimens. Warren recognized calcifications in the intact breast as early as 1927. Carlos Maria Dominguez, a Montevideo pathologist, histologically correlated calcifications in genital tumors demonstrated by radiography. In 1930 he published illustrations of x-ray tissue specimens with coarse type calcifications in uterine fibroids but only photomicrographs of finer calcifications in epithelial carcinomas. In 1935 he extended the study to the breast and published radiographs of calcifications in both fibroadenomas and "adenocarcinomas." This study had been encouraged by the reports of Espaillat (1933) and Ledoux-Lebard et al. (1933) on the use of x-ray examination of the breast.

Leborgne, also of Montevideo and a student of Dominguez, published (1943) on breast duct injection (already practiced with some danger in the United States [Reis, 1930]) and on breast calcifications in South America (1949) and in the United States (1951). His illustrations showed widespread dense coarse calcifications, which he described as "grains of sand," but not the tiny calcifications more frequently associated with carcinoma. His resolution was estimated as 0.2 mm particle size (compared with our 0.05 mm) owing to short target-film distance, long object-film distance, scattered radiation with poor collimation, poor positioning, high kilovoltage, and faster film (80 mas compared with our early 1800 mas). As Leborgne became more interested in duct injection and removal of papillomata, his investigation of breast calcifications declined. All these workers were, of course, hampered by the lack of the exquisite radiographic quality possible on fine-grain industrial x-ray film with a high-milliamperage and low-kilovoltage x-ray technique.

Clinical Mammography Contribution

The introduction of clinical mammography in 1956, with the detection of nonpalpable breast cancers, provided a welcome alternative to the unrewarding extension of surgical treatments in vogue at the time. The first report of a series of 19 clinically unsuspected breast cancers in 1960, and an additional 53 in 1962 (Egan), stimulated surgical exploration of minimal radiographic abnormalities with demonstration of noninvasive and locally invasive but irrefutably curable breast cancers. Many of these "mammographic"

cancers with only a small area of clustered calcification without mass were in young women with small, dense, nodular breasts. This consistent demonstration of unsuspected curable cancers unleashed an avalanche of inquiries about screening for breast cancer and, on the basis of this original work, led to selecting the beginning age of 35 years for screening for breast cancer.

One oncologic surgeon, frustrated by advanced breast cancers of the premammography era, prodded me with the potential of calcifications in the breast: If a carcinoma's presence is represented by 1000 or more calcifications, why not 100 or 10 or even fewer? As small clusters were spotted, problems of localization and study under the microscope opened up another challenge for me—localization and breast specimen radiography.

With the introduction of a mammographic technique capable of fine radiographic detail (resolution of a diameter of six red blood cells or smaller structures), the finding of calcifications in the breast led to repeated radiologist-pathologist altercations. The pathologists admitted that calcifications did occur in the breast, originally found as the microtome blade was dulled, especially by a calcifying fibroadenoma, but they strongly insisted that this did not occur nearly so frequently as indicated by x-ray. Then it was realized that the microtome fragmented and dislodged the smaller calcifications and that the commonly used acid fixatives and stains dissolved the fine calcifications remaining in the 7 μ thick histologic preparation. Once the suggestion to use less acid fixatives was followed, the pathologist learned that calcifications occurred many times more frequently than was demonstrated on the mammograms. Von Kossa's stain was perfected for even better demonstration of the calcifications.

In no aspect of mammography is the necessity for maximum radiographic detail so important as in the demonstration of the minute flecks of calcifications. Coarse calcifications may call attention to an area, but it is the much finer interspersed ones that really elevate the suspicion of malignancy. A good rule of thumb is that if a coned-down view brings countless additional fine flecks into view, the lesion is probably cancer (Fig. 27–1). These tiny calcifications may be clearly visible on extremely fine-grain film but not identified on grainier emulsions, i.e., those with a grain size as large as these minuscule

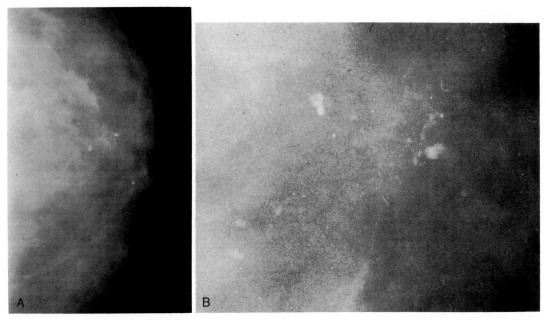

Figure 27–1. Coarse and fine calcifications. A 35-year-old woman with painful and clinically nodular breasts. Mammography: Several coarse calcifications with the suggestion of interspersed fine ones (*A*). Coned-down view of the area showing many fine calcifications (*B*). After localization and biopsy, an intraductal carcinoma was demonstrated.

calcific deposits of carcinoma. Each mammogram must be searched with a hand magnifying lens with optimal lighting lest calcifications be overlooked.

Higher kilovoltage, lack of collimation and scattered radiation, shortened target-film distance, film-screen receptors, electrostatic processes, overly darkened films, and magnification mammography cause disappearance of the smaller breast calcifications (Fig. 27–2). Muntz (1977) estimates that the minimal diameter of calcification observed on mammograms varies as the fourth root of dose, other things being equal. It is true that the size of potentially visible calcifications of benign and malignant breast diseases ranges from 0.05 mm to several centimeters, but only the larger particles will be appreciated on technically poor studies. It is just as obvious that the poorer the quality of mammography the fewer the interspersed finer calcifications that will be appreciated. The finer the calcifications, the greater their importance (Fig. 27–3).

With our use of xeroradiography of the breast, when a cluster of several coarse calcifications was noted, a coned-down view on fine-grain film was made of the area. If no interspersed fine calcifications were seen, the patient was observed. If fine calcifications were interspersed with the larger ones seen on xeroradiography, localization and biopsy was done. Martin and Wolfe (1973), using only xeroradiography, found one of 11 biopsies for calcifications not associated with a mass to be cancer, while our film studies detected a cancer for each three or four biopsies.

The unequaled clarity of breast calcifications on nonscreen fine-grain film mammograms signaled such a diagnostic potential that as early as the 1950s, we had categorized them into distinct types: six malignant and four benign. There is much overlapping in the characteristics of benign and malignant breast calcifications. An attempt to break down the calcifications into the two broad types of malignant and benign is helpful however.

PATHOPHYSIOLOGY OF BREAST CALCIFICATIONS

Formation

Differential points in diagnosis of breast calcifications are size, shape, and density. Ductal epithelial cells, later to produce intraductal or ductal carcinoma, still retain the potential for metabolism of calcium, as the mother cells did in milk formation. Contin-

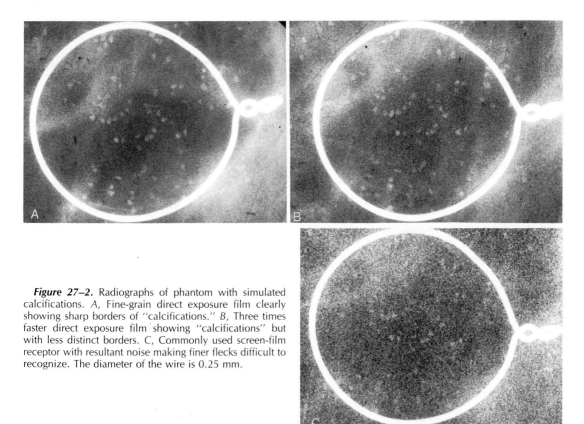

Figure 27–2. Radiographs of phantom with simulated calcifications. *A,* Fine-grain direct exposure film clearly showing sharp borders of "calcifications." *B,* Three times faster direct exposure film showing "calcifications" but with less distinct borders. *C,* Commonly used screen-film receptor with resultant noise making finer flecks difficult to recognize. The diameter of the wire is 0.25 mm.

ued secretion of calcium ions produces supersaturation, and calcium salts are precipitated. The gradual building-up of deposits of calcium produces wide variations in size and density: from very faint to moderately dense and from microscopic size to 2 to 3 mm or larger. With such a range in density and size many of the particles will be uncountable. These same epithelial cells are active in benign processes when, at times, the precipitation may be related to short-term episodes resulting in a more equal density and size of the calcium flecks. For example, the round calcifications of similar size and density with lobular distribution in sclerosing adenosis are formed during the florid phase of this process. Since ductal epithelial hyperplasia provides the link between normal and cancerous cells progressing through ductal hyperplasia, in situ carcinoma, and invasive carcinoma, indistinguishable deposits of calcification must be anticipated in noncancerous and cancerous processes.

Varied physiologic processes probably are involved in the deposition of calcification in the breast. Frequently noted are discrete mi-

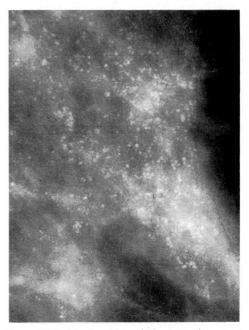

Figure 27–3. The finer the calcifications, the more important. Intraductal and infiltrative comedocarcinoma in a 56-year-old woman studied for thickening in this breast. These calcifications are unusually fine for comedocarcinoma, magnified in this reproduction.

croscopic flecks of calcification within a group of viable carcinoma cells unassociated with ducts and cellular or necrotic debris. These calcific deposits may occur in any duct carcinoma and need not be related to acinous or pseudoacinous arrangements of the carcinoma cells.

Large secreted calcific deposits are demonstrated in the intraductal carcinoma shown in Figures 27–4 and 27–5. The lining duct cells secrete calcific products into the lumen with precipitation into varying-sized, granular-appearing deposits of calcific salts. As these approach 50 μ in size they become radiographically demonstrable as macrocalcifications. In Figure 27–5 a large deposit of calcification, fragmented by the microtome blade, fills the lumen of a duct still lined by viable carcinoma cells (solid arrow). In a nearby duct (hollow arrow) the lining cells are no longer viable, with death perhaps caused by pressure necrosis. The process continues (Fig. 27–5), and finally there is only calcification in a vague shadow of a previous duct.

Our observations (Egan, 1964) that the calcifications of concern to the radiologist are

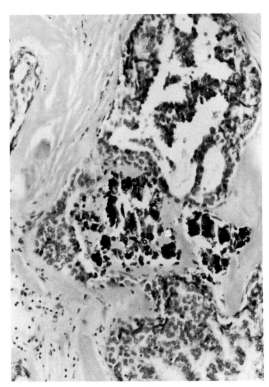

Figure 27–5. Another section from the same breast seen in Figure 27–4. Progressive disorganization of the lining duct cells can be seen (center) as well as the complete loss of lining cells, with the retained shadow of a duct to the right of center. These calcifications have resulted from secretory activity of the lining epithelial cells without associated necrotic debris.

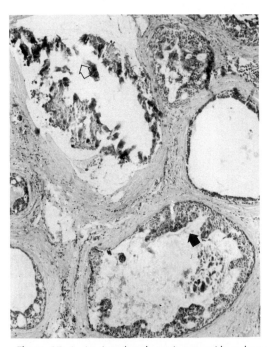

Figure 27–4. An intraductal carcinoma with a large calcification, shattered by the microtome, can be seen filling the lumen of a dilated duct (solid arrow). The cells are viable and only disturbed by sectioning in one small area superiorly. A similar calcification is seen, but the lining cells are disorganized and probably nonviable (open arrow).

the result of an active secretory process and not the result of mineralizaton of cellular debris and degenerate cells differ from those of Levitan et al. (1964) who concluded that all mammographically visible calcifications of carcinoma were formed in an area of comedocarcinoma, were granular, and were products of cellular and necrotic debris.

Ahmed's (1975) ultrastructural studies support our observations. He demonstrated that initially the calcifications were needle-like crystals within the tumor cells. He concluded that these crystals were secreted by an active secretory process and coalesced to form dense deposits in which the crystalline structure became obscure. He noted calcifications in stroma adjacent to tumor cells but not in stromal collagen or elastic fibers. His finding of a 5:3 calcium:phosphorus ratio was consistent with hydroxyapatite, $Ca_3(PO_4)_3OH$. Price and Gibbs (1978) agreed with the concept of the active secretory process of calcium deposits, demonstrated the extrusion of such particles into the interstitial tissues, and suggested that all calcifications are the result of hyperplastic, atypical, or carcinoma cells.

Galkin et al (1977) found by electron microscopy, x-ray microanalysis, secondary ion mass spectrometry, and crystallography, in addition to the well-known calcium-phosphorus compounds, some x-ray opaque particles containing other elements and at times no Ca or P. A particle could contain Ag, Mo, Cl, or I. Little significance can be placed on this finding to date.

Relation to Cancer

There is a continuum of progression of normal ductal epithelial cells into hyperplasia, into atypical forms of cells, into metaplasia, into intraductal carcinoma, and finally, breaching the basement membrane of the ducts, into invasive carcinoma. In the past few years a body of pathologists, but by no means all pathologists, have established and agreed on specific criteria for the diagnosis of intraductal carcinoma based on ductal epithelial cell changes. All criteria may not be clearly present, leaving many gray areas in diagnosis. Most students of breast diseases consider intraductal carcinoma (1) as having already broken through the basement membrane although not in the area of histologic study, or (2) as having an extremely high potential for metastasis. Also, all duct carcinomas arise from ductal epithelial hyperplasia even though all ductal hyperplasia does not proceed to intraductal carcinoma.

Intraductal carcinoma is envisioned as being associated with calcification. This stems from the usual discovery of fine stippled calcifications on mammography. Study of a large number of whole-organ breast preparations bore out the association of intraductal carcinoma with calcifications as paralleling that of invasive duct carcinoma: 60 per cent of intraductal carcinomas had calcification on mammography; 80 per cent on radiographs of thin breast sections; and at least 90 per cent on histopathologic study. Of course, the last-named calcification on 7 μ thick preparations was not the same as that recognized on radiography. Fifty μ sized particles seen by x-ray would be shattered by the microtome blade except, at times, the softer large calcifications of intraductal comedocarcinoma, which would be cut by the blade.

The concept of considering two types of intraductal carcinoma provides (1) distinction of potentially less aggressive intraductal comedocarcinoma from more aggressive solid intraductal carcinoma; (2) association of calcifications and types of calcifications with breast carcinomas; and (3) explanation of formation of calcification in the breast by at least two means.

Intraductal Comedocarcinoma

Intraductal comedocarcinoma is characterized by distention of the ducts with thick grumous material containing a large amount of calcification (Fig. 27–6). This is a more indolent tumor and may fill a quadrant or most of the breast with no or minimal invasion. Most of these lesions have multiple sites in multiple lobes, and they are frequently bilateral. This suggests a large area or base for formation of the carcinoma rather than a wide spread of the tumor from a single site via the ducts. This carcinoma is often associated with Paget's disease of the breast, as it has the propensity to grow along the ducts, the path of least resistance, to reach the summit of the nipple. This prolonged process may require years to become clinically evident, since Paget's disease of the nipple may be present for years before a palpable mass in the breast is noted.

Intraductal Solid Carcinoma

The "solid" intraductal carcinomas are those of distended ducts with closely packed viable cancer cells and finer calcifications (Fig. 27–7). A cribriform pattern is often present. A variant arrangement of these cells reminds one of "Roman bridges" and "flippers of dolphins." These ducts may be surrounded by thick cuffs of periductal fibrosis and/or lymphocytes, hypothetically a defense mechanism. Light microscopy of H & E stains may fail to show carcinoma cells beyond the ducts, while electron microscopy may readily demonstrate such a bridge of the basement membrane (Ozzello, 1971). Also, with light microscopy only a small portion of this diffuse multifocal disease is studied, and, with an occasional axillary lymph node metastasis, it is best to consider this process invasive. Some of these deposits of carcinoma do not demonstrate calcification.

Invasive Carcinoma

No intraductal carcinoma can produce a gross breast mass until infiltration occurs. In these noninvasive lesions, calcification must

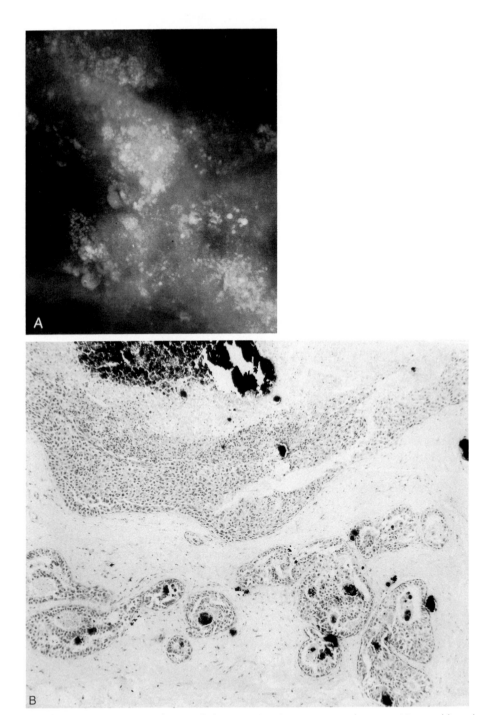

Figure 27–6. Intraductal comedocarcinoma calcifications. Routine mammography on a 44-year-old graduate nurse demonstrated areas of calcification not associated with a mass. *A*, Note the uncountable nature and wide range in density of these coarse and fine, varying sized calcifications. There was microinvasion in only a few areas. Magnified 6 ×. *B*, Modified von Kossa stain showing the intraductal calcifications of varying sizes.

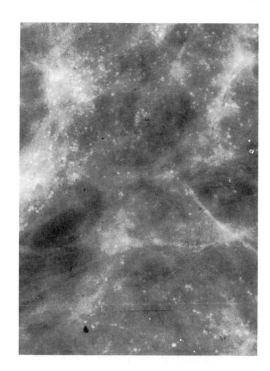

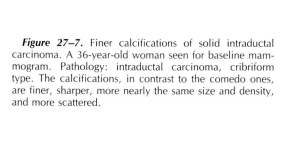

Figure 27–7. Finer calcifications of solid intraductal carcinoma. A 36-year-old woman seen for baseline mammogram. Pathology: intraductal carcinoma, cribriform type. The calcifications, in contrast to the comedo ones, are finer, sharper, more nearly the same size and density, and more scattered.

be seen on the mammogram for recognition of tumor.

In the two patterns of calcification deposition, whether primarily in necrotic debris in comedocarcinoma, secretory in solid intraductal carcinoma, or in subsequent invasive carcinoma, the components are usually characteristic. The patterns of calcification may be seen singly or in combination (Figs. 27–8 to 27–11).

The calcifications in comedo lesions tend to be larger and highly variegated, to have indistinct borders, to occur in a lobular pattern, and to be associated with limited fibroglandular distortion. They are seen with multiple deposits in one or both breasts or as a coalescence of such deposits to occupy a large portion of the breast. They produce malignant calcifications of the type that has been labeled bizarre or heterogeneous.

Those deposits associated with the solid intraductal carcinoma or its invasive form are

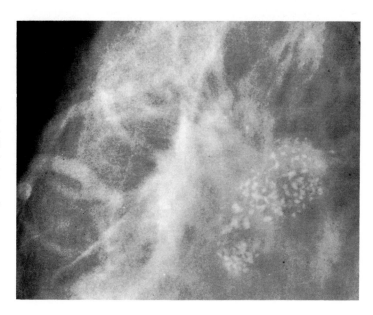

Figure 27–8. Coned-down view of intraductal comedocarcinoma calcifications. A 46-year-old woman with nodular breasts. Even though there is marked variation in size and shape of the calcifications the density remains rather consistent. Localization, diagnosis, and modified radical mastectomy resulted in apparent cure of this breast; the opposite breast requires yearly follow-up studies.

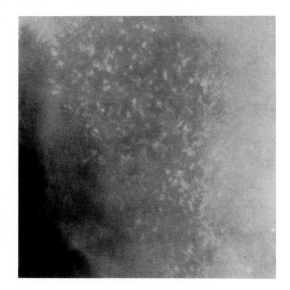

Figure 27–9. Large area of intraductal comedocarcinoma. A 42-year-old woman whose mother had breast cancer. Clinically: fibrocystic disease. Mammography: greatly variable size, shape, and density of clustered calcifications not associated with a mass. Magnified 6 ×. Despite the large area there is no suggestion of a pseudomass.

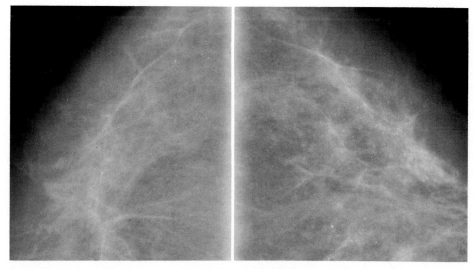

Figure 27–10. Intraductal (solid) carcinoma with pseudomass. There are tiny calcifications in the upper quadrant of the left breast. Despite the small size and the lack of invasion there is reaction in the surrounding tissues to the carcinoma in the form of increased density. The comedo type seldom produces a pseudomass.

smaller, of rather uniform density, and sharply outlined. They occur often as a single tight cluster and even before invasion may be associated with periductal architectural distortion. An associated infiltrative duct carcinoma is usually highly infiltrative and may have scirrhous elements. In such a lesion the calcifications are diffuse throughout the mass (Fig. 27–12).

In the combined types, the comedo calcifications are adjacent to (Fig. 27–13), or may be surrounded by, a rather markedly invasive lesion containing the solid carcinoma type calcifications. It is difficult to determine whether in the periphery the comedocarcinoma became highly invasive, producing the different form of calcification, or whether morphologically different carcinomas arose contiguously. At any rate, the lesion must be considered highly aggressive.

The coexistence of two separate types of ductal carcinoma most probably explains this pattern. Frequently the two types of carcinoma are present in the same breast in separate sites. Widespread comedocarcinoma could easily occur at the site of the solid duct carcinoma. On the other hand, as histologically pure comedocarcinoma is a less frequent

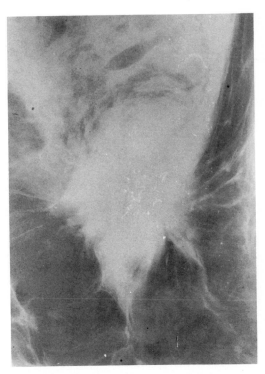

Figure 27–12. Fine calcifications of solid duct carcinoma better demonstrated. A whole-organ slicer section on a 66-year-old woman with clinical and radiographic carcinoma. The radiograph shows a highly invasive scirrhous duct carcinoma with central fine, faint calcifications. Histologic studies showed that the same type of calcifications above the lesion were in intraductal solid carcinoma and not associated with a mass.

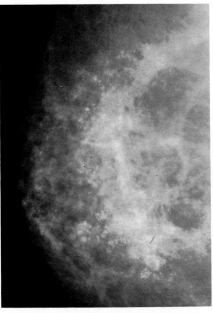

Figure 27–11. Widespread comedocarcinoma. A 61-year-old woman seen for a routine clinical examination for a thickening in both breasts. Mammography: diffuse calcifications of varying sizes, shapes, and densities without a definite mass, although there are areas of coalescent densities that could be considered pseudomasses.

duct carcinoma, one could advance the less likely hypothesis that this intraductal comedocarcinoma, to produce varied combined patterns, is a precursor of other types of breast carcinoma.

RADIOLOGIC-HISTOLOGIC CLASSIFICATION OF BREAST CALCIFICATIONS

The aim of placing intramammary calcifications into benign and malignant categories was never finalized owing to excessive overlapping of their characteristics. As long as clustering was present, radiograph differentiation could never be made. Subsequent attempts at radiographic-histologic classification may prove to be of value. Such a classification has to be based on calcium deposit size, location, and morphology. The size has been arbitrarily divided into (1) greater than 50 μ diameter (macrocalcifications) that may be seen by x-ray; (2) 7 μ or

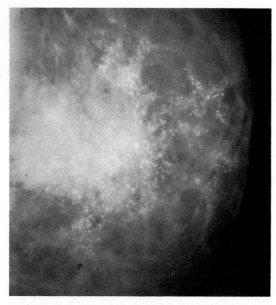

Figure 27–13. Combined patterns of comedo and solid duct carcinomas. A 68-year-old woman with a breast mass for several weeks. Clinically: suspicious breast mass. Mammography: a moderately invasive 3 × 4 cm dense mass of carcinoma containing innumerable faint fine calcifications. This mass is surrounded by comedocarcinoma type calcifications without a mass. Pathology: combined carcinomas—duct cell with productive fibrosis and comedocarcinoma that is primarily intraductal.

less in size (microcalcifications) that may be contained in the usual light microscopic preparation; and (3) 8 to 50 μ diameter (mostly microscopic but may not be seen on the 7 μ preparations as a result of being dislodged or fragmented). The location may be intraductal or extraductal; the calcifications may be associated with necrotic or cellular debris or associated only with viable cells. The morphologic characteristics may be laminated or nonlaminated.

Macrocalcifications

Arbitrarily these are greater than 50 μ in size, as smaller ones in dense breasts are not resolved radiographically. These calcifications are visible to the naked eye or by use of 2 × magnifying hand lens.

Granular. These relatively soft, amorphous calcifications are usually associated with intraductal detritus and cellular debris and may be partially the result of secretion. They are not shattered by the microtome blade and are common in comedocarcinoma (Fig. 27–14) and ductal ectasia. Even when seen with duct carcinoma (scirrhous, simplex, and so

forth) they are most likely related to comedocarcinoma.

Hard. These are hard calcifications that are at least partially shattered by the microtome blade. They are similar to the granular type but are infrequently seen entirely in 7 μ preparations. The pathologist must be sure that he is viewing the same area that interests the radiologist. Meticulous selection of the proper tissue for microscopic study is best accomplished by careful comparison with the thinly sliced biopsy specimen. The origin is intraductal (Fig. 27–15), less often associated with intraductal debris, and this same type of calcification may be seen in extraductal locations.

Psammomatous. This type includes all other visible discrete calcifications on the mammograms. It may be associated with fat necrosis, plasma cell mastitis, old hemorrhage, calcifying necrotic areas, or fibroadenomata.

Microcalcifications

Microcalcifications are generally much smaller than 50 μ in size and usually less than 7 μ, as this is the thickness of the usual light microscopy preparations.

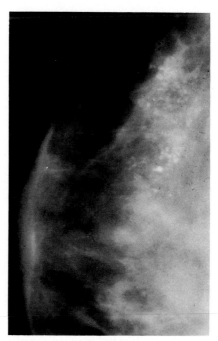

Figure 27–14. Soft, amorphous granular type calcifications. These are primarily in the ducts with invasive comedocarcinoma in a 72-year-old woman studied for a vague lump in her breast.

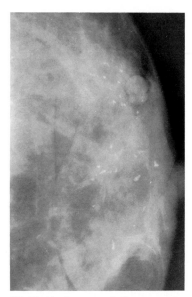

Figure 27–15. Hard macrocalcifications. This 64-year-old woman had a serous discharge from the nipple with a clinical subareolar carcinoma. This proved to be plasma cell mastitis. The calcifications were both intra- and extra-ductal.

Psammomatous. These are laminated and usually found in interstitial areas. They may be in the duct wall, in the lumen, in a pseudolumen of malignant glands, or in fibrous tissue.

Nonpsammomatous. This group includes all other nonlaminated microscopic calcifications and usually is associated with fibrocystic disease.

MALIGNANT BREAST CALCIFICATIONS

Criteria

The calcifications typical of carcinoma must satisfy three criteria:

1. They must be relatively fine.
2. They must be uncountable. While staring at an area of the breast with a hand lens, one gets the impression of more and more individual flecks popping into view (Fig. 27–2).
3. They must be confined to a measurable area. On the two views obtained at right angles, the calcifications cannot be diffused on either view but are confined to a definite area.

Types

Malignant breast calcifications may be described and placed into the following cate-gories and may or may not be associated with a mass.

Sandlike. These calcifications are sharp and slightly elongated and have the appearance of uncountable grains of salt sprinkled about a measurable area of the mammogram (Figs. 27–3, 27–7, and 27–9). The flecks are all similar in size and shape. A variation of this type is further elongation, in which the length may be several times the diameter but the flecks still retain a sharp outline.

Bizarre, Heterogeneous. This pattern could be likened to a jumble of the alphabet. No two flecks have the same shape. They appear curled, irregularly elongated, and re-curved or present other variegated shapes (Fig. 27–16). A variation is branching duct calcification, which may be seen in carcinoma but more often is seen in benign conditions.

Coarse, Smooth. The dense particles have the appearance of spilled droplets of mercury, being homogeneously dense and rounded but varying in size. With the hand lens, many intervening calcifications, which are less well formed and less dense, come into view (Fig. 27–17).

Lacy, Wavy. Tiny wavy veils of indistinct calcifications are entwined in the carcinoma. The true laciness is best appreciated with the hand lens, but some areas are dense enough to be seen without the lens. This kind of calcification has also been identified in axillary lymph nodes containing metastic carcinoma of the breast (Fig. 27–18).

Faint, Rounded. None of the calcifications appears dense or sharply outlined against the background density. Similar in size and shape to the coarse and smooth type of calcifications, these faint and round calcifications differ in their lack of density. This type may be seen with mucin-producing carcinoma (Fig. 27–19).

Packed Ducts. These densities are not calcific but may be confused with calcifications of carcinoma. Packed ducts are included to point out their possible value in the diagnosis of carcinoma. Viewed with a hand lens, the mammograms of carcinomas reveal small opacities, which are also round and almost calcific in density within the confines of the lesion. These minuscule opacities are composed of ducts tightly packed with carcinoma cells. Because the ducts are seen on-end, they appear denser than the surrounding carcinoma, the cells of which have more tendency to grow along and be confined within the ducts. All the opacities are of near-equal

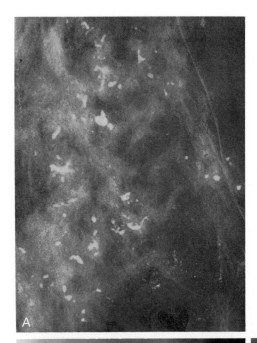

Figure 27–16. A, Variegated calcifications in an intraductal carcinoma in a 46-year-old woman who complained of painful breasts. B, Mammogram performed on a 43-year-old woman whose mother had breast cancer. The various-shaped calcifications are better seen in the 6 × blowup of the area (C), as a type of variegated calcification in comedocarcinoma.

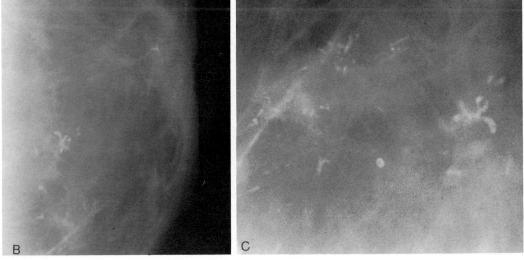

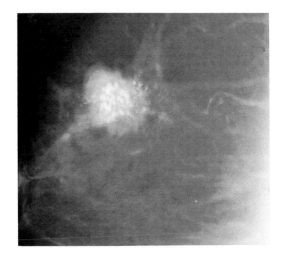

Figure 27–17. Coarse and smooth calcifications of carcinoma in a 61-year-old woman with a nodule for two weeks. Pathologically: 2 cm ductal carcinoma.

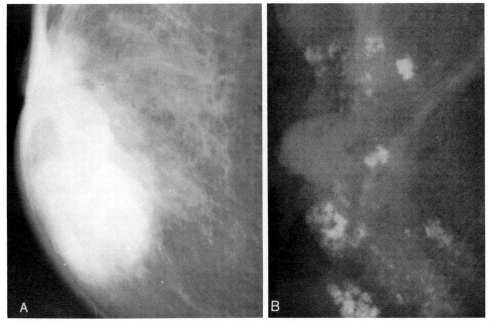

Figure 27–18. A, Lacy calcifications of carcinoma in a 64-year-old woman with a bleeding nipple. The faint vein-like calcifications reproduce poorly. *B,* Almost-lacy pattern of calcifications in a comedocarcinoma in a 46-year-old woman seen on a check-up mammogram. Variation in density is marked.

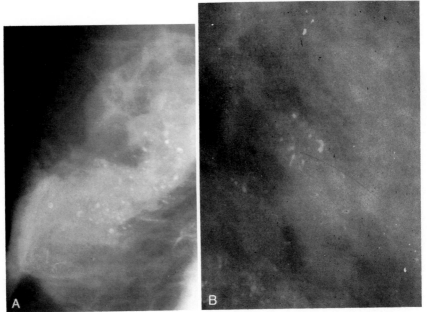

Figure 27–19. A, Faint, rounded calcifications in a 71-year-old woman studied for nipple retraction of seven months' duration. The diagnosis of a mucin-producing carcinoma was suggested from the mammogram, on which the calcifications appeared less dense. B, Blowup (6 ×) of a coned-down area showing the very faint, rounded calcifications of a comedocarcinoma. The patient was a 63-year-old woman studied for a nipple discharge in the opposite breast.

density but are uncountable. Staining the microscopic sections for calcium fails to reveal particles of calcium. Ductal hyperplasia, in which the ducts are packed with hyperplastic epithelial cells, has less tendency to produce similar discrete opacities.

BENIGN BREAST CALCIFICATIONS

Benign, noncancerous breast calcifications may be conveniently separated into ductal and those not associated with the ducts. Calcification is such an important diagnostic sign that when the exact etiology is not apparent and the appearance is similar to a malignant variety, it is better to label the lesion as most likely malignant. Improved quality of the mammograms does demonstrate more borderline calcifications. This allows an improved differentiation of other clusters, with an overall maintenance of cancer to noncancer biopsy ratio and identification of many more early cancers.

Ductal Calcifications

Benign calcifications in the ducts and duct walls often are readily recognized. They usually appear as (1) tiny scattered sharp flecks (Fig. 27–20); (2) ringlike round or oval densities (Fig. 27–21A); (3) parallel bands (Figs. 27–21B and 27–22); (4) complete opacification of a few branching ducts or one of several lobules of the gland (Fig. 27–22); or (5) a Y-shaped or branching configuration as the calcification follows a bifurcating duct for a short distance (Fig. 27–23).

Duct calcifications are seen so frequently that they could easily fall into the category of a normal finding. Even so, they must reflect some degree of abnormality of secretion or absorption of secretions.

Many times the calcifications associated with fibrocystic disease, although often diffuse throughout both breasts, occur in localized clumps that are indistinguishable from malignant calcifications. Sclerosing adenosis has a lobular distribution, but so does lobular carcinoma in situ. The small mulberry arrangement of fine calcifications of a papilloma may be signaling a transformation into an intraductal carcinoma. Subareolar fibrosis and duct ectasia frequently produce fairly closely spaced flecks in the subareolar area (Figs. 27–24 and 27–25). It is of some help that they are usually quite sharp, although small, are localized to the subareolar area, and are bilateral and symmetric. But at times there are an associated subareolar density,

Text continued on page 473

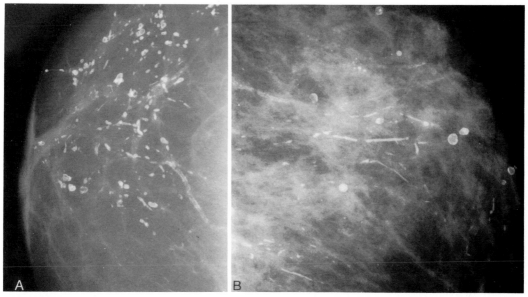

Figure 27–20. *A,* Several types of benign ductal calcifications in a 62-year-old woman studied for possible mass. A firm 2 cm area was biopsied and showed sclerosis and calcifications in fibrocystic disease. The arterial wall calcifications are parallel and intermittent, often appearing fragmented. *B,* Various benign calcifications in the same breast. Almost all are intraductal: The large rounded ones are partially calcified entrapped secretions; the small dense rounded ones are more solidly calcified, whereas those elongated with parallel sides, thin strands, intermittent rounded ends, and branching are merely various ways and extent of calcification of intraductal material. Arterial calcification is also seen.

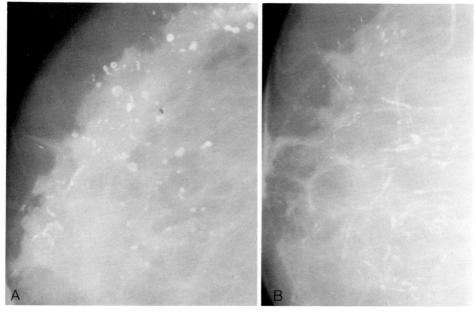

Figure 27–21. *A,* A better example of calcifications of secretory disease. The rounded deposits with a less dense center in a 72-year-old woman seen for routine follow-up mammograms. These spherical calcifications result from secretions being trapped within the ducts that calcify. *B,* Another form of elongated rodlike calcifying debris in the ducts in a 65-year-old woman seen for annual checkup.

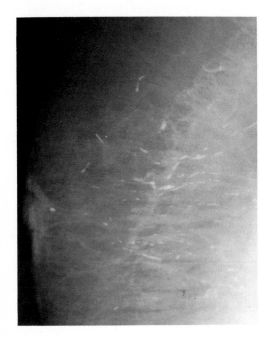

Figure 27–22. Elongated needle-like duct calcifications in a 62-year-old woman with an intermittent watery nipple discharge followed for six years. The polarization of these calcifications is the best clue that they are benign.

Figure 27–23. Opacification of part of the duct system filled with calcifications in a 72-year-old woman seen for routine checkup.

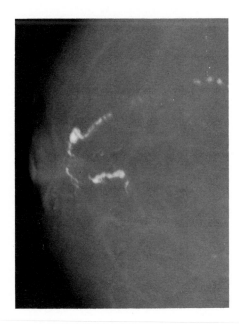

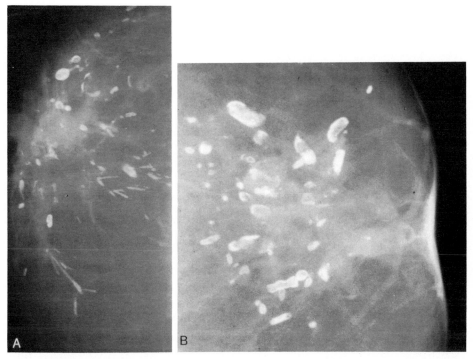

Figure 27–24. A, Benign ductal calcifications in a 63-year-old woman with a subareolar mass and nipple discharge. The Y, or branching, calcifications follow bifurcating ducts. B, Several types of benign breast calcifications. A 72-year-old woman with soreness in this breast. Clinically: vague subareolar changes with nipple retraction. Mammography: calcifications in subareolar fibrosis and secretory disease.

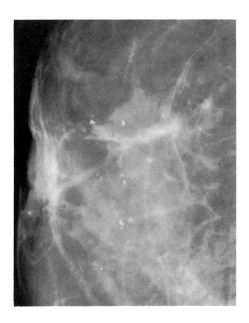

Figure 27–25. Sharp, benign calcifications in subareolar fibrosis in a 74-year-old woman with a subareolar mass, bloody nipple discharge, and nipple retraction for one year. Pathologically: fibrotic type fibrocystic disease, intraductal papillomata.

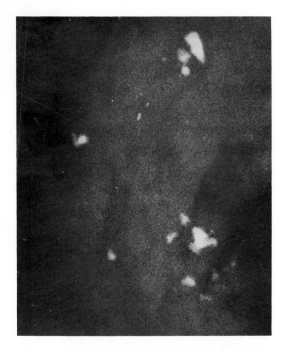

Figure 27–26. Coarse ductal calcifications of fibrocystic disease in a 47-year-old woman seen for a baseline mammogram. In a dense nodular breast, routine mammograms showed a group of calcifications. The coned-down view failed to show fine interspersed calcifications suggestive of cancer. Pathologically: fibrocystic disease. Magnified 6 × .

nipple retraction, and clumps of calcifications indistinguishable from carcinoma. The fine linear intraductal calcifications that are needle-like are usually uniformly elongated compared with the more variable carcinoma calcifications. Ring calcifications of old secretory disease can be clumped but characteristically have a lucent center. Several round or oval equally dense flecks, even though clustered, are less suspicious if on a coned-down view there are no interspersed finer flecks (Fig. 27–26).

The typical calcifications of fibrocystic disease are rounded, nearly uniform in size, nearly equal in density, and diffusely scattered throughout both breasts (Fig. 27–27).

Figure 27–27. Typical calcifications of diffuse fibrocystic disease in a 47-year-old woman with a nodule in her breast. Both breasts showed a similar process. Pathologically: fibrocystic disease. Magnified 6 × .

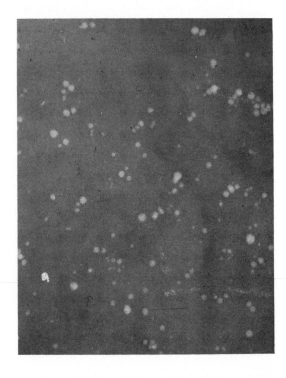

Radiographic studies with good detail can demonstrate the lobular arrangement of calcifications in sclerosing adenosis (Fig. 27–28). However, these lesions cannot be clearly differentiated from carcinoma. Localization and removal for histologic studies is still required.

Nonductal Calcifications

The very beginning calcifications of a fibroadenoma may be fine and closely arranged. Usually at this stage there is enough fat present to outline the mass, and these calcifications may be safely watched if the typical lobulated fibroadenoma is recognized (Fig. 27–29).

The amorphous plaques of calcification in fibroadenomata (Fig. 27–30) are probably the least confusing of all general types of calcification but are not always proved (Fig. 27–31). The parallel calcifications that are readily recognized as being in the walls of an artery are among the most common benign calcifications.

Foreign bodies in the breast, including parasites, produce localized or diffuse calcifications. These could also include particles resulting from the chemical inflammation interstitially of subareolar fibrosis, fat necrosis, and hemorrhage.

The usual cyst of fibrocystic disease rarely calcifies (Fig. 27–32). Calcifications in the cyst wall are generally associated with some unusual cyst contents (Fig. 27–33).

Systemic disease producing hypercalcemia could possibly cause the laying down of calcifications (Fig. 27–34A) or other anomalies (Fig. 27–34B).

Artifacts such as powder on the skin or some skin changes may mimic intramammary calcifications.

One cannot be overcautious about disregarding what may appear at first glance to be benign calcifications (Figs. 27–35 and 27–36).

Borderline Calcifications

Definition

Borderline calcifications of the breast not associated with a mass became one of the greatest problems to the radiologist. These nonspecific calcifications may be defined as characteristic neither of the fine, stippled, uncountable flecks in carcinoma nor of the

Text continued on page 478

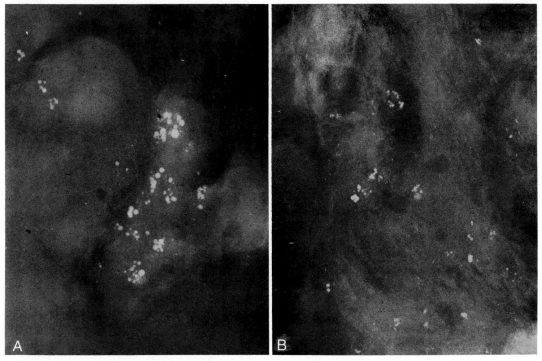

Figure 27–28. Calcifications in sclerosing adenosis. *A,* A 45-year-old woman with painful breasts. The calcifications are rounded and in a lobular distribution, but many are tiny. *B,* Similar problem in a 48-year-old woman with a baseline mammogram. Both lesions require localization and removal. Magnified 6 ×.

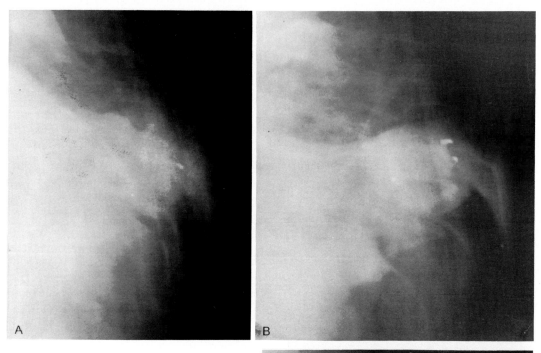

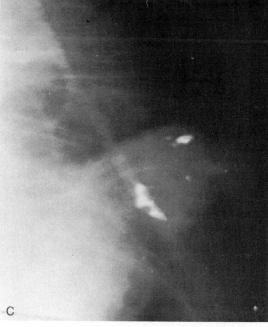

Figure 27–29. Calcifying fibroadenoma. *A,* Poorly outlined mass with one fleck of calcification in a glandular breast of a 28-year-old woman. *B,* Mass better outlined by fat three years later; three flecks of calcifications. *C,* After another three years.

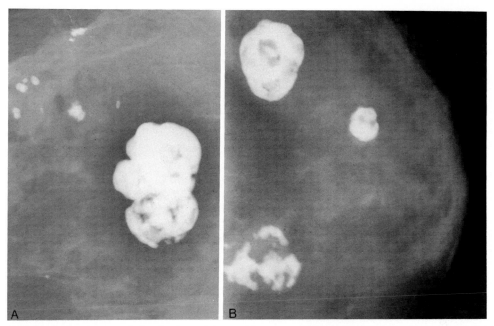

Figure 27–30. *A,* Amorphous calcification in an 80-year-old woman with a hard mass, clinically carcinoma. Faint mass lesion remains nearby. *B,* Calcifying fibroadenomata in a 72-year-old woman. The top two have central calcifications; the lower one has peripheral calcification in a faint mass.

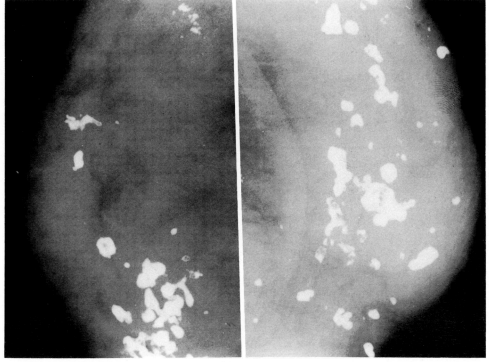

Figure 27–31. Dense amorphous breast calcifications. This 66-year-old woman had a biopsy for some clinical abnormality. The histopathologic studies revealed fibrocystic disease but no explanation for the masses of calcification. We always suspect these are the residual finding of old degenerated fibroadenomata.

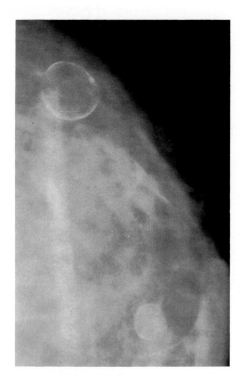

Figure 27–32. Calcifying cysts of fibrocystic disease in a 21-year-old woman. Six such cysts could be identified in this breast and four in the opposite breast. The largest (above), was biopsied and contained clear amber fluid; the calcium was identified in the cyst wall microscopically.

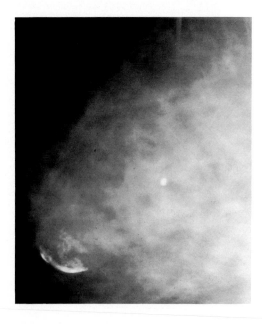

Figure 27–33. Calcifying cystic structure in the breast. The patient, a 49-year-old woman, was studied for a questionable mass in the opposite breast. After localization by mammography, the 1.5 cm lesion (above), was palpable. Biopsy revealed a 1.5 cm cyst containing soft brown granular material, marked surrounding fibrosis, and calcifications in the cyst wall.

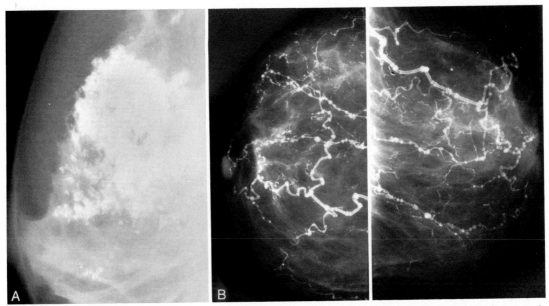

Figure 27–34. *A,* Hypercalcemia of the breast. A 29-year-old woman who, after treatment for Hodgkin's disease in the chest, developed a mass in the breast next to a radiation field. Treatment with ampicillin did not help. She developed a highly invasive carcinoma in the left breast. Modified radical mastectomy; 16 of 20 axillary lymph nodes with metastases. Cerebral, bone, and liver metastases were followed by death. Study of this right breast revealed calcification in the stroma. The diagnosis was hypercalcemia. *B,* Arterial calcifications. A 50-year-old woman with burning in her breast for three weeks. Nodular breasts clinically. Mammography: calcified arteries with numerous small aneurysms. She was being treated for uremia associated with polycystic kidneys; no known vascular lesions.

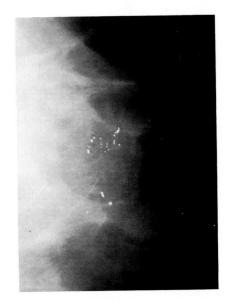

Figure 27–35. Metallic fragments from lead screen. Routine baseline mammogram on a 47-year-old woman. Most of these densities are obvious artifacts, but they can be very small and re-examination with another film holder may be necessary (one of the disadvantages of screen-film receptors).

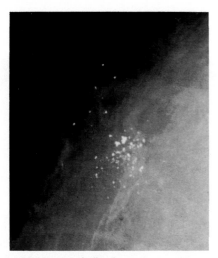

Figure 27–36. Fine bullet fragments mimicking breast calcifications. A 61-year-old woman, with a bullet wound over 10 years before, examined for large pendulous breasts. The metallic fragments are clustered for the most part, and many intervening ones are tiny. Special tangential views located the foreign bodies within the breast and not on the skin.

coarse, dense, amorphous deposits of benign diseases. These confusing concretions needed extensive study for elucidation, as they defy simple categorization. Initially, one third of the biopsies were in situ or minimally invasive carcinomas; one third were severe ductal hyperplasia, papillomatosis, or sclerosing adenosis, and one third were borderline histopathologically. With increasing experience with these borderline lesions most pathologists now agree on the diagnosis of intraductal carcinoma and benign processes. Continuing lack of agreement surrounds lobular hyperplasia, lobular neoplasia, and lobular carcinoma in situ.

Size

Most calcific particles seen by the radiologist are over 50 μ in size and will be shattered or dislodged by the microtome in preparation of the 7 μ thick histologic sections (Figs. 27–21 and 27–22). An exception is the softer calcification occurring in intraductal detritus of comedocarcinoma. Small calcifications in the histologic preparations may be present in an area distant from the area of concern as a product of generalized epithelial hyperplasia.

Problems

Endless errors by surgeons in the removal of nonpalpable but x-ray–suspicious breast tissue for the pathologist necessitated estab-

lishment of a strict routine for mapping the calcifications in the breast with their precise localization. In many instances the calcifications were not removed but remained visible on subsequent mammograms. As these radiographically suspicious areas look and feel no different from adjacent breast tissue, the pathologist often selected the wrong area to be studied. On occasion, if the calcifications were mounted, x-ray showed them in a part of the block not used for permanent sections. X-ray of all available tissues, including the residual breast, at times failed to demonstrate calcifications, indicating that they must have been discarded, probably in squaring up the block to obtain satisfactorily esthetic sections.

The pathologist's merely noting calcifications in his preparation does not guarantee that he is studying the area of concern. The pathologists' reaction to these borderline x-ray changes and their unfamiliar new role outside their isolated retreats was later described by Gallager (1974) as "most unsettling." Such errors were not unique to the 1950s but were repeated at Emory University, as recounted by Powell (1967), when in 1964 we instituted biopsy there for nonpalpable lesions before eventually finalizing a procedure to obviate these pitfalls.

Our routine continues the use of permanent sections for microscopy and has been outlined under the discussion of specimen radiography.

EMORY UNIVERSITY STUDY OF BREAST CALCIFICATIONS

Background

As we studied biopsy specimens with fewer and fewer calcifications, we became uncomfortably aware of our inability to categorize them into the rather clear-cut "pathognomonic" flecks of malignant disease of our earlier experience. The participating surgeons were not discouraged by the demonstration of one curable cancer by use of three or four biopsies but instead readily encouraged the search for these early cancers.

This presented the first clinical experience with clustered calcifications in the breast not associated with a mass. The radiologically demonstrable calcifications were discounted, observed, or investigated depending upon the clinical evaluation, most often reflecting inexperience due to lack of precedence. These avenues of patient care thus thrust upon the radiologist unsanctioned, but unique, opportunities to follow the course of breast calcifications. The gamut of clinical settings was provided for observation of the indolence of some of these carcinomas to development of inoperable carcinoma at the site of the unmolested cluster of calcifications not associated with a mass. Unlike the situation today, litigation in such cases was non-existent, as investigation of these findings in the breast was definitely not an established medical procedure.

In an attempt to see how well we differentiated calcifications in the breast as the only finding, we reviewed the Emory University material dating from 1963 and subject to five-year follow-up. Out attention was focused on the incidental finding of three or more clustered calcifications. This number was later changed to five flecks when we found no cancer by investigating only three specks.

Material

During this period 8000 women were referred from the oncologic breast clinic for mammography for a specific breast complaint, for follow-up of a breast complaint, or as part of a routine medical examination. All data forms were completed independently and prospectively: history by the technologist, physical examination by the oncologic surgeon, and mammography by the radiologist.

After 42,888 clinical and radiographic studies of the breast, there were 1487 operable cancers and 6667 benign lesions histologically confirmed (Table 27–1). Biopsy of 895 breasts

TABLE 27–2. Clustered Calcifications Not in a Mass as a Mammographic Finding With Over Five Years' Follow-Up

	Calcifications	
Breast Lesion	Clustered	Scattered and Clustered
Cancer		
Lobular in situ	5	13
Intraductal	56	16
Ductal	47	22
Benign		
Biopsied	161	285
Not biopsied	149	141
Total	418	477

for borderline (not obvious cancer) clustered calcifications not in a mass and subject to 5 to over 15 years' follow-up demonstrated 446 benign lesions and 159 primary operable carcinomas (Table 27–2). The rate of one carcinoma for each four biopsies for clustered calcifications was the usual average over the years, not unlike the rate extending back to the 1950s. Had all clusters been biopsied the rate would have been only six biopsies to find one of these early cancers. Nearly one half of the calcifications as well as the carcinomas were in women aged 40 to 49 years (Table 27–3). Two thirds were in dense glandular tissue (Table 27–4), with an uneven distribution of histologic types of carcinomas in these denser breasts (Table 27–5). Fatty and minimally glandular breasts made up one third of the women studied. The presence of two thirds of these carcinomas in denser breasts (two thirds of the women) and the 54 per cent incidence of the carcinomas in women under age 50 years strongly indicate the value of mammography to study denser breasts in the below-50 age group.

Procedures

Removal for Histologic Study

At Emory University from 1963 into the 1970s preoperative localization was done by mapping the calcifications on a diagram with the nipple as a landmark. Generally, a fairly large segment of tissue was removed, being larger from the larger breasts. Since smaller segments were desired to reduce deformity of the breasts and since in over 10 per cent of cases more than one specimen was required, we returned to the procedure of needle localization with radiopaque dye developed in the 1950s at the M.D. Anderson

TABLE 27–1. Recorded Calcifications Not in a Mass, With Their Arrangement and Their Association With Breast Cancers Subject to Five-Year Follow-Up

Calcification Arrangement	Number	Benign	Malignant
Scattered	2251	275	104
Clustered	741	214	106
Scattered and clustered	615	232	51
Single	501	57	41
Total	4108	778	302
Total Breast Examinations	42,888	6667	1487

TABLE 27–3. Age Distribution of Women With Clustered Calcifications Not in a Mass

Age	% of Women	No. of Carcinomas				% of Benign	% Without Biopsy
		LCIS	ID	D	Total CA		
30–39	37.3	1	10	10	21	18	14
40–49	40.9	10	35	21	66	40	52
50–59	15.4	5	24	23	52	24	14
≥ 60	6.4	1	4	15	20	18	20
Total	100.0	17	73	69	159	100	100

Hospital and Tumor Institute. Even so, at least 5 per cent of the cases required more than one specimen.

Radiographic Study

Single or scattered calcifications not in a mass were frequently recorded but were never the indication for biopsy. A cluster was defined as five or more calcifications in an area usually no larger than 0.5 × 0.5 cm.

The intact biopsy specimen was radiographed in the Breast Imaging Center using very fine-grain industrial film at 12 to 20 kvp. The presence of calcification was confirmed, and comparison with the mammograms ensured that the proper area of the breast had been removed. The biopsy specimen was sliced thin and carefully placed on cleared x-ray film, properly identified, and x-rayed again. The deposits of calcium were precisely pinpointed for the pathologist.

For a period, radiography of the biopsy specimen included double loading of a fast film with the fine-grain film emulsion. With hand processing, development time was cut in half for a quicker viewing of the calcifications. Incidentally, on the denser emulsion, when fully developed, the very fine calcifications were erased. With the advent of screen-film receptors the clarity of the radiographs was reduced, and again the fine calcifications were lost in the receptor mottle.

As calcifications are always visualized better in the small biopsy specimen compared with the intact breast, this system is sufficient to determine whether the calcifications were removed.

The characteristics of the calcifications were studied on the mammograms and on the radiographs of the intact biopsy specimen and the thinly sliced breast sections by a hand magnifying lens, by a dental 10 × x-ray enlarger, and by mounting areas of the radiographs in 2 × 2 inch slide mounts and enlarging 60 × by projection onto a screen. In many cases a 0.5 × 0.5 cm area of a radiograph was enlarged photographically as a negative and a contact print made.

The benign and malignant calcifications were associated with number, density, borders and shape, size and spatial arrangement, background tissues, age of women, histologic types of tumor, temporal alterations, and unilaterality or bilaterality. They were also studied for any increase in number in the specimen radiograph over the mammogram in an attempt to simulate their evaluation in a clinical setting (Tables 27–3 to 27–10).

Results

Clusters of more than ten calcifications were found in 84 per cent of the cancers, 54 per cent of the benign biopsied lesions, and

TABLE 27–4. Glandular Patterns of Breasts With Clustered Calcifications Not in a Mass

Pattern	% of Women	No. of Carcinomas				% of Benign	% Without Biopsy
		LCIS	ID	D	Total CA		
Fatty	20.6	0	16	21	37	14	17
Minimal glandular	13.1	0	6	11	17	4	11
Diffuse glandular	37.4	2	19	11	32	28	35
Dense fibronodular	28.9	15	32	26	73	54	37
Total	100.0	17	73	69	159	100	100

TABLE 27–5. Numbers of Carcinomas With Clustered Calcifications Not in a Mass Related to Age of Women, Breast Patterns, and Histologic Types of Tumor

Breast Pattern	Type CA	Age in Years 30–39	Age in Years 40–49	Age in Years 50–59	Age in Years ≥60
Fatty	LCIS	0	0	0	0
	ID	5	7	2	2
	D	5	3	8	5
Minimal glandular	LCIS	0	0	0	0
	ID	0	2	4	0
	D	0	3	1	7
Diffuse glandular	LCIS	1	2	0	0
	ID	0	7	10	2
	D	3	3	4	1
Dense	LCIS	1	8	5	1
Fibronodular	ID	5	19	8	0
	D	2	12	10	2
Total		22	66	52	20

19 per cent of nonbiopsied breasts (Table 27–6). The age of the women, the relative amount of fibroglandular tissue, or an isolated cluster of calcifications vs one associated with scattered calcifications was not helpful in differentiating benign and malignant breast diseases. The pattern of scattered calcifications alone was usually found in benign conditions.

Very fine calcifications associated with widely varying sized flecks were often found in carcinoma. Calcifications with a wide range in density, from very faint to dense, were more frequent in carcinoma but often seen in benign disease. Relatively fine calcifications, when widely variable in shape, were a clue to carcinoma.

The number, density, size, and shape of the calcifications did not distinguish between benign and malignant lesions (Tables 27–6 to 27–9).

For a period there was a marked increase in number and finer particles seen in the radiographs of the thinly sliced breast specimen using very fine-grain nonscreen film, as compared with the mammogram. The increase was such that it was thought to represent carcinoma and not a benign process. Upon observation of a larger number of cases, this did not hold up, as there was too much overlap with benign and malignant lesions (Table 27–10). Calcifications are increased as a result of better radiography, but an especially large increase still highly favors carcinoma.

Treatment at the time of initial demonstration of calcifications resulted in 88 per cent survival (Table 27–11). With treatment after periods of observation of two to five years (mean 3.1 years) without appearance of a mass, there was 89 per cent survival. Once a mass was associated with the calcifications, the survival was reduced to that of a similarly staged infiltrating duct carcinoma (Table 27–11).

The few breasts in which several calcifications (fewer than five) increased to a suspicious number (more than five) infrequently

TABLE 27–6. Clustered Calcifications Without a Mass in 0.5 × 0.5 cm Area

Calcification Number	No. of Carcinomas LCIS	No. of Carcinomas ID	No. of Carcinomas D	No. of Carcinomas Total CA	% of Benign	% Without Biopsy
≤ 5	0	0	0	0	4	69
6–10	6	19	5	30	44	12
11–15	3	11	12	26	28	9
16–25	2	14	16	32	10	10
26–50	2	19	29	50	2	0
> 50	4	10	7	21	12	0
Total	17	73	69	159	100	100

TABLE 27–7. Density of Clustered Calcifications Not in a Mass (1–4, Increasing Density)

Density	No. of Carcinomas				% of Benign	% Without Biopsy
	LCIS	*ID*	*D*	*Total CA*		
1–2	4	16	10	30	12	37
1–3	11	57	54	122	48	11
2–3	0	0	5	5	26	49
3–4	2	0	0	2	14	3
Total	17	73	69	159	100	100

TABLE 27–8. Size of Clustered Calcifications Not in a Mass

Size (mm)	No. of Carcinomas				% of Benign	% Without Biopsy
	LCIS	*ID*	*D*	*Total CA*		
0.05–1.0	8	41	20	69	82	49
0.05–2.0	9	22	49	90	16	23
1–3	0	0	0	0	2	22
2–3	0	0	0	0	0	6
Total	17	63	69	159	100	100

TABLE 27–9. Shape of Clustered Calcifications Not in a Mass

Shape	No. of Carcinomas				% of Benign	% Without Biopsy
	LCIS	*ID*	*D*	*Total CA*		
Punctate	6	29	16	51	64	9
Round	6	3	0	9	14	71
Linear, bizarre	0	0	2	2	4	9
Variable	5	41	51	97	18	11
Total	17	73	69	159	100	100

TABLE 27–10. Cancers With Calcifications, Not in a Mass, Having Increased Calcification in Specimen Radiographs Over Mammogram*

Increase	% of Carcinoma			% of Benign
	LCIS	ID	D	
none	20	8	0	31
2 times	60	7	25	52
3–4 times	0	35	50	11
5 times	20	50	25	6

*Expressed as percentage of the total number of each type of cancer.

produced a mass during observation. These women still had nearly 90 per cent ten-year survival.

Bilateral involvement with cancer calcification, whether as the second primary simultaneously, as one primary simultaneously, or as both primaries simultaneously, had little effect on prognosis (Table 27–12).

Calcifications in Risk Scheme

The addition of numerous risk indicators to the digitalized x-ray appearance of the breast calcifications, all being subjected to a strong discriminant analytic procedure, resulted in a much improved differentiation of malignant and benign calcifications. This approach has far exceeded our attempts to refine and digitalize calcification characteristics using a microdensitometer.

Policy Development

Our aggressiveness in pursuing breast biopsies during the establishment of clinical mammography was tempered by the individual surgeon's previous experience with non-palpable breast cancer and his surgical tenets. Biopsy of six to ten suspicious breast nodules to demonstrate one operable cancer was acceptable surgical practice, but a policy of biopsying three to four clusters of unsuspected calcification to detect one curable cancer had to be established as a plausible routine. Mutual aims of the surgeon and the radiologist evolved through tedious and varied learning processes, with each new experience often a cliffhanger. All clusters of calcifications were of concern to the radiologist, and he was uneasy until their removal. In retrospective analysis, biopsy of all clusters of calcifications without mass in this group of women would have produced an acceptable biopsy rate, one cancer in six biopsies, even in clinical practice and surely prospectively in a mass screening program. Based on this finding, today we think that the best policy is to biopsy all clusters if they can be localized on both mammographic views (Fig. 27–37). If bilateral clusters were found, the more worrisome cluster is biopsied first, or, occasionally, bilateral biopsies are done at the same time.

During the early stages of this study the typical calcifications of advanced comedocarcinoma were "practically pathognomonic" of cancer, whereas literature on borderline calcifications was nonexistent. Today our more aggressive routine policy, practiced over at least the past 20 years, to biopsy all clusters of calcifications is gaining wider acceptance. With changes in surgical attitudes and the enormous impetus from the American Cancer Society–National Cancer Institute Breast Cancer Detection Demonstration Projects designed to search for Stage 0 or Stage I cancers, the more widespread use of this approach should improve overall results with breast cancer.

TABLE 27–11. Clustered Calcification Without Mass Studied on Initial Discovery, After Increase in Calcification, or After a Mass Formed in the Cluster

Time of Biopsy	No.	Lobular In Situ		Intraductal		Duct		Total
		No.	% N.E.D.	No.	% N.E.D.	No.	% N.E.D.	% N.E.D.
Initial discovery	119	12	100	55	100	51	78	88
After calcification increased*	23	5	100	18	86	0	0	89
After mass appeared	17	0	0	0	18	18	86	86

*Axillary lymph nodes free of tumor at modified radical mastectomy.
N.E.D. = No evidence of disease.

TABLE 27–12. Occurrence of Cancer With Calcification Not in a Mass as a Single Primary or as One of Bilateral Cancers

Carcinoma	No.	Lobular In Situ		Intraductal		Duct		Total
		No.	% N.E.D.	No.	% N.E.D.	No.	% N.E.D.	% N.E.D.
Unilateral	121	10	100	55	100	56	74	88
Bilateral								
as 1st primary	0	0	0	0	0	0	0	0
as 2nd primary	27	2	100	14	82	11	100	91
simultaneous	11*	5	100	4	100	2	100	100

*Clustered calcifications in one breast only.
N.E.D. = No evidence of disease.

TRENDS IN BIOPSY RATES AT EMORY UNIVERSITY

The history of calcifications not in a mass at Emory University (from 1965) can be illustrated by the patients referred from the oncologic clinic, the biopsies for borderline calcifications, and the benign and malignant lesions. Prior to that date biopsies for calcium were sporadic. In 1965 we were just instituting routine specimen radiography patterned after the procedure done previously both at M.D. Anderson Hospital and in Indianapolis. Its use doubled during the following year and waxed and waned until 1975. During this year there was great publicity about the breast cancers of the wives of the President and the Vice President of the United States. Many breast biopsies were forced on surgeons, partly because of increased fear but primarily because of patients bringing in poor-quality mammograms. Either our Section of Mammography was too rushed to do repeat mammography or the surgeons just proceeded to perform biopsy on artifacts. Also, many radiologists were just beginning mammography by using xeroradiography with its increased number of artifacts. In 1969 and 1971 the biopsy rates as well as the percentage of carcinoma were at the lowest

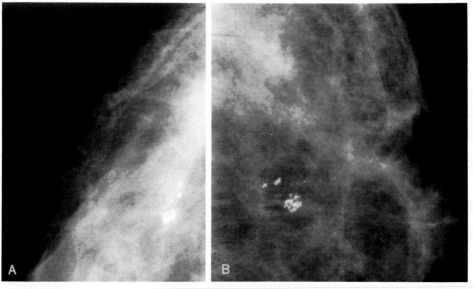

Figure 27–37. Coalescent comedo calcifications that suggest a "benign" type. A 54-year-old woman gravida 5, para 5; one sister with breast cancer; baseline study. Two previous biopsies in this breast were benign. Mammography: Craniocaudad (A) and mediolateral (B) views show primarily dense, closely packed calcifications with suspicious intervening small ones. After localization, biospy and modified radical mastectomy: 6 × 7 mm area of 90 per cent intraductal and 10 per cent invasive comedocarcinoma; all 16 axillary lymph nodes were free of tumor. The patient was living and well nine years later.

levels despite the sharpest rise in the number of patients.

In 1976 there was a strong negative response following the radiation cancer scare generated by the Consensus Meeting on Screening by the National Institutes of Health in September. The percentage of women with cancer declined from 1974 to 1977 and then began a marked increase in 1978. This corresponded to the low biopsy rate and high rate of carcinoma in 1967, 1968, and 1971. The 1978 variation could be explained by reluctance to use mammography before the age of 50 years. Below that age over one-half the carcinomas with calcifications without a mass occurred. The fall in the biopsy curve is readily explained by the sharp drop in patients from the Emory University Oncologic Clinic in 1977 and 1978.

The decision to biopsy or not to biopsy a certain group of calcifications without a palpable mass is made by the radiologist. The surgeons follow suit. Since 1965 almost all the mammograms have been read by one radiologist. This lack of parallelism of the curves in Figure 27–38 is unexplained.

WORKING HYPOTHESES

It was possible to form some working hypotheses:

Clustered calcifications not in a mass indicate a high risk of breast carcinoma.

Certain characteristics of these calcifications are increased number, variability in texture from very fine to rather coarse, and variable density from almost imperceptible to fairly dense; an increased number in the specimen radiograph also provide clues to the presence of carcinoma.

There is such a broad overlapping of the calcifications in fibrocystic disease and carcinoma that the mammographer cannot confidently exclude carcinoma. He must then participate in the team effort to localize for removal and to ensure that the proper tissue is carefully studied by the pathologists (Figs. 27–37 and 27–39 to 27–43).

An indolent phase of breast cancer probably exists while there is x-ray evidence of only calcification without mass. Some of these lesions may regress, but it is indisputable that many do not. There is a variable

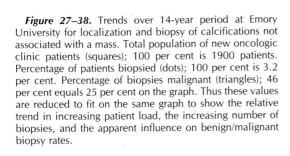

Figure 27–38. Trends over 14-year period at Emory University for localization and biopsy of calcifications not associated with a mass. Total population of new oncologic clinic patients (squares); 100 per cent is 1900 patients. Percentage of patients biopsied (dots); 100 per cent is 3.2 per cent. Percentage of biopsies malignant (triangles); 46 per cent equals 25 per cent on the graph. Thus these values are reduced to fit on the same graph to show the relative trend in increasing patient load, the increasing number of biopsies, and the apparent influence on benign/malignant biopsy rates.

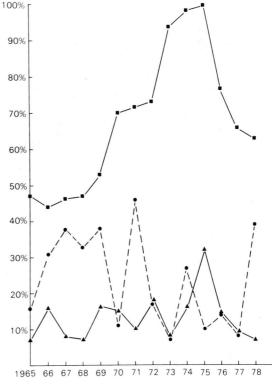

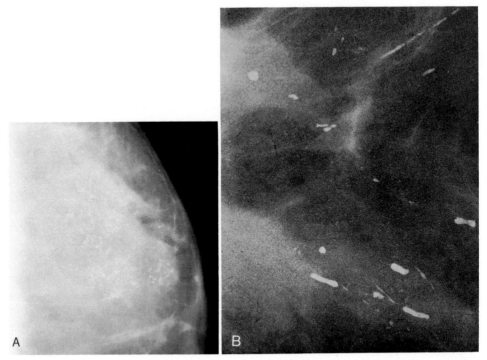

Figure 27–39. *A,* Sandlike calcifications of carcinoma in a 72-year-old woman with a lump in her breast. Pathologically: 2.5 cm comedocarcinoma; axilla free of disease. *B,* Dense needle-like intraductal calcifications of a minimally invasive duct carcinoma in a 42-year-old woman with a nodule in the opposite breast. Magnified 6 ×.

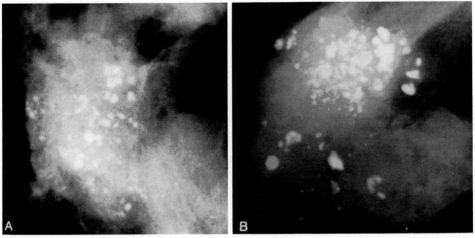

Figure 27–40. Similarity of benign and malignant calcifications radiographically. *A,* A 35-year-old woman with painful breasts. The calcifications were associated with mammary dysplasia, lobular hyperplasia, apocrine metaplasia, ductal hyperplasia, and cysts (no atypia). *B,* Similar radiographic findings in a 39-year-old woman having a physical examination checkup. Pathologically: comedocarcinoma with a few isolated areas of minimal invasion; no positive axillary lymph nodes. Some of the calcifications are larger and denser but some are smaller than in *A*. Magnified 6 ×.

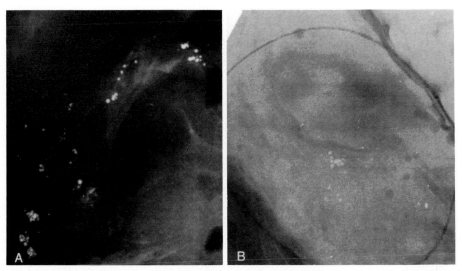

Figure 27–41. A, Calcifications in a lobular distribution, suggesting benign nature. Pathologically: adenosis. B, Calcifications also in a lobular distribution. Pathologically: intraductal comedocarcinoma.

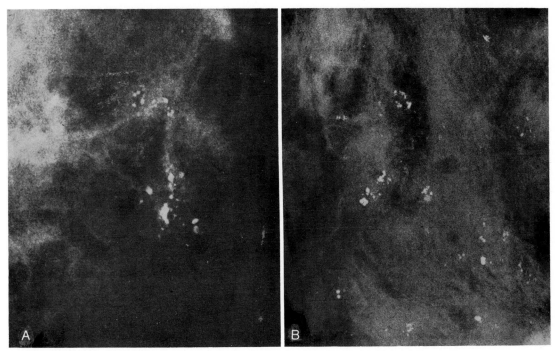

Figure 27–42. Wide variation in size and shape of malignant (A) and benign (B) calcification at 6 × magnification; 50 μ sized particles readily demonstrated.

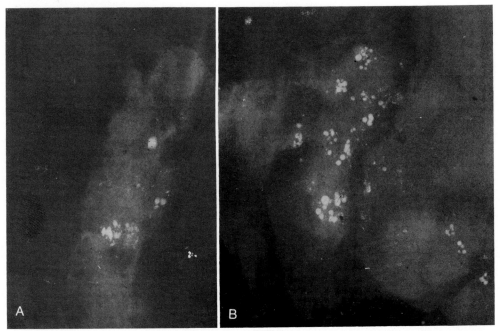

Figure 27–43. Variation in density of malignant (*A*) and benign (*B*) calcifications (6 × magnification).

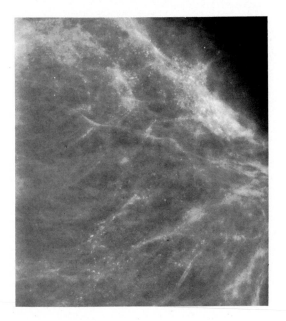

Figure 27–44. Calcifications being followed for years. A 46-year-old woman who had bilateral breast biopsies for calcifications not associated with a mass eight years before. Only fibrocystic disease was demonstrated. She has been followed yearly since, without change in the breast calcifications.

and probably extensive phase of indolence with clusters of calcifications without a mass of x-ray. Once a mass appears, aggressiveness of the tumor is intensified and the survival rate is drastically depressed from the expected 95 to 98 per cent ten-year cures with calcifications of carcinoma without a mass.

Since a high percentage of cancerous masses in the breast contain radiographically demonstrable calcifications, one could assume that many of the clusters of calcifications in the dense breasts may be within masses not demonstrable by x-ray. But they are not found associated with a mass by palpation at surgery or in the biopsy specimen, by thinly slicing the specimen, or by histopathologic study. Light miscroscopy may demonstrate microinvasion or limited invasion but not invasiveness sufficient to produce a distinctive mass. A large comedocarcinoma, perhaps occupying one quadrant of the breast, without a true radiographic mass, often presents with an asymmetric thickening without a true delineated mass.

The calcification associated with neoplastic diseases of the breast results from an active secretory process of the ductal epithelial cells in addition to mineralization of cellular debris and degenerate cells.

Our previous observation of the develop-

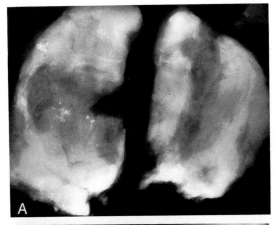
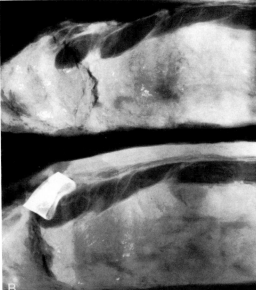

Figure 27–46. A and B, Numerous foci of calcifications. A 48-year-old woman with nodularity of both breasts. Mammography showed innumerable foci of clustered calcifications, not associated with a mass, in the right breast. The radiographs of the slicer sections (B) and the original biopsy specimen (A) show representative areas of these calcifications. Pathology: multiple foci throughout the whole-organ study of intraductal papillomatosis, sclerosing adenosis, lobular carcinoma in situ, and ductal hyperplasia, all associated with calcifications. Modified radical mastectomy; all 22 axillary lymph nodes free of tumor. The patient was alive and well 17 years later.

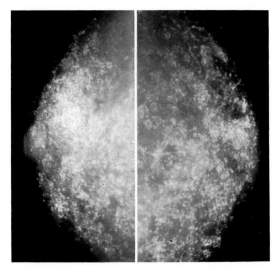

Figure 27–45. Unusual type of breast calcification. A 40-year-old Oriental woman who had lived for the past ten years in the San Francisco area after moving from China. A breast abnormality had been noted on her chest film. Mammography: no apparent etiology for the calcifications. Pathology: papillomatosis, duct ectasia; no explanation for the calcification.

ment of 32 carcinomas in areas of clustered calcification, and our inability in retrospect to differentiate with confidence benign and malignant clusters, lead us to our present concept that clusters of calcifications by x-ray cannot safely be observed but need careful histopathologic evaluation (Figs. 27–44 to 27–46).

REFERENCES

Ahmed A (1975): Calcification in human breast carcinomas: ultrastructural observations. J Pathol 117:247.

Dominguez CM (1930): Investigacion radiografica y quimica sobre el calcio precipitado en tumores del aparato genital femenino. Bol Soc Anat Pathol 1:217.

Dominguez CM (1930). Estudio radiologico de los descalcificadores. Bol Soc Anat Pathol 1:175.

Dominguez CM (1935). Estudios Cancerologicos: la radiografia de la mamma dinamica. Anales del Departmento Cientifico de Salud Publica, II:71.

Egan RL (1960): Experience with mammography in a tumor institution. Evaluation of 1,000 studies. Radiology 75:894.

Egan RL (1962): Fifty-three cases of carcinoma of the breast, occult until mammography. Am J Roentgenol 88:1095.

Egan RL (1964): Mammography. Springfield, IL, Charles C Thomas, pp 99 and 304.

Egan RL (1964). A Guide to Mammography. Washington, DC, Dept HEW, USPHS.

Espaillat A (1933): Contribution à l'étude radiographique du sein normal et pathologique. Thèse de Paris, No 417, Librairie Paris.

Galkin BM, Feig SA Patchefsky AS, Rue JW, Gamblin WJ, Gomez DG, Marchant LM (1977): Ultrastructure and microanalysis of "benign" and "malignant" breast calcifications. Radiology 124:245.

Gallager HS (1974): Panel presentation on cancer of the breast. American College of Surgeons 60th Clinical Congress, Miami Beach, October 22.

Leborgne R (1951): Diagnosis of tumors of breast by simple roentgenography: Calcifications in carcinoma. Am J Roentgenol 65:1.

Ledoux-Lebard R, Garcia-Calderon J, Espaillat GA (1933): Etude radiographique de la glande mammaire. Bull Soc Radiol Med 21:418.

Levitan LH, Witten DM, Harrison EG (1964): Calcifications in breast disease: mammography-pathologic correlation. Am J Roentgenol 92:29.

Martin JE, Wolfe JN (1973): Panel discussion, 12th Annual Mammography Seminar, San Diego, March 5–9.

Muntz EP, (1977): In Logan WW (ed): Breast Carcinoma: The Radiologist's Expanded Role. New York, John Wiley & Son's.

Murphy MA, Deschryver-Kecskémeti K (1978): Isolated clustered microcalcifications in the breast: radiographic-pathologic correlation. Radiology 127:335.

Ozzello L (1971): Ultrastructure of the human mammary gland. In Sommer SC (ed): Pathology Annual 1971. Chicago, Appleton-Century-Crofts, p 37.

Powell RW (1967): Surgeons look at mammography. In Proceedings of the Sixth Annual Mammography Conference, San Juan, Puerto Rico, p 194.

Price JL, Gibbs NM (1978): The relationship between microcalcifications and in-situ carcinoma of the breast. Clin Radiol 29:447.

Reis E (1930): Diagnostic lipoidal injection into milk ducts followed by abscess formation. Am J Obstet Gynecol 20:414.

Rogers JV, Powell RW (1972): Mammographic indications for biopsy of clinically normal breasts: correlation with pathologic findings in 72 cases. Am J Roentgenol 115:794.

Salomon A (1913): Beitrage zur pathologie und klinik der mammacarcinome. Arch Klin Chir 101:573.

Warren SL (1930): A roentgenographic study of the breast. Am J Roentgenol 24:113.

28

Multicentric Breast Carcinoma

BACKGROUND

The multicentric nature of breast carcinoma has attracted increasing interest in the past two decades. Yet there has been inadequate stimulus to establish clear-cut definitions and to lessen variable reported frequencies. Distinct, separate lesions may be established by including epithelial atypias and in situ lesions within the immediate vicinity of the main tumor mass or by the extreme of insisting on a separation of at least 5 cm of normal breast tissue from the reference carcinoma. In the pioneering work of Cheatle and Cutler (1931), the emphasis was on development de novo of foci of carcinoma in situ at a distance from the primary tumor rather than on intraductal spread of the lesions. Thus, these investigators found it necessary only to demonstrate a segment of intervening noncancerous ducts to establish separate multicentric foci. We had adopted this concept prior to our report in 1969 (Egan et al., 1969). Later Gallager and Martin (1969) substantiated this theory. Qualheim and Gall (1957) did not specify a necessary distance for separation of foci. Fisher et al. (1975, 1976) and Schwartz et al. (1980) did random quadrant samplings, indicating that this would provide sufficient separation for multicentricity. Morgenstern et al. (1975) and Rosen et al. (1975) were more concerned with residual tumor following an excision type biopsy than with establishing independent foci of carcinoma.

The variability of the reported frequency of multicentric breast carcinoma no doubt is related to the definition as well as the thoroughness of study of the whole breast. Qualheim and Gall (1957) reported that 85 of 157 breasts studied had multiple tumors. Gallager and Martin (1969a) reported a 45 per cent frequency of multicentric invasive foci among 47 primary invasive carcinomas and (1969b) a 75 per cent frequency in 34 breasts, counting atypias and in situ nearby changes as separate foci. In his series, Lagios (1977) found 18 of 85 cases (21 per cent) to have multiple tumors. On random quadrant sampling of 904 mastectomy specimens, Fisher et al. (1975, 1976) found multiple quadrants involved in 13.4 per cent, and Schwartz et al. (1980) in 49.2 per cent of 43 breast specimens.

Several histologic methods have been employed to demonstrate multicentric breast carcinoma: (1) generous biopsy samples of breast tissue taken from all quadrants of the breast, including that containing the primary cancer (Tellem et al., 1962; Morgenstern et al., 1975); (2) serial sections several mm thick of the whole breast examined macroscopically, with areas selected visually for microscopic study (Cheatle and Cutler, 1931); and (3) large blocks of the breast embedded in paraffin and a limited number of 8 to 20 μ thick subserial microscopic sections prepared (Qualheim and Gall, 1957). A macroscopic approach has been used: The breast specimen is frozen, sliced 1 mm to several mm

491

thick, fixed in formaldehyde, stained in hematoxylin, washed, stored in mineral oil, and viewed with a dissecting microscope (Ingleby and Gershon-Cohen, 1960). Another method consists of cleaned, formalin-fixed whole mounts stained with hematoxylin, mounted in plastic, and viewed through a dissecting microscope (Wellings et al., 1975).

EMORY UNIVERSITY WHOLE-ORGAN STUDY

Methods

A separate histopathology laboratory had been set up for this project. One pathologist and two technologists were required full-time for five years to complete the studies. So much breast tissue was processed that two microtome blade sharpeners were kept in use during the entire working day.

Tissue Selection and Preparation

A correlated clinical, radiographic, and pathologic approach to study whole-organ breast was developed at Emory University. It consisted of freezing the breast, slicing it in serial sections, and doing radiography of the slicer sections (Egan et al., 1969; Egan, 1970; see also Chapter 11). Areas for microscopic studies were selected by examination of the radiographs. With low kvp nonscreen radiography demonstrating resolution of 50 μ sized particles, or smaller, this approach probably came the closest to ''whole-organ'' study. All nonfatty tissues by x-ray were studied by light microscopy, since it was soon learned that completely fatty tissues on these radiographs contained no detectable glandular tissue. Avoiding mounting areas of pure adipose tissue allowed technically easier, more meticulous, and better-quality preparations. To us this proved to be a faster, less expensive, and more thorough approach than subserial sectioning. Also, it did not depend on chance to include all areas of pathology (Egan, 1970) or to appreciate fully the three-dimensional aspects of a lesion and its relationship to the breast (Fig. 28–1). This technique has become readily reproducible (Richardson, 1975; Lagios, 1977).

To avoid air pockets and distortion of tissues by partial slicing or cutting into the breast, intact specimens were needed for worthwhile radiography. These were obtained following needle biopsy and diagnosis, following positive axillary lymph node biopsy with positive clinical or x-ray findings in the breast, or following strong clinical and x-ray findings in the breast, especially in surgically poor-risk patients. On some occasions, specimens were obtained following simple mastectomy (prophylactic and/or diagnostic), following a radical mastectomy for carcinoma, or prior to prosthetic implant of the breast. Breasts containing a carcinoma detected by a cluster of calcifications not associated with a mass were routinely biopsied, the wound closed, and paraffin block studies carried out; in one to two days a mastectomy was done.

The axillary portion of the mastectomy specimen was first removed to prevent delay in histologic staging for possible additional treatment; then the whole breast was frozen overnight. The breast was neatly sliced into about 20 to 40 sections 5 mm thick in the plane of the mediolateral mammogram. The carefully laid-out and numbered slices were x-rayed with 12 kvp; no filtration was added to the beryllium window x-ray tube; and long target-film distance and extremely fine-grain industrial film with hand processing were used. The slicer radiographs were reviewed by the pathologist and radiologist. Each area of identifiable glandular tissues and suspected pathology was selected, fixed, and embedded in paraffin. Slides 7 μ thick were prepared, stained by various and appropriate stains, and studied both with the naked eye and by light microscopy (Egan, 1970). All cases were reviewed on at least three occasions in conference, with the radiologist, pathologist, and surgeon spending at least two to three hours on each review. Usually two weeks of preparation was needed for the pathologist to prepare a case for review.

Definition of Histologic Types and Multiple Sites

The carcinomas were classified by the number of distinct histologic types and the number of sites, implying to some degree the sites of origin. Mucoid carcinoma was limited to tumors having islands of cells floating in pools of mucus. The intracystic papillary carcinoma contained a papillary growth within a blood-filled cyst, with or without invasion into the breast tissue. Medullary carcinoma, lobular carcinoma, lobular carcinoma in situ, tubular carcinoma, and ade-

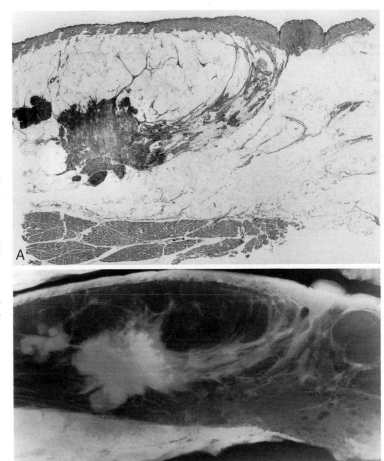

Figure 28–1. Medium-sized microscopic study of central portion of breast; main mass of cancer and nearby nodule of cancer are readily seen. *A*, Haphazard selection of additional cuts may or may not have demonstrated the area connecting the tumor masses precisely shown on the radiograph. *B*, Combined team approach is indispensable in breast studies. Mounting of the microscopic section alongside the radiograph of the same area provides ready comparative studies.

nocarcinoma (not otherwise specified) were separate entities. Invasive duct carcinoma was considered as four types: (1) infiltrating duct; (2) comedo; (3) scirrhous, with prominent desmoplastic reaction; and (4) simplex or no special type (NOS). Borderline changes were considered noncancerous.

Multicentricity was based on definite separation grossly with noncancerous breast tissue intervening: radiographically seen in Figure 28–2. The separation may have been apparent both radiographically and microscopically with grossly different morphology (Figs. 28–3 to 28–6). There were separate and histologically different tumor types (Figs. 28–7 and 28–8). Patterns of multiple areas of infiltrating carcinomas throughout much of the breast readily indicated multiple foci, often of the same histologic type (Figs. 28–9 to 28–11). A number of those many foci may have been histologically dissimilar (Fig. 28–

6). The widely scattered clusters of carcinoma type breast calcifications on the mammograms indicated separate foci of carcinoma (Fig. 28–12). The separation of these foci of stippled calcifications was best appreciated on the slicer-section radiographs (Fig. 28–13). Sometimes separate foci were found only after long searching (Fig. 28–14). In most cases, however, there was a dominant nodule palpable that became the reference tumor, and smaller foci were found peripheral to it (Figs. 28–15 to 28–17).

Some cases posed problems in the determination of whether separate foci were present. Intraductal carcinoma surrounded by or adjacent to duct carcinomas was one site and one type (Fig. 28–12). With a highly invasive carcinoma, nearby or contiguous intraductal carcinoma was considered merely a part of the infiltrating lesion, but if at a reasonable separation, it was a second focus (Fig. 28–

Text continued on page 508

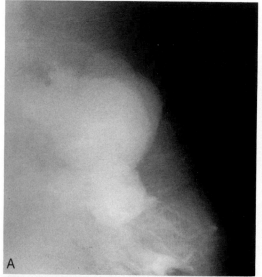

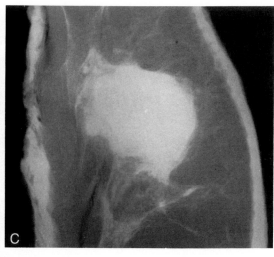

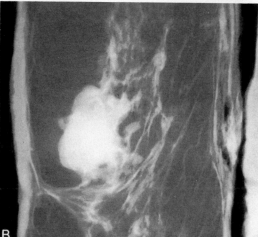

Figure 28–2. Two intracystic papillary carcinomas. A 78-year-old woman with a mass and nipple retraction that appear contiguous on the mammogram (*A*). Slicer section of the inferior smaller mass is near the nipple in section 11 (*B*). The larger mass was far laterally in slicer 18 (*C*).

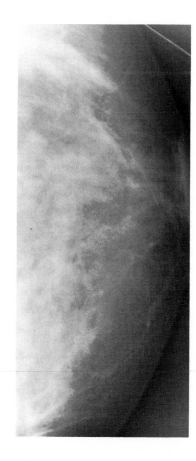

Figure 28–3. Two separate invasive duct carcinomas with intervening intraductal carcinomas. A 58-year-old woman with a breast lump UOQ that is clinically carcinoma. Mammography: two small carcinomas deep on the extreme edges of the mammogram recognized primarily by trabecular retraction (the upper about 8 mm and the lower about 5 mm in size). Severe ductal hyperplasia. Pathology: two lesions, both intraductal and infiltrating duct carcinoma with productive fibrosis, Grade III, with the intraductal components, both comedo and solid, extending into sub-nipple ducts. Modified radical mastectomy; five Level I and one Level II of 21 lymph nodes contained metastases. Two years later the patient was free of disease.

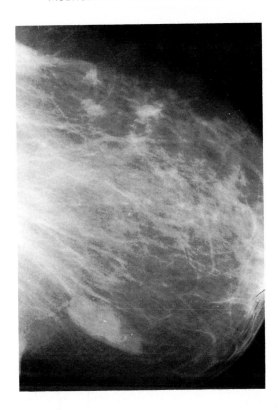

Figure 28–4. Multiple sites of carcinoma. A 74-year-old woman studied for a lump in her breast. Mammography: severe ductal hyperplasia; four separate spiculated carcinomas in the upper breast measuring 3 × 2, 3 × 3, 3 × 4, and 12 × 15 mm in size; a benign 1.4 × 3.3 cm mass in the lower breast. Pathology: five distinct deposits of duct carcinoma; many sites of intraductal carcinoma; sclerosing fibroadenoma. Radical mastectomy; 8 of 24 axillary lymph nodes at all levels with metastases. Widespread metastases 18 months later.

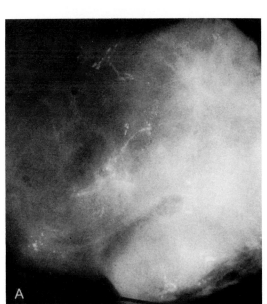

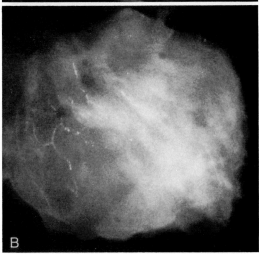

Figure 28–5. Multifocal intraductal and microinvasive breast carcinomas. A 45-year-old woman undergoing baseline studies for clinically nodular breasts. Mammography: bilateral ductal hyperplasia with at least two separate areas of clustered calcifications. A–B, Specimen radiographs of the two areas: comedo type calcifications following some ducts, areas of clustered punctate calcifications, and what may be tiny flecks of interstitial calcifications. Pathology: multifocal intraductal carcinoma with comedo, micropapillary, and solid patterns. Modified radical mastectomy; at least two areas of microinvasion of carcinoma; atypical ductal hyperplasia; 19 axillary lymph nodes free of tumor. The patient was alive without disease three years later.

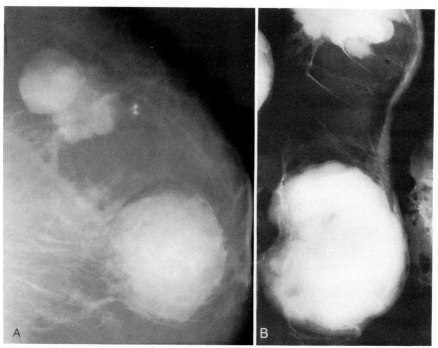

Figure 28–6. Morphologically different carcinomas. This 67-year-old woman presented with a self-discovered mass in this breast. She had had a radical mastectomy for carcinoma of the opposite breast five and one-half years previously for infiltrative duct carcinoma. The mammogram (*A*) and slicer section radiograph (*B*) show two separate breast carcinomas with different growth patterns. The whole-organ mount (*C*) shows two well-circumscribed carcinomas. The lower lesion was histologically a well-differentiated adenocarcinoma. The upper lesion was a well-circumscribed, lobulated tumor with focally infiltrative border; histologically (*D*) it was carcinoma simplex, quite different from the lesion on the left.

Illustration continued on opposite page

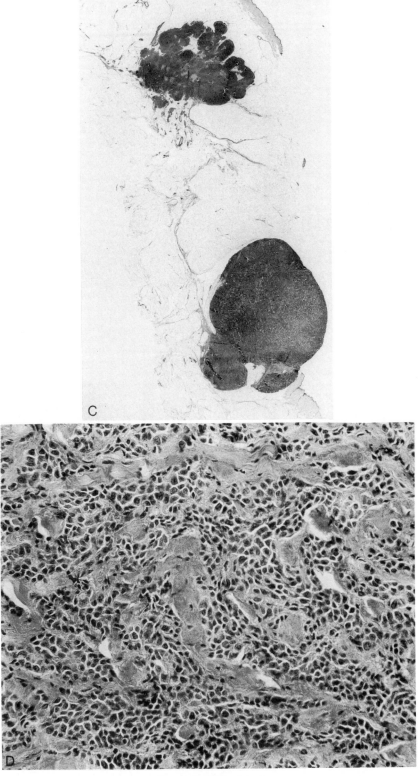

Figure 28–6 Continued

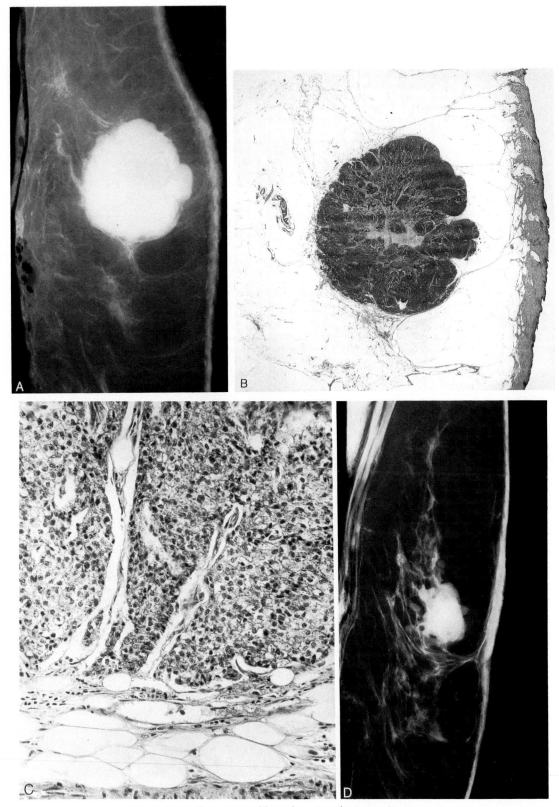

Figure 28–7. Illustration and legend continued on opposite page

Figure 28–7. Histologically different carcinomas. The patient, a 66-year-old woman, had noted a breast lump for three weeks in the upper outer quadrant. Clinically, the mass was 8 cm in size; it was positive on the mammograms. *A*, Slicer section radiograph of 2 × 2.6 cm circumscribed breast. Note the rather smooth but focally lobulated border. On the mammogram, definite skin thickening was present; on this study there is a question of skin thickening over the lesion, but this is difficult to judge owing to retraction of the skin following sectioning. *B*, Whole-organ mount section of the carcinoma. The lobulated peripheral projections are clearly seen. The tumor is highly cellular and is well circumscribed. *C*, High-power view of the tumor. Note the well-circumscribed border in the lower portion. *D*, Slicer section radiograph of 1 cm circumscribed carcinoma close to the nipple but remote from the carcinoma in the same breast as *A–C*. The lesion was not palpable but was readily identified on the mammograms. *E*, Photomicrograph of the second lesion. This demonstrated an intracystic papillary carcinoma. There was no demonstrable infiltration beyond the thick wall of the cyst.

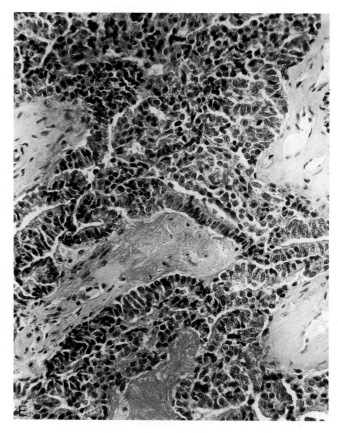

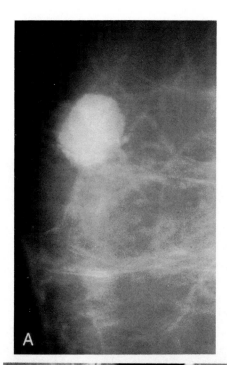

Figure 28–8. Medullary and numerous sites of intraductal carcinoma. An 80-year-old woman with a clinically suspicious mass in the breast. *A,* Mammography showed a circumscribed 1.4 × 1.8 cm carcinoma in a fatty breast. *B,* Slicer radiograph: a coarsely spiculated, mostly circumscribed mass, with distant glandular activity in many areas. Pathology: medullary carcinoma with lymphoid stroma; eight distant sites of intraductal carcinoma. Modified radical mastectomy; all five axillary lymph nodes free of tumor. The patient lived over 11 years without evidence of breast cancer.

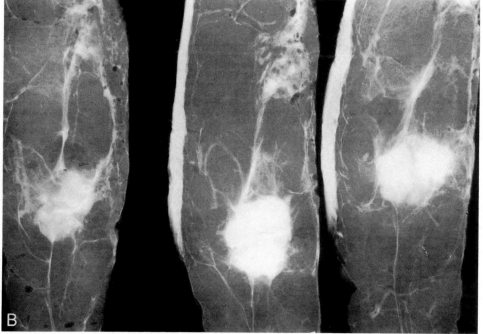

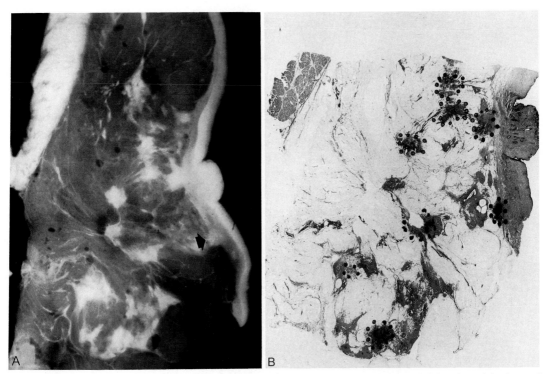

Figure 28–9. Coalescing carcinomas. This 45-year-old woman had noted an ulceration of the skin of the breast for several months. Slicer section radiograph through the nipple showed numerous foci of infiltrating duct carcinoma (white areas). *B*, Whole-organ mount section corresponding to the radiograph. Histologically the numerous and separate darker-staining areas indicated by ink dots were infiltrating duct carcinoma. The mass invading the skin (arrowhead) is clearly shown. Most of the 33 slices of the breast had a similar pattern of small cancers without a reference, or larger, mass.

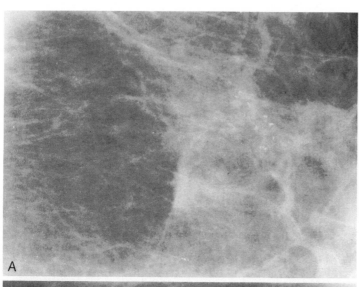

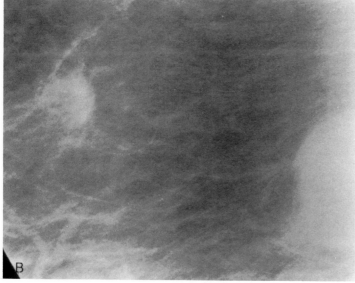

Figure 28–10. Multifocal carcinomas, all quadrants. A 73-year-old woman seen for check-up of a known breast mass of nine months' duration, clinically suspicious, in the UOQ of a large breast. Mammography (craniocaudad [A] and mediolateral [B]): LOQ at the chest wall, 3.5 cm circumscribed carcinoma; 7 × 9 mm carcinoma UIQ; comedocarcinoma LIQ. Pathology: multifocal (in all quadrants) sites of intraductal and duct carcinoma and intraductal and comedocarcinoma. Modified radical mastectomy; all 22 axillary lymph nodes free of tumor. The patient was alive and well three years later.

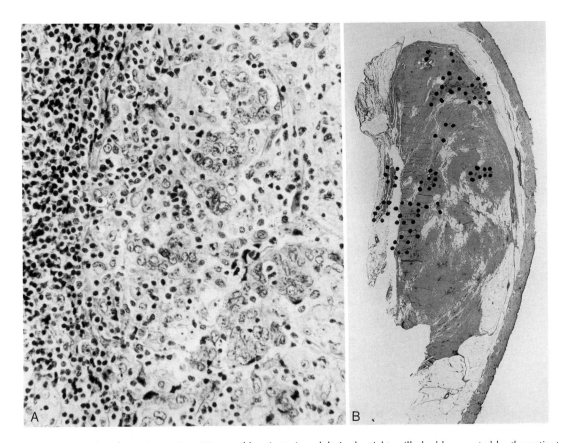

Figure 28–11. Occult carcinoma in a 57-year-old patient. A nodule in the right axilla had been noted by the patient; biopsy revealed undifferentiated malignant tumor in a lymph node (above). Several pathologists who were consulted thought that it was most likely metastatic carcinoma, probably originating in the breast. Clinically the breasts were nodular, but otherwise normal; mammograms revealed a calcification pattern of carcinoma. *B,* Representative whole-organ mount shows compact fibroglandular tissue, referred to as fibroplasia. The dense staining areas between ink dots indicate distribution of intraductal carcinoma. Whole-organ studies revealed widespread intraductal carcinoma. Carcinoma is noted particularly at the periphery of the fibroglandular tissue. No mass was noted; no area of infiltration was demonstrated despite careful whole-organ study. Note periductal fibrosis.

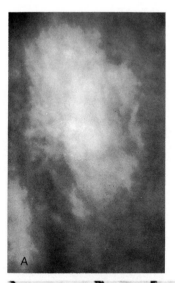

Figure 28–12. Foci of carcinoma calcifications. This 65-year-old woman complained of heaviness in her breasts. Clinically they were nodular without a dominant nodule. A, Mammogram showed four distinctly separated areas of fine faint calcifications. Some had a lacy appearance. B, Photomicrograph of the highest lesion showed highly invasive scirrhous carinoma. Two low axillary lymph nodes contained metastatic breast carcinoma.

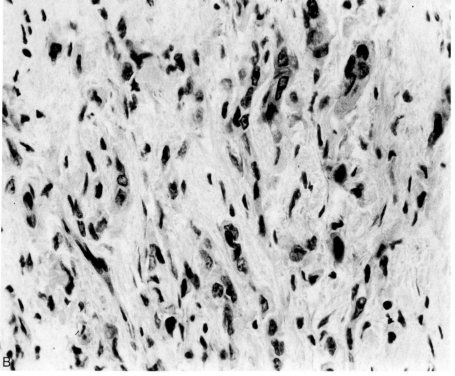

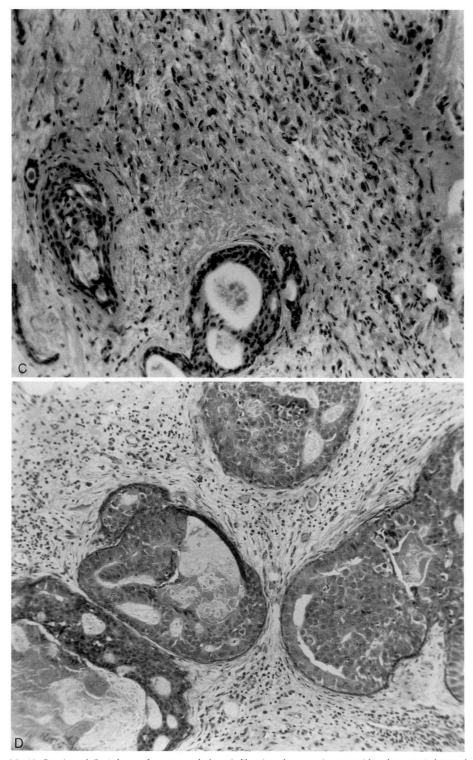

Figure 28–12 *Continued C*, A lower focus revealed an infiltrating duct carcinoma with a lesser scirrhous element. *D*, This photomicrograph was representative of many areas in the breast, with only noninfiltrating ductal carcinoma identified. These areas were usually associated with flecks of calcifications seen on the radiographs of the slicer sections.

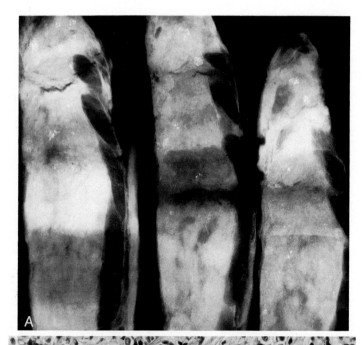

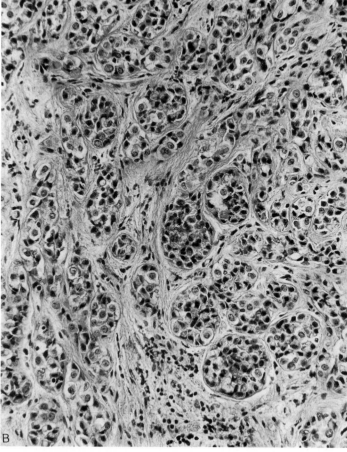

Figure 28–13. Numerous clusters of calcifications. This 48-year-old woman had bilateral breast nodularity. Routine mammograms showed numerous foci of calcifications in the right breast; clinically this was a nonpalpable and unsuspected breast cancer. *A,* Radiographs of three slicer sections of right breast show numerous clusters of fine calcifications in dense fibroglandular tissue: slices 10, 16, and 19 (nipple 13). *B,* Photomicrograph of typical area from the breast. Numerous scattered foci of lobular carcinoma in situ (as shown), corresponding to the areas of clustered calcifications on the radiographs of the specimens, were demonstrated.

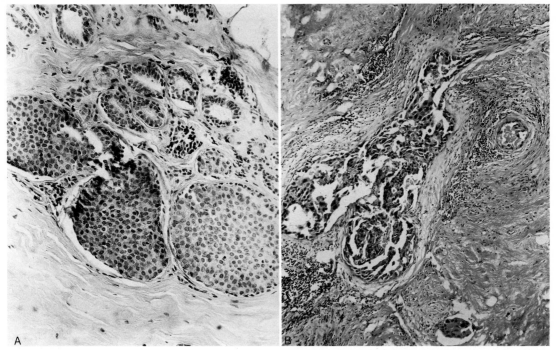

Figure 28–14. A and B, Two foci of intraductal carcinoma. The patient was the 53-year-old aunt of a mammography technologist. She was asymptomatic but asked for routine mammography. The breasts were clinically normal; mammograms showed an area of suspicious calcifications. Biopsy revealed a very small area of borderline lobular carcinoma in situ. A subcuticular mastectomy was done preparatory to insertion of a breast prosthesis. A whole-organ mastectomy specimen of this breast was carefully studied; only two areas showed intraductal carcinoma in situ (as above) in several ducts.

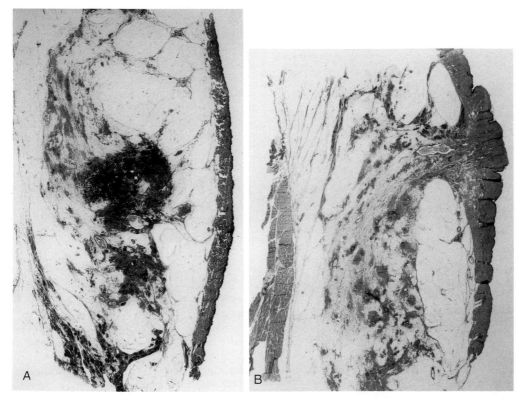

Figure 28–15. Reference tumor and distal foci. A 53-year-old woman with a mass in the breast for three days, clinically a 4 × 5 cm rather well-circumscribed carcinoma. A, Slicer section through the main mass of comedo duct carcinoma; the scattered dark-staining areas are also intraductal and comedo duct carcinoma. B, The section through the nipple shows numerous small and coalescing deposits of the same type of carcinoma, representative of the 23 slicer sections of this breast that contained fibroglandular tissue.

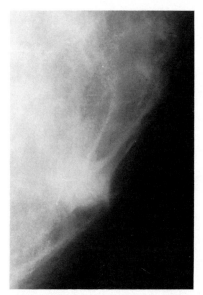

Figure 28–16. Duct and intraductal papillary carcinomas. A 47-year-old woman with a breast lump for one month, clinically a benign mass; one maternal aunt with breast cancer. Mammography: 8 × 10 mm moderately invasive carcinoma, with many punctate calcifications; straightening of trabeculae. Pathology: duct carcinoma with nearby but separate focus of intraductal papillary cribriform carcinoma. Modified radical mastectomy; all 16 axillary lymph nodes free of tumor. The patient was living without disease seven years later.

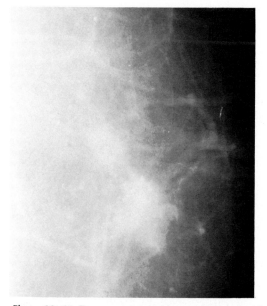

Figure 28–17. Two separate carcinomas. A 56-year-old woman who had a mammography checkup that showed an indefinite mass that was suspicious clinically. Mammography: 1 × 1.2 cm and 5 × 6 mm moderately invasive carcinomas; increased vascularity. Pathology: two distinct and separate foci of infiltrating duct carcinoma, 5 mm and 1 cm in diameter; the larger with moderate desmoplasia.

18). On the radiograph, sites often appeared quite distinct but were less so on the histologic preparation (Fig. 28–19).

The phenomenon of breast cancer causing fibrosis, scarring, and retraction with collapse of the breast tissue is poorly appreciated. This readily produces contraction of many separate foci of carcinoma into one mass (Figs. 28–20 to 28–22). Such a lesion was considered unicentric unless distinct and well-separated foci were demonstrable. If this happened frequently, these highly invasive (obvious multiple) foci would skew results on prognosis for a unicentric lesion of one histologic type.

Other lesions may be multicentric but by definition must be considered unicentric. These probably include satellite nodules that arise de novo but expand into contact with the larger mass of reference tumor (Fig. 28–23). At times the pathologist is hampered by the inability to identify the source of the tumor cell as ductal or lobular. If so, when one area appears to be of lobular origin and another area to be of ductal origin, the conclusion can be that the tumor is a multifocal lesion of one histologic type (Fig. 28–24) or two different types (Fig. 28–25). However, lobular carcinoma in situ in the same duct system as intraductal carcinoma represented to us a single focus of in situ duct carcinoma.

Distinctly different histologic types of carcinoma may be demonstrated in a single mass to be unicentric with multiple histologic types of carcinoma (Figs. 28–26 to 28–30). In situ and intraductal lesions and those carcinomas with microinvasion without a demonstable mass were considered of zero volume or size.

Subjects

There were complete studies on 161 whole breasts on 156 patients from May 3, 1965 to September 23, 1969; all patients were subject to more than ten-years of follow-up. These included: 15 with benign disease, one bilateral study; one male; two lost to follow-up; four simultaneous bilateral primaries; three initial primaries only; 13 second primaries only; and 118 unilateral breast primaries. The 118 cases of unilateral primary carcinoma were examined as a group, as it was difficult to estimate the effect of the contralateral primary carcinoma on prognosis.

Text continued on page 516

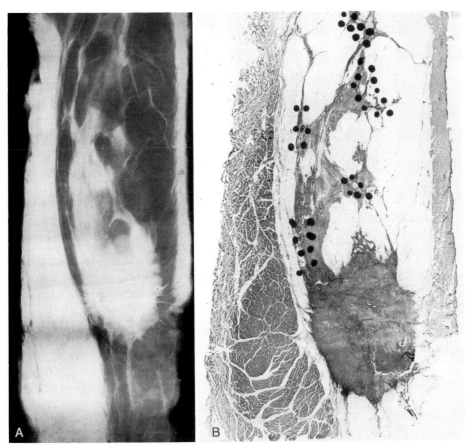

Figure 28–18. Reference tumor and almost contiguous foci. *A*, Routine radiograph of whole-organ slicer section of the breast shows a highly infiltrative 2 × 3 cm carcinoma containing numerous small flecks of calcium. Fine trabeculae are retracting the skin and muscle toward the lesion. *B*, Photograph of whole-mount breast section corresponding to the radiograph. It illustrates a dominant mass of scirrhous carcinoma (bottom) with spiculated border and local retraction about the mass but without demonstrable invasion of the skin or retromammary structures. On top there are at some distance from the main mass multiple sites of intraductal carcinoma (black dots). The contiguous one would not be a separate focus, but the upper ones would be.

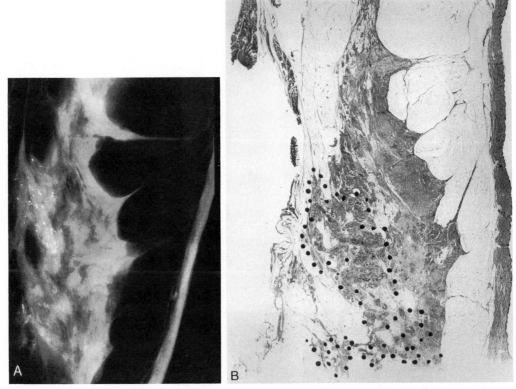

Figure 28–19. Foci of calcifications. *A,* Radiograph of whole-breast slicer section shows two areas of typical calcifications of breast carcinoma. The areas were apparently separate radiographically. *B,* Whole-mount breast section with calcium stain shows no distinct interval of breast without calcifications. The calcium stains as dark flecks (outlined by ink dots). No distinct mass is noted.

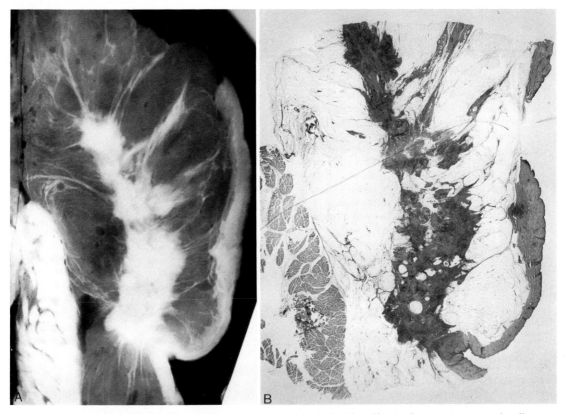

Figure 28–20. Coalescence of foci. *A,* Slicer section radiograph of a highly infiltrative breast carcinoma. This illustrates coalescence of a number of separate foci to produce a more dominant mass with skin retraction. *B,* Whole-organ mount section of the tumor. This illustrates multiple foci of infiltrating duct carcinoma coalescing to form more solid masses of tumor. There are at least three separate larger masses of tumor being formed.

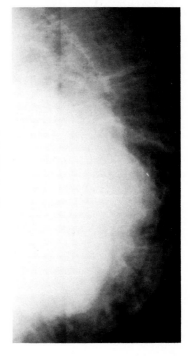

Figure 28–21. Coalescence of three duct carcinomas into one huge mass. A 69-year-old woman with breast masses for an indefinite period. Clinically: carcinoma filling most of the breast with deep fixation. Mammography: the appearance of at least three carcinomas, 2.5 × 3, 2.2 × 2.5, and 2.5 × 2.5 cm, collapsing into one large mass of carcinoma, still radiographically operable. Pathology: intraductal and duct carcinoma. Radical mastectomy; a mass 4.5 × 6 × 7 cm in size extending into but not through the pectoral muscles; 1 low of 22 axillary lymph nodes with metatasis. No recurrence three years later.

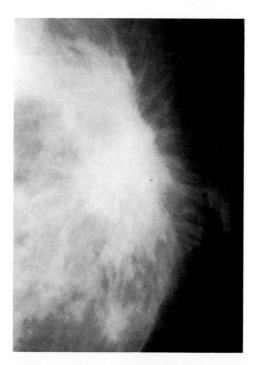

Figure 28–22. Probably contracting carcinomas. A 54-year-old woman with a lump for three months that was clinically cancer. Mammography: 2.2 × 3.5 cm highly invasive central carcinoma. Pathology: duct carcinoma with fibrosis; main mass 3 cm in diameter; separate foci of similar tumor in the upper outer and lower outer quadrants. Modified radical mastectomy; 6 of 18 low and 0 of 4 midaxillary lymph nodes with metastases. The patient was alive without disease five years later.

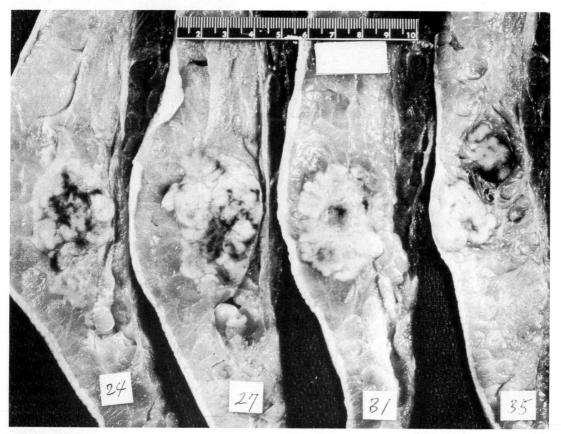

Figure 28–23. Reference tumor and satellite foci. Photograph of several whole-organ slicer sections of a breast. There is a large infiltrating duct carcinoma with several satellite masses of carcinoma. There was metastasis to 1 intramammary and 3 of 22 axillary lymph nodes. Slices 24 through 35 represent a 6 cm thickness of breast tissue. A carcinoma growing to such a length could easily expand to come into contact with nearby, at one time separate, nodules of tumor.

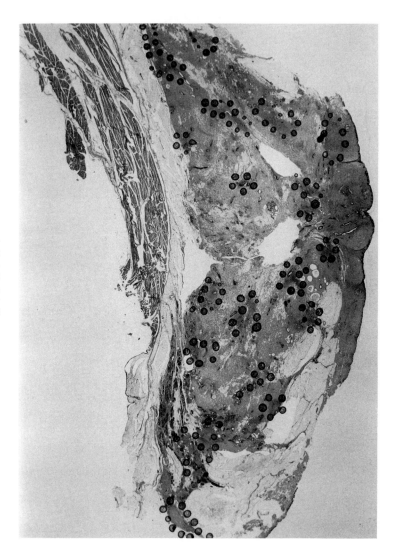

Figure 28–24. A case of diffuse infiltrating scirrhous carcinoma that can be of either ductal or lobular origin. This 41-year-old woman had noted a lump in her breast for several months. Numerous foci of carcinoma are outlined by ink dots to demonstrate the diffuse nature of the carcinoma.

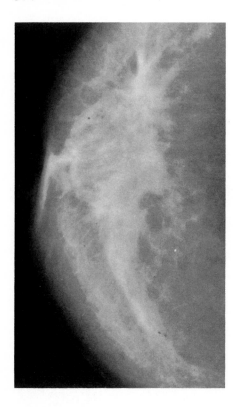

Figure 28–25. Multifocal, different types of carcinoma. A 51-year-old woman had mammograms for a clinical breast nodule that was highly suspicious. Mammography: central density extending into all quadrants, more highly invasive superiorly; areolar changes. Pathology: LOQ, scirrhous ductal and papillary noninfiltrating carcinomas; all other quadrants, scirrhous ductal and lobular carcinomas (no lobular carcinoma in situ). Modified radical mastectomy; 2 low of 22 axillary lymph nodes with tumor. The patient was alive and well three years later.

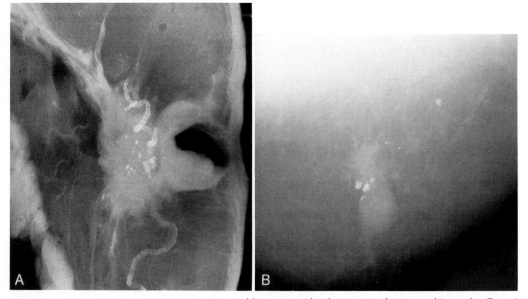

Figure 28–26. A, Two contiguous tumors. A 75-year-old woman with a breast mass for "several" months. Two sisters had breast cancer. Clinically a 6 × 7 cm carcinoma with skin thickening. The slicer radiograph shows a circumscribed thick-walled cyst and typical fine calcifications of intracystic papillary carcinoma and a contiguous highly invasive carcinoma containing fine and quite coarse calcifications. Histologically this was believed to be two separate lesions, as no intracystic carcinoma elements could be found in the lesion on the left. Also, there was intraductal carcinoma with at least one area of minimally infiltrating duct carcinoma. B, Similar case of contiguous tumors, medullary and scirrhous duct.

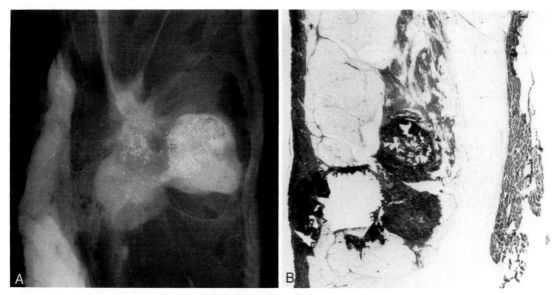

Figure 28–27. Three contiguous tumors. A 67-year-old unmarried woman, 22 years post menopause with a breast mass found by her sister three months previously. Clinically a 7 × 8 cm carcinoma with skin fixation. *A,* The slicer radiograph through the solid portion of two separate intracystic papillary carcinomas shows an intervening highly invasive carcinoma. The fine calcifications are typical of this lesion. (These are obscured on the mammograms owing to the density of the lesion.) *B,* Histologically both foci of intracystic papillary carcinomas were infiltrating. Some sections of the center lesion appeared to be infiltrating duct carcinoma, but this is not likely since they were surrounded by an intracystic papillary carcinoma pattern. (This section is at a slightly different level than the radiograph, and the wall of the upper cystic lesion is fragmented.)

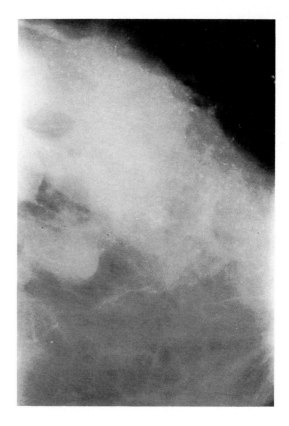

Figure 28–28. Multiple carcinomas in the same quadrant. A 34-year-old woman with a breast lump for one year. Clinically: lump LOQ of the right breast. Mammography (craniocaudad view): four circumscribed discrete masses 1.2 to 3 cm in size LOQ, with comedo duct carcinoma throughout most of the LOQ. Sonography: markedly distorted echo pattern with four solid masses LOQ. Pathology: four duct carcinomas with intraductal, cribriform, and solid patterns and intraductal and comedo carcinoma diffusely, all in LOQ. Modified radical mastectomy; one of ten Level I and one of one Level II lymph nodes with metastases. The patient was alive and well two years later.

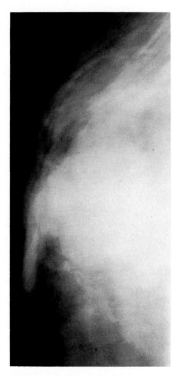

Figure 28–29. Multiple types of carcinoma at one site. A 58-year-old woman with a lump for "several" months; clinically cancer. Mammography: 1.6 × 2 cm moderately invasive carcinoma filling most of the central portion of the breast. Pathology: intraductal and duct carcinoma with productive fibrosis, intraductal comedo, comedo duct, and cribriform carcinoma at the same site. Modified radical mastectomy; 6 of 19 axillary lymph nodes at Levels I and II with metastases. The patient died of widespread disease three years and seven months later.

Results

Factors Affecting Prognosis

Of the 118 primary carcinomas limited to unilateral disease, distinct multiple sites of carcinoma were present in 72 cases (60 per cent), multiple histologic types in 29 (25 per cent), and multiple sites or multiple types in 82 (69 per cent) (Table 28–1). The cases in the four classifications (Table 28–2) relating to sites and types of carcinoma were rather evenly distributed in Stage I and Stage II, yet there was a decidedly better prognosis in carcinoma with a unicentric site and single histologic type (Table 28–1). Volume of tumor in the single-site, single-type carcinoma had no striking effect on the survival rate (Table 28–3). With multiple sites and types of tumor the trend was poorer prognosis with all characteristics and especially when associated with greater volume. With 26 carcinomas of less than 0.5 ml volume, survival was 92 per

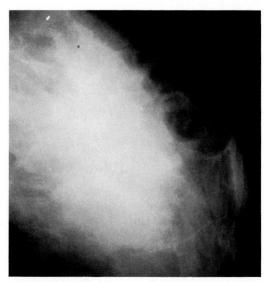

Figure 28–30. Duct and comedo carcinoma in same mass. A 36-year-old woman seen for baseline study for fibrocystic disease with a questionable change in the left breast centrally. Mammography: large irregular asymmetric area, increased vascularity, and minimal thickening of the areola; one 3 mm intramammary lymph node toward tail of breast (not shown). Sonography: cyst in fibrocystic disease. Pathology (in addition to the fibrocystic disease): mixed; both intraductal and infiltrating duct and comedo carcinomas. Modified radical mastectomy; 1 low axillary lymph node positive out of 1 intramammary and 13 axillary lymph nodes. The patient was alive without disease three years later.

cent, whereas with 21 cancers greater than 10 ml (approximately equivalent to 2.5 cm diameter), survival was 29 per cent. Even in larger tumors with unicentricity and of a single type, survival remained at 75 per cent.

A poor prognosis was associated with the presence of clinical signs of carcinoma. Prognosis was not significantly associated with calcifications or intramammary lymph nodes (Table 28–3). Intramammary lymph nodes were present in 34 of the breasts (29 per

TABLE 28–1. One Hundred Eighteen Unilateral Primary Breast Carcinomas by Number of Sites and Histologic Types

	Number	% of Total Cases
Single site		
Single type	36	31
Multiple types	10	8
Multiple sites		
Single type	53	45
Multiple types	19	16
Total	118	100
Multiple sites/types	82	69

TABLE 28–2. Classification of the 118 Unilateral Breast Primary Carcinomas into Number of Sites and Histologic Types, Stage of Disease, and Ten-Year Survival

Class[a]	No.	% 10-Year Survival	Stage 0		Stage I		Stage II	
			% in Stage	% Survived	% in Stage	% Survived	% in Stage	% Survived
Ms	53	66	11	100	45	79	43	43
Mm	19	47	0	0	53	70	47	33
Us	36	78	8	100	58	81	33	67
Um	10	50	0	0	70	71	30	0
Total	118	65	8	100	52	74	40	40

[a]M = multiple sites; U = unicentric site; single (s) or multiple (m) histologic types.

cent), and of these, 11 (32 per cent) contained metastatic carcinoma. Calcifications suggestive of carcinoma noted by x-ray was present in 79 breasts (67 per cent).

The prognosis of the 19 patients with a positive family history of breast cancer was not significantly different. A single focus of one histologic type of carcinoma had a high rate of survival in all age groups, even beyond 70 years, which was in contrast to that of multiple sites and multiple types of carcinoma. Stage II carcinoma and tumors with a volume greater than 10 ml retained good prognosis in unicentric, single-type lesions in the various age groups. More indolent tumors occurring with duct carcinoma would have poorer prognosis (Table 28–4).

Mortality in the single-site, single-type carcinoma was approximately 2.5 per cent per year, while tumors with multiple sites and types produced a family of curves with a higher mortality (Figs. 28–31 and 28–32). If these multiple site and type carcinomas included a scirrhous element, the mortality approached 25 per cent per year.

Study Problems

These primary operable breast carcinomas represented approximately one half of the total 284 carcinomas treated by the Emory University Oncologic Clinic during this period. Lack of consecutive cases, due to technically poor or incomplete studies or the necessity for incision biopsy, precluded a statistical report. Yet they were representative to the degree that more of the carcinomas were Stage 0 or Stage I, were less than 2 ml in size and over one third were in women less than 50 years of age. Thus, any definite trend could be significant.

We relied on the Cheatle and Cutler (1931) definition that as long as normal ducts histologically separate tumor sites, each tumor had developed de novo. Radiography frequently was helpful in demonstrating connection of tumor masses or the presence of normal, usually adipose, tissue between deposits of carcinoma (Egan, 1970). Qualheim and Gall (1957) stated, "If serial sections were taken instead of the one or two samples utilized, the incidence of multifocal lesions would be significantly increased." We did not examine all breast tissue histologically, but incorporation of exquisitely detailed radiography assured a near-complete breast study. Structureless or fatty areas on the radiograph of the slicer sections, unlike those on the mammograms, contained no tissue of histologic interest. Avoiding large areas of adipose tissue permitted thinner and more

TABLE 28–3. Ten-Year Survival (Surv.) in the Four Classifications of Sites and Types of 118 Unilateral Carcinomas: Total Tumor Volume, Detection, Radiographic Calcification, and Intramammary Lymph Nodes

	Volume (ml)								Calcifications				Intramammary Lymph Nodes					
	<2		>2		Clin + X-ray +		Clin − X-ray +		None		Present		0		−		+	
Class	No.	Surv. (%)	No.	Surv. (%)	No.	Surv. (%)	No.	Surv. (%)	No.	Surv. (%)	No.	Surv. (%)	No.	Surv. (%)	No.	Surv. (%)	No.	Surv. (%)
MS	27	85	26	46	40	55	13	100	19	63	34	65	38	71	11	55	4	50
Mm	7	71	12	33	12	33	7	71	2	0	17	53	15	60	2	0	2	0
Us	22	82	14	71	30	73	6	100	13	77	23	78	26	73	6	83	4	100
Um	5	60	5	40	9	44	1	100	5	60	5	40	5	60	4	50	1	0
Total	61	80	57	49	91	57	27	93	39	67	79	63	84	65	23	57	11	55

Minus sign (−) = nodes without tumor; + = with metastasis.

TABLE 28–4. Histologic Types of Carcinoma and Distribution in the 118 Unilateral Carcinomas

Class	Intra-ductal	Lobular Carcinoma In Situ	Comedo	Duct	Scir-rhous	Medul-lary	Lobular	Mucoid	Adeno	Intracystic Papillary	Tubular
Ms	3	1	2	30	14	1	2	0	0	0	0
Us	1	1	0	20	7	5	2	0	0	0	0
Mm*	0	1	10	10	4	1	0	2	3	3	1
Um*	0	0	2	2	3	2	1	3	0	2	0
Total	4	3	14	62	28	9	5	5	3	5	1

*All associated with duct carcinoma.

diagnostic sections of fibroglandular tissues. Many of the areas of in situ or microinvasive carcinoma would have gone undetected by palpation and inspection of incomplete subserial sectioning.

Separate sites of carcinoma occurred as multiple foci in one quadrant, in two or more quadrants, or throughout the entire breast. Multiple histologic types occurred in a similar distribution with single or multiple foci. Aggressiveness of the lesions spanned the gamut from indolent intraductal comedocarcinoma to highly invasive scirrhous carcinoma.

Many separate sites of invasive carcinoma could be seen coalescing to produce a single large focus of tumor. Unless distant foci were demonstrated, this was considered unicentric, since peripheral growth could not be confidently excluded. Some larger, or mixed, unicentric carcinomas may have developed in this manner. Categorizing different cell types of contiguous carcinomas was difficult. Commonly, one histologic type of carcinoma in the breast manifested a different cell type in axillary lymph node metastasis or with intramammary spread. Since separate deposits of different cell types are frequently demonstrated in the same breast, one would prefer to consider that the axillary metastasis came from a similar occult tumor in that breast. This problem necessitated the category Um. Coalescence of foci of tumor and/or collapse of breast tissues could explain: (1) an invasive intracystic papillary carcinoma adjacent to a duct carcinoma, instead of invasion of the intracystic papillary carcinoma in the form of duct carcinoma; (2) a mixture of comedo and duct carcinoma; and (3) a focus of simplex, scirrhous, and lobular carcinoma as a unicentric lesion.

Multiple separate sites of carcinoma in 60 per cent of the cancerous breasts studied suggest that breast cancer is a multicentric, and often a whole-organ, disease. Of the 118 cases of unilateral carcinoma the number with multicentricity would be as great as 75 per cent if multiple histologic types were included. A precise and uniformly accepted definition of multicentricity of origin and location as well as delineation of different histologic types of breast carcinoma is needed. These histologic characteristics of breast carcinoma may well reflect the biologic nature of the tumor and host resistance. This series is so small that stratification results in cells with small numbers. There are no other

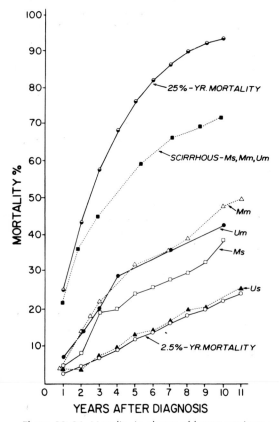

Figure 28–31. Mortality in classes of breast carcinoma compared with the slower rate of 2.5 per cent per year and the more rapid rate of 25 per cent per year.

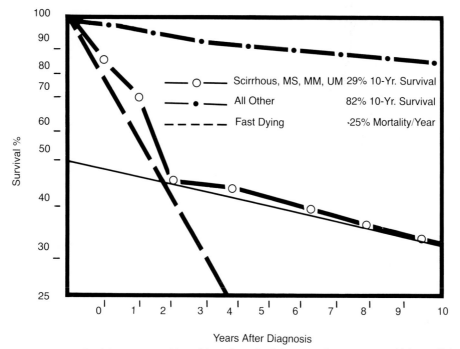

Figure 28–32. More rapidly dying women with multicentric and scirrhous carcinoma curve, which parallels that of the fast-dying (25 per cent per year of Fox) women with breast carcinoma.

similar series with this degree of search for direct comparison. Yet it is hoped that these observations may be sufficiently striking to arouse further investigation.

The study design of requiring intact breasts for whole-organ preparations precluded consecutive cases. Ninety-one were moderately advanced operable carcinomas, both clinically and radiographically positive. Twenty-seven were nonpalpable tumors with the diagnosis delayed until permanent histologic preparations could be carefully studied. The incidence of histologically positive axillary lymph nodes in the series was 34 per cent compared with an overall incidence of 17.8 per cent of all Emory University operable breast carcinomas.

Although one third of the cancerous breasts contained intramammary lymph nodes and two thirds of these contained metastatic deposits, little connection of these nodes with prognosis could be observed. However, the multiplicity of sites and/or histologic types retained a very strong influence on prognosis despite the presence or absence of metastasis to intramammary lymph nodes.

Extremes in Prognosis

Fox (1979) has calculated that about 40 per cent of newly diagnosed breast cancer pa-tients would die at an exponential rate of 25 per cent per year. This mortality rate is similar to that of women with untreated breast cancer from the Middlesex Hospital in the late nineteenth and early twentieth centuries. The remaining 60 per cent of the women with breast cancer would die at the rate of 2.5 per cent per year. Using the present data one can select these two groups. The mortality curve of women with unicentric single-type carcinoma superimposes on the 2.5 per cent mortality curve, and the mortality rate of the remaining women (multiple sites and types of carcinoma) with an element of scir-rhous carcinoma approximates the 25 per cent annual rate. Some additional factors could help establish an even greater than 25 per cent annual mortality rate.

Clinical Applications

Assignment of prognosis of breast cancer based on size, even though staged, often is difficult. "Minimal" breast cancer as defined by Gallager and Martin (1971) encompasses lobular carcinoma in situ; noninvasive intraductal carcinoma, and invasive carcinoma, either lobular or ductal, forming a mass no greater than 0.5 cm in diameter. The term, whether defined as less than 0.5 cm or less than 1 cm in size, may be meaningless and misleading. Forty of the 118 unilateral carcinomas that were Stage I and 1 cm or greater in size had a 74 per cent ten-year survival rate, whereas 16 Stage II "minimal" carcinomas had as poor a prognosis as the larger carcinomas (45 per cent compared with 40 per cent). This alerts us to be wary of using "minimal" to connote assuredly curable cancer and realize that there are other prognostic factors besides size and stage.

The perplexing heterogeneity of survival of breast cancer patients could strongly influence clinical trials. The stratification of women into at least unicentric and multicentric carcinoma may well establish better treatment policies. Unicentric Stage II carcinoma had a mortality rate of 27 per cent, whereas the multicentric mortality rate was 65 per cent, a 2.5-fold difference (Table 28–2). With use of these microscopic characteristics at the time of diagnosis, the biologic importance of the carcinoma can be established for better understanding these diverse survival rates and for establishing logical treatment planning. The parameters of sites and types of breast cancer added to the prognostic factors suggested by Fisher et al. (1978) should greatly improve their discriminant analysis in predicting mortality.

The practicality of applying this tedious, time-consuming, and expensive whole-breast study clinically can be questioned. A complete laboratory, two technologists, and one pathologist full-time with five years to study fewer than 200 breasts, plus a great deal of time of the radiologist and surgeon, and much clerical assistance, could be tolerated only under research conditions. However, during thorough routine breast studies, multiple histologic types of carcinoma are demonstrated. The knowledge that multiple sites of breast cancer are common and are of great significance in prognosis may stimulate more thorough breast studies. Lagios (1977) has shown good results with a much less extensive procedure in his radiographic-pathologic routine study of breast cancer that requires only the added services of one technologist. Schwartz et al. (1980), studying four sections from each breast quadrant and four sections from the retroareolar area, demonstrated an incidence of 49.2 per cent multicentricity of cancer in 43 breast specimens.

The several cases shown in Figures 28–33 to 28–38 indicate that multiple sites and/or multiple histologic types of breast cancer can be demonstrated both radiographically and histologically in a clinical setting. Alerting the pathologist to the probable presence and location of multiple breast carcinomas may stimulate his search of the specimen more carefully and thoroughly.

The presence of multiple sites of comedocarcinoma, and most likely other types of carcinoma, indicates an increased risk of malignancy in the opposite breast. Prophylactic mastectomy is not indicated at present, as there is usually an extended period of development of the contralateral primary, during which calcifications can be recognized radiographically prior to any mass formation.

In the past, most lesions secondary to the reference tumor were considered satellite nodules. This would suggest metastasis or spread of the reference carcinoma within the breast. Such dissemination of grossly apparent carcinomatous nodules then connotes a greater risk for similar spread throughout the body. Our observations indicate that separate carcinomas arise de novo and have the same potential for metastasis as any breast carcinoma of similar size and type. With a second distant tumor 0.5 cm in size, as in Figures 28–34 and 28–35, one should anticipate many other, perhaps smaller, lesions in those breasts instead of the single second focus in each case.

OBSERVATIONS

The presence of multiple sites and multiple histologic types of breast carcinoma signals a poor prognosis. These findings demote age of the patient, stage of disease, volume of tumor, and other clinical features to lesser indicators of prognosis. Multiple sites of breast carcinoma in 60 per cent of cancerous breasts suggest that this disease at times is multicentric in origin and could be a whole-organ process. Intramammary lymph nodes are commonly present in the breast, but metastatic disease to these nodes per se has no significant prognostic value.

More extensive breast studies add valuable information about the multiple sites and histologic types of breast cancer. Without prohibitive cost and effort a routine could be established to include histologic search for multiple sites and/or types of breast cancer.

The presence of a high percentage of multiple sites of carcinoma in a breast harboring a reference tumor appears pertinent to treatment planning regarding the role of subtotal

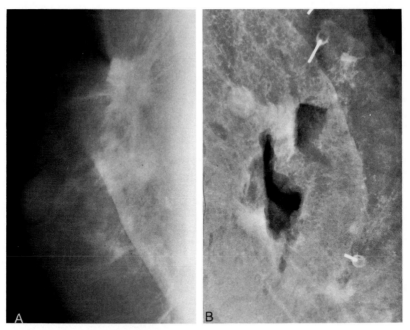

Figure 28–33. A and B, Multiple sites of carcinoma. A 65-year-old woman who found a lump in her breast that was clinically suspicious. Mammogram shows at least four separate sites of carcinoma. The radiograph of the specimen shows at least four sites of carcinoma despite two excisional biopsies. There is also a large round mass, presumably an intramammary lymph node. Pathology: three separate infiltrating duct carcinomas; two separate intraductal comedocarcinomas; several intramammary lymph nodes contained tumor, axillary lymph nodes were free of tumor. The patient died four years later of metastatic disease.

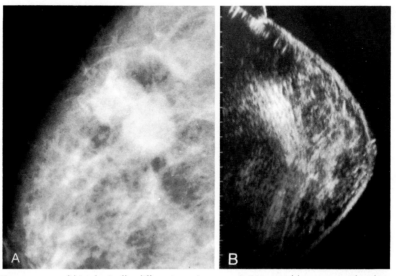

Figure 28–34. Two masses of histologically different carcinomas. A 63-year-old woman with a breast lump and skin dimpling. A, The mammogram shows a 1.6 cm spiculated mass and a nearby 1.2 cm more circumscribed mass of carcinoma. B, Breast sonography shows an irregular hypoechoic area, upper slightly inner quadrant, with skin flattening. Pathology: an infiltrating duct and a less aggressive infiltrating tubular carcinoma; separate primary lesions; nodes free. Two years later no evidence of disease.

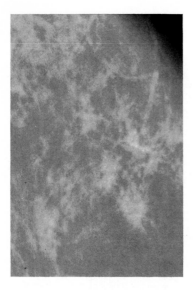

Figure 28–35. Multiple clusters of calcification. A 58-year-old woman seen for baseline mammogram, which showed five separate sites of clustered calcifications associated with vague increased densities. Pathology: All the sites of calcification were associated with intraductal comedocarcinoma, considered separate primary tumors. The opposite breast is in a high-risk category with multiple sites of comedocarcinoma on a background of ductal hyperplasia.

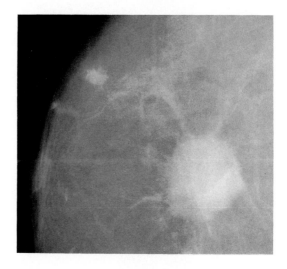

Figure 28–36. Two separate primary carcinomas. A 77-year-old woman with a breast lump for six months. Clinically: a 4 × 5 cm carcinoma. Mammograms: 2.5 and 0.5 cm carcinomas. Pathology: two separate infiltrating duct carcinomas with axillary lymph node metastasis.

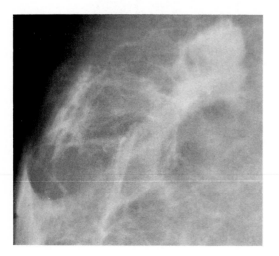

Figure 28–37. A mass and a cluster of calcifications of carcinoma. A 71-year-old woman with a breast mass that was clinically suspicious. Mammograms: 1.5 × 3.5 cm mass, the upper portion circumscribed and the lower portion spiculated. Anterior to this mass is a cluster of stippled calcifications. Pathology: Infiltrating comedocarcinoma with marked desmoplasia in part of it. A separate area of intraductal comedocarcinoma.

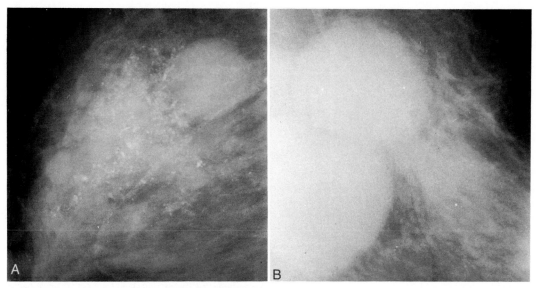

Figure 28–38. A and B, Bilateral intracystic papillary carcinoma with comedocarcinoma. A 77-year-old woman with a large firm mass UIQ of the left breast. Mammography: one 3.5 and one 4.5 cm dense homogeneous mass of intracystic papillary carcinoma on the left and a similar 2.5 cm lesion on the right surrounded by a 4.5 × 6.5 cm comedocarcinoma. Bilateral modified radical mastectomy with all nodes free of tumor.

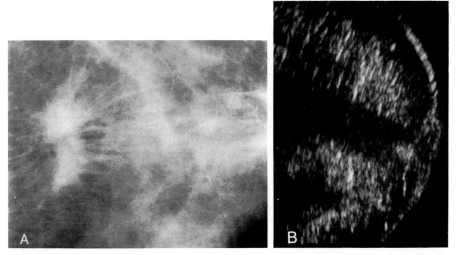

Figure 28–39. A and B, Two small highly invasive contiguous carcinomas. A 46-year-old woman with breast tenderness for a year, during which time she developed a deep mass and skin dimpling. Mammography: two adjacent 7 × 8 and 5 × 9 mm highly invasive carcinomas containing fine stippled calcifications. Sonography: large irregular nearby anechoic area that extends to and deforms the skin and is associated with a 2 cm band of deep shadowing. Pathology: intraductal and duct carcinoma with a scirrhous element. Modified radical mastectomy; 0 of 13 Level I and one of three Level II nodes with metastasis. The patient was living and well two years later.

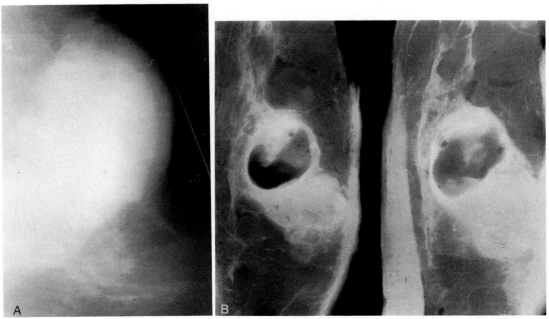

Figure 28–40. Two types of carcinoma producing a single mass. *A*, Mammography: 3.2 × 5.5 cm lobulated, homogeneously dense, circumscribed mass; intracystic papillary carcinoma vs sarcoma. *B*, Whole-organ slicer radiograph: The intracystic lesion appears to be confined within its irregularly thickened wall; adjacent is a circumscribed invasive carcinoma containing fine and coarse calcifications.

mastectomy, or lumpectomy, as the sole treatment for carcinoma of the breast. The ease of eradication of minute, often microscopic, foci of carcinoma by radiotherapy after the removal of the main mass of tumor lends credence to lumpectomy and radiotherapy as an alternate treatment of less advanced breast carcinoma. However, the concept of multicentricity of breast carcinoma provides the greatest single rationale for maintaining total mastectomy as the prevalent surgical procedure for this malignancy.

Confusion relating to the practical significance of multicentricity stems largely from the wide variation in its frequency as reported in the literature, based on varied definitions of multicentricity, different methods of examination of the breast specimen, and thoroughness of the sampling techniques.

Coalescence of two or more sites of breast carcinoma, e.g., highly invasive duct carcinomas, may produce a single mass of one cell type. In estimating prognosis, this could mistakenly be considered a unicentric tumor. This process also clearly demonstrates the phenomenon of breast contracture with carcinoma (Fig. 28–39).

In the last quarter of a century, intraductal carcinoma has catapulted in frequency from the highly unusual working diagnosis to now account for over one fourth (a 20-fold increase) of all currently accessioned breast carcinomas. This, of course, reflects the increasing use of mammography in the clinical evaluation of the breast. Concomitantly, increased survival has promoted bilateral primary breast carcinomas, as well as multicentricity, into a vastly greater problem in management of the patient.

The concept of breast carcinoma as a diffuse process of the entire epithelial system, both as multicentric foci and bilateral disease, is now accepted in pathology and oncology.

CASE HISTORY

First of bilateral simultaneous primary carcinomas. A 67-year old woman with a breast lump "for months" that was clinically suspicious. Mammography was done (Figure 28–40). Pathology: two distinct breast carcinomas within a mass: one intracystic papillary, noninvasive; one circumscribed duct carcinoma. Radical mastectomy; one of 24 axillary lymph nodes contained metastasis. Ten years later the patient developed another primary lobular carcinoma in the opposite breast. Cardiac death ensued nine months later in the absence of breast cancer.

With such diverse cell type carcinomas, it seems more appropriate to assume that each arose de novo rather than to assume a transformation from one type to another in the same area of the breast.

REFERENCES

Cheatle FL, Cutler M (1931): Tumors of the Breast: Their Pathology, Symptoms, Diagnosis and Treatment. Philadelphia, JB Lippincott.

Egan RL (1964): Mammography. Springfield, IL, Charles C Thomas, pp 129, 245.

Egan RL (1970): Mammography and Breast Diseases. Baltimore, Williams & Wilkins, p 19.70.

Egan RL, Ellis JT, Powell RW (1969): Team approach to the study of diseases of the breast. Cancer 23:847.

Fisher ER, Gregorio RM, Fisher B, et al (1975): The pathology of invasive breast cancer. A syllabus derived from findings of the National Surgical Adjuvant Breast Project (Protocol No. 4). Cancer 36:1.

Fisher ER, Gregorio RM, Fisher B (1976): Prognostic significance of histopathology. In Stoll BA (ed): New Aspects of Breast Cancer II. Chicago, Year Book Medical Publishers.

Fisher ER, Swamidoss S, Lee CH, et al (1978): Detection and significance of occult axillary node metastases in patients with invasive breast cancer. Cancer 42:2025.

Fox MS (1979): On the diagnosis and treatment of breast cancer. JAMA 241:489.

Gallager HS, Martin JF (1969a): The study of mammary carcinoma by mammography and whole organ sectioning: early observations. Cancer 23:855.

Gallager HS, Martin JF (1969b): Early phases in the development of breast cancer. Cancer 24:1170.

Gallager HS, Martin JF (1971): An orientation to the concept of minimal breast cancer. Cancer 28:1505.

Ingleby H, Gershon-Cohen J (1960): Comparative Anatomy, Pathology and Roentgenology of the Breast. Philadelphia, University of Pennsylvania Press.

Lagios MD (1977): Multicentricity of breast carcinoma demonstrated by routine correlated serial subgross and radiographic examination. Cancer 40:1726.

Morgenstern L, Kaufman PA, Friedman NB (1975): The case against tylectomy for carcinoma of the breast. The factor of multicentricity. Am J Surg 130:251.

Qualheim RE, Gall EA (1957): Breast carcinoma with multiple sites of origin. Cancer 10:460.

Richardson PJ (1975): The radiographic examination of sliced surgically resected breasts. Radiography 41:37.

Rosen PP, Fracchia AA, Urban JA, Schottenfield D, Robbins GF (1975): "Residual" mammary carcinoma following simulated partial mastectomy. Cancer 35:739.

Schwartz GF, Patchesfsky AS, Feig SA, Shaber GS, Schwartz AB (1980): Multicentricity of nonpalpable breast cancer. Cancer 45(12):2913.

Tellem M, Prive L, Meranze DR (1962): Four-quadrant study of breast removed for carcinoma. Cancer 15:10.

Wellings SR, Gensen HM, Marcum RG (1975): An atlas of sub-gross pathology of the human breast with special reference to possible precancerous lesions. J Natl Cancer Inst 55:231.

29

Bilateral Breast Carcinomas

CHAPTER OUTLINE

Noncarcinomatous breast malignancies are sufficiently uncommon that bilaterality is so rare as to scarcely need comment.

BACKGROUND

High-resolution mammography is at present one of our best methods of studying bilateral, and particularly second breast, carcinomas. The gross radiographic appearance of the carcinomas, either primary or metastatic, is so typical that the differential by x-ray examination is usually clear-cut. In premammography days it was convenient for the surgeon to consider any change in the second breast as a manifestation of metastasis and to refer the patient to a radiotherapist, the first breast carcinoma usually being so advanced that it most likely was lethal. The effectiveness of wide-field three-dimensional mammography in early detection of the second primary lesion and in differentiation into primary and metastatic breast carcinoma has forced a readjustment in traditional modes of thinking about bilateral breast carcinoma.

Pivotal new concepts are that (1) breast cancer is not a local phenomenon but a diffuse disease of mammary duct epithelium; (2) noninvasive and minimally invasive cancers do exist and may be detected and treated with present surgical procedures, yielding unprecedented cure rates; (3) these high cure rates provide greater opportunity for a second primary cancer to develop; (4) breast specimen radiography is mandatory to carry out proper localization of these minimal cancers for histopathologic studies; (5) the effectiveness of frozen-section study of these early carcinomas should be re-evaluated; and (6) bilateral breast carcinomas should be recognized and differentiated into primary vs metastasis without delay for proper treatment of the patient. Since multicentric cancers are often present in one breast (82 of 118 of our whole-organ studies), the opposite breast as a paired organ should receive more attention in terms of harboring an additional primary carcinoma.

The survival of patients with breast cancer had been slowly extended so that Kilgore (1921) in his earlier report on second breast cancers noted that 75 per cent of the second cancers arose in 22 per cent of the patients who had negative axillary lymph nodes at the time of the original mastectomy. In 1956 he reported that 10 per cent of the patients with Stage I cancer developed a second primary within 15 years, whereas only 5 per cent of Stage II patients developed a second cancer. Most series are hampered by short-term follow-up, incomplete data, and simply too few cases.

At the New York Academy of Sciences in the early 1960s, my attempt to convince the thousand or so physicians in attendance that our data reflected a potential improvement of 150 per cent by simply caring for the opposite breast was negatively received. However, as survival and cure rates continue to improve, especially with the use of mammography, the increasing importance of this approach is reflected by reports of series in the literature. With greater knowledge of the natural history of breast cancer, more precise and consistent histopathologic diagnoses, and more meticulous patient follow-up, the increased risk of a second primary can be better estimated in subgroups of patients surviving one primary breast cancer. Fewer reports of metastasis to the opposite breast are encountered. This, no doubt, reflects interruption of the cancer before it achieves large size and distant metastasis. But one would like to relate this change to greater awareness of the disaster of not treating properly the breast with a second primary cancer.

Our data are at variance with other reports, such as the classic by Robbins and Berg (1964) (Table 29–1), since all our patients have been studied by mammography. In fact, in that report these authors predicted that mammography "would seem to be a significant source of help" in detecting the second breast primary.

THE SECOND CARCINOMA

Pathologic Features

The pathologist may be unable to differentiate primary vs metastatic carcinoma. The biopsy specimen represents a small area of the breast and may not include the optimal tissue. He infrequently has the opportunity to study tissue from both breasts simultaneously. Different histologic types of carcinoma may be present in the same breast, and these types may produce altered patterns upon metastasis. An in situ component may not be in the sampled tissue.

A carcinoma with multiple sites may be multicentric in origin, may have one site of origin and multiple metastatic sites via lymphatics, may have secondary deposits via the lymphatics from a carcinoma of the opposite breast superimposed on the primary cancer, or may be entirely metastatic deposits from the opposite breast. Ducts containing noninfiltrating carcinoma may be completely engulfed by invasive carcinoma. Variations of these findings contribute at times to the difficulty in histopathologic differentiation between combinations of primary and metastatic carcinoma in both breasts.

Metastatic Carcinoma

A number of pathologic findings do serve as criteria for differentiation of primary cancer vs metastasis in the second breast. Metastases from one breast to the other are

TABLE 29–1. Mammographic Features of Primary and Metastatic Beast Carcinoma

Feature	Primary Carcinoma	Metastatic Carcinoma (From Opposite Breast)
Mass	Usually present	Not present
Calcifications	Present in 40 per cent	Not present
Skin thickening	None, local thickening or diffuse thickening	Could be none, but usually diffuse thickening
Background stroma	Usually clear or only patchy densities	Diffuse increase in density
Multiple nodules	May be present	No distinct nodules present
Opposite breast	May be normal, may contain a primary or metastatic carcinoma	Contains a primary carcinoma or the breast is absent
Axillary lymph nodes	Present, if diffuse cancer is depicted	May be present, usually not identified
Retraction	Nearly always present, about the mass, skin, or nipple	Not present
Edema	If present, very advanced cancer	Present and may be the first sign

largely intralymphatic and are most often in the fat that surrounds the breast parenchyma proper. Since the spread is usually across the sternum via the lymphatics, the earliest involvement will be in the medial portion of the breast. Less often there is retrogressive spread from ipsilateral axillary nodes containing metastatic tumor from the contralateral breast; then the earlier changes will be noted in the fat of the tail of the breast.

Metastases tend to be multiple, diffusely involving a segment of the breast or the whole breast; these are often seen only microscopically. Spread is more expansile without gross mass formation. Most likely the cellular morphology will resemble the most aggressive part of the primary carcinoma. Intraductal carcinoma could be an incidental finding in a breast with metastatic carcinoma, to confuse the diagnosis of metastasis. Insistence upon a histologically different carcinoma to fit the criteria of a second primary is unwise, as most breast carcinomas are duct cell and the second primary would also by all odds be a duct cell carcinoma.

Second Primary Carcinoma

Second primary carcinomas, by contrast, occur in the breast parenchyma and most often in the upper outer quadrant but not in the fatty portion of the tail (or in the subcutaneous fat medially). Usually there is a single gross lesion that may be fairly well circumscribed and moderately or highly invasive but with a finely infiltrative border and a crablike or stellate pattern of growth; or the lesion may be highly infiltrative with a scirrhous pattern. Satellite nodules may be present. Intramammary lymphatic spread may occur, not unlike spread from the opposite breast. Nearby in situ carcinoma is strong evidence to establish the diagnosis of a second primary carcinoma.

Mammographic Features

Mammography affords a graphic means of recording gross changes simultaneously in the entirety of both breasts as frequently as desired without disturbing either breast. The growth patterns of carcinoma are so clearly depicted that primary carcinoma may be readily differentiated from metastatic carcinoma (Table 29–1).

Metastatic Carcinoma

Spread of breast carcinoma to the second breast directly across the sternum via the lymphatics produces quite distinct mammographic findings (Figs. 29–1 and 29–2). There is a diffuse edematous appearance to the second breast (especially in the subcutaneous tissue), lack of sharpness of the trabeculae, increased density of the breast, and blurred vein margins. There is diffuse thickening of the skin, with loss of the thin penciled line below the skin. Swollen subcutaneous lymphatics may be apparent. No mass or typical calcifications are present. These changes correspond closely to the histopathologic criteria.

The advanced second primary carcinoma that produces a breast so dense and skin so thick on the mammogram that the primary mass or calcification is obscured does present a problem in differentiation from metastatic disease radiographically (Fig. 29–3). Such a

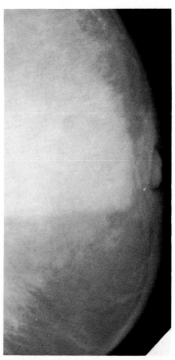

Figure 29–1. Nonsimultaneous bilateral carcinomas, with the second representing metastasis from the first. This 62-year-old woman had a radical mastectomy for a Stage II (large axillary nodes) carcinoma 18 months prior to this mammogram. Mammograms of this breast were normal at that time; during radiotherapy, at six months and one year follow-up visits, clinically this breast was normal (no interval mammograms). This mammogram shows typical metastatic breast carcinoma.

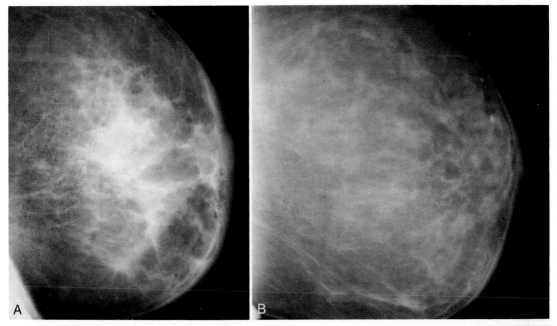

Figure 29–2. Simultaneous bilateral carcinomas with the one in the second breast being metastatic from the first breast. Mammogram of the left breast (*A*) reveals a clinically and mammographically advanced carcinoma. The larger pendulous right breast (*B*) was clinically normal but mammographically showed metastatic carcinoma: diffuse density throughout the breast, edematous appearance of breast tissues, and diffuse thickening of the skin without a demonstrable mass, even though a good study. (Proved by needle biopsy.)

lesion is inoperable, and clinical evaluation for treatment would not differ.

Second Primary Carcinoma

With the characteristic pattern of a primary carcinoma, there is no necessity to postulate that this pattern has resulted from a blood-borne metastasis from the carcinoma in the opposite breast.

The small, clinically unsuspected carcinoma in the right breast in Figure 29–4 satisfies all the radiographic characteristics of a

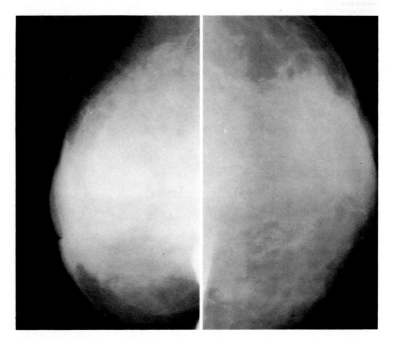

Figure 29–3. Bilateral simultaneous clinically recognized primary carcinomas of the breast. The one in the right breast is primarily subareolar in location, with stippled calcification in the mass. The one in the left breast has less mass component and a diffuse appearance that could suggest a metastasis. The stippled calcification that extends to the base of the breast identifies it as a second primary, however. The patient is a 60-year-old woman with a 5 cm mass in one breast and a 3.5 cm mass in the opposite, both clinically carcinoma.

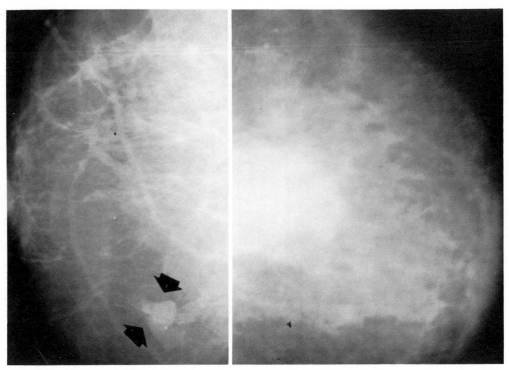

Figure 29–4. Bilateral simultaneous primary breast carcinomas, with the second primary not suspected clinically. The 63-year-old woman presented with a suspicious lump in the left breast, but a clinically normal right breast contains a typical-appearing carcinoma (arrowheads): mass, stippled calcifications, spiculation, and distortion of the nearby tissue.

primary carcinoma; it should be considered so. With the unsuspected second breast primary carcinoma, without mammography, the patient will have treatment only to the breast with the palpable lesion. It is not known how long it may be before the second lesion becomes clinically evident. If it were within two years, the second cancer would be considered a metastatic deposit, but if it were after five to ten years, it would probably be considered a second primary carcinoma.

Bilateral simultaneous primary carcinomas may be differentiated clinically (Fig. 29–3).

Some pathologists feel that different histologic types of simultaneous carcinoma in both breasts may be some evidence that each represents a separate primary lesion. An interval of time between the detection of the lesion in each breast may also be evidence of primary carcinomas of the breast by radiographic detection (Fig. 29–5) or by clinical detection (Fig. 29–6). The absence of positive axillary lymph nodes on the side of the second lesion may be evidence of a second primary carcinoma.

Clinical Features

Bilateral simultaneous breast carcinomas, and second primary vs metastasis, present

problems in clinical decisions. The discovery of the second malignancy, particularly in the absence of distant metastasis, also forces crucial decisions in treatment planning. The clinical differentiation of primary vs metastasis in the opposite breast must depend on the abiliity to palpate abnormal masses in the

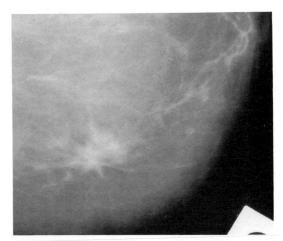

Figure 29–5. Nonsimultaneous bilateral primary carcinomas. This second carcinoma was clinically unsuspected in a 64-year-old woman during routine follow-up mammography three years after her previous mastectomy. She is living and free of disease six years following her second radical mastectomy (no mammogram was done prior to the first surgery).

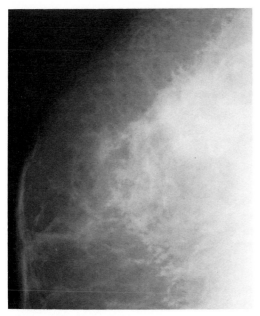

Figure 29–6. Nonsimultaneous bilateral breast carcinomas. This second carcinoma was clinically suspected, as the patient had noted a lump for several months. Although her original cancer had been treated four years previously, she did not present for interval follow-up. Last seen four years after the second radical mastectomy, she was clinically free of disease. (No mammograms were made of the original lesion.)

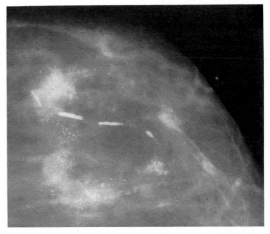

Figure 29–7. Second nonsimultaneous primary carcinomas. A 79-year-old woman being followed 30 years post mastectomy for infiltrating duct carcinoma of the opposite breast. Clinically: normal breast. Mammography: several areas of stippled calcifications without a true mass. Pathology: comedocarcinoma with microinvasion. Modified radical mastectomy; all 19 axillary lymph nodes free of tumor. The patient was alive and free of disease six years following the second mastectomy.

breast, select certain tissues for histopathologic study, and set an arbitrary time interval between the recognition of clinical abnormality in each breast.

Since with mammography early breast carcinoma may be detected prior to signs and symptoms, there will be an increased cure rate for this initial carcinoma. The patients will be expected to live longer and to have a greater chance of developing a second breast carcinoma (Fig. 29–7).

patient with one breast carcinoma has many times the likelihood of developing a second carcinoma as compared with the general population.

A sampling of series of bilateral primary breast carcinomas is presented in Table 29–2. Most of the series had a similar incidence of second primary carcinomas. However, at Emory University with the use of mammography, there was a two to seven times greater incidence of simultaneous primary carcinomas. This greater percentage of simultaneous primary carcinomas at Emory University emphasizes the contribution of mammography in finding the second cancer at an earlier date.

EMORY UNIVERSITY SERIES

Out of a total of 2289 patients with breast carcinoma, 341 had carcinoma in both breasts. The carcinoma in the second breast was primary in 261 and metastatic in 80 patients. Of 2200 patients who entered this series with a previous mastectomy for carcinoma, 271, or 12 per cent, developed a carcinoma in the opposite breast, 75 per cent being primary and 25 per cent metastatic lesions. In the latter group of patients the incidence of the second carcinomas was at the rate of 9 per 1000 primary and 3 per 1000 metastatic carcinomas. This indicates that the

M.D. ANDERSON SERIES

In one series of The University of Texas M.D. Anderson Hospital and Tumor Institute, mammographic studies were available on 278 patients who had had a previous radical mastectomy for proven carcinoma of the breast. Of these, 28 patients developed a carcinoma in the opposite breast during follow-up periods ranging from 1 month to 16 years. Thus, of these patients with one carcinoma of the breast, 10 per cent developed or had at the time a carcinoma in the opposite breast. Radiographically, of this 10 per cent, 20 per cent (eight patients) had metastatic

TABLE 29–2. Bilateral Primary Carcinomas of the Breast

Series	Total Patients With Breast Carcinomas	Total Patients With Second Primary Carcinomas	Per Cent With Second Primary Carcinomas	Patients With Simultaneous Primary Carcinomas	Per Cent of Bilateral Carcinomas With Simultaneous Primaries	Per Cent of Total Carcinomas With Simultaneous Primaries
Berge and Ostberg	687	77	11.2	6	7.2	0.9
Emory	2209	261	11.8	58	22.2	2.6
Haagensen	626	36	5.7	5	13.9	0.8
Herrmann	418	31	7.4	3	9.7	0.7
Leis et al.	611	49	8.0	2	4.0	0.3
Lewison and Neto	490	42	8.6			
Robbins and Berg	1458	91	6.2	4	4.4	0.27
Slack et al.	2734	52	1.9	0	0	0

disease and 70 per cent (20 patients) had second primary carcinomas. Considering all 278 patients, and remembering that the majority had moderately advanced initial lesions and had a follow-up period of less than six and one-half years, 7 per cent of all patients had or developed a primary carcinoma in the opposite breast; 3 per cent had, upon initial radiographic study and proved by biopsy, bilateral simultaneous carcinomas. Of the total bilateral lesions of carcinoma, almost 75 per cent were radiographically separate primary carcinomas of the breast. This varied rather sharply from Haagensen's reported cases from his personal series (Haagensen, 1956): bilateral and simultaneous carcinomas, 0.4 per cent; bilateral but successive, 1.9 per cent; and total bilateral carcinomas of the breast, 2.3 per cent. His observation, that simultaneous involvement of the breast is rare, is not borne out in this study. In fact, simultaneous carcinoma of the breast is of such frequency that study of the opposite breast is necessary for sound treatment planning.

This variation of clinical and radiographic frequency of bilateral carcinomas of the breast may be explained by the following: The presence of 18 of 21 simultaneous second primary carcinomas in this series was suspected only on the basis of mammography; 11 out of 28 successive bilateral carcinomas were detected by mammography. This would indicate that mammography is of much more value than clinical examination in detecting the second primary carcinoma of the breast at an earlier stage of growth.

Patient Features

Age

The median age at diagnosis of bilateral simultaneous primary carcinomas was 57.5 years. The youngest patient was only 21 years of age, while the oldest was 86 years (Fig. 29–8).

With the nonsimultaneous bilateral primary carcinomas, the median age was 54.0 years at diagnosis of the first lesion and 57.8 years at diagnosis of the second carcinoma. The youngest woman was 21 years old at the time of the first carcinoma and 31 at the second; the oldest woman was 81 and 86 years of age, respectively. With the second lesion as metastasis, the interval between the two carcinomas was longer than with primary carcinomas. This was true as well for the inflammatory metastatic carcinomas (Table 29–3).

The occurrence of the first and second carcinomas in the different age groups is indicated in Table 29–4.

Symptoms

The history of the patients, their symptoms, and their fate after diagnosis are recorded in Tables 29–5 and 29–6. Approximately one half of the patients were premenopausal at the time of diagnosis of the first primary carcinoma, but only one third were premenopausal with the diagnosis of the second primary.

Almost all the patients had signs and symptoms with the first primary carcinoma, but one half of the second primaries were

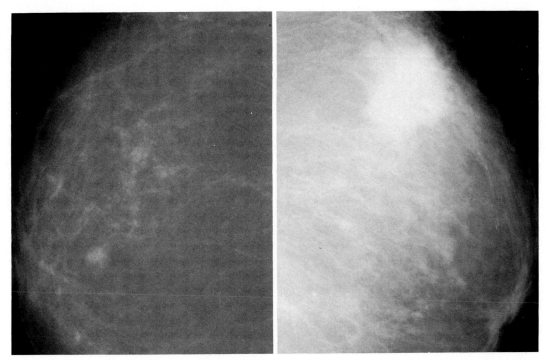

Figure 29–8. Bilateral simultaneous primary carcinomas. An 86-year-old woman with a clinically suspicious lump in the left breast; no abnormality on the right. Mammography: 2.2 × 2.8 cm moderately invasive carcinoma with a satellite nodule in the left breast and a 3 × 3 mm carcinoma containing fine calcification on the right. Bilateral extended simple mastectomies; all lower nodes recovered were free of tumor. Four years later, the patient is doing fine.

detected by routine check-up examinations (Figs. 29–9 and 29–10). Since few of the remaining signs (such as nipple discharge) or symptoms (such as pain) are necessarily

TABLE 29–3. Age and Interval of Bilateral Breast Carcinoma

Type of Carcinoma	Age at First Carcinoma	Age at Second Carcinoma
Simultaneous primaries		
Median age	57.5	57.5
Youngest patient	21	21
Oldest patient	86	86
Nonsimultaneous primaries		
Median age	54.0	57.8
Youngest patient	21	31
Oldest patient	81	86
Primary with metastasis		
Median age	48.9	54.6
Youngest patient	25	26
Oldest patient	68	70
Inflammatory with metastasis		
Median age	58.5	63.4
Youngest patient	39	42
Oldest patient	50	81

reasons for biopsy, x-ray must be assumed to be greatly responsible for biopsy and diagnosis in many others (Figs. 29–11 and 29–12). A lump was present in 87 per cent of the first primary carcinomas and in only 39 per cent of the second primary carcinomas; 46 per cent of the second carcinomas were found on routine checkup, again indicating the value of close follow-up during at least the first six years after mastectomy.

Tumor Size and Stage

The known size of the primary carcinomas is recorded in Table 29–7. Only 10 per cent of the first primary carcinomas were less than

TABLE 29–4. Primary Bilateral Breast Carcinomas With the First and Second Occurrence Indicated for Each Age Group

Age Group (Years)	Number of First Cancers	Number of Second Cancers
20–40	20	21
41–50	47	60
51–60	35	65
Over 60	56	115
Total	158	261

TABLE 29–5. Symptoms of Bilateral Breast Carcinoma Patients

Symptom	First Primary Carcinoma	Second Primary Carcinoma
Lump in breast found		
by patient	177	66
by physician	49	35
Nipple discharge	10	11
Pain	4	12
Routine check-up	4	121
Nipple retraction	9	8
Thickening	0	4
Enlargement	4	4
Axillary nodes	4	0

1 cm in size, whereas over one third of the second primary carcinomas were less than 1 cm. The two primary simultaneous or non-simultaneous carcinomas were more apt to be near-equal in size (Fig. 29–13) unless one was clinically unsuspected. The second non-simultaneous carcinomas were considerably smaller than the first and had fewer axillary lymph node metastases.

The levels of axillary lymph node involvement are noted in Table 29–8. The location of the tumors within the breast are shown in Table 29–9.

Histologic Types

Most of the carcinomas were of the duct cell type histologically (Table 29–10). However, there were the other various histologic types of carcinoma. The incidence of these as well as their multiplicity was not significantly different from the occurrence in the single breast cancers. As usual, the less aggressive and more curable carcinomas did allow more time for a second primary to appear.

TABLE 29–6. Fate Following Diagnosis of Second Primary Carcinoma

Years After Diagnosis of Second Primary	Dead		Alive	
	Cancer	Other	No Disease	With Cancer
0–1	12		4	1
1–2	5		5	
2–3	4	1	5	3
3–4	3		4	1
4–5			5	1
5–6			4	
6–7	2		3	
7–8			2	
8–9			1	
14–15			1	
Total	26	1	34	6

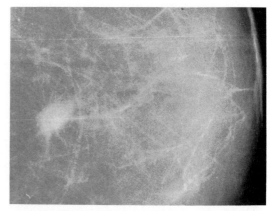

Figure 29–9. Second primary breast carcinoma. A 78-year-old woman being followed for a right mastectomy six years previously, with a clinically normal remaining breast. Mammograms: a 7 × 11 mm moderately invasive second primary carcinoma containing stippled calcification in a fatty breast. Pathology: duct carcinoma with mild fibrosis; modified radical mastectomy; 19 axillary lymph nodes free of tumor. No evidence of disease six years later.

Occurrence

The 261 primary carcinomas in the contralateral breast occurred in the following circumstances: 102 times in patients seen subsequent to a mastectomy; 19 times with the

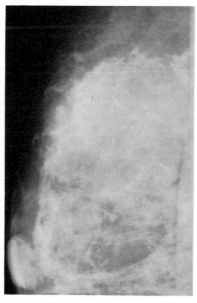

Figure 29–10. Second nonsimultaneous primary carcinoma. A 66-year-old woman with a clinically suspicious mass in the remaining breast following a radical mastectomy for carcinoma of the opposite breast six years before. Mammography: poorly defined, moderately invasive 3 cm carcinoma. Pathology: infiltrating duct carcinoma. Modified radical mastectomy; all 21 axillary lymph nodes free of disease. The patient was free of disease 18 months later.

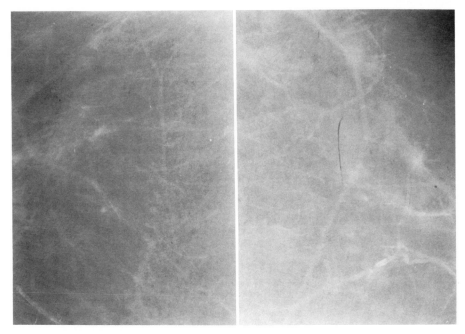

Figure 29–11. Bilateral nonpalpable primary breast carcinomas. A 70-year-old woman with a clear nipple discharge on the right and a central thickening on the left. Mammography: Poorly defined asymmetric central density (right) and 4 × 5 and 3 × 4 mm suspicious areas (left). Pathology: Right central collecting duct system showed papillary intraductal carcinoma in a setting of severe intraductal papillomatosis and atypia; 14 lymph nodes normal; left two masses, infiltrating duct carcinomas; all axillary lymph nodes free of tumor. No evidence of disease five years later.

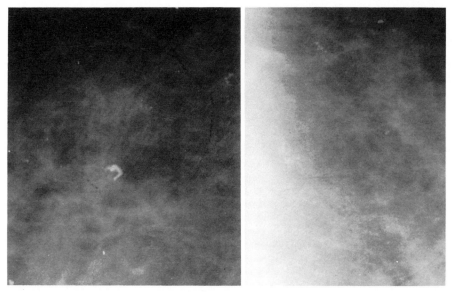

Figure 29–12. Simultaneous bilateral nonpalpable breast carcinomas. A 67-year-old woman whose sister had breast cancer. Mammography: Above the coarse benign calcification centrally are two areas of stippled calcification, one associated with a pseudomass (right); two similar areas of calcification centrally on the left. Localization and biopsy; infiltrating duct carcinoma (right) associated with severe papillomatosis and focal areas of atypia in all quadrants; three separate areas (largest 0.9 cm in diameter) of infiltrating duct carcinoma (left) with components of comedo and scirrhous patterns, severe papillomatosis, and areas of intraductal tumor of cribriform type. Axillary lymph nodes free of tumor after bilateral modified radical mastectomies.

TABLE 29–7. Known Pathologic Size of Bilateral Primary Breast Carcinomas

Carcinoma	No Mass	<1.0 cm	1.1–2.0 cm	2.1–5.0 cm	≥5.1 cm
Simultaneous					
right breast	23	7	13	12	2
left breast	20	6	16	16	0
Nonsimultaneous*					
1st primary	11	9	38	39	4
2nd primary	42	35	68	47	7

*Of those who entered series, 102 had had one breast removed.

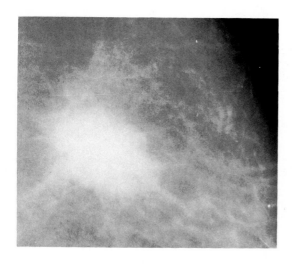

Figure 29–13. Second primary nonsimultaneous carcinoma following a Stage II lesion. A 56-year-old woman, who had a radical mastectomy for a 1.8 × 2.3 cm Stage II duct cell carcinoma five years previously, presented with a firm mass of two weeks' duration in the remaining breast. Mammograms: 1.7 × 2.3 cm moderately invasive carcinoma. Pathology: duct cell carcinoma with reactive fibrosis. Modified radical mastectomy; all 20 axillary lymph nodes free of tumor. No evidence of disease five years later.

TABLE 29–8. Level of Axillary Metastases in Bilateral Primary Carcinomas and of Primary Carcinomas with Metastasis to the Opposite Breast

Carcinoma	No Axillary Metastasis	Level I ≤ 3 Nodes	Level I > 3 Nodes	Level II	All Levels	Not Studied	Total
Simultaneous primary							
right breast	39	5	2	2	4	6	58
left breast	42	4	0	3	2	7	58
Nonsimultaneous							
1st primary	57	12	1	12	9	10	101
2nd primary	132	14	3	11	10	33	203
Primary with metastasis	3	2	0	2	4	3	14

TABLE 29–9. Location of Bilateral Breast Carcinomas

Carcinoma	UOQ	UIQ	LOQ	LIQ	Central	Diffuse	Total
Simultaneous primary							
right breast	30	10	8	3	4	3	58
left breast	29	12	4	2	8	3	58
Nonsimultaneous							
1st primary	56	12	10	11	10	2	101
2nd primary	112	33	17	17	13	11	203
Primary with metastasis	6	2	1	1	0	4	14

TABLE 29–10. Histologic Types of Bilateral Primary Breast Carcinomas in 261 Patients

Carcinomas	Scirrhous	Intraductal	Duct Cell	Medullary With Lymphoid Stroma	Infiltrating Lobular	Lobular In Situ	Intracystic Papillary	Duct With Other	Miscellaneous
Simultaneous									
right breast	2	9	26	1	2	4	0	11	2
left breast	5	7	27	1	3	5	2	6	2
Nonsimultaneous									
1st primary	18	8	50	3	3	2	1	11	6
2nd primary	30	23	99	2	7	13	2	15	12
Total	55	47	202	7	15	24	5	43	22

carcinoma on the initial mammogram and development of the second lesion during follow-up; 58 times with simultaneous bilateral primary carcinomas (Figs. 29–14 and 29–15), and 79 times (nonsimultaneous) in patients who developed two carcinomas after initial normal bilateral mammograms. Eighty-four per cent (218) of the second primary carcinomas occurred within the sixth year of the diagnosis of the first. Sixteen per cent (43) occurred after six years (Fig. 29–1) and spread evenly up to 23 years (Table 29–11).

The longest span between appearance of the two primary carcinomas was 23 years, at ages 50 and 73; the shortest interval was seven months. In the Emory University series there was no second primary cancer within six months of the diagnosis of the first carcinoma in those patients studied by mammography. It is assumed that, in many cases, mammography detected the second primary carcinoma six months prior to its becoming clinically evident. All the second simultaneous primary breast carcinomas were detected by mammography.

Of the women with metastatic carcinomas, 37 had undergone mastectomy prior to being seen, 38 presented with a primary carcinoma and then developed metastasis, and 5 had simultaneous carcinomas when first seen.

ROLE OF MAMMOGRAPHY

Robbins and Berg (1964) reported a second primary carcinoma in 6.2 per cent of the total patients with breast carcinoma, 0.27 per cent of which were simultaneous. At Emory University there were bilateral primary carcinomas in 12 per cent of the total breast cancer patients, with bilateral simultaneous primary carcinomas in 2.6 per cent of this total—a tenfold increase in simultaneous primary carcinomas. At 20-year follow-up, the Emory University Study should have additional second carcinomas and one may postulate that less advanced disease allows better cure and greater opportunity to develop the second carcinoma. Mammography, by providing recognition of more simultaneous bilateral breast carcinomas, leads to earlier treatment of the second carcinoma. Mammography was much more efficient in detecting the second carcinoma than clinical examination and prophylactic mastectomies practiced by Leis (Leis et al., 1965), and more efficient than Urban's (1967) bilateral breast biopsies, producing 31 bilateral carcinomas in 281 patients. However, in this latter series, if 18 noninfiltrating lesions (many lobular carcinoma in situ) were excluded, the two methods were even less comparable to mammography in detecting the second carcinoma.

Mammography, by placing more of the clinically unsuspected carcinomas in the simultaneous group, apparently removes many potential clinical nonsimultaneous carcinomas from discovery in years 1, 2, and 3 after the first carcinoma; thus, it levels out the discovery of these second cancers over the first six years. This is at variance with

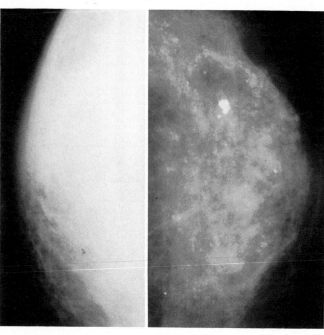

Figure 29–14. Bilateral primary breast carcinomas, one inoperable. A 58-year-old woman who referred herself for "painful, smaller breasts, indented one week." Clinically: diffuse disease in right breast, no inflammation; normal left breast. Mammograms: diffuse involvement of right breast; if carcinoma, inoperable. In left breast, several areas of comedocarcinoma calcifications without mass. Pathology: needle biopsy of right breast; duct carcinoma. After irradiation to right breast plus chemotherapy, the carcinomas were still controlled at four years.

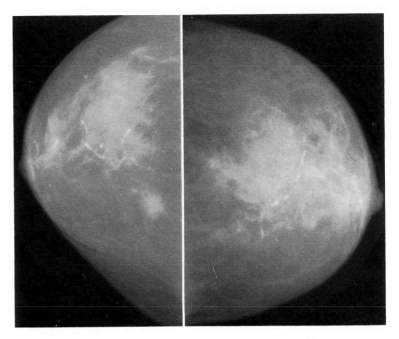

Figure 29–15. Bilateral simultaneous primary breast carcinomas. A 77-year-old woman with a left breast lump for one week. Clinically: normal right breast; suspicious 4 cm mass in left breast. Mammography: 2 × 2.5 cm moderately invasive carcinoma (left) and 1 × 1.2 cm carcinoma (right). Pathology: bilateral infiltrating duct carcinomas. Bilateral modified radical mastectomies; all axillary lymph nodes free of metastasis. The patient was alive and well eight years later.

nonmammographic studies carried out by Robbins and Berg (1964) and by Haagensen (1971). The 84 per cent of the second primary carcinomas that occurred within six years of the first carcinoma compares with 54 per cent and 39 per cent, respectively, of these two series (Table 29–2). Also, at Emory University 22 per cent of the primary carcinomas were simultaneous, compared with 4 per cent and 13 per cent, respectively, in these two series.

Since 84 per cent of the second primary carcinomas at Emory University were detected within the sixth postmastectomy year and the remaining 16 per cent were scattered evenly up to 23 years, mammography is helpful in predicting the lessened risk for the second primary carcinoma after the sixth year of follow-up.

In the series shown in Table 29–2 there was only a slight difference in the percentage of total bilateral carcinomas, except in that of Slack et al., but there was a substantial increase in the percentage of simultaneous carcinomas at Emory University in which mammography was employed.

TREATMENT

Treatment consisted of a complete or modified radical mastectomy, usually a radical mastectomy if there was extensive axillary lymph node metastasis.

Pack (1951) advocated prophylactic simple mastectomy of the opposite breast following radical mastectomy for cancer of the first breast, based on his observation that 7 per cent of the patients treated successfully for the first cancer would develop a primary cancer in the opposite breast. Farrow (1956) advocated prophylactic mastectomy only in certain patients, whereas Leis performed this procedure on all selected women who submitted to it (Leis et al., 1965). He found seven unsuspected cancers in 66 patients so treated. Herrmann (1973) contended that

TABLE 29–11. Yearly Number of Second Primary Breast Carcinomas in Three Series

Series Total	Years After First Operation																								
	0*	1†	2	3	4	5	6	7	8	9	10	11	12	13	14	15	16	17	18	19	20	21	22	23	24
Emory University 261 (Contemporary data)	58	30	31	28	22	24	25	8	2	1	2	1	3	1	5	1	3	2	5	3	0	3	1	1	1
Haagensen (1971) 36	5	0	3	3	1	0	2	4	3	2	3	2	2	2	3	1									
Robbins and Berg (1964) 91	4	10	14	6	4	4	7	1	6	4	3	7	3	2	2	0	3	4	2	1	3	0	1		

*Simultaneous.
†Within first year, 7 to 12 months following first primary.

prophylactic mastectomy was totally unwarranted. In his series of 418 patients operated upon for carcinoma of the breast, 28 patients had nonsimultaneous and 3 patients had simultaneous, bilateral primary operable carcinomas. If routine prophylactic mastectomy had been performed, 198 or 47.3 per cent would have undergone a useless mastectomy. We have found no condemning evidence that mammography is unreliable in following the second breast.

Yet, none of the cited authors, except Herrmann, spoke of using mammography in this manner; as late as 1974 (Berge and Ostberg) mammography was not considered of value with this breast problem.

PROGNOSIS

There was an even spread in size with the simultaneous bilateral carcinomas, both by x-ray and by gross pathology, with 75 per cent less than 2 cm for the right side compared with 72 per cent for the left side. In the nonsimultaneous group, only 57 per cent of the first carcinomas (by pathology) were less than 2 cm, while 73 per cent of the second primaries were less than 2 cm. Only 20 per cent of the first primary carcinomas were less than 1 cm (Table 29–7), compared with 76 per cent of the second. Based on size alone, the second carcinoma should have a better prognosis.

Some carcinomas bilaterally were highly invasive (Fig. 29–16), some were circumscribed (Fig. 29–17), and one highly aggressive and the other indolent (Fig. 29–18). Bilateral multicentric, multiple histologic types of carcinomas could influence the prognosis (Fig. 29–19). The first primary carcinoma may be the cause of death, complicating the estimate of value of treating the second primary (Fig. 29–20).

However, this was not as clear-cut with axillary lymph node metastases. Of simultaneous primaries, 67 per cent were without axillary metastasis. The first and second nonsimultaneous primaries had 55 and 63 per cent, respectively, axillae free of metastasis. This discrepancy between size of the second primary carcinoma and extent of axillary lymph node metastasis at the time of its detection is complicated by the inability to assess the possible contralateral axillary lymph node metastasis and distant metastasis (relating to prognosis) from the first primary carcinoma.

Four years after diagnosis of the second primary breast carcinoma is the dividing point in prognosis (Table 29–6); 25 of the 27 deaths had occurred by then, and only one patient with cancer was living beyond four years. The living patients without evidence of disease were spread evenly up to eight years after diagnosis of the second primary. Fifty per cent of the patients were alive 1 to 15 years following the second primary carci-

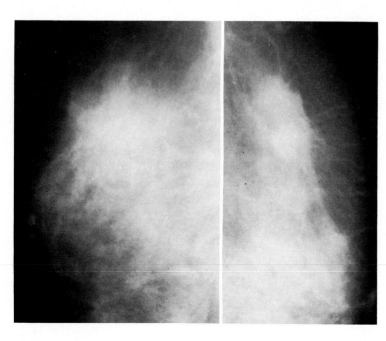

Figure 29–16. Bilateral simultaneous aggressive carcinomas. A 57-year-old woman with a right breast lump clinically suspicious for a circumscribed carcinoma. Mammograms: right breast, 2 × 2 cm highly invasive carcinoma containing stippled calcifications; left breast, 1.5 × 2 cm highly invasive carcinoma containing stippled calcifications with increased vascularity. Pathology: bilateral duct carcinomas with scirrhous elements; bilateral modified radical mastectomies, 0 of 12 nodes with tumor (left) and one of six with tumor (right). Both breasts had marked changes histologically of dysplasia, fibroadenomatosis, ductal hyperplasia, sclerosing adenosis, papillomatosis, and apocrine and cystic changes. Four years later the patient was free of disease. Comment: These severe changes of fibrocystic disease masked the real nature of the left carcinoma clinically.

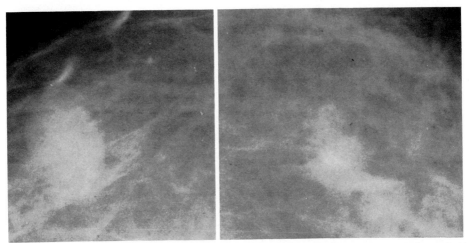

Figure 29–17. Bilateral circumscribed simultaneous primary carcinomas. A 49-year-old woman with a palpable mass in the right breast. Mammograms: right breast, 1.2 × 1.8 cm circumscribed carcinoma with increased vascularity; left breast, 7 × 10 mm similar mass of carcinoma. Pathology: bilateral duct carcinomas. Bilateral modified radical mastectomies; all axillary lymph nodes free of tumor. Four years later there was no evidence of disease.

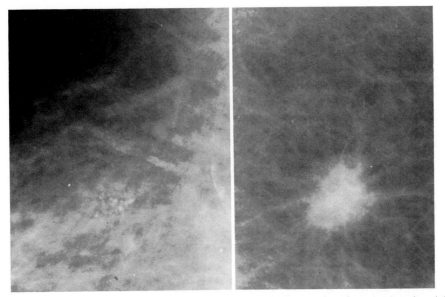

Figure 29–18. Bilateral simultaneous breast carcinomas, one highly infiltrative, the other microinvasive. A 79-year-old woman with a clinically suspicious left breast lump. Mammograms: right breast, area of comedocarcinoma calcifications without definite mass; left breast, 7 × 10 mm highly invasive carcinoma. Pathology: On the right, there is intraductal comedocarcinoma with minimal invasion and, on the left, duct carcinoma with marked fibrosis. Bilateral modified radical mastectomy; both Stage I lesions. When death occurred two years later, the patient was free of carcinoma.

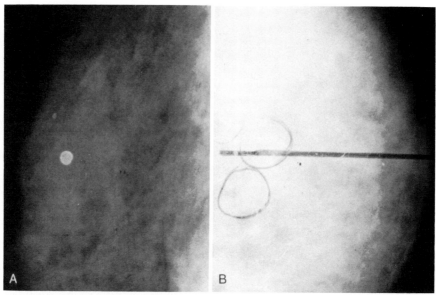

Figure 29–19. Bilateral primary carcinoma of multiple histologic types. A 61-year-old woman with firm right breast mass for three or four months. *A,* Mammograms: large, irregular, asymmetric mass centrally extending into the UOQ right breast. Pathology: 6 × 5 × 2.7 cm lobular carcinoma with a 5 mm papillary carcinoma nearby. Right radical mastectomy; 24 lymph nodes free of tumor. On follow-up three years later, suspicious calcifications were noted in the left breast (*B*). Pathology: In 1 sq cm, prominent intraductal carcinoma with lobular extension and small foci of invasion was present. The invasive carcinoma was predominantly papillary, with central necrosis associated with calcifications. Four years later, the patient was free of disease.

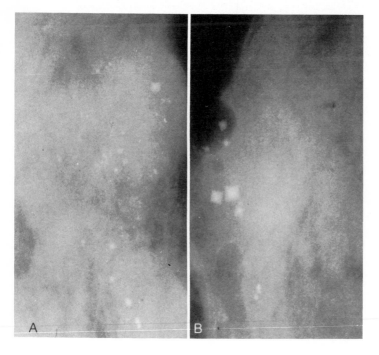

Figure 29–20. Nonsimultaneous (duct, then lobular in situ) bilateral primary carcinomas. A 50-year-old woman who eight years before had had right radical mastectomy for Stage II comedo and duct carcinoma. Mammogram: Coarse and fine calcification suspicious for comedocarcinoma of the left breast, seen in two different specimen radiographs (*A* and *B*). Pathology on elective complete mastectomy: Lobular carcinoma in area of, but not related to, the calcifications. Severe fibrocystic disease. Death occurred from disseminated disease five years following the second mastectomy.

noma, and 24 per cent were alive four years after the second primary carcinoma.

CASE HISTORY

This 46-year-old woman, seen for baseline mammograms, had nodular breasts with some questionable abnormality in the right breast. There was no family history of breast cancer. Bilateral mammograms and sonograms were obtained (Fig. 29–21).

The mammogram of the right breast (A) showed a spiculated mass containing stippled calcifications (arrow). This was in the area of a firmer nodularity clinically. The sonogram of this breast (B) showed an irregular, jagged, hypoechoic mass (arrow) with distorted surrounding tissue and consistent with carcinoma, although without demonstrable attenuation of the beam. Routine mammogram of the left breast (C) demonstrated an irregular, spiculated, moderately invasive carcinoma (arrow) in the upper quadrant near the chest wall. The sonogram of the left breast (D) revealed an irregular, bilobed, jagged 1.2 cm mass (arrow) with some architectural distortion, indicating the presence of carcinoma. In both breasts with the single-sector scans there was definite shadowing.

The pathology was bilateral infiltrating duct carcinomas with an element of desmoplasia. After bilateral modified radical mastectomies, all axillary lymph nodes (18 on the right and 20 on the left) were found to be free of metastasis. In the three years of follow-up the patient has remained free of disease. Sonography in patients having nodular breasts with coalescent areas of ductal hyperplasia provides considerably more confidence in treatment planning.

CASE HISTORY

Second nonsimultaneous primary carcinoma. A 72-year-old woman who had a left radical mastectomy plus irradiation two and a half years before for a duct carcinoma Stage II, and left chest wall recurrence two years later, presented with a right axillary lump.

Mammography (Fig. 29–22) showed a 1.8 × 2.4 cm highly invasive carcinoma with early diffuse skin thickening, marked increase in vein size, axillary masses including a 1 cm lesion just above the reference mass, and a second primary carcinoma in the tail of the breast. Pathology: (tail of breast and lower axillary resection) duct carcinoma in tail of

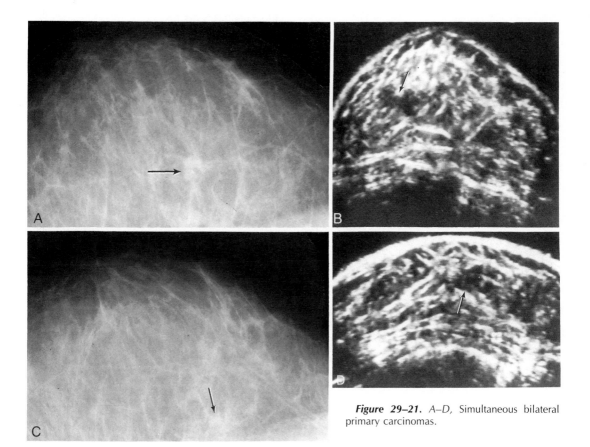

Figure 29–21. A–D, Simultaneous bilateral primary carcinomas.

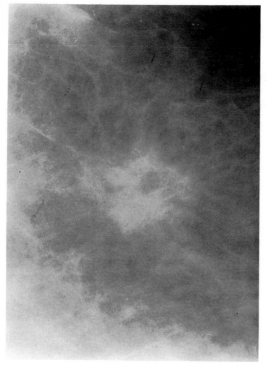

Figure 29–22. Second primary carcinoma.

breast and axillary lymph node, no in situ component. Comment: With the advanced and diffuse disease clinically the breast mass could not be separated from the lymph nodes. Further histopathologic study revealed invasive carcinoma with productive fibrosis. The axillary lymph node spread could have possibly been from the left breast primary, but this is less likely to contralateral low axillary lymph nodes near an ipsilateral primary carcinoma. Ten months later death ensued from liver and widespread metastatic carcinoma.

CASE HISTORY

During a routine examination by an Emory University gynecologist, a questionable nodule was noted in the upper outer quadrant of the left breast of a 39-year-old woman, gravida 1, para 1; she had nursed for three months. There was no family history of breast cancer. She was being followed for endometriosis and a nodular thyroid.

Mammograms dated 3/7/66 revealed dense fibroglandular tissue bilaterally with a 1.5 cm cyst in the upper outer quadrant of the left breast. After several weeks the cyst disappeared. On 10/21/71 the patient required a panhysterectomy. Repeat mammograms, taken on 12/14/72 while she was being followed in the oncologic breast clinic for fibrocystic disease, were normal. On 1/7/74 the next set of mammograms done for nodular breasts showed that a cluster of calcifications not associated with a mass had

appeared in the upper inner quadrant of the right breast. It was interpreted as "calcification pattern of carcinoma" (Fig. 29–23).

Apparently the woman was referred back to her primary care physician without notification to her or her physician about the radiographic comedocarcinoma. In May 1977 by breast self-examination she noted a mass in the upper inner quadrant of the right breast. This was confirmed by her family physician and had appeared since his examination one year previously. Mammograms taken on 5/31/77 showed a 1.5 cm moderately invasive carcinoma in the upper inner quadrant of the right breast in the area of the previous calcifications (Fig. 29–24). As there were two additional separate areas of calcifications indicating multifocal lesions, the radiologist suggested an increased risk in the opposite breast.

Study of the right radical mastectomy specimen on 6/8/77 revealed a 2.5 × 2.2 × 2 cm focus of duct carcinoma with fibrosis; nearby foci of intraductal carcinoma, both comedo and papillary, in the upper inner quadrant; and multiple foci of intraductal papillary carcinoma in other areas of the upper inner quadrant and in the lower outer quadrant (Fig. 29–25). Two of 16 axillary lymph nodes were positive. The surgery was followed by cobalt radiotherapy, then by chemotherapy beginning on 9/8/77.

A routine mammogram of the left breast on 6/13/79 showed scattered calcification thought to be associated with the fibrocystic disease. On 6/18/80 a cluster was present in the upper inner quadrant, not reported (Fig. 29–26A). On 6/4/81 the calcifi-

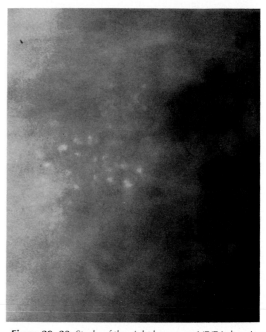

Figure 29–23. Study of the right breast on 1/7/74 showing the "calcification pattern of carcinoma" in the upper inner quadrant.

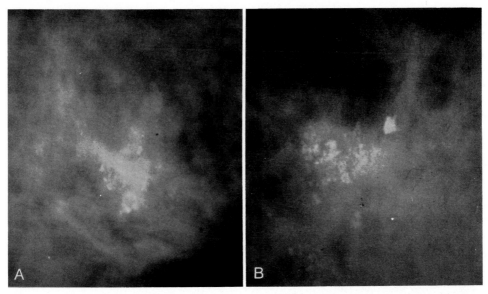

Figure 29–24. Mammogram of the same right breast on 5/31/77 showed a density with increased calcifications at the site of the calcifications noted 40 months previously. *A*, Radiographically invasive carcinoma. At least two other foci of calcifications of comedo intraductal carcinoma were present. One area (*B*) was in the LOQ.

cations were still not associated with a mass but were reported as probable carcinoma (Fig. 29–26*B*). Following localization and biopsy specimen radiography, the pathologic diagnosis was intraductal carcinoma without evidence of invasion (Fig. 29–27). Study of the modified radical mastectomy specimen showed other foci with similar pathology.

By 1974 the patient was still only 46 years old, not yet at the magical age of recommended yearly mammograms (NIH/NCI, 1977). More than three years was required for the carcinoma to grow to clinical recognition despite its presence being shown by mammography. The indolent nature of many breast carcinomas provides a lengthy curable period. However, in this case a large mass was produced, fibrosis was present, multiple foci and multiple histologic types had been formed, and metastasis to axillary lymph nodes from an inner quadrant lesion had occurred. All these findings signal a poor prognosis (Egan et al., 1980; Egan, 1982). Such an oversight of abnormal mammographic findings was unfortunate. Conceivably this could have resulted from three separate physicians being involved in patient care for many problems, one of which was the opposite breast with its questionable status eventually resolved.

With the second primary carcinoma, annual mammograms had been omitted despite the radiologist's indicating increased risk; then another year was lost by not promptly calling attention to the presence of clustered calcifications. The prognosis for this lesion, if it were the only carcinoma, would be good; but finding a minimally invasive second primary does not improve the guarded prognosis imparted by the first invasive primary.

CASE HISTORY

Simultaneous bilateral multifocal primary carcinomas. A 56-year-old woman presented with a mass in the left breast; the right breast was clinically normal. Mammography (Fig. 29–28) showed two nearby masses (*A*, right). One was a 1 × 1.5 cm poorly defined mass containing comedocarcinoma type calcifications; the other mass, inferiorly, was similar but smaller. Dense spiculated carcinoma, 1.5 × 2.5 cm, suggesting highly invasive duct carcinoma (left); large diffuse area without true mass but comedocarcinoma calcifications. Sonography revealed a large, poorly defined, hypoechoic area, nonhomogeneous internal echoes, marked architectural distortion, and slightly decreased through-transmission (right). On the left there is a large irregular area, almost anechoic, with marked shadowing—a highly invasive carcinoma. Nearby less severe changes in the sound beam suggest a less aggressive carcinoma. Pathology: intraductal and early invasive comedocarcinoma, multifocal and diffuse (right). A modified radical mastectomy was performed; all 16 lymph nodes were free of tumor. Duct carcinoma with scirrhous element, multifocal and diffuse (left); modified radical mastectomy. Three low nodes of a total of 24 lymph nodes were positive. Death from a stroke occurred three months later; there was no evidence of cancer.

OBSERVATIONS

Mammography is extremely valuable in finding and differentiating a second primary

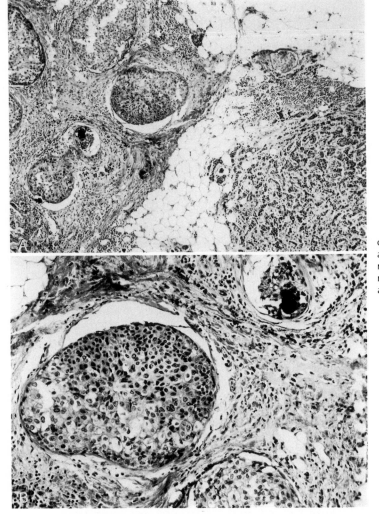

Figure 29–25. Pathology: multifocal carcinoma, invasive duct with fibrosis and intraductal comedo, × 20. *A,* Representative photomicrographs of the main mass of tumor in the UIQ and another focus. *B,* From the LOQ, × 50.

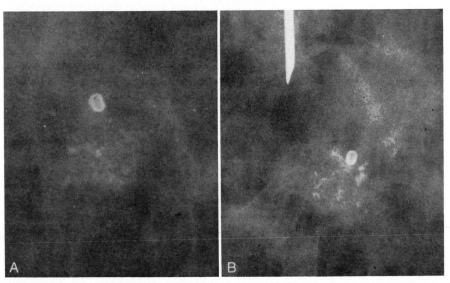

Figure 29–26. *A,* Left breast on 6/18/80 with a cluster of suspicious calcifications. *B,* Same area on 6/4/81, still without an associated mass requiring needle localization.

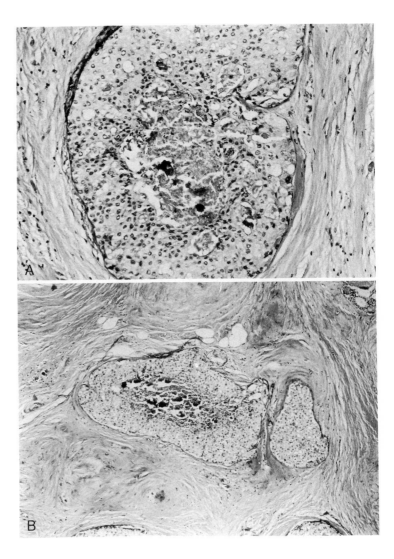

Figure 29–27. Second primary carcinoma in the opposite breast in 1981. *A*, Intraductal carcinoma with calcification in the center of the duct and others completely surrounded by viable carcinoma cells, e.g., upper centrally. *B*, Another focus of intraductal carcinoma with surrounding heavy fibrotic reaction with collagen.

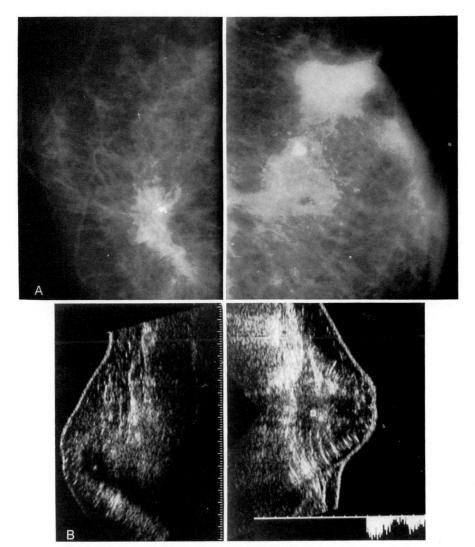

Figure 29–28. A–B, Bilateral multifocal simultaneous primary breast carcinomas.

carcinoma from metastasis. Carcinoma in the opposite breast is usually a second primary carcinoma; it is not necessarily metastasis; and it should be treated accordingly. If the second primary carcinoma is properly treated, there should be at least 150 per cent increase in the survival rate. The second primary carcinoma has a specific natural history: Almost all the second primary carcinomas were detected within the sixth postmastectomy year, indicating that close follow-up during this period is mandatory. Four years after the diagnosis of the second primary breast carcinoma, prognosis is extremely good.

Failure to detect a breast carcinoma for earliest possible treatment is the bane of the mammographer. This may be due either to not recognizing changes in the mammogram or to failing to communicate diagnostic changes. A case is presented to illustrate both situations.

A uniform system of compiling data in bilateral breast carcinomas is needed. Single series have limited numbers of patients, varying periods and types of follow-up, and different criteria for diagnosis and fail to consider properly in situ cancers, among other variables. Leis et al. (1965), in presenting an extensive review of the literature, found that the incidence of simultaneous second primary carcinoma varied from 0.1 to 2.0 per cent, with a median of 0.7 per cent, and that the incidence of nonsimultaneous second primary carcinoma varied from 1.0 to 12 per cent, with a median of 3.2 per cent.

Haagensen (1986) revised his data on bilateral primary breast carcinomas. Of 1992 women with breast carcinoma, 7.9 per cent had bilateral primary carcinomas, with 1.0 per cent of the total carcinomas being simultaneous primaries. This compared with the eightfold ratio of total second primaries vs simultaneous primaries noted in Table 29–2, showing no increased detection of simultaneous primary carcinomas based primarily on clinical examination of the breast.

REFERENCES

Berge T, Ostberg G (1974): Bilateral carcinoma of the female breast. Acta Clin Scand *140*:27.

Egan RL (1972): Mammography, 2nd ed. Springfield, IL, Charles C Thomas.

Egan RL (1976): Bilateral breast carcinomas: Role of mammography. Cancer *38*:931.

Egan RL (1982): Multicentric breast carcinomas: Clinical-radiographic-pathologic whole organ studies and 10-year survival. Cancer *49*:1123.

Egan RL, McSweeney MB, Sewell CW (1980): Intramammary calcifications without an associated mass in benign and malignant diseases. Radiology *137*:1.

Farrow JH (1956): Bilateral mammary cancer. Cancer *9*:1182.

Haagensen CD (1956): Diseases of the Breast, 1st ed. Philadelphia, WB Saunders, p 344. Ibid (1971), 2nd ed. Ibid (1986), 3rd ed, p 444.

Herrmann JB (1973): Management of the contralateral breast after mastectomy for unilateral carcinoma. Surg Gynecol Obstet *136*:777.

Kilgore AR (1921): Incidence of cancer in second breast; after radical removal of 1 breast for cancer. JAMA 77:454.

Kilgore AR, Bell HG, Ahlquist RE (1956): Cancer in the second breast. Am J Surg *92*:156.

Leis HP Jr, Mercheimer WL, Black MM, DeChabone A (1965): The second breast. NY State J Med *65*:2460.

Lewison EF, Neto AS (1971): Bilateral breast cancer at the Johns Hopkins Hospital—A discussion of the dilemma of contralateral breast cancer. Cancer *28*:1297.

NIH/NCI (1977): Consensus Development Meeting on Breast Cancer Screening. Bethesda, MD, September 14–16.

Pack GI (1951): Argument for bilateral mastectomy. Surgery *29*:929.

Robbins GF, Berg JW (1964): Bilateral primary breast cancers. Cancer *17*:1501.

Slack NH, Bross IDJ, Nemoto T, Fisher B (1973): Experience with bilateral primary carcinoma of the breast. Surg Gynecol Obstet *136*:433.

Urban JA (1967): Bilaterality of cancer of the breast. Biopsy of the opposite breast. Cancer *20*:1867.

Breast Cancer in Young Women

30

BACKGROUND

Breast cancer is rare prior to age 20 years; under 25 years it is infrequent, but after 30 years there is an increased frequency that continues steadily with advancing age (Egan, 1975). Haagensen (1986) reported 0.2 per cent of total breast cancers under age 25 years, 1 per cent under age 30 years, and 4.3 per cent under age 35 years. The controversies that abound over diagnosis and management of breast cancer and the importance of the breast as a sexual symbol strongly affect younger women. Research into the influence of younger age on the course and prognosis of breast cancer has suggested the following: none (Berkson et al., 1957; Alderson et al., 1971); worsened (Sistrunk and MacCarty, 1922; Bloom, 1964; Langlands and Kerr, 1979); or improved (Merller et al., 1978; Redding et al., 1979). Opinions range more diversely on the effects of pregnancy, lactation, and subsequent pregnancy (Haagensen and Stout, 1943; Cheek, 1953; White and White, 1956; Rissanen, 1968; Egan and Egan, 1984b).

Even with rather classic signs or symptoms of breast cancer, younger women too frequently are observed rather than having a diagnosis aggressively pursued. The rationalization may be based on the lower incidence of breast cancer in younger women (even though this is the leading cause of death in women aged 40 to 44 years); the added expense; the "radiation hazard" of mammography; and the fact that mammography is at times less accurate in the dense nodular, less fatty breast.

The more hopeful attitudes about breast cancer following improved results by using mammography to lessen delays in detection and overcome hesitant treatments in women over age 50 years have not been extended to these younger patients. A higher frequency of axillary lymph node metastasis and more aggressive histologic types of tumor are cited to explain poorer prognosis in young, pregnant, and lactating women (Bloom, 1964; Langlands and Kerr, 1979). Our experience has convinced us that none of the resultant dilemmas should interfere with an optimistic and unhesitant pursuit of the diagnosis and treatment of breast cancer in this "neglected group of women" aged 34 years or less. Actually, with their potentially greatly increased life expectancy, they should be more vigorously treated. This potential of adding a greater number of years of useful life to women is perhaps the greatest contribution of mammography. But this use of mammography depends on its systematic use. The ideal is proper selection by risk factors.

FREQUENCY AND AGE DISTRIBUTION

Over a 20-year period, 27, 472 women were followed with prospectively gathered epidemiologic, clinical, and radiologic data with 58,665 breast examinations; 8053 excision biopsies produced 2209 malignant and 5844 benign (excluding cyst aspirations) histologically proved lesions (see Table 35–1). Approximately one fourth of the mammograms were performed on women aged 34 years or less. Biopsies were done on 1921 (24 per cent of the total biopsies) young women having prebiopsy mammography to demonstrate 139 (6.3 per cent of the total) primary operable cancers.

A review of all Emory University Pathology Department breast biopsies during the same period showed 307 recorded breast cancers in 290 women 34 years of age or younger (Table 30–1). The age at diagnosis of 279 primary operable breast cancers is shown in Table 30–2. In this series, the number of primary operable breast cancers in women under age 35 years approximated the number of breast cancers in the 71 to 75 year group and was similar to the number of breast cancers encountered after about age 77 years.

This incidence of breast cancer in young women is noteworthy, as very few oncologists ignore a breast complaint when a woman passes menopause. Yet, in the young age group, in which treatment of a curable cancer would provide long years of useful life, the diagnosis of breast cancer is too infrequently entertained. Limited experience with cancer in these younger women by the referring physicians tends toward a reversal from the higher biopsy rate for breast cancer required in our institution. Neither clinical practice provides a ready solution to this enigma. This limited experience is well exemplified by Haagensen (1986), who encoun-

TABLE 30–2. Age at Diagnosis of Young Women With 279 Primary Operable Breast Cancers

	Age in Years						
	18	19	21	23–25	26–28	29–31	32–34
Number of women	1	1	4	26	38	89	120

tered only 256 cancers in breasts of young women during a 40-year period in a busy practice limited to breast diseases. Nevertheless, this does not condone apathy toward breast cancer in young women. The relative increase in cancer in the young in our series most likely reflects the type of referrals (less obvious serious problems) and the use of mammography, despite its curtailed use in younger women.

PRESENTING COMPLAINTS

In these young women there was no great difference in presenting complaints, risk factors, or discovery of a lump from those of other age groups. Mass was the presenting complaint in 77 per cent of the cases (94 per cent of these being discovered by the patient), with discharge, thickening, pain, axillary adenopathy, and change in breast size equally making up the other 23 per cent of the primary complaints (Figs. 30–1 to 30–4). A family history of breast cancer was recorded in each case: mother, five times; sister, two times; maternal grandmother, six times; and maternal aunt, four times. The youngest patient was 18 years of age; the mean age was 30.6 years for the women with breast cancer who were under age 35 years. Young women's breasts were often similar to those of older women (Figs. 30–5 and 30–6). Pregnancy and lactation were more common, however (Fig. 30–7), than in older women.

CLINICAL EXAMINATION

Physical findings in young women did not differ significantly from those in older women with breast cancer. More nodular, glandular, and firmer breast tissue was more difficult to evaluate clinically than the softer breasts usually associated with older women. At the initial examination, physical examination failed to detect only 14 of 103 cancers (13.6 per cent) diagnosed at that time in the young, while the overall failure of detection

TABLE 30–1. Types of 307 Breast Cancers in 290 Women 34 Years of Age or Less

Occurrence	Number	Cancer Type
Operable		
Primary	274	Breast Carcinoma
	3	Cytosarcoma phylloides
	1	Hodgkin's disease
	1	Fibrosarcoma
Inoperable		
Inflammatory	7	Breast carcinoma
Metastatic	10	From opposite breast
	11	From distant focus
		8 Melanoma (1 bilateral, 3 males)
		2 Hodgkin's disease
		1 Lymphosarcoma

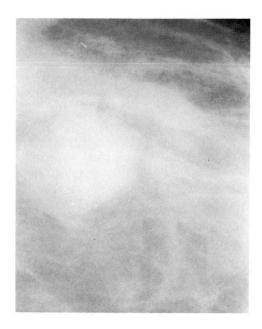

Figure 30–1. Mass of intraductal carcinoma, microinvasion only. This 34-year-old woman noted a lump that was firm to palpation. Mammography: 2 × 2.3 cm smooth-bordered, lobulated, almost encapsulated mass, which in this age group suggests medullary carcinoma. Pathology: a poorly defined 2 cm mass of firm fatty, fibrous, and gray tissue. Histologically the mass was filled with intraductal carcinoma with only focal invasive areas. After modified radical mastectomy a very small amount of residual intraductal carcinoma was seen at the superior margin of the mass. All 17 axillary lymph nodes were free of disease, and there was no evidence of disease five years later.

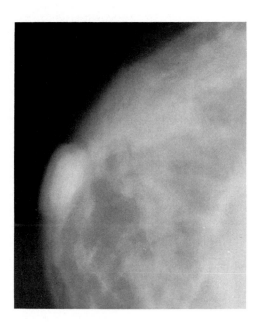

Figure 30–2. A benign mass clinically and radiographically is carcinoma in a young breast. A 29-year-old woman with a nodule in nodular breasts. A benign dominant mass clinically and by x-ray was biopsied. Pathology: one site of infiltrating duct carcinoma, 1.5 × 2 cm in size, part of the border smooth, part infiltrative. Modified radical mastectomy; all 34 axillary lymph nodes free of tumor. The patient was free of disease 12 years later.

Figure 30–3. Anaplastic duct carcinoma in the young. A 33-year-old woman with thickening UOQ of each breast, no masses. Mammography: 7 × 9 mm moderately invasive carcinoma UOQ left breast. Pathology: anaplastic duct carcinoma; all 22 nodes negative for tumor; modified radical mastectomy; no evidence of disease three and one-half years later.

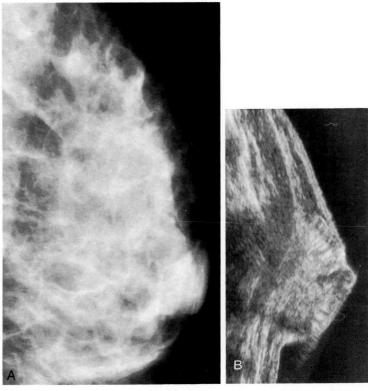

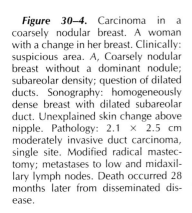

Figure 30–4. Carcinoma in a coarsely nodular breast. A woman with a change in her breast. Clinically: suspicious area. *A,* Coarsely nodular breast without a dominant nodule; subareolar density; question of dilated ducts. Sonography: homogeneously dense breast with dilated subareolar duct. Unexplained skin change above nipple. Pathology: 2.1 × 2.5 cm moderately invasive duct carcinoma, single site. Modified radical mastectomy; metastases to low and midaxillary lymph nodes. Death occurred 28 months later from disseminated disease.

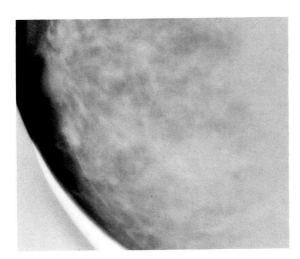

Figure 30–5. Infiltrating duct carcinoma Stage II, in huge breast. A 31-year-old woman with a self-discovered breast mass for at least seven months. Clinically: huge nodular breasts; palpable nodule was considered a cyst. Mammography: large breast, severe dense ductal hyperplasia, 3 × 3.5 cm moderately invasive carcinoma, operable. Pathology: infiltrating duct carcinoma, scirrhous type; also area of noninfiltrating papillary carcinoma. Radical mastectomy; 12 of 12 Level I, 0 of 7 Level II, and 1 of 4 Level III nodes with metastases. The patient is living and free of disease after six years.

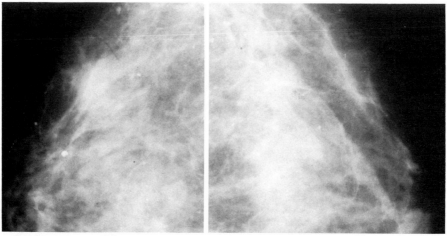

Figure 30–6. Carcinoma in the dense elderly breast. An 81-year-old woman with a question of a mass in nodular breasts. Xeroradiographic studies dated 3-26-78, 9-26-78, and 11-6-79 (13 months previously) did not demonstrate a lesion. Mammography: 1 × 1.5 cm moderately invasive carcinoma, upper quadrant of right breast, with prominence of Cooper's ligaments. Pathology: duct carcinoma; 0 of 19 nodes positive. Modified radical mastectomy; free of disease three years later.

was 22.0 per cent (see Table 30–5). At the same time, 36 of 139 total cancers in the young, or 26 per cent, remained to develop under observation, while overall that rate was 7.8 per cent. This probably does indicate a difficulty with younger breasts in the masking phenomenon of prevalent cancer to be-

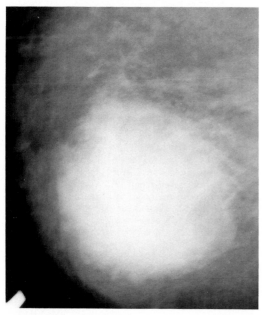

Figure 30–7. Demonstration of a carcinoma in a lactating breast. A 32-year-old white female who noted a lump in the breast for one year. She had been lactating for one year with normal clinical examinations during this period. Clinically: 5 × 6 × 4 cm discrete mass. Mammography: 6 × 7 cm circumscribed carcinoma in a lactating breast. Pathology: 5 × 6 cm adenocarcinoma of the breast.

come incident cancers. The increased rate of diagnosis or detection of cancers by clinical examination simply reflects the high selection of more positive cases for mammography. Fewer than one half of the young women with cancer had mammography preoperatively, whereas almost all older women with breast cancer had a preoperative mammogram.

We considered findings on physical examination sufficient for biopsy within six weeks following the initial examination as a positive diagnosis. A benign mass, usually diagnosed as a cyst or fibroadenoma, was considered equivocal but did not always undergo immediate investigation (Fig. 30–8).

Emory University Clinic physicians may have provided only initial diagnosis and treatment, with follow-up being available through referring physicians. Incomplete data did occur outside the Emory Breast Imaging Center despite the willingness of the referring physicians to cooperate. Many deceased patients' data may have been incomplete because their records were retired or became accessible only through the referring physician. At least diagnosis of malignancy and cause of death were recorded in each of our cases. Initial treatment and length of survival were missing in some cases.

MAMMOGRAPHIC EXAMINATION

Of 307 of the breast cancers in young women in the series, mammograms were

TABLE 30–3. Use of Mammography in 307 Breast Cancers in Young Women

| Mammography | Number | |
	Total Cancers	Primary Cancers
Preoperative	150	139
Postoperative	59	56
Never	98	91
Total	307	286

available on 209. In the primary operable cancers there were preoperative mammograms on 139 and postoperative mammograms on 56; on 91 patients, no mammograms were performed (Table 30–3).

The glandular pattern was available on all 209 women having pre- or postoperative mammography. The mammographic parenchymal pattern was fatty in 11 breasts, densely near-homogeneous in 18, and coarsely nodular or dense glandular in 43; 137 showed average density composed of lobules with fat or fibrofatty tissue. This is not an extreme variation from patterns of other age groups (Egan and McSweeney, 1979).

Most mammograms were of high quality, especially in breasts with fat or average-density tissue. Yet, in the dense breasts, usually nodular and more difficult to evaluate clinically, mammography was often lifesaving—by demonstration of calcifications, an asymmetric density, or changes in vascularity, skin, or breast architecture. Mammography for the primary cancers was considered technically inadequate in five cases: three with a benign mass diagnosed and with a positive physical examination, and two with the physical examination also negative. The demonstration of such a high percentage of the cancers or of a mass or disease process in these younger women attests to the efficiency and value of mammography (Table 30–4).

However, with total reliance on a positive mammographic cancer diagnosis, 19 per cent of the cancers present on the initial examination would not have been biopsied (Table 30–5). The more subtle, less definite mammographic findings should be carefully weighed with clinical findings to determine the most appropriate course of investigation and treatment planning. When the decision was based on clinical judgment, 15 per cent of younger women had breast biopsies, with 7.2 per cent of the biopsies revealing cancer (Egan, 1975). This is hardly greater than chance, as nearly 14 false positive biopsies preceded each carcinoma, and that carcinoma usually at an advanced stage. Thus, complete reliance on physical findings is also hazardous to these young women.

The recent practice of following mammography of dense breasts or dense areas of the breast tissue with breast sonography has proved a valuable supplemental imaging technique (Figs. 30–8 and 30–9) (Egan and Egan, 1984a,b). This should be an added incentive for using sonography in young women, in whom there is greater likelihood of encountering dense tissue by x-ray. Ultrasound employed in four young cancer patients was positive or suspicious (Fig. 30–4) in all four. In one case it was the only positive diagnostic modality.

DELAYS IN DIAGNOSIS

Of the 139 primary cancers having prebiopsy mammography, some were not demonstrated on mammography, all of these being in dense, fibroglandular breasts (Table 30–4). All but five had clinical findings leading to investigation. Clinical examination was difficult in these younger patients. In 15 cases clinical examination was equivocal upon first examination, then after delays of from one month to over two years a cancer was proved at the site of the original complaint. Diagno-

TABLE 30–4. Initial Examination on 286 Primary Cancers (No Record of Clinical Examination in 29)

| Clinical Examination | X Ray Examination | | | | |
	+	−	Benign Disease	Not Done	Total
+	67	0	8	32	107
−	22	5	0	8	35
Benign disease	0	0	37	35	72
No diagnosis*	0	0	0	43	43
Total	97	5	37	118	257

*Examined but no diagnosis recorded.

TABLE 30–5. Methods of Detection and Age at Detection of 2209 Primary Operable Breast Cancers During First Examination on Young Women*

Detection	Age in Years at Breast Cancer Detection						
	0–30	*31–34*	*35–39*	*40–54*	*≥55*	*Total*	*Per Cent*
Rad +, PE −†	5	9	22	179	270	485	22.0
Rad +, PE +	32	30	64	440	809	1375	62.2
Rad −, PE +	8	19	12	80	58	177	8.0
Rad −, PE −	12	24	8	82	46	172	7.8
Total	57	82	106	781	1183	2209	100.0

*On subsequent examination 172 cancers were detected (Rad −, PE − on first examination).
†Rad + = mammographically cancer; − = no cancer; PE + = clinical examination suspicious; − = not suspicious.

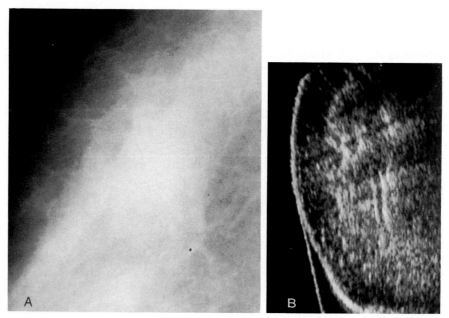

Figure 30–8. Moderately invasive carcinoma in a 34-year-old woman. Mass and pain in the right breast for several months; mass aspirated three weeks before; bilateral breast biopsies three and six years previously. *A,* Mammography: density UOQ, disturbed architecture, overlying prominent Cooper's ligaments, stretching of ducts leading to nipple. *B,* Sonography: rather well-demarcated solid mass, nonhomogeneous internal echoes, with borderline increased through-transmission; suggestive of medullary carcinoma. Pathology: duct carcinoma. Modified radical mastectomy; all 19 axillary lymph nodes free of disease. No evidence of disease 18 months later.

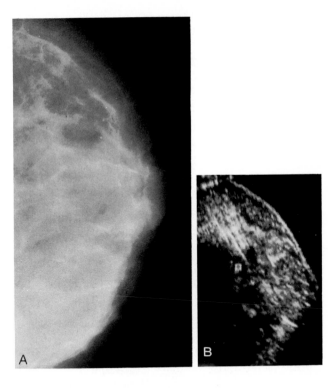

Figure 30–9. Sonography helpful in the young. A 33-year-old woman seen for a baseline mammogram, being followed for a right nipple discharge; a right breast mass had appeared two months previously. This was clinically a fibroadenoma. *A,* Mammography: dense nodular breasts only. *B,* Sonography: nonhomogeneous high-level echoes throughout. One cm hypoechoic solid mass that persisted; margins indistinct and irregular; suspicious. Pathology: 7 mm duct carcinoma with mild scirrhous element. Modified radical mastectomy; all 19 axillary lymph nodes free of tumor. The patient was alive without disease two years later.

sis was delayed in 55 per cent of the cancers, usually more than three months from the appearance of signs or symptoms (Table 30–6).

Delays in diagnosis and treatment were due equally to the patient and the physician, with worsened prognosis associated with longer delay. Five women were given antibiotics from one to five months; one patient was treated for an abscess, including antibiotics, for over one year; and three had inadequate incisional biopsies with delays of 7, 9, and 14 months; all were adequately reassured except for one who went shopping for a diagnosis. Greater length in delay paralleled the more advanced disease at the time of treatment (Table 30–6). There were more Stages 0 and I primary breast carcinomas

TABLE 30–6. Delay in Diagnosis and Treatment Caused by Patient (PT) or Physician (MD) in 103 Primary Cancer Patients Having Complete Historical Information

Delay in Months	Total No.	5-Years Survival Alive N.E.D.	5-Years Survival Alive N.E.D.	% Alive N.E.D.
0–1	MD 16*	6	6	75.0
	PT 31	17	9	83.8
1–6	MD 16†	5	5	62.5
	PT 18	9	3	66.7
7–12	MD 6‡	2	1	50.0
	PT 4	0	2	50.0
13–24	MD 6§	1	1	33.3
	PT 4	0	1	25.0
24	MD 1	0	0	0.0
	PT 1	0	0	0.0
Total	103	40	28	62.9

*One treated with antibiotics; others observed.
†Four treated with antibiotics.
‡One wrong area biopsied; one benign biopsy.
§One treated as abscess; one wrong area biopsied.
N.E.D. = no evidence of disease.

TABLE 30–7. 270 Primary Carcinomas, Mammography, Survival, and Stage*

Stage	Mammography	Total No.	No. Alive	% Survival
Stages 0, I	Preoperative	82	75	91
	Postoperative	20	15	75
	Never	17	11	65
Stage II	Preoperative	47	17	36
	Postoperative	15	9	60
	Never	12	5	41
Stage III	Preoperative	10	3	30
	Postoperative	4	1	25
	Never	7	1	14
Unknown	Postoperative	17	8	47
	Never	55	3	5

*Survival = Alive, N.E.D.

when mammography was used preoperatively, with better follow-up of the patients (Table 30–7). Although mammography was valuable in improvement of the survival rates in Stages 0 and I, it did not influence the survival with Stages II and III cancers.

One of the most significant differences in carcinoma in young women was that even with these advanced tumors physical examination, in many cases with an accompanying radiographic abnormality, was not positive enough to suggest biopsy in more than one half the lesions. Our general policy has been to have prebiopsy mammography on all suspected cancerous lesions. In this age group this was done in only 28 per cent of the cancers, suggesting an even lower level of suspicion of cancer. Physical examination in our patients over 60 years of age with breast cancer has been suggestive enough to biopsy

the carcinoma in two thirds of the cases (Table 35–9).

The impression is gained that the more conscientious the physician caring for these young patients, the more apt mammography is to be used. For instance, the postmastectomy women having mammography survived longer than those who never had the study. Procrastination on the part of the patients to do something about their health problems may be strongly influenced by their physicians' indirectly contributing to delay in treatment. The physicians' active roles in delays included ignoring women's breast complaints ("It's just a milk duct") and treating a lump with antibiotics.

The seemingly worse prognosis associated with physician delay may be partly due to the patient's delay. Her tendency to minimize her condition may signify an underestimation of the total length of compounded delay in these young breast cancer victims.

HISTOLOGY

Histologic types and aggressiveness of tumors were similar to all other age groups except that there was a tendency toward intraductal carcinoma and medullary carcinoma (Fig. 30–10; Table 30–8). This would be expected, since one of the more frequent means of detecting cancer in the young woman is the demonstration of calcifications on mammography. These are usually not associated with a mass and remain intraductal; medullary carcinoma of the breast is a disease of younger women. Owing to lack of

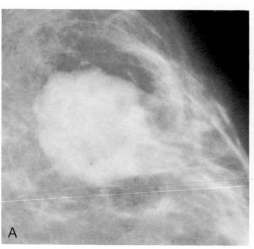

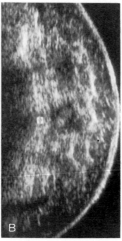

Figure 30–10. Medullary carcinoma with lymphoid stroma. A 33-year-old woman with a breast mass; aspiration attempted, no fluid. Clinically: a 4 × 5 cm breast mass enlarging over the past six months. Finally, mammography (A): 3 × 3.5 cm circumscribed carcinoma with stretching of superficial fascia, suggesting medullary type. B, Sonography: circumscribed hypoechoic area, variable internal echoes surrounded by high-level echoes, prominent Cooper's ligaments, skin flattening (without compression). Pathology: medullary carcinoma with lymphoid stroma. Modified radical mastectomy; all 21 axillary lymph nodes free of tumor. The patient was free of disease two years later.

ML

TABLE 30–8. Histologic Types of 279 Primary Operable Breast Carcinomas

Type	Number
Noninfiltrating duct	13
Intraductal papillary	2
Intraductal comedo	13
Noninfiltrating lobular	2
Infiltrating duct (3 with lobular)	75
Infiltrating comedo (3 with duct)	13
Scirrhous duct	22
Medullary (7 with duct)	36
Adenocarcinoma	8
Papillary	5
Lobular	2
Colloid (5 with duct)	10
Unknown	78
Total	279

TABLE 30–9. Size of 279 Primary Operable Breast Cancers (Largest Diameter)

Size (cm)	Number
0	7
≤1	18
1.1–2.0	49
2.1–5.0	76
5.1–10.0	5
Diffuse	4
Unknown	120
Total	279

secondary signs, this tumor may grow to 2 cm or larger before it is detectable, accounting for the increased size in many of the young patients' cancers (Table 30–9). Yet 45 per cent of the cancers were less than 2 cm in size, some not being associated with a mass; 14 per cent were less than 1 cm in size. This indicates that early, assuredly curable lesions can be found and treated. In the young these also include lobular carcinoma in situ (Fig. 30–11) and cystosarcoma phylloides (Fig. 30–12).

Despite the larger than usual size, approximately one half of the cancers were histolog-

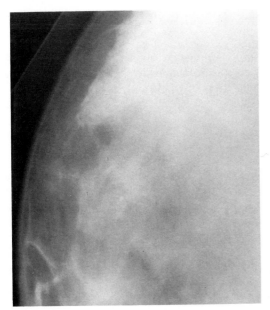

Figure 30–11. Solitary focus of lobular carcinoma in situ; patient's fears led to biopsy. A 34-year-old woman with breast complaints of pain and feeling lumps. Clinically: nodular fibrocystic disease. The xeroradiography report had indicated no disease. The patient insisted upon mammography, which showed an asymmetric vague 1.5 × 2 cm area in the UOQ and prominence of a Cooper's ligament, which was interpreted as a cyst vs a fibroadenoma (this study was done prior to sonography). A thickening could be localized to the area. The area was removed and contained a focus of lobular carcinoma in situ. Worries led to insistence on removal of the breast. Pathology (complete mastectomy): no further in situ lesions; none of 8 axillary lymph nodes recovered contained metastases. Six years later no evidence of disease.

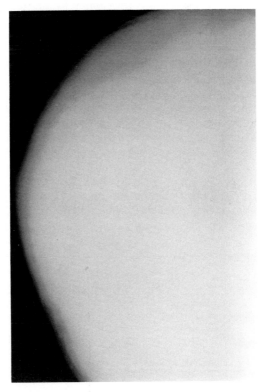

Figure 30–12. Cystosarcoma phylloides, malignant. A 31-year-old woman with an enlarging left breast. By history, three years previously an 8 × 15 giant fibroadenoma had been removed from this breast. Mammography: dense, homogeneous, slightly lobulated tissue filling the breast and compressing any normal tissue beyond recognition. Pathology: 10 cm hard central mass, malignant cystosarcoma phylloides. Modified radical mastectomy; all 31 axillary lymph nodes free of tumor. No evidence of disease 12 years later.

TABLE 30–10. Axillary Lymph Node Metastasis in 279 Primary Operable Breast Cancers

Positive Axillary Lymph Nodes	Number
0	93
≤ 3 low	25
Low + mid	16
Mid only	3
All levels	22
Unknown	120
Total	279

ically free of axillary lymph node metastasis (Table 30–10). On available information 42 per cent of the operable cancers had spread to all levels of axillary lymph nodes, indicating vast room for improvement in detection and treatment.

TREATMENT

In addition to the unusual size of these cancers and their rampant metastasis as primary operable cancers in our clinic, there is a diverse array of treatment modalities used in these young women (Table 30–11). The usual treatment for breast cancer is simply a modified radical mastectomy in most of the cancers in all ages that are free of nodal metastasis.

PROGNOSIS

Prognosis with breast cancer in young women is often distinctly better than in older

women; e.g., the detection of calcifications not associated with a mass (Fig. 30–13) or the more frequent presence of medullary carcinoma with lymphoid stroma (Fig. 30–14). However, detection of calcifications and treatment without delay of early phases of mass-producing carcinomas are highly dependent on mammography. This is unfortunate, as there remains the reluctance to use mammography in these "forgotten women."

The prognosis of most breast carcinomas in young women is similar to that of older women, being related to nodal status, histologic types, and multicentricity. The occasional small carcinoma, usually duct, may be widespread, just like a similar tumor in older women (Fig. 30–15). The disaster of allowing a breast carcinoma in a young woman to proceed to an inflammatory stage is no different than in other age groups (Fig. 30–16). The diffuse noninflammatory breast carcinoma is just as lethal in young women (Fig. 30–17).

Axiomatically, the prognosis of breast cancer, particularly in young women, is intimately related to the use of mammography to (1) detect breast cancer at a curable stage and (2) interrupt observation of the clinical course as it progresses to a lethal stage before institution of treatment (Figs. 30–18 and 30–19).

MISCELLANEOUS GROUPS

There were two simultaneous bilateral primary breast carcinomas before age 35 years

TABLE 30–11. Primary Surgical Procedures in 203 Primary Breast Cancers

Surgery	Number	Survival A	Survival M	Survival D	% Survival (N.E.D.)
Biopsy*	15	5	0	10	33
XRT	2	0	0	2	0
XRT, chemo	6	0	3	3	0
Simple mastectomy	3	2	0	1	66
XRT, chemo	1	0	1	0	0
Radical mastectomy	36	26	0	10	72
XRT	13	4	2	7	31
Chemo	3	1	2	0	33
XRT, chemo	9	1	4	4	11
Modified radical mastectomy	56	43	6	7	77
XRT	5	2	1	2	40
Chemo	3	0	3	0	0
XRT, chemo	9	1	4	4	11
Surgery unknown	24	0	0	24	0
Missing data	18	0	0	18	0
Total	203	85	26	92	42

*Includes seven inflammatory carcinomas.
XRT = radiotherapy; chemo-chemotherapy.

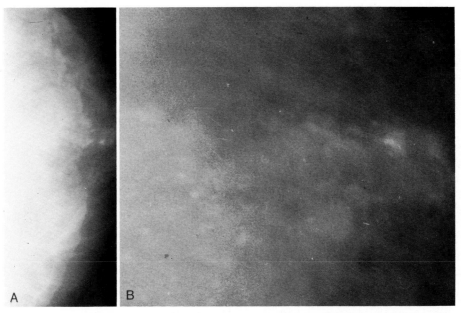

Figure 30–13. Calcification of carcinoma as the only sign in a young dense nodular breast. A 34-year-old woman with an intermittent bloody discharge for four months. *A*, Mammogram: central calcification without mass. *B*, Enlargement to show calcifications in the major subareolar ducts. Pathology: intraductal and minimally invasive comedocarcinoma (no Paget's disease). Modified radical mastectomy; all 19 axillary lymph nodes free of tumor. Similar lesion developed in contralateral breast five years later. The patient was alive without disease 14 years after first diagnosis.

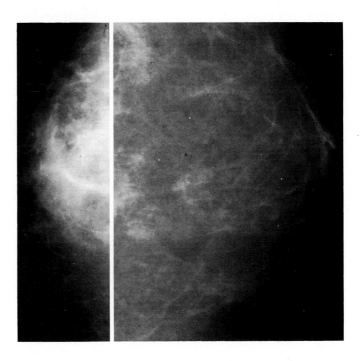

Figure 30–14. Medullary carcinoma with lymphoid stroma; clinically confusing. A 28-year-old woman, no family history of breast cancer, gravida 2, para 2, with lump in upper right breast for two months. Clinically: observed through menstrual cycle, then on antibiotics for six weeks with no improvement. Subsequent mammography: right breast smaller, denser than left with 1 cm poorly defined mass highly suspicious of malignant change rather than an inflammatory process. Pathology: medullary carcinoma with lymphoid stroma. Modified radical mastectomy; a total of 11 axillary lymph nodes, all free of tumor. The patient was alive without disease three years later.

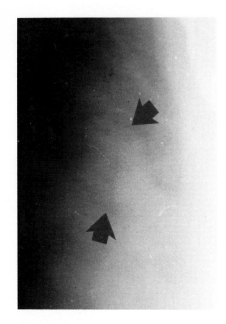

Figure 30–15. Carcinoma in the young. A 33-year-old woman, being followed clinically for fibrocystic disease, who developed a dominant nodule. Mammography: 0.5 cm poorly defined mass in a dense breast. Pathology: The carcinoma was 5 mm in size, consisting of both duct and intraductal carcinoma. Radical mastectomy; all nodes free of tumor. The patient died six years later with extensive disease.

Figure 30–16. Inflammatory carcinoma. At age 26 years and again at age 27 years this woman had removal of a clinically suspicious area UOQ of the right breast that proved to be fibrocystic disease. At age 29 years she noted a mass in the UOQ of the left breast. Since it seemed similar to the two previous ones on the right and there was no family history, she was reassured. She also called attention to asymmetry of the breasts, with the left being larger and firmer. After six months, in addition to this finding a pinkish hue was noted in the skin. A few days later initial mammography revealed diffuse disease on the left consistent with diffuse inoperable breast cancer. An open biopsy demonstrated duct, intraductal comedo, and intraductal papillary carcinoma. Tumor cells were demonstrated in the deep lymphatics, subcutaneous fat, and dermis compatible with the clinical diagnosis of inflammatory carcinoma. Despite radiotherapy and chemotherapy, she died 26 months later with widespread disease.

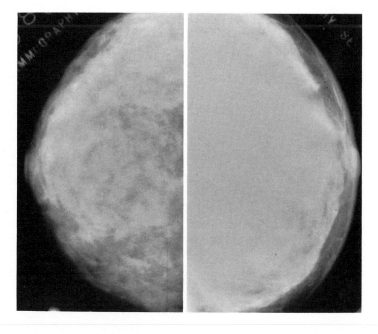

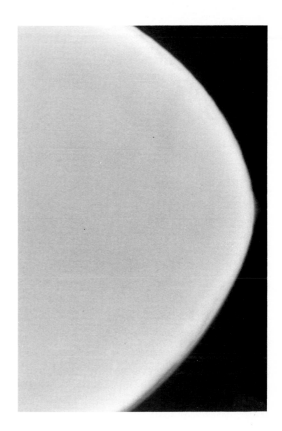

Figure 30–17. Diffuse breast carcinoma. This 31-year-old woman, gravida 3, para 2, with no family history of breast cancer, had a fibroadenoma removed from this breast four years before. She continued to complain of fullness and lumpiness of the breast but was told she had nodular fibrocystic disease with some induration about the biopsy scar. At some unknown point the breast became fuller, firmer, and heavier; three to four weeks previously she had complained of a mass. Clinically there was asymmetric enlargement and fullness but no dominant nodule. Mammography: homogeneously dense breast, diffuse skin thickening compatible with diffuse inoperable breast cancer. Pathology: incision biopsy; duct cell carcinoma involving the skin, subcutaneous tissues, breast, and permeation of lymphatics. Radiotherapy and chemotherapy. Death occurred 17 months later with disseminated disease.

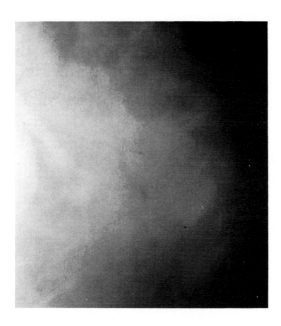

Figure 30–18. Adenocarcinoma in a young breast. A 33-year-old woman with a clinically benign lump being observed for five months. Mammography: a 1.2 × 1.8 cm lobulated mass centrally on the left that looks like a fibroadenoma but is a dominant mass in nodular breasts. Pathology: expansile adenocarcinoma with an intraductal papillary component. Modified radical mastectomy; one of ten low axillary nodes with micrometastasis, nine midnodes free of tumor. The patient was alive without disease four years later.

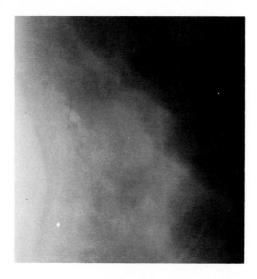

Figure 30–19. Circumscribed carcinoma in the young breast. A 32-year-old woman, gravida 1, para 1, with no family history of breast cancer; on birth control pills for seven and one-half years; breast lump less than a week. Clinically: being followed for advanced fibrocystic disease. Mammography: 1.3 × 1.4 cm circumscribed, homogeneous mass in the upper inner quadrant of the left breast in dense nodular fibroglandular tissues. Since it could not be seen on the craniocaudad view the surgeon had to rely on the patient's localization. Pathology: 2.2 cm expansile papillary carcinoma with marked lymphatic permeation. Modified radical mastectomy; all 14 recovered axillary lymph nodes free of tumor. Chest wall recurrence in operative site four months later, death occurred 13 months later from disseminated disease.

and nine nonsimultaneous bilateral primary carcinomas, with four second primaries occurring as long as 12 years after the first and after age 35 years (Table 30–12).

There were 11 cases of primary breast carcinoma related to pregnancy and lactation: pregnant, three; lactating, three; postpartum, five; with six alive, one with metastasis, and four dead. Of the living women, two had delays of one and two months prior to treatment, while the four dead women had delays of 5 to over 30 months (Table 30–13). The lesion with metastasis was an intraductal lesion (by light microscopy) requiring dye injection and specimen radiography.

Nineteen women had reconstruction of the breast following mastectomy for 21 breast carcinomas, with 14 alive and free of disease (67 per cent), four with metastasis, and one dead of disease (Table 30–14). One patient living and free of disease at 62 months had one positive low axillary lymph node. All the dead women had at least one positive node. (Reconstruction should not be done when axillary lymph nodes contain metastasis.)

Seven primary inflammatory carcinomas

TABLE 30–12. Ages at Appearance of 11 Bilateral Primary Cancers, Tumor Type(s), Treatment, and Survival After the Second Primary

Age at First Primary	Age at Second Primary	Interval (years)	Tumor Type	Treatment	Survival After Second Primary (months)
21			duct, ID	rad. mast.	
	23	2	ID, pap. ID	mod. rad.	N.E.D. 60
25			med.	rad. mast.	
	32	7	duct, med.	rad. mast.	N.E.D. 257
27			duct, ID	mod. rad.	
	38	11	duct, ID	mod. rad.	N.E.D. 60
28			duct, scirrhous	rad. mast.	
	30	2	duct	rad. mast.	metas. 118
31			"pleomorphic" CA	rad. mast.	
	43	12	ID	rad. mast.	N.E.D. 169
32			duct	rad. mast.	
	33	1	ID	mod. rad.	dead 131
32			duct	mod. rad.	
	32	0	duct	mod. rad.	metas. 26
32			duct	mod. rad.	
	35	3	duct, scirrhous	mod. rad.	metas. 52
33			duct, inflammatory	biopsy only	
	33	0	duct, inflammatory	biopsy only	dead 5
34			ID, duct, scirrhous	rad. mast., XRT	
	37	3	LCIS	simple mast.	dead 60
35			ID, duct, scirrhous	rad. mast.	
	36	1	ID, duct, scirrhous	biopsy, XRT	dead 30

TABLE 30–13. Eleven Breast Cancers Associated With Pregnancy

Status at Diagnosis	Age	Tumor Type	Stage	Treatment	Delay in Diagnosis	Survival (months)
Term-pregnant*	32	duct	I	rad. mast.	none	A—22
7 mo. pregnant	34	duct, mucoid	II	mod. rad.	MD 3 mo.—abscess	D—30
6 mo. pregnant	28	comedo	II	rad.	SD 3 wk.	D—14
lactating	28	duct	I	mod. rad.	SD 1 mo.	A—1
lactating	31	duct, adeno	I	mod. rad.	SD 1 mo.	A—47
lactating	35	duct, LCIS	II	simple mast. XRT, chemo	SD 6 wk.	A—95
5 wk. post partum	31	duct, scirrhous adeno	II	rad.	SD 7 days	D—36
2 mo. post partum	33	duct, med.	II	XRT	SD 3 mo., MD aspirated, no fluid	D—10
21 mo. post partum	33	ID	0	rad.	MD 6 mo., I & D, antibiotics	A—100
1 mo. post lactation	33	duct, med.	0	rad. mast.	SD mass, termination of pregnancy, MD 5 mo.	A—173
2 mo. postlactation	28	ID, duct	I	mod. rad.	MD 2.5 years biopsy FCD and negative mammograms	A—12

*Found upon admission for cesarean section.
MD = physician; SD = self-discovered; D = dead of disease; A = alive.

TABLE 30–14. Breast Reconstruction Following Mastectomy (19 patients, 21 Cancers)

Age	Type Tumor	Stage	Treatment	Survival (months)
21 and	ID, duct	II*	simple	alive 62
23	ID, ID pap.	0	radical	alive 60
26	ID, duct, scirrhous	I	mod. rad.	alive 41
27	duct	II	mod. rad.	metas. 57
28	ID, duct	I	mod. rad.	alive 29
28	duct	I	radical	alive 48
31	duct	I	mod. rad.	alive 24
31	med	I	mod. rad.	alive 36
31	duct	II	rad., XRT	dead 36
31	duct, mucoid	II	mod. rad., chemo	metas. 28
32	duct	I	mod. rad.	alive 52
32	lobular	I	radical	alive 105
32	ID, comedo	I	mod. rad.	alive 11
32 and	duct	II	mod. rad.	metas. 55
35	ID, duct, scirrhous	I	mod. rad.	(metas?)
33	ID	0	simple	alive 5
33	duct	I	radical	alive 125
33	med.	I	mod. rad.	alive 25
33	duct	II	mod. rad., chemo	metas. 86
34	duct	II	mod. rad.	alive 36
34	med.	I	mod. rad.	alive 153

*Miminal microinvasive.
Alive = free of disease.

TABLE 30–15. Data on Seven Primary Inflammatory (Inflam) Carcinomas and Five Primary Sarcomas

Cancer Type	Age (years)	Mammography	P.E.	Survival (months)	Complaint-Delay	Type Carcinoma
Inflam*	33	postop	+	D-5	SD-1 mo.	duct
Inflam	35	postop	+	D-11	no hist.	duct
Inflam	24	none	+	D-134	MD-6 mo.	duct 1 + node
Inflam	34	none	+	D-1	SD-6 mo.	duct
Inflam	32	none	+	D-13	no hist.	duct
Inflam	33	none	+	A-1	SD-0, delay	duct (pt. shopping for dx)
Inflam	25	+	+	D-36	SD 1–6 mo.	duct with lobular extension of duct
Hodgkin's	31	+	+	D-12	SD 5 wk. swelling	+ ax. nodes
Cystosarc	24	+	+	A-13	SD, trauma, asp. RX	− ax. nodes
	30	+	−	A-22	SD mass 5 mo.	− ax. nodes
	28	+	+	D-36	SD mass 6 wk.	− ax. nodes
Fibrosarcoma	30	postop	+	A-171	MD on routine	− ax. nodes

D = dead of disease; M = metastasis; A = alive.

and five sarcomas fared as shown in Table 30–15.

CASE HISTORY

Three years' delay; guarded prognosis.

One month after her twenty-sixth birthday Mrs. D.D. noticed a lump in the UOQ of her right breast. Her maternal grandmother had died of breast cancer. She was gravida 3, para 3, and had nursed her last child for four months, stopping three months prior to the discovery of the lump. Her physician checked her breasts and diagnosed fibrocystic disease. Two other physicians in the same clinic told her not to worry, but her complaints continued. Approximately 33 months after discovery of the mass her obstetrician ordered a mammogram. This was negative, and she was told again not to worry. This all transpired in Wisconsin.

She sought another opinion, and two months later a mammogram was obtained (Fig. 30–20).

Pathology: intraductal and infiltrating duct carcinoma; three of 15 Level I and two of ten Level II

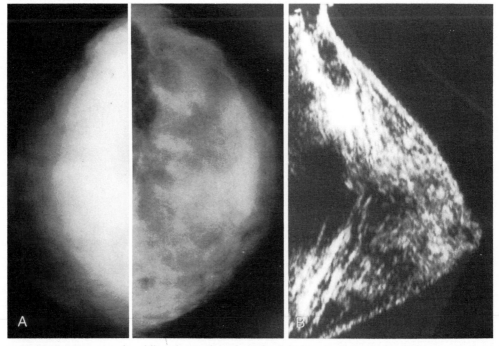

Figure 30–20. A, Mammography: diffuse density throughout the right breast with local skin thickening, very suspicious asymmetry; a glandular left breast. B, Sonography: disrupted architecture, hypoechoic upper and outer breast, bulging of the skin, axillary adenopathy, shadowing and irregular mass suggesting invasive carcinoma (note transverse scan).

nodes with metastases. Two years following the modified radical mastectomy the patient was still free of disease.

A guarded prognosis is related to the nearly three years' delay in detection and treatment. Sonography helped localize the carcinoma and added confidence to its investigation.

CASE HISTORY

Unrelated bloody nipple discharge led to detection of carcinoma.

This 33-year-old Montana horse (appaloosa) rancher noted a spontaneous bloody discharge from her right nipple. There was no history of breast cancer in the family. Her family physician recommended that she have the breast problem investigated at the Mayo Clinic.

During the medical work-up there she was told that she would have mammography, a new x-ray examination of the breast and that she was in good hands, since the radiologist there has studied with the developer of the new technique. As she insisted she wanted to be studied by the developer of mammography, she checked out of the Mayo Clinic and came to Emory University Clinic.

Mammography (Fig. 30–21) demonstrated a 3 × 4 cm area of uncountable punctate calcifications in the right breast. Localization, biopsy, and specimen radiography revealed intraductal and duct carcinoma. A right radical mastectomy (some surgeons were still doing an occasional one in 1966) specimen was submitted for whole-organ study. All 22 axillary lymph nodes were free of tumor. Five distinct sites of intraductal and duct (mostly comedo) carcinoma were demonstrated. The etiology of the bloody nipple discharge was a papilloma of a major duct and was unrelated to the carcinoma.

The patient returned annually for 14 years for checkup of the operative site, mammogram of the left breast, and a festive lunch with old friends from the breast imaging center.

CASE HISTORY

Nonsimultaneous bilateral primary carcinomas at ages 33 and 38 years.

A right mastectomy was performed for a Stage I duct carcinoma at age 33 years. This breast was reconstructed at age 34 years, and at that time a biopsy was performed on the left breast. At age 38 years routine mammography, following aspiration of a cyst, was done (Fig. 30–22).

Localization and biopsy: intraductal and comedocarcinoma. Modified radical mastectomy; all 16 axillary lymph nodes were free of tumor. The patient was free of disease three years following the second nonsimultaneous primary carcinoma.

Follow-up of the remaining breast after mastectomy for carcinoma is just as essential in young women as in older women.

OBSERVATIONS

At Emory University only 49 per cent of the women under age 35 years who were diagnosed and treated for breast cancer had prebiopsy mammography. This is in sharp contrast to almost 100 per cent mammography on the women over age 50 years diagnosed and treated for breast cancer at this institution. These data and the established practice of prebiopsy mammography on all

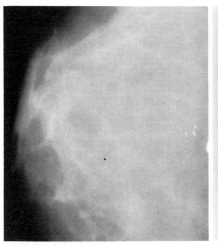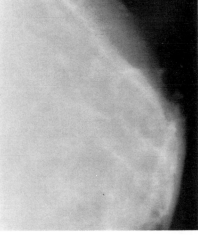

Figure 30–21. Calcification of carcinoma in the breast of a young woman. Mammography: deep and centrally in the right breast is a cluster of coarse mixed with fine calcification, poorly seen, suggesting carcinoma. Localization and specimen radiography required.

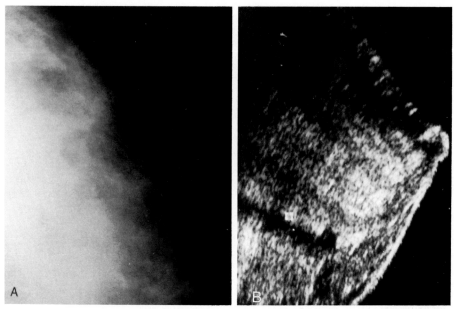

Figure 30–22. Nonsimultaneous second primary carcinoma. *A,* Mammography: faint stippled calcification of comedo-carcinoma in the UOQ of the left breast, 2 cm above and 2 cm deep to the nipple. *B,* Sonography: high-level echoes throughout the breast representing active glandular tissue. A persistent 0.5 cm irregular hypoechoic area with shadowing, invasive carcinoma.

women clinically suspected of breast cancer lead one to conclude that breast cancer in the young is clinically suspected in less than one-half the cases. Such an estimate would be a maximum, as physician delays in diagnosis are disregarded.

The use of preoperative mammography in 69 per cent of the Stages 0 and I cancers was associated with a 91 per cent survival rate compared with a 65 per cent survival at the same stages without its use. It was readily apparent that the cancers in these young women at treatment were comparatively advanced, with 44 per cent (or more realistically, 58 per cent, including the unknowns with a high death rate) being Stage II or III. This compared with less than one fourth in those stages in our total population of all age groups.

An additional 19 per cent of the young women had postmastectomy mammography during follow-up for cancer. Consistently the survival rate was less than with premastectomy mammography but also improved over those never having mammography in all stages of breast cancer. This, no doubt, relates to patient selection but also may suggest more meticulous and conscientious care of the patients.

In the recorded size of the cancers in young women, 16 per cent were 1 cm or less and 53 per cent were greater than 2 cm. Also, 74 per cent of the cases had three or fewer low axillary lymph nodes, and 14 per cent had metastasis to all levels of axillary lymph nodes. The 120 unknown cases most certainly would make these data more formidable. Four of 11 women with breast cancer associated with pregnancy died of their disease; they represented four of five women with Stage II duct carcinomas. The incidence of inflammatory carcinoma as 2.3 per cent of the total cancers in the young does not differ from the overall incidence of inflammatory carcinoma of 2.4 per cent at Emory University.

From our data there is no strong evidence that a cancer in the young woman, or one associated with pregnancy, is "faster growing," is "more lethal," or has an increased "incidence" when compared with all age groups. However, our previously reported data (Egan, 1981) have proved that breast cancers are more frequent in older women with less glandular breasts. Cancers in glandular breasts are more difficult to detect by mammography and are more likely to remain prevalent than cancers in fatty breasts. Incident cancers in dense breasts have a poorer prognosis than those detected in more fatty breasts with comparable histologic staging, suggesting more advanced disease in dense breasts at detection.

In a series of 864 breast cancers in 7123

women, 56 per cent of the cancers occurred in less dense breasts, making up 37 per cent of the population; 44 per cent of the cancers were in dense breasts in 63 per cent of the population. From 6 to 36 months' follow-up on noncancerous breasts the incidence of breast cancer was eight times greater in dense breasts, but after that time the incidence became similar. This indicates that many incident cancers are simply overlooked prevalent cancers masked by dense breasts (Carelile et al., 1985).

Despite an equal percentage of cancers classified histologically as Stage II, the mortality among those in dense breasts was almost double that of those in less dense breasts. Fisher et al. (1978) demonstrated overlooked axillary lymph node metastases in one quarter of cases studied by the routine technique used by most pathologists and confirmed the fallibility of this approach. The assumption must be that there is a significant difference in actual stage of the cancers at diagnosis that is escaping histologic recognition.

No difference in the size of the tumor affecting staging (large tumors with no metastatic axillary nodes), histologic type (more scirrhous cancers), or location (upper inner quadrant with greater chance of unknown internal mammary node metastasis) could be demonstrated to explain the difference in mortality in the dense breasts. Cancers are merely more advanced in dense breasts at the time of radiographic recognition, and our histologic staging is insensitive to some of the changes of this advanced disease.

From our experience we feel justified in concluding the following:

There is no reason to ignore breast cancer in the young. These cancers are no different and are just as lethal if allowed to advance to Stage III as in any age group. At present mammography is the most valuable weapon against cancer in all age groups, and its greatest value is in the younger patients: less than 1 per cent false positive rate to detect 90 per cent of the breast cancers, and usually at a much earlier stage. This detection rate can be improved if x-ray is complemented with ultrasound imaging. Early detection of breast cancer in the young woman can add many, many years of useful and normal life. Our data suggest that care must be exercised in selecting the patient for breast reconstruction or prosthesis. Also, cautious hesitancy is necessary in labeling breast cancer in young women as being unduly fast-growing or excessively lethal. There are more plausible reasons for our inferior results in these women.

REFERENCES

Alderson MR, Hamlin I, Staunton MD (1971): The relative significance of prognostic factors in the breast carcinoma. Br J Cancer 25:646.

Berkson J, et al (1957): Mortality and survival on surgically treated cancer of the breast: a statistical summary of some experience at the Mayo Clinic. Proc Staff Meet Mayo Clinic 32:145.

Bloom HJG (1964): The natural history of untreated breast cancer. Ann NY Acad Sci 114:747.

Carlile T, Kopecky KJ, Thompson DJ, et al (1985): Breast cancer prediction and the Wolfe classification of mammograms. JAMA 254:1050.

Cheek JH (1953): Survey of current opinions concerning carcinoma of the breast occurring during pregnancy. Arch Surg 66:664.

Egan RL (1975): Breast biopsy priority: Cancer versus benign pre-operative masses. Cancer 35:612.

Egan RL (1981): So-called mammographic risk patterns. In Schwartz GF, Marchant DJ (eds): Breast Diseases: Diagnosis and Treatment. New York, Elsevier North Holland.

Egan RL, Egan KL (1984a): Detection of breast carcinoma: comparison of automated water-path whole-breast sonography, mammography and physical examination. AJR 143:493.

Egan RL, Egan KL (1984b): Automated water-path full-breast sonography: Correlation with histology of 176 solid lesions. AJR 143:499.

Egan RL, McSweeney MB (1979): Mammographic parenchymal patterns and risk of breast cancer. Radiology 133:65.

Fisher ER, Swamidoss S, Lee CH, et al (1978): Detection and significance of occult axillary node metastases in patients with invasive breast cancer. Cancer 42:2025.

Haagensen CD (1986): Diseases of the Breast, 3rd ed. Philadelphia, WB Saunders, p. 406.

Haagensen CD, Stout AP (1943): Carcinoma of the breast; criteria of operability. Ann Surg 118:859, 1032.

Langlands AO, Kerr GR (1979): Prognosis in breast cancer; the effects of age and menstrual status. Clin Oncol 5:123.

Merller B, Ames F, Anderson GD (1978): Breast cancer in 3558 women: age as a significant determinant in the rate of dying and causes of death. Surgery 83:123.

Redding WH, Thomas JM, Powles TJ, Ford HT, Gazet JC (1979): Age and prognosis in breast cancer. Br Med J 2:1495.

Rissanen PM (1968): Carcinoma of the breast during pregnancy and lactation. Br J Cancer 22:663.

Sistrunk WE, MacCarty WC (1922): Life expectancy following radical amputation for carcinoma of the breast. A clinical and pathologic study of 218 cases. Ann. Surg 75:61.

White TT, White WC (1956): Breast cancer and pregnancy: report of 49 cases followed five years. Ann Surg 114:384.

31

Breast Carcinoma Developing Under Observation

BACKGROUND

The lack of recognition of a clinically apparent breast lesion requiring an immediate biopsy creates an uncomfortable position for the radiologist. But overlooking a breast cancer, with contribution to subsequent delay in institution of treatment, is the bane of the mammographer. These latter primary lesions having a previous no-cancer mammogram have been recognized for several decades and have been termed "carcinoma under observation." In the BCDDP they were labeled "interval cancers." These especially filed cases have provided long-term interest as an ego-buster and as a potential of developing radiographic signs of earlier breast cancer.

Discovery of more subtle signs of breast cancer has been disappointing, as on review in none of the cases were changes sufficient for a suspected lesion. In all cases, regardless of the length of time since the last normal mammogram, the studies were considered false negatives. This philosophy obviated the necessity for speculation of the time frame for the genesis of recognizable breast cancer. An arbitrary interval of greater than six months from the last normal mammogram was assigned to distinguish a lesion from a prevalent tumor.

INCIDENCE

In the Emory University data base of 2209 primary operable breast cancers were 250 primary breast carcinomas developing under observation during a 20-year interval (11.3 per cent of the total cancers). In the BCDDP approximately 50 per cent of the more than 4000 breast cancers developed within a maximum of four years following normal clinical and mammographic examinations. Lack of breast imaging experience during the first screening year of the 29 projects and the use primarily of the more cumbersome xeroradiography of the breast no doubt accounted for much of this difference in the BCDDP.

METHODS OF STUDY

With our use of xeroradiography of the breast in the BCDDP, study of an unexplained smudge, altered trabeculae, or an area of several flecks of calcification was supplemented with a coned-down view using nonscreen industrial film. This markedly reduced not only the number of "interval" cancers but also the necessity to recall patients in three to six months. At the same time, better and more aggressive care of the patients resulted, e.g., three biopsies of clustered calcifications not associated with a mass yielded one cancer, whereas with the sole use of xeroradiography, 12 biopsies for such

TABLE 31–1. Months to Confirmation of Cancers Under Observation

No. Months	% of Total
6–12	37.8
13–24	13.5
25–36	24.3
37–48	5.4
49–60	5.4
61–84	5.4
≥85	8.1

calcifications were needed to demonstrate one cancer (Martin and Wolfe, 1973).

Our subjects with cancers developing under observation had had 1 to 15 previous no-cancer mammograms. There was wide variation in time between the no-cancer and cancer mammograms—1 to 12 years (Table 31–1). The average number of visits for women who never developed cancer was 5.9, while the average number of visits for those developing cancer under observation was 3.3 (Table 31–1). These cases were filed separately as a constant reminder of the shortcomings of mammography and as a hope that they would provide clues to the x-ray diagnosis of earlier cancer. Since the mammograms were the ultimate in state of the art and had been carefully, but objectively, interpreted, they provided no new signs.

The signs of cancer under observation were usually similar to those of any relatively early cancer but more easily recognized on comparative studies: a new mass; a new density, localized or diffuse; a new area of altered architecture; progressive retractive phenomenon; or a new cluster of calcification or increase in number to five or more of an old grouping of calcifications. Comparative studies usually provided easier differential diagnoses, but not always.

New Mass

Just as in all radiology, comparative mammograms that provide interval changes are the source of our most subtle diagnoses. Once the woman reaches breast cancer age, any mammographic change, except clear-cut physiologic aging, is important. A new nodule, whether cystic or solid, even in a nodular breast must be explained.

The appearance of a new breast mass on the mammogram is the most common indication of developing cancer. Since few tiny, or beginning, cancers are overlooked in fatty breasts, the most frequent site of the nodule is on the background of active or nodular breast tissue (Fig. 31–1). In this case, advanced ductal hyperplasia was present throughout both breasts without an area of concern that could be pinpointed. Obviously then, the carcinoma developed in an area of

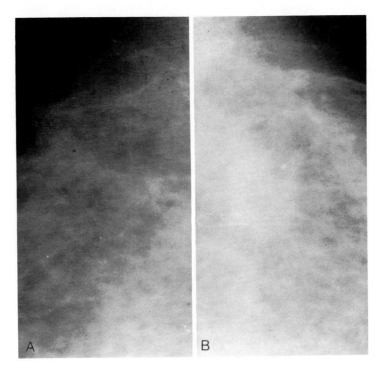

Figure 31–1. Carcinoma developed in ductal hyperplasia during routine follow-up examination. A 55-year-old woman with known ductal hyperplasia by mammography for six years, last mammogram 27 months previously. Mammography: the coalescence of the process to form a 1.5 × 1.5 cm mass of carcinoma UOQ of the left breast (*B*) occurred within that period. The previous mammogram (*A*, printing reversed for comparison) showed nothing suspicious in the area. Pathology: duct carcinoma, foci of intraductal carcinoma; modified radical mastectomy. All 18 axillary lymph nodes free of tumor. No disease five years later.

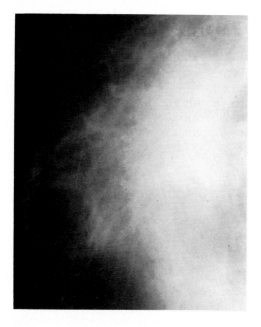

Figure 31–2. Duct carcinoma appeared after a period of seven years. A 41-year-old woman with a breast mass, clinically cancer. Mammography: A 1.8 × 2.2 cm highly invasive carcinoma, with increased vascularity, just below the level of the nipple, had occurred since the most recent study seven years ago. Pathology: poorly differentiated duct carcinoma associated with fibrocystic disease. Modified radical mastectomy, 2 of 10 Level I and 2 of 11 Level II nodes positive for metastases. The patient was free of disease three years later.

ductal hyperplasia. If the carcinoma was present on the last prior mammogram 27 months before diagnosis, it was masked by this proliferative process. At times the carci-

noma may become quite large before it is diagnosed (Fig. 31–2), yet have a favorable prognosis. The woman in Figure 31–3 had a similar interval between mammograms and

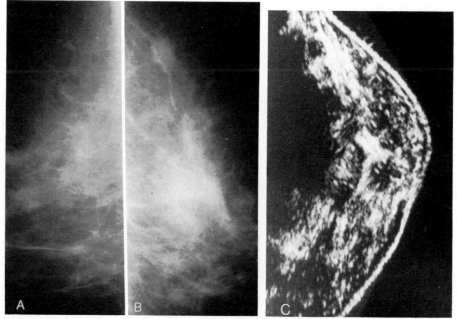

Figure 31–3. Appearance of advanced carcinoma and a positive intramammary lymph node in seven years. A 62-year-old woman with soreness of the left nipple and an intermittent bloody discharge. Clinically Paget's disease was suspected. Two left circumareolar biopsies, the last three years ago; fibrocystic disease. *A,* Last mammogram seven years ago. *B,* Centrally, a poorly defined new density, 1.6 × 2 cm, with stretching of the major ducts into prominence and nipple retraction. There is a 6 × 9 mm intramammary lymph node superiorly, also as a new density. *C,* Sonography: irregular hypoechoic area with nonhomogeneous internal echoes, surrounding architectural distortion, and flattening of the skin. Pathology: intraductal and invasive comedocarcinoma in three quadrants; positive intramammary lymph node; Paget's disease of the nipple; severe papillomatosis. Modified radical mastectomy; 7 of 21 axillary nodes with metastases. Nine months following seven months of chemotherapy, lung metastasis. Four months later liver and bone metastases appeared.

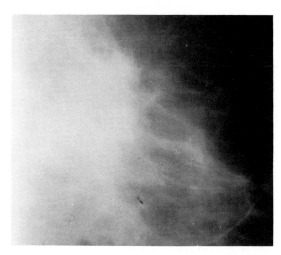

Figure 31–4. Carcinoma developing under observation. A 48-year-old woman with a sore area in the breast, clinically suspicious. A mammogram and clinical examination five years previously were within normal limits. Mammography: 1.9 × 2.9 cm moderately invasive carcinoma, an entirely new development. Pathology: duct carcinoma with focal fibrosis, foci of solid and comedocarcinoma at a distance from the reference lesion. Modified radical mastectomy; all 49 axillary lymph nodes (Levels I and II) free of disease. The patient was alive and well four years later.

tumor size but a grave prognosis. Women develop multiple types and sites of carcinoma under observation (Fig. 31–4).

New Density

The new density may be masslike (Fig. 31–5), a faint density (Fig. 31–6), or a new vague nodule in a nodular breast (Figs. 31–7 and 31–8).

Distorted Architecture

Sometimes the main interval change is an area of distorted architecture that may or may not be associated with some increase in density of the area. At any rate, the change is the important clue (Fig. 31–9).

Progression of a Change

Retractive Phenomenon

In addition to retraction of the breast parenchyma to produce altered architecture, there may be retraction of the ducts, skin, nipple, fascia, and nipple and/or areola. In Figure 31–10 a degree of straightening of the ducts with fixation of the nipple was present on the previous mammogram, but it was bilaterally symmetric and no investigation of either subareolar area was carried out. Three years later there was marked obvious progression only on the left caused by a garden-variety carcinoma.

Calcifications

Although our policy is that five or more clustered calcific flecks not associated with a mass are required to recommend biopsy, calcifications are still considered an increased

Figure 31–5. Duct carcinoma in ductal hyperplasia. A 67-year-old woman seen for a routine checkup; most recent previous mammogram six years before was without abnormality. *A,* Mammography: marked ductal hyperplasia and subareolar fibrosis; 1.1 × 1.5 cm spiculated density with fine strands extending for several centimeters, classic mass of carcinoma. *B,* Sonography: irregular hypoechoic area, skin flattening, shadowing. Note pinpoint rounded anechoic areas indicating ductal hyperplasia. Pathology: duct carcinoma with desmoplasia (scirrhous element). Modified radical mastectomy; no metastasis in 19 axillary lymph nodes. The patient was free of disease two years later.

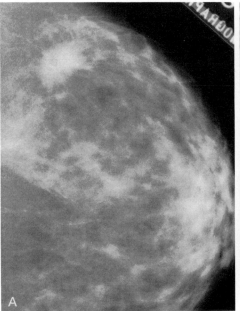

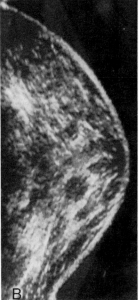

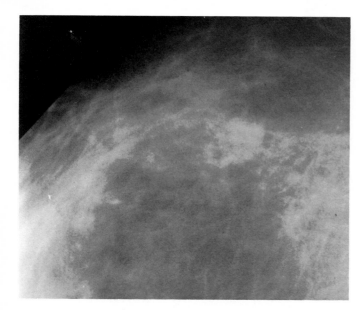

Figure 31–6. Coalescence of ductal hyperplasia into a mass of carcinoma. A 56-year-old woman seen for checkup of ductal epithelial hyperplasia found on mammography two years before. This area appeared on the mammogram in the interval. Localization and biopsy resulted in a diagnosis of intraductal carcinoma; all 16 axillary lymph nodes were free of tumor following modified radical mastectomy. The opposite breast is being followed four years later with no evidence of disease.

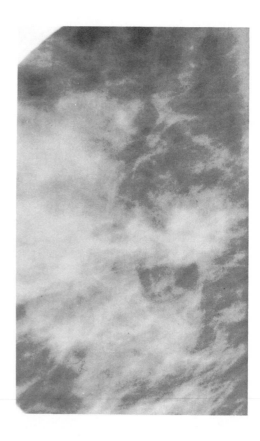

Figure 31–7. Carcinoma developed in breast being followed for cysts. A 51-year-old woman had one maternal aunt with breast cancer. At the time of first mammogram at age 48 years she had three previous breast biopsies (two on left and one on right) for fibrocystic disease. At age 50 years she had a second mammogram for a left cyst that was aspirated. A routine checkup mammogram the following year for nodular breasts showed the appearance of this mass in the UIQ of the right breast. Pathology (needle aspiration and biopsy): duct carcinoma with fibrosis. Modified radical mastectomy; all 19 axillary lymph nodes were free of tumor. The patient was alive and well three years later.

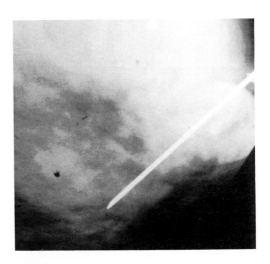

Figure 31–8. New density of carcinoma under observation. A 53-year-old woman for checkup; clinically nodular breasts. Mammography (compared with the most recent study of nine years before): a 6 × 7 mm new density in area of needle tip (black dot). Pathology: tubular carcinoma, well differentiated. Modified radical mastectomy; all 15 axillary lymph nodes free of tumor. The patient was alive and well two years later.

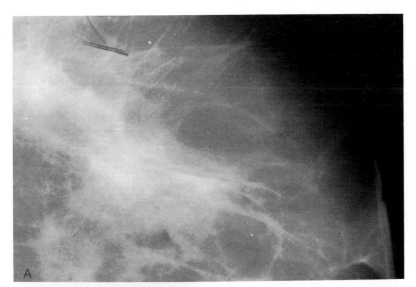

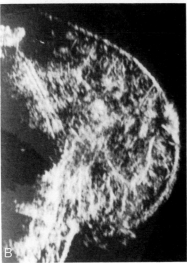

Figure 31–9. Lobular carcinoma developed under observation. A 57-year-old woman with slowly inverting nipple on the right; no mass clinically. *A,* Mammography: two areas of contracted breast tissue, each about 8 mm in size, producing retraction toward the masses, straightening of the trabeculae and Cooper's ligaments, shortening of the major subareolar ducts with retraction of the nipple, distortion of the superficial layer of superficial fascia, and increased vascularity. These two carcinomas had appeared since the most recent study four years previously. *B,* Sonography: homogeneous low-level disorganized echoes usually associated with fatty breasts; distortion of the trabeculae; hypoechoic area. Pathology: infiltrating lobular carcinoma. Modified radical mastectomy; all 18 axillary lymph nodes free of disease. The patient was alive and well three years later.

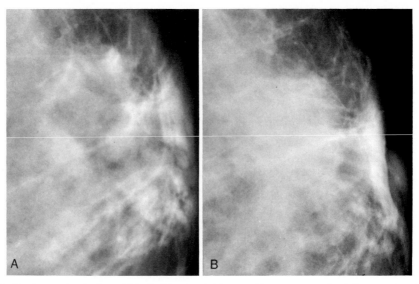

Figure 31–10. Carcinoma developing within three years. A 51-year-old woman seen for follow-up; two biopsies on left and five biopsies on right breast during the past 23 years. Clinically: lump UOQ of the right breast. Mammography: *A,* Nodular breasts; dilatation of major subareolar ducts; symmetric. At age 54 years there was a palpable mass near the nipple. *B,* A 2.5 × 3 cm moderately invasive carcinoma subareolar in location. Pathology: intraductal and duct (NOS) carcinoma. Modified radical mastectomy; all 43 lymph nodes free of tumor. The patient was alive and well five years later.

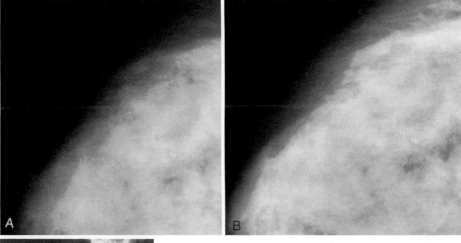

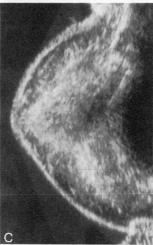

Figure 31–11. Intraductal carcinoma that developed under observation. A 73-year-old woman being followed for dense ductal hyperplasia. The last preceding mammogram (*A*) showed only a few scattered coarse calcifications; the larger one was a conglomerate of several small ones. A follow-up mammogram 16 months later (*B*) revealed the appearance of very faint tiny calcifications throughout much of the upper quadrant of the breast. *C,* Sonography: normal fibroglandular breasts with active tissue (typical sonographic pattern of ductal hyperplasia). Localization and biopsy: intraductal carcinoma. Modified radical mastectomy; widespread intraductal carcinoma; no demonstrable infiltration; all of 13 axillary lymph nodes free of tumor. The patient was free of tumor three years later.

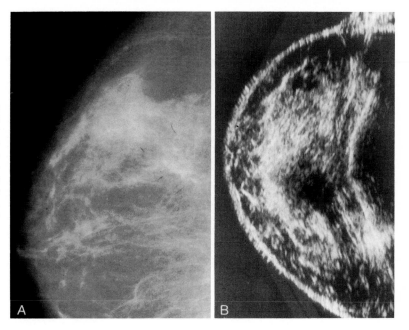

Figure 31–12. Fat necrosis as a new density. A 55-year-old woman seen for postmastectomy (four years) checkup. *A*, Mammography: 1.5 × 1.5 cm poorly circumscribed new density since last annual mammogram. *B*, Sonography: irregular, hypoechoic lesion; carcinoma. Pathology: fat necrosis. No history of trauma could be elicited.

risk, and follow-up is desired. With increase in the number of calcifications, carcinoma is suspected (Fig. 31–11). Intraductal carcinoma may well have been present at the time of the prior study.

Differential Diagnosis

Lesions in the breast that are confused with cancer may also be recognized as interval changes on the mammograms. Extreme care must be given these lesions, as most of them are rarities compared with the more frequent cancer (Fig. 31–12).

Miscellaneous Lesions

Nonsimultaneous second breast primary carcinomas frequently develop under observation. The woman's concern about breast cancer is heightened, she has frequent clinical checkups, and there is an increased risk (Fig. 31–13).

The carcinoma may be occult (Fig. 31–14).

Sarcomas also develop under observation (Fig. 31–15).

Additional carcinomas may develop while observing some already present (Fig. 31–16).

A carcinoma may develop and then be observed for a period (Fig. 31–17).

Figure 31–13. Second nonsimultaneous primary breast carcinoma. A 77-year-old woman being followed for an operable breast carcinoma four years before. In the clinically normal remaining breast the mammogram showed a 3 × 6 mm new density that proved to be a Stage I duct carcinoma. A cardiac death occurred eight months following the modified radical mastectomy for this carcinoma.

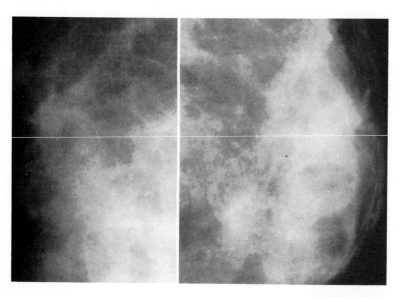

Figure 31–14. Truly occult carcinoma producing only asymmetry. A 47-year-old woman with a lump in the tail of the left breast for two weeks; previous biopsy UOQ this breast one year ago for benign disease. Clinically the lump was a fibroadenoma. Mammograms: asymmetric area above left nipple; increased vascularity with a 1 cm low axillary lymph node (not shown). Biopsy of the tail of breast lump proved duct carcinoma in an intramammary lymph node. Sectioning of the modified radical mastectomy specimen pinpointed a 0.5 cm primary intraductal and ductal carcinoma corresponding to the radiographic abnormality. A mammogram one year before our study was reported as normal, which was our initial impression before recognition of the subtle changes.

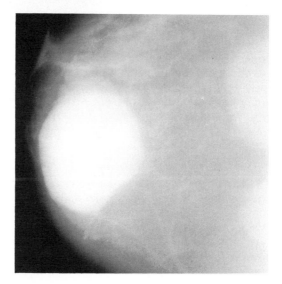

Figure 31–15. Lymphoma of the breast under observation. A 57-year-old woman being followed for lymphoma who developed a mass in the right breast. Clinically: a 3 × 4 cm firm movable breast mass in the subareolar area. Mammography: three homogeneous circumscribed nodules measuring 2.9 × 3.1, 1.6, and 2.7 cm (not present on the most recent mammogram two and one-half years before); lymphoma suspected on the basis of the appearance and history. Pathology (needle aspiration of the palpable mass): lymphoma. Decreased to approximately 1½ inches in size with a subsequent remission of the lymphoma.

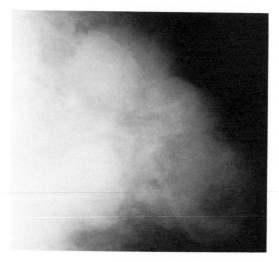

Figure 31–16. Intracystic papillary carcinoma developing under observation. A 78-year-old woman who had a right mastectomy for 1.5 cm duct carcinoma, Stage I; left breast clinically normal. Follow-up mammogram one year later; normal left breast. One year later she returned with a history of a mass for six months. Mammography: 1.8 and 2 cm masses, radiographically intracystic papillary carcinomas. Thirty months later, mammography (above) showed three lesions 1.5, 2.0, and 2.8 cm in size. Pathology: intracystic papillary carcinomas. Left radical mastectomy; all 17 axillary lymph nodes free of tumor. The patient was last seen ten years following second mastectomy, alive and free of disease.

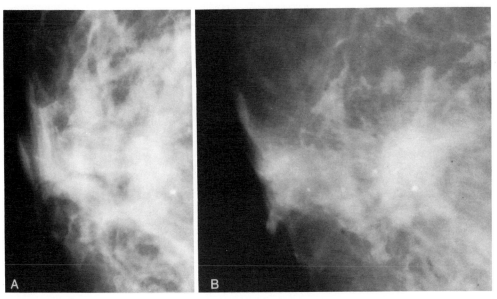

Figure 31–17. Slowly surfacing carcinoma. A 73-year-old woman with a breast lump for two weeks. Clinically: 1 × 1.5 cm mass UIQ requiring biopsy. Mammography: nodular breasts with a 6 mm poorly defined subareolar carcinoma (*A*). Four months later, nonpalpable carcinoma still present; patient elected not to return owing to family sickness. Three years later, still clinically normal breasts; mammographic cancer 1 cm in size. Two years later, inverted nipple, clinically subareolar fibrosis. Mammography: 1 × 1.5 cm spiculated carcinoma with secondary changes (*B*). Pathology: 2 cm scirrhous carcinoma. Modified radical mastectomy; 5 (Levels I and II) of 24 axillary lymph nodes with metastases. Two years later, distant metastases.

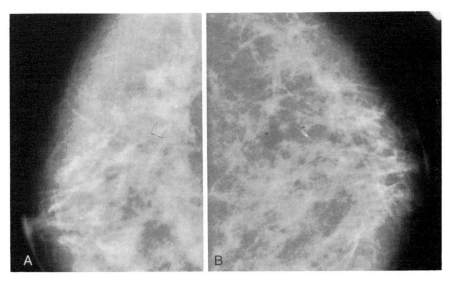

Figure 31–18. *A* and *B*, Mammograms show advanced ductal hyperplasia with asymmetric density and calcifications in the upper outer quadrant of the right breast.

CASE HISTORY

This 60-year-old woman had five normal yearly mammograms as part of our BCDDP. One maternal aunt and both grandmothers had breast cancer. From age 46 to 53 years she took birth control pills, had a hysterectomy at age 53 years, and then intermittently took Premarin. Her physician did annual follow-up examinations and recommended a mammogram at age 60 years. Several months elapsed before this was done.

We noted a new and asymmetric density with fine calcifications in the UOQ of the right breast against the background of severe ductal hyperplasia (Fig. 31–18). (Our final BCDDP recommendation of yearly mammograms for this ductal hyperplasia in addition to her usual clinical examination had been ignored.)

A note from her surgeon: "No lesions were palpable preoperatively, even at surgery I could not feel a nodule, so a quadrant resection was done." This showed intraductal and duct carcinoma, so small that there was insufficient tissue for estrogen receptors. The patient, her husband, and the family doctor discussed therapeutic options for primary breast cancer, and a modified radical mastectomy was decided upon.

After surgery the remaining breast was found free of tumor as well as 31 axillary lymph nodes. Two years later her surgeon "was still expecting a good result."

REFERENCE

Martin JE, Wolfe JN (1973): Panel discussion. 12th Annual Mammography Seminar, San Diego, March 5–9.

32

The Breast Following Surgery and Radiotherapy

BACKGROUND

The extent of tissue manipulation, amount of tissue removal, and degree of restorative surgical procedures vary widely from simple needle aspiration of a cyst to an extended radical mastectomy. The breast studied during or after radiotherapy invariably has had some surgical procedure even if only a diagnostic needle biopsy. The changes in the breast immediately following surgery or radiotherapy are greatly influenced by the healing process and by any interference with that process, such as infection.

The degree of altered breast architecture, fibrosis, scarring, retraction, and pseudomass formation dictates the confidence in interpretation of the mammograms following surgery and radiotherapy. The element of time is most helpful, since little may be gained from immediate surgical re-exploration of the breast unless there has been an obvious omission, such as not removing the suspicious mass or cluster of calcification. In practice many postoperative changes may produce highly suspicious changes of malignancy, such as an abscess, on the mammogram or diffuse hemorrhage on sonography.

Some of the more usual diagnostic, treatment, and prophylactic procedures that provide breast tissue for study are listed. Many may be combined, as they produce similar changes.

SURGICAL PROCEDURES

Diagnostic

Needle Aspiration

Percutaneous needle aspiration of a cyst or cellular aspiration for diagnostic purposes may leave only minimal changes. Our policy has been to have annual mammograms on women who have had a cyst aspirated or repeated cyst aspirations. Depending on patient scheduling, the mammogram may be obtained prior to or after cyst aspiration. If mammography follows needling of the cyst, the radiologist must be aware of the order of events, as the procedure often produces increased vascularity that can be misleading (Fig. 32–1).

With more vigorous and frequent needling of the breast, as sometimes occurs with a thick-walled cyst, the breast may be ecchymotic and show hemorrhage and skin thickening on the mammograms. The area of hemorrhage is characteristically homogeneously dense asymmetrically, owing to the diffuse deposition of hemosiderin (Fig. 32–

581

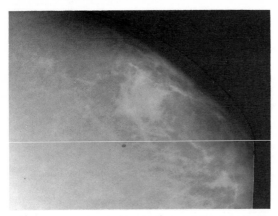

Figure 32–1. Local skin thickening following needle aspiration of a cyst. A 45-year-old woman who has had repeated cyst aspiration, one a few hours prior to study. Mammograms: small area of skin thickening in the area of needling that was no longer present on follow-up mammograms one year later. The veins in this breast were increased in size.

2). The entire breast may be involved and the thin penciled radiolucent line beneath the skin obscured. A quadrant or a half of the breast only may be opacified; then the borders of the lesions are indistinct and extend into the subcutaneous tissue (Fig. 32–

3). Unless complicated by infection, the breast returns to normal appearance in two to three weeks. The skin changes are usually less marked than those following incision of the breast.

Incision and Excision Biopsy

Breasts biopsied because of benign lesions have been followed with mammography during their postoperative course. Immediately following the biopsy, there is a diffuse density, noncircumscribed, not unlike a moderately infiltrative carcinoma; no calcification is present (Fig. 32–4). There is rather rapid resorption of the density and, if no infection supervenes, the breast reverts to normal appearance in 10 to 14 days. The uncomplicated biopsy rarely leaves significant intramammary scarring but may produce recognizable changes in the breast architecture. The usual biopsy rarely leaves recognizable changes in the skin unless the area is in a tangential view on the mammogram. The healed skin scar may be slightly raised clinically, but there is usually no radiographic evidence of skin thickening.

Where numerous large biopsies or quad-

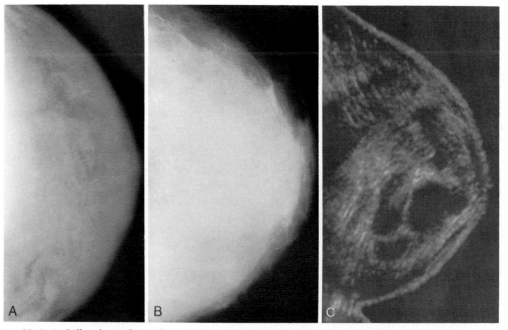

Figure 32–2. A, Diffuse breast hemorrhage. A 35-year-old woman with a mass in the breast following biopsy ten days previously; biopsy showed fibrocystic disease. Clinically: large mass in the breast. Mammography: diffuse density in breast without definable parenchyma; suspected trauma, hemorrhage, and hemosiderin deposition. Pathology: fibrocystic disease and marked hemosiderin deposition representing hemorrhage. B, Diffuse density of the breast following five needle aspiration attempts. Clinically: breast nodules, ecchymosis. Mammography: dense, almost homogeneous, breast; suspected interstitial hemorrhage (by history). C, Sonography: multiloculated cysts; diffuse high-level homogeneous echoes suggesting diffuse hemorrhage. Cyst aspiration and disappearance of the nodules.

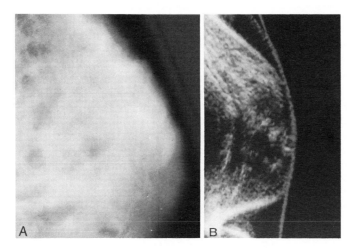

Figure 32–3. Hematoma following aspiration attempt. A 35-year-old woman who had a recent cyst aspiration attempt. Clinically: lump UOQ, ecchymosis; suggestive of hematoma. *A,* Mammography: asymmetric density centrally, dense fibroglandular tissue. *B,* Sonography: large hypoechoic central area. Pathology: fibrocystic disease with hematoma.

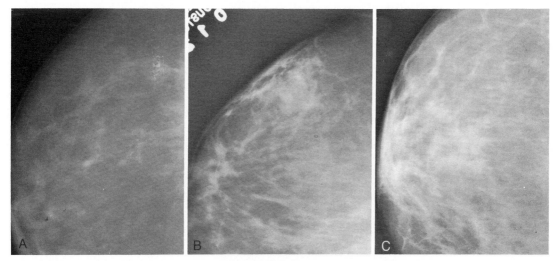

Figure 32–4. A, Breast following biopsy for a benign lesion. A 37-year-old white female with a lump in the breast for two months. Clinically: 2 cm mass above areola. Mammography (prebiopsy study): ductal dilatation, minimal fibrocystic disease, no dominant mass. Pathology: fibrocystic disease. *B,* Mammography (one week following biopsy): diffuse 2 cm density with thickening of the overlying skin. *C,* Mammography (two weeks after biopsy): no residual abnormality in the breast or skin in the area of biopsy.

rant removal have occurred, there may be seen a smooth depression in the overlying skin, without skin thickening (Fig. 32–5). In one case, six months following breast biopsy, a 1.5 cm linear deposition of tiny flecks of calcification was seen immediately beneath the skin. The absence of significant mammographic change in the skin or breast following biopsy makes radiographic study of the scarred breast indispensable; carcinoma in such a breast must be quite advanced to be appreciated clinically.

If infection complicates the biopsy procedure, extensive changes may be apparent on the mammograms for varying periods of time. The infection may be reflected as an ill-defined area of mastitis (Fig. 32–6). Localized areas of inflammatory disease may follow biopsy, with the more circumscribed changes of an abscess. A distinct finding in four cases in which the infection was localized following biopsy and the overlying skin was thickened was the laminated appearance of the skin (Fig. 32–7). This is an important differential point. If no history of the previous procedure is available, the infected biopsy site and the overlying thickened skin will suggest carcinoma; yet laminated skin thickening has not been encountered with carcinoma.

Treatment

Benign Conditions

Excision Biopsy. Excision of a benign breast mass produces changes similar to those of an excision biopsy. A lesion removed from the skin of the breast is no different from other skin lesions.

However, surgery in the subareolar area may produce marked changes. Excision of a single duct for a bleeding papilloma and the more extensive apple-core procedure for removal of the entire major duct system are examples. Unlike the filling-in of a large void in the breast tissues following a near-complete quadrant biopsy, there is little tissue to fill in the subareolar area; also, there is an increased element of infection with severance of the major ducts. The mammographic changes may resemble subareolar fibrosis, a chronic breast abscess, or even a malignant process (Fig. 32–8).

Malignant Conditions

The following are the most frequent therapeutic surgical procedures for breast cancer: standard (or Halsted) radical mastectomy; modified radical mastectomy; quadrantectomy with axillary dissection; quadrantectomy; partial mastectomy; segmental mastectomy; tylectomy; lumpectomy.

Many surgical procedures for breast cancer include the complete removal of all breast tissues as well as the axillary contents so that soft tissue x-ray examination of the residual chest wall on the side of the mastectomy is noncontributory. After some procedures, such as lumpectomy or UOQ lumpectomy with contiguous axillary dissection, mam-

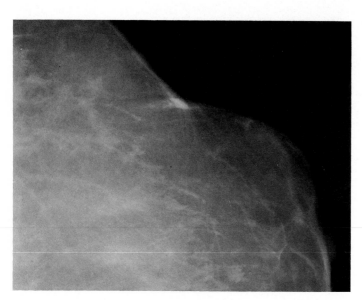

Figure 32–5. Deformity of the breast following biopsy. A 62-year-old white female who had a cyst removed from the breast five months previously. Clinically: deformity of the breast, questionable skin retraction. Mammography: deformity of the breast and retraction of the skin without thickening following removal of a large quantity of breast tissue. Followed for two years, no change.

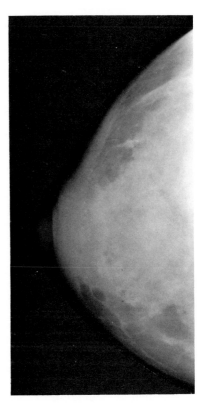

Figure 32–6. Breast abscess following breast biopsy. A 39-year-old white female who, two weeks previously and elsewhere, had an adenocarcinoma that appeared to be clinically benign removed from the breast. Clinically: diffuse induration in the breast. Mammography: diffuse central density, several tiny air pockets, breast abscess following biopsy. Preoperative irradiation followed by radical mastectomy was the treatment of choice for the patient who had previous biopsy that revealed carcinoma.

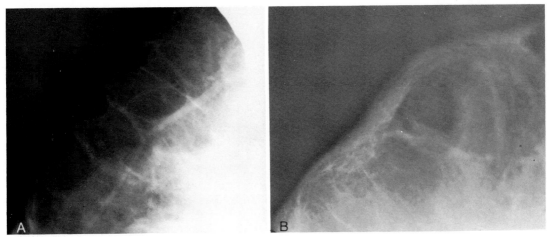

Figure 32–7. A, Biopsy of the breast complicated by infection. A 38-year-old white female with a breast lump for eight months. Clinically: suspicioius palpable nodule. Mammography: minimal fibrocystic disease, otherwise normal. Pathology: fibroadipose tissue. *B,* Breast six weeks later. Clinically: obvious carcinoma, mass fixed to skin with matted axillary nodes. Mammography: laminated thickening of the skin, localized, no underlying mass; inflammatory disease. Pathology: chronic inflammatory changes with foreign body granulomatous reaction.

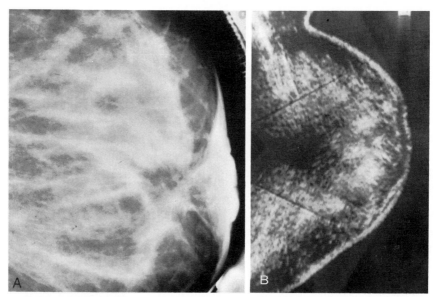

Figure 32–8. Subareolar fibrosis following surgery. A 28-year-old woman who had the major duct system removed (apple-core procedure) three months earlier for persistent nipple discharge. *A,* Mammography: areolar thickening, fixation of the nipple, subareolar distortion and density. *B,* Sonography: hypoechoic subareolar area, flattening of the areolar skin. No significant change on follow-up.

mograms may clearly show the status of the remaining tissues and often foretell a recurrence (Figs. 32–9 to 32–11). Still other surgery, such as debulking or toilet procedures or even partial mastectomy, may produce such loss and distortion of tissues that x-ray studies are of no value.

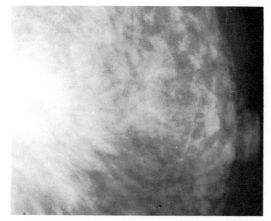

Figure 32–9. Carcinoma with lumpectomy as treatment. An 85-year-old woman with a breast lump that was clinically cancer. Mammography: 1.5 × 2 cm moderately invasive central carcinoma. Pathology: duct carcinoma. The mass was only excised, as she had extensive cancerosarcoma of the uterus and severe basal cell carcinomas of the head and neck. Mammogram (shown) postlumpectomy: large area of irregular density, a normal immediately postoperative appearance.

Reconstruction or Prosthesis

Occasionally patients who have had reduction mammoplasties are seen (Fig. 32–12). Ordinarily these procedures consist of removal of varying amounts of breast tissue. If the amount removed is small, very slight or no abnormality will be noted on the mammogram. Removal of large amounts of breast tissue, as in quadrant biopsy, may result in deformity of the breast (Fig. 32–5). Removal of the nipples may have been carried out; this will be most confusing if the radiologist is unaware of the procedure.

Reconstructive procedures most often are accompanied by augmentation prostheses. Body tissues, such as omental fat, have been used. The earlier aim, especially after a radical mastectomy, was merely the provision of a mound of tissue that would hold the brassiere up and keep it from sliding. The alternative was the removal by simple mastectomy of the remaining large, heavy, pendulous breast to return balance to the woman and relieve back strain.

Most prosthetic breast procedures consist of addition of some relatively inert material to or behind the breast to increase its volume. One practice has been the insertion of varying amounts of polyurethane foam sponge into the retromammary space. For several

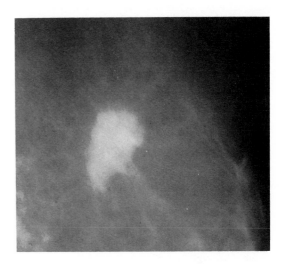

Figure 32–10. Lumpectomy for carcinoma in cardiac patient. A 69-year-old woman with a breast lump for two weeks; no family history; severe cardiac decompensation. Clinically the lesion was malignant. Mammography (preoperative): 1.2 × 1.7 cm moderately invasive carcinoma (poor film is due to poor patient cooperation). Lumpectomy as definitive treatment. Pathology: duct carcinoma with a scirrhous element.

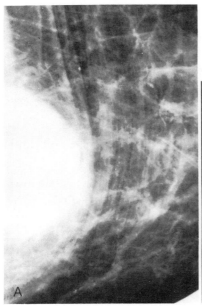

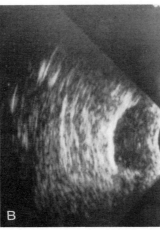

Figure 32–11. Circumscribed lesion as duct carcinoma. A 79-year-old woman with a mass for one year that was clinically 5 cm in diameter. *A*, Mammography: well-circumscribed, homogeneously dense 4.5 cm mass; at the patient's age, an intracystic papillary carcinoma. *B*, Sonography (real-time): demarcated, slightly irregular mass with nonhomogeneous internal echoes; potentiation of posterior border; suggestive of sarcoma. Pathology: fleshy, lobulated circumscribed duct carcinoma. Only tumorectomy was performed owing to the patient's ill health; she was alive and apparently free of disease 18 months later.

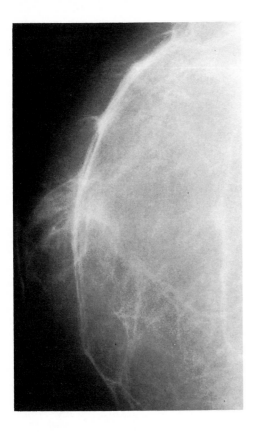

Figure 32–12. Reduction mammoplasty. A 53-year-old woman who had reconstruction of the left breast following mastectomy for an intraductal carcinoma and a reduction mammoplasty on the right breast. Mammography: little fibroglandular tissues are apparent; the superficial layer of superficial fascia became more apparent following mammoplasty. The woman was still pleased with the results six years later.

months after installation, air may be seen retained in the foam, which allows immediate recognition; the procedure may be complicated by infection (Fig. 32–13). The breast tissue, usually scanty in amount, will be seen crowded into the subareolar area. Eventually the entire prosthesis and breast become homogeneously dense (Fig. 32–14). Increased convexity of the breast outline, lack of breast tissue in a moderate-sized organ, and identification of suture material along the inframammary crease provide the clues to the operative procedure.

For several years, liquid silicone was introduced into the breast by a series of injections to enlarge the breast. Massage distributed it more evenly and broke the liquid into smaller globules. The material slowly left the breast, requiring reinjection to maintain a buxom appearance. Owing to concern about its possible harmful effects, this practice was outlawed and largely abandoned (Figs. 32–15 to 32–18).

Liquid silicone within impervious sheets of silicone, or foam-type plastic within impervious sheet plastic, has been used for augmentation of the breast size or replacement following subcuticular mastectomy (Fig. 32–19). The former was smooth anteriorly, allowing the skin to move in relation to the prosthesis, but was rough posteriorly, providing adherence to the chest wall. The latter was rough overall, with adherence to the entire periphery by the chest wall and skin.

A variation of the silicone-filled bag was the use of saline within the bag. This was softer to the touch. Some devices were equipped with a nozzle by which the amount of saline could be varied. However, the nozzle moved about under the skin and was difficult to find by palpation. Another variation was the silicone-filled bag with an anterior layer of saline, again, more breastlike to palpation.

For about ten years, silicone type prostheses have been used for augmentation of the breast, particularly by plastic surgeons. During this period there has been sporadic interest in reconstructing the breast following surgery for breast cancer using the silicone bag type prosthesis.

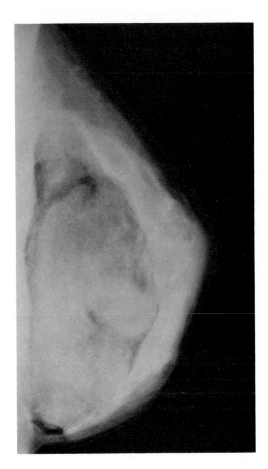

Figure 32–13. Infected breast prosthesis. A 39-year-old white female, six months following insertion of a cosmetic type of breast prosthesis and two months following drainage of 100 ml of clear fluid. Mammography: small amount of breast tissue pushed anteriorly by partially aerated infected breast prosthesis.

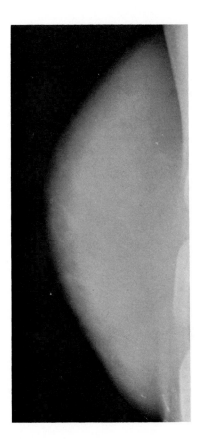

Figure 32–14. Older breast prosthesis. A 28-year-old white female, several months following insertion of a polyurethane foam breast prosthesis for cosmetic purposes. Mammography: homogeneous, very dense breast tissue; suture material at inframammary crease. The results were excellent, both surgically and esthetically.

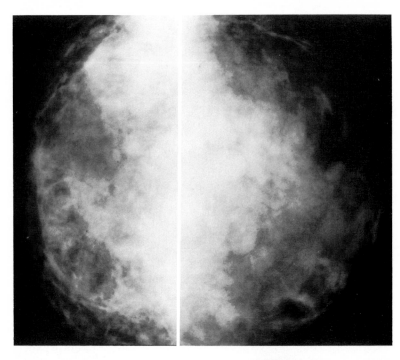

Figure 32–15. Liquid silicone droplets in the breast. A 28-year-old woman with pain in the right breast; bilateral liquid silicone injections four years before; brassiere size increased from 34AA to 36C. Mammography: diffuse rounded masses of liquid silicone measuring up to 1.2 cm in size. The dense intervening breast tissue is due to fibroglandular tissue in the young breast, minute droplets of silicone, and fibrous reaction to the silicone. Increasing firmness of the breasts; otherwise no change during 11 years' follow-up.

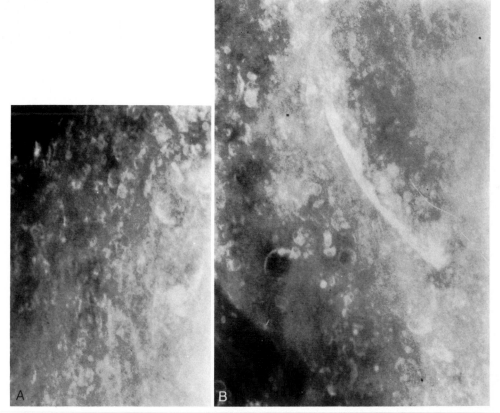

Figure 32–16. Liquid silicone injection of the breast. A 40-year-old woman who had liquid silicone injections of her breasts seven years before. Clinically the breasts were nodular, but otherwise they were normal in texture. Mammography: diffuse small deposits of silicone bilaterally. *A* and *B*, Blowup of two areas (the largest cystic area on the left is 2.5 mm in diameter) of the breast showing these cystic areas, irregular globules, and linear deposits of liquid silicone. The arrangement of the injected liquid silicone varies with different women.

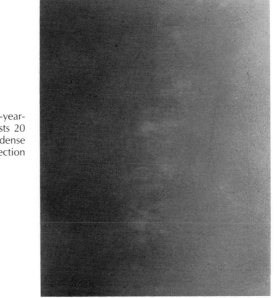

Figure 32–17. Residual liquid silicone in the breast. A 41-year-old woman who had bilateral silicone injections in her breasts 20 years ago in Japan. Most of the radiographic density is due to dense fibroglandular tissue. The only evidence of the silicone injection are the faint densities near the base of the breast.

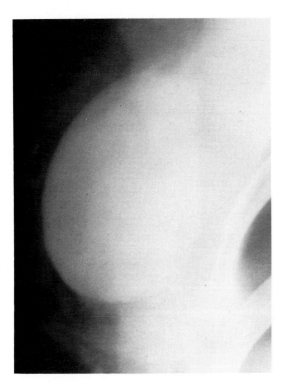

Figure 32–18. Liquid silicone injection. A 35-year-old woman seen for routine follow-up. Reportedly, while in Taiwan she had liquid silicone injected behind the breasts into the retromammary space, where it remained well confined.

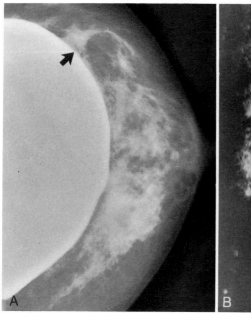
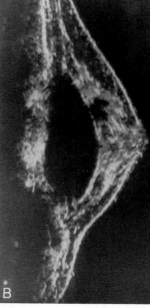

Figure 32–19. Augmentation prosthesis followed by carcinoma. A 37-year-old woman who had bilateral augmentation prosthesis seven years before developed a mass above the nipple. *A,* Mammograms: bilateral augmentation prosthesis in good position. A 1 cm moderately invasive carcinoma inferiorly on the right resting on the prosthesis. *B,* Sonography: normal-appearing right breast prosthesis. An irregular hypoechoic mass indenting the surface of the prosthesis. Pathology: duct carcinoma. Modified radical mastectomy; all 18 axillary lymph nodes free of metastases. No evidence of disease two years later.

Prophylactic Mastectomy

Complete

Prior to mastectomy for cancer the oncologic surgeon may suggest to the woman an alternative to the complete loss of the breast. After the chest wall healed and the pathologist had an opportunity to review the resected tissues, a new breast could be reconstructed, including nipple and areola. At the same time the sagging remaining breast could be rebuilt to a more cosmetic form. Often, when the woman finds that she can live happily with only one breast, she never seeks this procedure. However, if she should, at Emory University the oncologic surgeon would do a complete mastectomy, which would be followed by reconstruction by the plastic surgeon.

More recently, there have been intense efforts by the plastic surgeons to restore a fully formed breast with nipple and areola. The most esthetic procedure consists of placement of a flap of posterior pectoral muscles over the silicone prostheses on the anterior chest wall, the muscle in turn covered by skin with a fashioned nipple and areola.

Subcuticular

There has also been interest in prophylactic removal of the breast by subcuticular mastectomy, followed by insertion of the prosthesis. This has proved of particular value in the reluctant women who have severe borderline

changes in their breasts due to ductal hyperplasia, sclerosing adenosis, or minimal lobular carcinoma in situ and in cases in which one pathologist feels that the changes are benign and another pathologist believes that

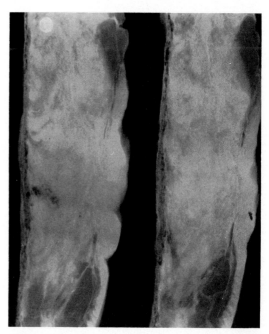

Figure 32–20. Dense fibroglandular tissue and marked fibrocystic disease. A 54-year-old woman with nodular (confusing clinically) breasts and with numerous biopsies showing atypia. With a strong family history of breast cancer and the difficulty of follow-up by mammography, she elected prophylactic mastectomies. No malignancy found.

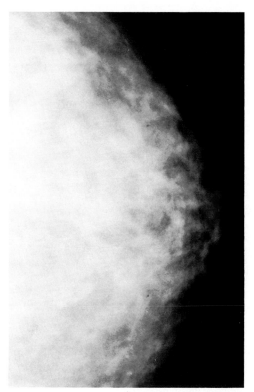

Figure 32–21. Ductal epithelial hyperplasia being followed by mammography. A 58-year-old woman who had a right mastectomy ten years before for carcinoma. Mammography shows many areas of concern. However, without interval change, no area can be pinpointed for biopsy.

the lesion is malignant (Figs. 32–20 and 32–21). This approach also supplies the pathologist with more tissue for study.

The oncologist's applications of the subcuticular mastectomy and prosthetic breast implantation at the Emory University Clinic had the advantage of having correlated clinical, radiographic, and pathologic whole-organ studies of his resected specimens in the well-equipped mammography-pathology laboratory at Emory University.

Considerable trepidation accompanied this procedure even when the mastectomy was performed by an oncologic surgeon and the reconstruction was done by the plastic surgeon. All the glandular tissue could not be removed: that left under the areola; that along Cooper's ligaments near the skin; and any aberrant extension of the gland (Figs. 32–22 and 32–23). This amount of residual glandular tissue could conceivably be the shock organ of the entire hormonal system of the woman.

Mammography is useful in all these procedures in outlining the prosthesis in relation to nearby tissues in its migration, rupture, or wrinkling. Ultrasound at times is even more useful.

Miscellaneous

Unusual surgical procedures may be carried out to preserve the breast contour (Fig. 32–24). In our twelve cases of Mondor's disease, little change on the mammogram was produced and surgery has not been performed; some cases have been biopsied when the retraction was confused with carcinoma. Pacemakers may be implanted in the breast (Fig. 32–25). Surgery on the chest wall that may or may not involve the breast may produce spontaneous lactation (Fig. 32–26). Biopsy of unilateral early ripening has been discussed.

RADIOTHERAPY

Benign Conditions

Today benign conditions are seldom treated by irradiation, but they have been in the past, with some long-term effects (Fig. 32–27). At one time irradiation was a popular treatment for postpartum mastitis.

Malignant Conditions

Definitive external radiotherapy has been used in inflammatory carcinoma following needle biopsy or in early-stage carcinoma following biopsy or with sufficient breast tissue remaining for mammography. This therapy may be supplemented by interstitial irradiation, chemotherapy, or hormone manipulation.

Mammographic Changes

During and after irradiation of the breast for cancer, a graphic serial record may be made. The response or lack of response and the recurrence or regrowth of the lesion may be measured more accurately by mammography than by clinical evaluation. Similarly, after systemic or hormone treatment measurement of the size and appearance of the breast lesion may be the only reliable factors for judging the response to treatment.

The changes most frequently noted during radiotherapy of the breast are (1) the overall density of the breast, (2) the mass itself, (3) skin thickening, (4) the appearance of calcification, and (5) recurrence of the tumor.

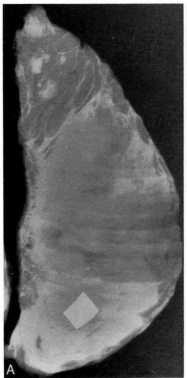

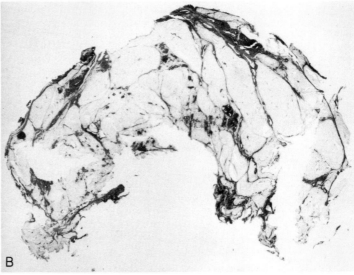

Figure 32–22. Subcuticular mastectomy specimen whole mount. A 45-year-old woman with numerous breast biopsies and marked changes of severe fibrocystic disease, including atypia. Thirty-six such sections clearly showed dissection of breast tissue inside the superficial layer of superficial fascia. *A*, radiograph of slicer section. *B*, H & E whole breast mount. Breast tissue could extend along Cooper's ligaments beyond the point of severance; there was, as always, residual breast tissue under the nipple and areola.

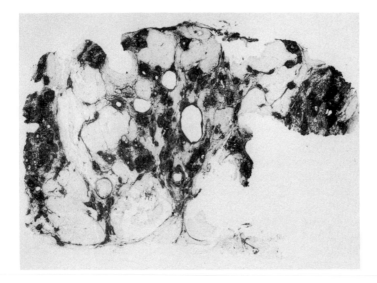

Figure 32–23. Subcuticular mastectomy specimen mount showing incomplete removal of the breast. A 38-year-old woman with nodular breasts, cancerophobia, and severe histologic changes. One edge of the specimen clearly shows that sharp dissection had been carried out through breast tissue, leaving some of that tissue on the chest wall.

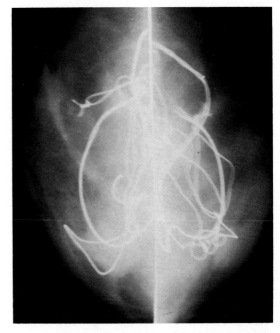

Figure 32–24. Wires used to shore up breasts. A 36-year-old woman gravida 1, para 1, 11 years post mammopexy. Following her only delivery 14 years before, the breasts began to sag. Decided to "have breasts wired up one year ago." She seemed pleased with the results. (The wires didn't prevent motion during radiography, however.)

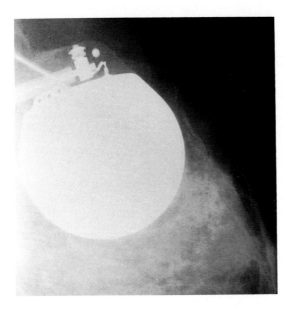

Figure 32–25. Cardiac pacemaker inserted in the left breast. This 6 cm diameter object is well concealed in the pendulous breast (with ductal hyperplasia) of a 67-year-old woman.

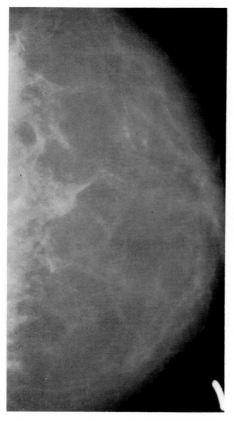

Figure 32–26. Syndrome of spontaneous lactation following chest wall trauma. An adult white female, one week after resection of pulmonary hamartoma, with pain at the T4–T8 level (thoracotomy site), began lactating normal milk. This changed to serous discharge with menstruation but returned to normal milk following menstruation.

Figure 32–27. A long-term effect of radiation on the breast. A 22-year-old female who had four radon seeds implanted in the left nipple area at age six months as treatment of a hemangioma. Clinically: small indurated left breast, right breast normal. Mammography: left breast small, dense, some distortion; four radon seeds. Pathology (of mastectomy specimen, insert lower right): primarily non-functioning fibroglandular tissue.

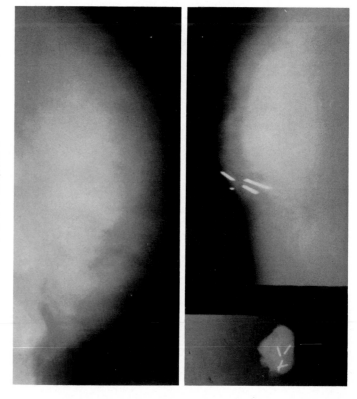

Density of the Breast. Radiotherapy is most often given to the intact breast for an inoperable cancer (Fig. 32–28). At that stage there are the usual diffuse changes of the breast producing varying degrees of overall increase in density of the structure. As therapy progresses there will be an increase in density of the breast, an edematous appearance to the structures, and in the subcutaneous areas an indistinctness of the trabeculae. This reaction reaches a peak sometime after a few weeks of therapy but may be quite marked at the six-week follow-up after completion of the four to five weeks of therapy. There will be continued clearing of the density but never to the precancerous state. Some increase in density will be retained owing to varying degrees of scarring, contracture, and fibrosis.

The mechanism of this increase in density is not completely known. It no doubt results from continued growth of and reaction to the tumor for a week or so. There is some contribution to the reaction to the ionizing radiation. Where one ends and the other takes over is difficult to determine. Surgery may have contributed little to the process, as only a needle biopsy may have been done.

With tumorectomy and radiation the breast is less dense initially. However, following surgery and a complete regimen of radiotherapy, there is an overall increase in density of the breast resulting from the trauma of the surgery and the reaction to radiotherapy. These changes are not nearly so marked, but can be quite marked with infection and severe individual response to ionizing radiation, as with treatment of the inoperable breast cancer.

Mass. The density of the breast harboring an inoperable breast cancer can mask the mass on x-ray, as noted in the discussion on inflammatory cancer of the breast or advanced noninflammatory breast cancer. As therapy progresses the mass, when apparent initially, becomes less distinct and less dense. On occasion the surrounding reaction may recede before appreciable response of the mass, making it more distinct. The persistence of a definite mass at the end of a full course of therapy indicates a need for additional radiation, e.g., 2000 rads, to the tumor through reduced fields in perhaps five days. The bed of a tumorectomy may simulate a mammographic mass and respond similarly to the true cancerous mass.

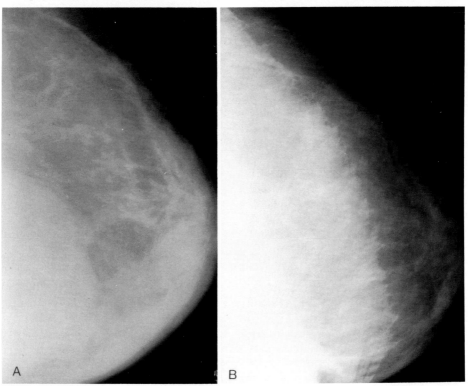

Figure 32–28. Response of breast carcinoma to protracted radiation therapy. A 61-year-old woman with a massive carcinoma proved by needle biopsy. *A,* Mammography (prior to biopsy): massive carcinoma with diffuse skin thickening. *B,* Mammography (six months later following radiation): Mass of carcinoma and most of the skin thickening have disappeared, leaving only an area of calcification not seen in the density of the carcinoma prior to treatment.

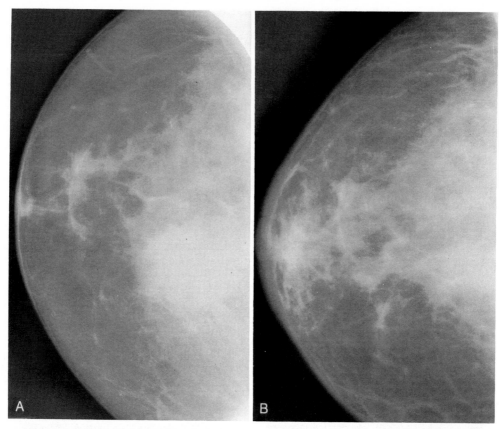

Figure 32–29. Lack of complete response of carcinoma to routine treatment with radiation. A 67-year-old woman admitted with a diagnosis of breast carcinoma, inoperable on the basis of skin involvement upon biopsy. *A*, Mammography (prior to treatment): highly infiltrative, inoperable 3.5 × 5 cm carcinoma. *B*, Mammography (after 14 weeks of irradiation to 5500 rads tumor dose): thickened skin and residual tumor on the basis of carcinoma rather than irradiation. An additional 2000 rads were then given through reduced fields to the tumor site. The breast was clinically free of disease four months later, but bone metastases had occurred.

Skin. Increased thickness of the skin of the breast is a sign of inoperability of a breast cancer and will be present at the onset of radiotherapy in those cases. Its response to radiation parallels that of the breast, as, in fact, the thickened skin contributes to the overall density of the breast. The skin changes subside similarly, always with some residual changes of thickening about the areola or a flattened area with contracture of the breast. The skin following tumorectomy and radiation also reacts similarly but to a lessened degree than with an inoperable breast cancer.

Calcification. Most breast cancers contain calcifications of some type. The flecks of carcinoma calcification are rarely seen in the inoperable breast cancer. As the density of the breast lessens and the size and density of the mass recede calcifications often become apparent in the mass and in other parts of the breast. These calcifications are not felt to be the result of radionecrosis and deposition of calcification in the detritus. Instead, they are merely a normal part of the tumor and become visible following response of the breast and the mass to radiotherapy. This would be comparable to demonstration by x-ray of the calcifications of an intracystic papillary carcinoma after the dense blood had been removed from it. The calcifications outside the area of the mass of tumor are merely the residual of other foci, often intraductal, of carcinoma. This phenomenon does not occur with tumorectomy and radiation.

Recurrence. Progression of any or all of the radiographic changes is of no concern even at the six weeks' checkup. However, after a few months, increase in any of them heralds an impending recurrence. An increased vascularity may be the first hint of trouble. Periodic mammograms are useful in early detection of recurrence so that treatment planning may be better executed (Fig. 32–29).

33

Indications and Applications of Mammography

BACKGROUND

With the present simple means of obtaining diagnostic mammograms, there is no valid reason for mammography, in any instance, to remain in the realm of attempted and discarded procedures. Mammography has long since advanced beyond an investigative procedure even for screening women under the age of 50 years. It has proved to be highly accurate and valuable in the diagnosis of normal, benign, and malignant conditions; it is safe, simple, acceptable, and reproducible; and it is effective in the diagnosis of cancer of the breast when used as a survey procedure before clinical signs and symptoms are present.

Surgeons introduced to mammography enumerated indications for its use. These reflected their long-held confidence in breast palpation but also controlled optimism for the detection potential of the new procedure (Table 33–1). Practical applications were noted, surgeons maintaining that the proper choice of surgical drapings and trays of instruments (either for simply excision biopsy or for radical mastectomy) paid for the procedure many times over. To eschew nonproductive and frustrating breast surgery would ease their already overburdened surgical schedule. Anesthesiologists were pleased to know whether intravenous agents for a simple procedure or intubation for an extended procedure would be required.

The indications for mammography that evolved from use of the technique stemmed from the clinician's search for the maximum evidence, or proof, of the existence (or nonexistence) of a breast lesion and its specific character (Table 33–2). A more positive diagnosis and a more exact knowledge of the extent and character of the disease aid in planning treatment, whether the treatment is to be surgery, radiation, observation, or systemic or local palliative procedures.

Mammography should not dictate treatment procedures, but it may provide in certain cases the small but vital amount of information necessary to avoid undesirable results. Indications for mammography more broadly encompass the presence of breast complaints or malignant disease, primary site

TABLE 33–1. Indications for Mammography by Surgeons in a Tumor Hospital in 1956

Give radiologist enough rope to hang himself
Determine type of surgical drapings
Identify additional signs of inoperability
Eliminate many benign biopsies
Determine type of anesthesia
Find few cancers missed by residents
Aid in treatment planning

TABLE 33–2. Early Clinical Indications for Mammography

Signs and symptoms of breast disease, whether evident or questionable
Breast changes sufficient to have led to previous biopsies
Strong familial history of breast cancer
Survey of the opposite breast after mastectomy
Breast difficult to examine clinically (lumpy or large and pendulous)
Cancerophobia
Adenocarcinoma, primary site undetermined
Provision of a baseline in asymptomatic patients for future comparison

undetermined. Specific applications are increasing, and many overlap. Many of the cases already presented exemplify various indications and applications of mammography; others are presented here more specifically.

EVALUATION OF SPECIFIC COMPLAINTS THAT BRING THE PATIENT TO THE PHYSICIAN

1. Nipple changes of retraction, discharge, or eczema present various problems (Figs. 33–1 and 33–2). The patient's history may be unreliable (Fig. 33–3). No abnormality may be palpable beneath the nipple. In such instances, the clinician cannot be sure that a deep-seated malignant tumor is present. Since there is often some degree of ductal dilatation and fibrosis beneath the nipple, palpatory findings may be confusing. Advanced subareolar fibrosis or duct ectasia may present problems to both clinician and radiologist. Nipple discharge, either serous or sanguineous, poses similar problems. Eczema of the nipple may be confusing even to the pathologist. Frequently, the mammograms will show clearly the nonspecific fibrosis or carcinoma causing nipple retraction, a dilated duct and/or intraductal papillomata, a carcinoma causing nipple discharge, or the centrally placed carcinoma of the breast that causes Paget's disease. The mammogram may supply the necessary bit of information for the clinician either to proceed unhesitantly with preparations for a radical surgical procedure or to follow a more conservative or localized therapeutic approach.

2. The vague symptoms referable to the breast—pain, tenderness (Fig. 33–4), or fullness—can be most disturbing and may be the first indication of serious disease. The negative mammogram of such a patient affords considerable assurance to the clinician. Even cancerophobic patients may harbor a carcinoma (Fig. 33–5).

3. Skin changes of thickening, redness, ecchymosis, flattening, or retraction often signal the presence of carcinoma (Fig. 33–6).

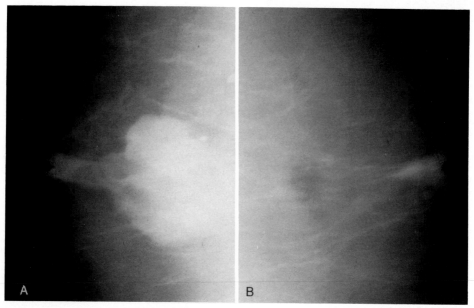

Figure 33–1. A and B, Bilateral nipple retraction. Retraction was present for years in this 63-year-old woman. Clinically there was a lump in the right breast. The mammograms show a 3 × 3.5 cm moderately invasive carcinoma, probably not producing the nipple retraction.

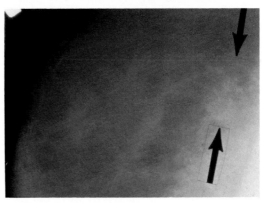

Figure 33–2. Clinically unsuspected carcinoma. A 1 × 1.5 cm carcinoma *(arrows)* clinically unsuspected was found in a 53-year-old woman presenting with a bloody discharge from the nipple of the opposite breast. Histopathologic studies proved the etiology of the bloody discharge to be benign in the opposite breast, but the lesion in this breast to be an unrelated carcinoma.

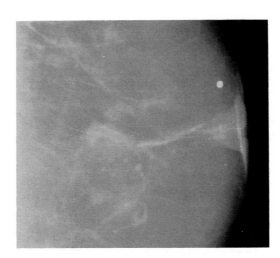

Figure 33–3. Nipple retraction of benign etiology. This 61-year-old patient insisted that the nipple retraction was recent and progressive. This complaint, coupled with a palpable subareolar thickening, alarmed the clinician. Mammograms of this fatty breast showed the nipple retraction with only minimal subareolar fibrosis. A five-year follow-up revealed no change; it is suspected the nipple retraction was of long duration.

Figure 33–4. Nonpalpable carcinoma. Vague tenderness in both breasts in this 64-year-old woman caused her to seek medical aid. The subsequently proved cancer was nonpalpable even after localization by mammography.

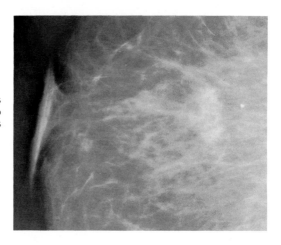

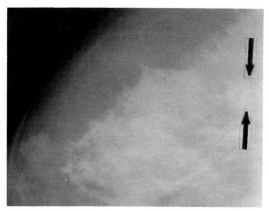

Figure 33–5. The patient presented with vaginal bleeding and breast pain. This 55-year-old woman presented with vaginal bleeding that proved to be due to a benign disease. She then complained of pain in the opposite breast. Her breasts were normal to palpation; she was labeled as cancerophobic. Mammograms did show a 1 cm faint area of stippled calcifications (between arrows) that proved to be breast carcinoma.

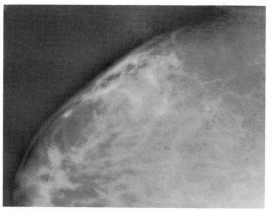

Figure 33–7. Healing breast abscess. The abscess in this 39-year-old woman was initially confused with carcinoma, both clinically and radiographically. The abscess was drained surgically; this represents clearing of the main mass on the mammograms with residual skin thickening as the pertinent findings. Drainage of pus does not always indicate benign breast disease; clearing of the mass on the mammograms was a most useful finding because, at this stage, clinical examination was still difficult.

Other less serious disease processes may be demonstrated to be etiologic factors: scleroderma morphea, localized inflammatory disease (Fig. 33–7), a hematoma, trauma, atrophy, or no significant lesion at all.

4. One frequently encounters a mass or masses in both breasts. When there is a dominant nodule in the breast, the accepted treatment is removal of the nodule for his-

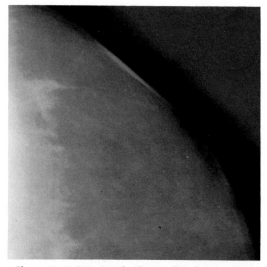

Figure 33–6. Cancer with adjacent skin change. A breast cancer of less than 1 cm produced a very early adjacent skin change of flattening. This 59-year-old woman complained of pain in her neck, back, and chest; all areas revealed osteolytic bone lesions; biopsy of the lesion in the cervical spine revealed metastatic adenocarcinoma. During one year of observation this breast lesion did not change appreciably.

topathologic study. There are times, however, such as in the first trimester of pregnancy, when general anesthesia is to be avoided if the lesion is clinically and radiographically benign. In the event of several breast masses, the mammograms outline a more definite approach in selection of the most suspicious masses for biopsy.

5. An extremely difficult problem to resolve is the questionable mass in the breast (Fig. 33–1). This problem is evidenced by conflicting clinical appraisals and by the occasional practice of surgical removal of normal breast tissue at biopsy. Mammography has definite value in the case of such questionable clinical findings, since the technique may reduce the number of biopsies or indicate that a biopsy should be done without loss of time.

6. Of clinical significance is the differentiation of primary carcinoma of the tail of the breast from enlarged axillary lymph nodes (Fig. 33–8). Errors in judgment have resulted in improper treatment. The mammogram may demonstrate clearly that the malignant lesion is within the axillary prolongation of the breast tissue, or it may demonstrate that the mass is clearly defined axillary lymph node unrelated to breast disease and that there is no malignant disease within the breast.

7. Providing the pathologist with the proper tissue specimen is mandatory for the correct histopathologic diagnosis. It is axiomatic that the carcinoma must be under the

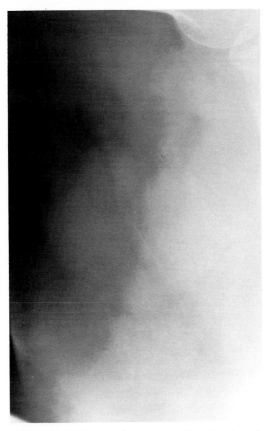

Figure 33–8. Masses of enlarged axillary lymph nodes that could not be clinically differentiated from carcinoma of the tail of the breast. The mammogram clearly indicates well-outlined masses of nodes rather than an infiltrative carcinomatous mass. The nonpalpable cancer deep in a pendulous breast is poorly demonstrated near the bottom of this axillary view.

microscope to be diagnosed. Generous tissue specimens can be obtained from the proper quadrant, yet the carcinoma may remain undisturbed, or a specimen may be removed from the wrong area of the breast (Fig. 33–9). Re-examination by radiography may show that the carcinoma remains and that re-exploration of the breast must be carried out to avoid a false sense of security on the part of the surgeon and patient.

SURVEY AND SCREENING FOR THE DETECTION OF BREAST CANCER IN HIGH-INCIDENCE GROUPS, OR IN SEARCH FOR THE PRIMARY SITE IN CASES OF KNOWN METASTATIC CANCER

1. Patients with a previous radical mastectomy for carcinoma have a higher incidence of clinically undetected carcinoma of the opposite breast. A number of other patients who could easily have been part of a survey program also had nonpalpable carcinomas demonstrated by mammography. Women who have had numerous breast biopsies for benign disease or who know other women with such experience ask for and submit to mammography as a screening procedure even though they reject physical examination. Thus, these women are not entirely lost to follow-up. In their minds such physical examinations only lead to further "useless biopsies" entailing anesthesia, operation, loss of time, and added expense. Mammography is invaluable in surveying patients with a strong family history of breast carcinoma and allaying the fears of the clinician regarding these patients.

2. Search for the primary site of a malignant tumor often is tedious, expensive, and unrewarding. A patient with axillary lymph nodes involved with adenocarcinoma may have an occult carcinoma of the breast. Histologic study of such nodes may result in an erroneous diagnosis of lymphoma, melanoma, or anaplastic squamous cell carcinoma (Fig. 33–10). Unless there is knowledge of the primary lesion in the breast, errors in treatment may result. In the presence of demonstrable localized or systemic malignant disease, mammography has eliminated prolonged, painful, and expensive diagnostic procedures, a thoracotomy, or biopsy of a metastatic bone lesion that often can only be labeled "metastatic adenocarcinoma" by the pathologist (Fig. 33–6).

3. Clinical evaluation of the huge pendulous breast may be impossible (Fig. 33–4). The more subcutaneous fat, even in a small breast, the more difficult is the physical examination, and yet the mammogram can be more precisely performed. Carcinoma in the massive and pendulous breast is difficult to diagnose clinically. In one patient a carcinoma reached a size of 13 × 17 cm before it was palpable. A physician, adept at initial physical examinations, often stated his reason for mammography as "breasts too large for physical examination."

4. In patients who have a mass in the breast accompanied by clinically or histologically positive axillary or supraclavicular lymph nodes, mammography has demonstrated the breast mass to be benign and unrelated to the systemic disease. Under these circumstances, failure to remove tissue from such a mass for histologic study delays

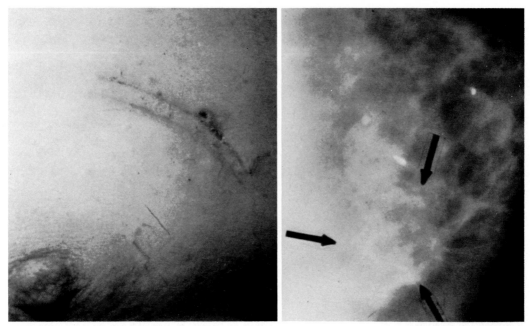

Figure 33–9. Biopsy scars and infiltrative carcinoma. This 39-year-old patient had had six biopsies of this breast and five biopsies of the other breast for benign disease. The healing scar of the most recent biopsy was the only clinical abnormality of this breast. Mammogram at the same time reveals in the same breast three calcifying and one noncalcifying benign masses and one infiltrative carcinoma (between arrows). Faint calcifications and skin changes aided in the diagnosis. The surgeons were most grateful for aid in examining this scarred breast.

establishment of the proper diagnosis and treatment.

5. Either proved or suspected carcinoma may exist in one breast and there may be a second primary carcinoma in the opposite breast (Fig. 33–11). If there is no knowledge of the second primary tumor, a radical mastectomy may be performed as a curative procedure. The second primary growth remains to become clinically manifest later (one

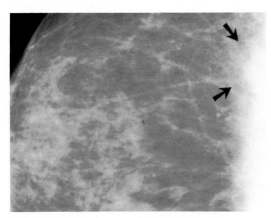

Figure 33–10. Erroneous diagnosis of lymphoma. This 55-year-old woman presented with axillary masses. Histopathologic studies were interpreted as lymphoma. This mammogram was obtained one year later, after a full course of radiotherapy to the region. The mammogram was made to determine whether radiation of the axilla had produced skin thickening. The deep, poorly reproduced carcinoma (arrows) was biopsied. The diagnosis was then changed from lymphoma of the axillary lymph nodes to carcinoma of the breast with metastasis to the axillary lymph nodes.

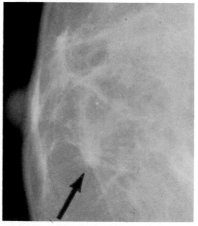

Figure 33–11. Simultaneous second primary carcinoma. A second primary carcinoma, clinically unsuspected, was found in the breast opposite the one containing a palpable primary carcinoma. This 2 × 4 mm carcinoma is one of the smallest true malignant masses we have detected by mammography. It was a typical spiculated mass containing stippled calcification. This 59-year-old patient had discovered the cancer of the opposite breast.

of four cases is still occult after 23 months), and hence the second lesion is often labeled metastatic. Mammography has shown simultaneous bilateral carcinomas to be present more often than suspected. In addition, mammography is the most logical single method of determining whether the second breast contains a primary carcinoma (Fig. 33–12) or a metastatic lesion (Fig. 33–13). With mammography, the primary mass may be studied in minute gross detail in relation to the entire organ. The diffuse nature of spread from the opposite breast is also quite apparent on the mammogram. The pathologist realizes his limitations in studying fragments of isolated tissue obtained by biopsy and is well aware that metastatic carcinoma may produce dissimilar patterns of growth. The existence of an interval between the demonstration of a carcinoma in one breast and the recognition of a malignant lesion in the opposite breast does not rule out simultaneous carcinomas that became clinically evident at different times (Fig. 33–13).

6. In clinically confusing axillary lymph nodes with apparently normal breasts, or even with histologically normal or benign lymph nodes, the breast may still contain a carcinoma.

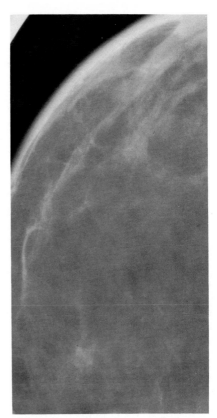

Figure 33–13. Metastatic breast carcinoma from the opposite breast. Typical appearance shows diffuse skin thickening, increased density, and edema of the glandular tissue without evidence of a breast mass. This 67-year-old woman had a radical mastectomy 18 months previously for advanced carcinoma; no mammograms were done at that time. This breast was clinically normal, but on the basis of mammography a biopsy of the skin was done. This was microscopically normal, but rebiopsy of masses growing through the biopsy site two months later showed carcinoma of the breast. (This section is representative of the entire huge breast without a primary site.)

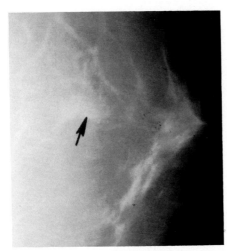

Figure 33–12. Nonsimultaneous demonstration of a second primary breast cancer. Two years prior to mammography this 53-year-old woman had a radical mastectomy for proven breast carcinoma. This, her first mammogram (done as a part of a routine follow-up), demonstrated a nonpalpable primary breast carcinoma. Conceivably, the carcinoma could have been present at the time of the first mastectomy.

AN AID IN CLARIFYING CONFUSING PALPATORY FINDINGS

1. The breast may be lumpy without having a dominant nodule. The radiologist may detect the dominant nodule or appreciate the secondary signs of carcinoma earlier than they are recognized clinically.

2. There may be evidence of fibrocystic disease with or without a dominant nodule. The objective radiographic findings in these breasts or changes during serial studies on mammography frequently aid in their evaluation. The changes of fibrocystic disease are graphically recorded in serial studies. The carcinoma hidden by fibrocystic disease may be nonpalpable but may be readily apparent

on the mammogram (Fig. 33–14). The patient who has had multiple biopsies for fibrocystic disease, perhaps during the third and fourth decades of life, tends to think that further biopsy specimens will also prove to be benign. In fact, the chance of developing malignant disease may be 20 to 30 times greater in the later decades than in the earlier ones. These patients accept mammography more willingly than further biopsy.

3. Several previous biopsies may have resulted in scarring and irregularities (Fig. 33–9). Previous surgical procedures seldom interfere with mammography, but they make evaluation of palpatory findings difficult and they exasperate the clinician.

4. Although there is little palpable disease, vague complaints may persist. Mammography helps allay the fears of the patient and clinician as well as providing assurance that no serious abnormality is present.

5. After aspiration of a cyst, it may be difficult to evaluate the breast for the presence of malignant disease. The presence of a cyst, established by aspiration of its contents, does not eliminate the possibility of coexisting malignant disease (Fig. 33–14).

6. Mammography is helpful for diagnosis of carcinoma during pregnancy and lactation (Fig. 33–15). Carcinomas often become quite large and advanced during pregnancy; difficulty of examination contributes to delay in detection. During these states the breast is

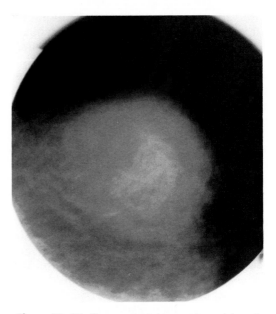

Figure 33–15. Overpenetrated spot view of lactating breast. View was made to show a large, well-circumscribed carcinoma in a dense lactating breast, six months after delivery. The patient was aware of a change in her breast during later pregnancy, but both she and her doctor attributed the changes to pregnancy. A recent rapid increase in size of the lump prompted the mammogram.

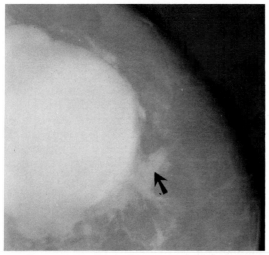

Figure 33–14. Large cyst clinically masking smaller carcinoma. This cyst would ordinarily have been aspirated. It was removed surgically; palpation of the wound was normal. By sharp dissection toward the nipple the carcinoma (arrow) was located and excised.

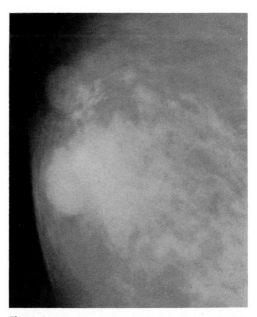

Figure 33–16. Mammogram of patient who was difficult to examine because of an exquisitely sore breast. Clinically there was a mass and associated, but limited, inflammatory carcinoma. The absence of diffuse skin changes of inflammatory carcinoma and the history of pain suggested infected cyst as the possible diagnosis from the mammograms. This was the diagnosis.

denser, but enough adipose tissue is present for radiographic demonstration of the lesion or secondary signs of carcinoma, which often are poorly elicited by physical examination.

7. Mammography can be used for examining patients with sore breasts (Fig. 33–16). Often such a patient will confide to the radiologist that her breasts are too sore for vigorous palpation. She is more hesitant to confide this to the surgeon. Such patients are willing to submit to radiographic examination. However, compression also poses problems with painful breasts.

8. Mammograms show that the upper quadrant mass is no more than an equivocal palpatory mass. The main body of glandular tissue of the breast lies in the upper and outer quadrants. As this is the last glandular tissue to be replaced by fat, palpation reveals an elongated or localized mass. Actually, however, it is normal glandular tissue outlined by fat in the breast.

9. Mammography is useful in diagnosing the subcutaneous "lump." The discrete lumps of fat under tension, entrapped between Cooper's suspended ligaments, disappear to palpation with severance of the ligaments. On the mammograms no distinct nodule is seen.

10. Mammography has been proved invaluable in selection of the proper site for biopsy, or when to biopsy (Figs. 33–17 and 33–18).

11. Mammography is often useful as an

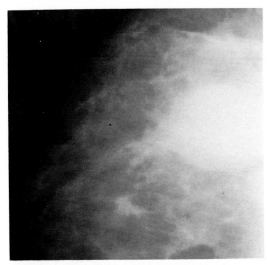

Figure 33–18. Mammographic diagnosis of cyst. A painless lump was discovered in the upper outer quadrant of the breast by this 56-year-old woman. Clinically it was described as a 4 cm mass suggestive of carcinoma. Mammograms suggested a cyst as the diagnosis, which led to the clinical decision to aspirate; clear amber fluid was removed and the lesion disappeared, thus establishing quickly not only the diagnosis but also adequate treatment.

aid to palpation. At times, when the lesion is demonstrated on mammography and its exact site is pinpointed, it then becomes palpable.

RESPONSE OF BREAST LESIONS TO THERAPY

1. Evaluation is possible after therapy for an inflammatory lesion or removal or aspiration of a cyst.

2. Following irradiation for carcinoma, a graphic serial record may be made. The lack of response or recurrence or regrowth may be measured more accurately than by clinical means.

3. After systemic therapy, changes in the size of a lesion or skin thickening may be more accurately measured; these changes may be the only available criteria for judging response to treatment.

IN TREATMENT PLANNING FOR BENIGN AND MALIGNANT DISEASE

1. When mammography indicates that the dominant nodule is benign, a more conservative regimen may be adopted (Fig. 33–17).

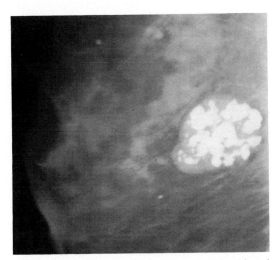

Figure 33–17. Calcifying fibroadenoma. A heavily calcifying fibroadenoma was found in an 86-year-old woman with a suspicious mass in the breast. Mammograms were so characteristic that no resection was done in this old and feeble patient.

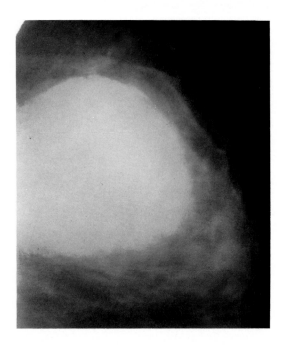

Figure 33–19. Carcinoma clinically found to be 10 cm and inoperable on the basis of large size. Mammograms revealed a well-circumscribed 6 × 7 cm mass without evidence of inoperability. The patient, a 63-year-old woman, had a breast lump for at least two months. A four-year follow-up after radical mastectomy was without evidence of disease despite the presence of low and midaxillary lymph node metastasis at the time of the mastectomy.

Figure 33–20. Diffuse thickening of skin of right breast associated with carcinoma indicates inoperability. A, The disease is so advanced that the mass of carcinoma is almost obliterated (arrow). B, The left breast is shown for comparison and to indicate that it is free of disease, excluding consideration of metastasis to this breast.

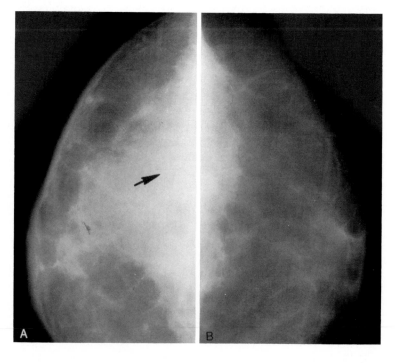

The fibroadenoma during the first trimester of pregnancy may be treated better when it is safer to give the patient anesthesia, after the first trimester or delivery.

2. When mammography indicates a recurrent lesion, whether in a breast previously biopsied and showing fibrocystic disease or whether a clear-cut cyst, the lesion may be more safely observed. Demonstration of a definite cyst on mammography may aid in the clinical decision to aspirate that cyst as a diagnostic and therapeutic procedure (Fig. 33–18).

3. Many circumscribed carcinomas, even though clinically large, may be treated by surgical resection rather than protracted radiation, as the growth pattern cannot be assessed by palpation (Fig. 33–19). The small, highly invasive carcinoma with its associated peripheral tissue reaction may feel as large as a circumscribed, less invasive carcinoma.

4. Errors in clinical judgment regarding the size of the lesion may be reduced by the use of mammography. Diffuse thickening of the skin seen radiographically, but not appreciated clinically, may have some significance as a radiographic sign of inoperability (Fig. 33–20).

5. In breasts in which the scars of numerous biopsies interfere with clinical examination, mammography may afford an extra objective evaluation that will minimize unnecessary amputation.

6. Evaluation of positive axillary adenopathy is incomplete without the knowledge of the presence or absence of disease in the contralateral breast; mammography often leads to the proper diagnosis. Establishment of the proper palliative treatment may be of extreme value.

7. The findings on mammography may be deemed sufficient evidence to proceed with a radical mastectomy without breast biopsy in the presence of proved adenocarcinoma of the axillary nodes and a definite carcinoma on the mammogram.

8. Mammography is invaluable as a direct approach to diagnosis of carcinoma of the breast in women with proven or suspected cancer. Much time, patient discomfort, and expense may be saved through this diagnostic procedure.

9. In numerous instances, mammography has been an extremely useful aid to the pathologists, who know only too well their difficulties in the diagnosis of breast lesions. In fact, it is difficult to judge whether it is the surgeons or the pathologists who are more appreciative of mammography as they become more experienced in the procedure.

If mammography accomplishes nothing more, it keeps the pathologist on the alert, thus avoiding serious errors. Despite the knowledge that mammography is fallible, the pathologist has erred in sufficient instances when he disregarded mammographic findings, that he gives his immediate problem great consideration before disagreeing with the radiologist. The radiologist frequently can alert the pathologist to the presence of an unusual lesion or the interesting features of a lesion (Fig. 33–21).

10. So little is known about the natural history of breast carcinoma that any aid is important. Mammography provides a permanent record of a lesion in relation to the surrounding tissue, the whole organ, and the axillary node–bearing area; this record

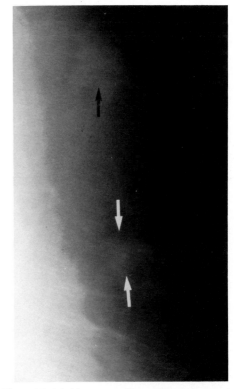

Figure 33–21. Mammographic evidence of two primary carcinomas in same breast. This 77-year-old woman complained of pain in her breasts, which were clinically normal. Both the surgeon (who was alerted to the presence of the carcinomas) and the pathologist felt that a cursory examination would not have demonstrated the smaller, somewhat soft lesion, a mucinous carcinoma (opposing arrows); the upper lesion was an infiltrative duct carcinoma (top arrow).

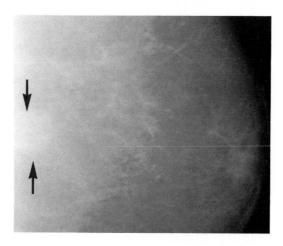

Figure 33–22. Deep carcinoma. A central, deep, non-palpable carcinoma was found in the breast of a 56-year-old woman complaining of "drawing in her breast." A mass of this size is readily palpable after sharp surgical dissection into the general area, although it cannot be palpated through the skin, fat, and fibroglandular tissues.

can be repeated as often as necessary without disturbing the lesion, thus allowing continued evaluation of the natural history of breast diseases.

Carcinoma of the breast in the young is uncommon; the youngest patient in our series was 18 years of age. A patient dying of widespread metastatic adenocarcinoma may have a primary carcinoma in the breast so small that it may be overlooked at postmortem examination, and the source of the disease may never be known. Presenting symptoms often are confusing but can be readily explained by mammography, because carcinoma of the breast may be present even though the breast remains clinically normal (Figs. 33–22 and 33–23).

Some carcinomas of the breast may remain latent for long periods of time, then, for one reason or another, manifest rapid growth. Several primary carcinomas of the breast in the same individual may grow at the same rate, spurring conjecture that each is more or less retarded in its growth by systemic body factors.

These applications are clear-cut, and many are practiced routinely in our institution. It must be reiterated that in no instance is the

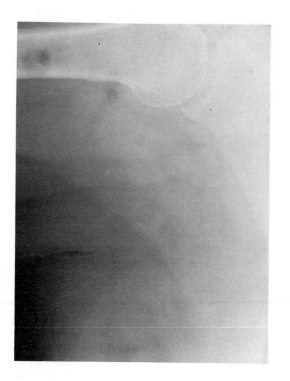

Figure 33–23. Occult carcinoma. The patient, a 56-year-old woman, had large axillary nodes, low back pain, and an osteolytic bone lesion in the innominate bone. This axillary view shows not only large nodes but also an osteolytic lesion of the shaft of the humerus. A 1.5 cm primary carcinoma was found deep in the pendulous breast.

radiologist attempting to dictate the treatment of the patient; he merely provides additional information on which the clinician may make his diagnosis.

POSSIBLE INDICATIONS

Other applications have evolved more slowly, are incompletely assessed, and hence are not incorporated in the treatment planning of each individual case. Some applications, no doubt, will be modified as experience increases. With this clearly in mind, we may consider some further possible indications, always remembering the limitations of mammography.

1. Mammography may be useful in the determination of type of anesthesia. Intubation may be carried out for a radical procedure and a simple anesthesia planned for biopsy of a benign lesion. The surgical draping may be similarly predetermined (Figs. 33–22 and 33–24).

2. Mammography may limit the number of biopsies under local anesthesia. Some surgeons believe that adequate exploration of the breast cannot be done if the patient is under local anesthesia and that the possibility of the presence of a malignant lesion must be considered. Other surgeons contend that, with practice, exploration, biopsy, and hemostasis are easily accomplished under local anesthesia. It is evident that outpatient biopsies are being and will continue to be performed in physicians' offices and in busy clinics; however, the number of biopsies of

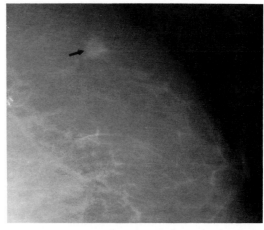

Figure 33–25. Use of mammography in the decision to do simple mastectomy. This 73-year-old woman presented with a clinically diagnosed carcinoma in the opposite breast. The nonpalpable carcinoma of this breast would be difficult to find at surgery in such a large breast, and the patient was not a good surgical risk. Following radical mastectomy for the clinically known carcinoma, a simple mastectomy was done on this breast, proving the presence of a simultaneous second breast carcinoma.

carcinoma of the breast in such places would be markedly reduced by the use of mammograms.

3. Mammography may be considered as the sole basis for radical operation. It must be emphasized that such a procedure is not condoned in our institution. Theoretically, avoiding a biopsy that may cut through cancerous tissue may prevent seeding of cancer cells, but no sensible radiologist would want the diagnosis based simply upon the mammogram until there is uniform accuracy in reading of the films.

4. The advisability of simple mastectomy may be determined by a mammogram. Radiographically, there are no established precancerous lesions. Dependence upon the radiologist for a decision to perform prophylactic simple mastectomy would be dangerous. With keen surgical judgment a mammogram may aid in deciding that a prophylactic mastectomy is the treatment of choice. Such instances include the presence of numerous nodules in the breast and mammographic demonstration of carcinoma in the remaining breast following a radical mastectomy (Fig. 33–25). Also included would be the poor surgical risk, especially when some delay would be anticipated in finding the carcinoma.

The radiologist cannot exclude the presence of early carcinoma when, on the mam-

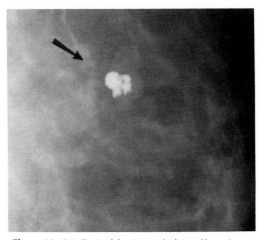

Figure 33–24. Typical benign calcifying fibroadenoma. The 39-year-old female patient presented with a breast lump (arrow) that was clinically suspicious.

mogram, numerous nodules are seen, some of which are irregular. A simple mastectomy may be considered when the pathologist, having studied several nodules and decided that they are either lobular hyperplasia or carcinoma in situ, thinks that no different decision will be made after studying the permanent tissue sections. The simple mastectomy will provide the pathologist with all the glandular tissue for study. In the event that a carcinoma is demonstrated elsewhere in the breast or on permanent sections, additional treatment may still be used.

After a radical mastectomy is completed for carcinoma, if there is a radiographic diagnosis of a nonpalpable carcinoma in the opposite pendulous breast, a simple mastectomy may be considered. Such a decision encompasses the knowledge that the pathologist probably will need the entire breast in order to find the carcinoma. Localization and specimen radiography is preferred.

Mammography has proved of inestimable value in selecting patients as candidates for prophylactic subcutaneous mastectomy and prosthetic implant and in studying the removed glandular tissue by the combined radiographic-pathologic approach.

SURVEYING THE GENERAL POPULATION FOR CARCINOMA OF THE BREAST

Breast cancers demonstrated only by mammography are usually small, with a low incidence of axillary nodes. Clinical Stage I breast cancer has a five-year survival rate of 82 per cent, as opposed to 42 per cent five-year survival with regional involvement, according to the American Cancer Society. Prior to mammography there were 637 patients with breast cancer at Emory University subject to a ten-year study; without axillary lymph node metastases, 89 per cent had five-year survival and 70 per cent had ten-year survival. With axillary metastases, the ten-year survival was only 30 per cent. Breast cancer demonstrated only by mammography and localized by radiography in the specimen for pathologic study has nearly 100 per cent survival if the opposite breast is properly treated.

It is difficult to classify women into truly symptomatic and asymptomatic groups for breast cancer. In 18,688 consecutive patient examinations there were biopsies in 436

TABLE 33–3. Results of Early Mammographic Screening Programs

Study	Year	Patients	No. Cancers	No. Cancers per 1000 Patients
Witten and Thurber	1964	5014	8	1.6
Wolfe	1965	3891	14	4.1
Stevens and Wergen	1966	1223	7	5.8
Permanente	1966	12,245	18	1.5
H.I.P. (Strax) et al.	1967	17,691	40	2.3

women with no complaint, in 65 with a chief complaint of pain, in 1777 with a complaint of mass, and in 357 with a complaint without a mass. Of this group, 222 were biopsied for a clinical mass. The percentages of benign biopsies varied (only 9 per cent) from 67 per cent (clinical mass) to 76 per cent (pain, mass, complaint without mass, no complaint).

Our original reports that mammography was the first procedure that consistently detected breast cancer prior to the appearance of signs and symptoms (Egan, 1963) attracted several visitors who later embarked on screening programs for breast cancer (Table 33–3). These survey programs verified that cancer of the breast could be discovered by mammography. The Wolfe, Witten, and Stevens rates of discovery (Table 33–3) could be considered "rock bottom," since the patients had gone through a cancer detection center and most high-risk and symptomatic patients were excluded, especially those of Stevens. As a group these studies indicate a discovery rate of 2.2 per 1000 compared with the usual rate of 1.0 per 1000 without mammography. In previous tables from the author's series as well as other radiologists, 10 per cent of patients having mammography and breast cancer had nonpalpable breast cancers. Ninety-two per cent of occult cancers at Emory University had no axillary node metastases.

Thus, the rungs of the ladder to a national screening program were being fashioned following a report on our national reproducibility study (Egan, 1963; Clark et al., 1965).

OBSERVATIONS

More encompassing indications for mammography can now be listed as routine.

Specific:
1. Before a decision to biopsy the breast.
2. Breast complaint.
3. Baseline x-ray study by age 30 to 35 years.
4. Questionable pathology before age 30 years.

General (Annual):
5. Age 35 years or older.
6. Personal history of breast cancer.
7. Strong family history of breast cancer.
8. Radiographic ductal hyperplasia.
9. Pathologic changes of atypia.
10. Follow-up of cystic disease.

As very important addition to better treatment planning and earlier diagnosis, mammography promises to be a helpful method for studying the natural history of breast cancer. At present, it is the only means by which a nonpalpable cancer can be demonstrated in the intact breast. This provides our only opportunity to study in vivo the events leading to the production of breast cancer, by noting at first retrospectively, then prospectively, subtle local changes (e.g., altered architecture) that proceed into a recognizable cancer. Similarly, borderline calcifications may be observed through various stages during which an associated mass of carcinoma developed that is still nonpalpable.

In 1980 a select body of oncologists, radiologists, surgeons, epidemiologists, physicians, and biostatisticians representing the National Cancer Institute responded to our proposed cooperative, national, rigidly controlled clinical program to determine the value of screening patients under age 50 years for breast cancer. Such a program had already established that mammography was a very valuable screening modality in those over age 50. This scientific body concluded that such a clinical controlled screening program was not needed in the under-50 age group. A sufficient body of scientific data already existed which determined that mammography was acceptable for breast cancer screening in those under age 50. This was quite an admission to gain from that august body.

Despite all the written and spoken words to the contrary, by far the most essential part of mammography is the radiograph of good technical detail. At a recent meeting of mammographers, representing the widest accumulated experience in the United States, there was unanimity in the following conclusions.

1. Alteration or substitution of any of the outlined technical conditions for mammography invariably results in loss of radiographic detail.

2. Each student beginning mammography should adhere strictly to those technical conditions and gain wide experience in what a satisfactory mammogram looks like. Only then may he vary the conditions if he so desires, as he is qualified to weigh the loss of radiographic detail against possible gains in other areas.

REFERENCES

Egan RL (1963): Reproducibility of mammography. A preliminary report. AJR *90*:356.

Griesbach WA, Eads WS (1966): Experience with screening for breast cancer. Cancer *19*:1548.

Stevens GM, Weigen JF (1966): Mammography survey for breast cancer detection. A 2-year study of 1,223 clinically negative asymptomatic women over 40. Cancer *19*:51.

Strax P, Venet L, Shapiro S, Gross S (1967): Mammography and clinical examination in mass screening for cancer of the breast. Cancer *20*:2184.

Witten DM, Thurber DL (1964): Mammography as a routine screening examination for detecting breast cancer. Am J Roentgenol *92*:14.

Wolfe JN (1965): Mammography as a screening examination in breast cancer. Radiology *84*:703.

Difficulties and Limitations of Mammography

34

BACKGROUND

The most obvious difficulty with mammography is that it is not 100 per cent accurate in the diagnosis of breast diseases, especially cancer at a stage in which the disease is entirely limited to the breast. The greatest source of error is improper radiographic technique; technique is 90 to 95 per cent of the procedure. The next important consideration is the density of the breast as related to that of the lesion. Interpretative error is a difficulty but is judged to be only 5 to 10 per cent.

Mammograms lacking in radiographic detail due to faulty technical factors should not occur. There are no short cuts in setting up the procedure; serious errors follow deliberate or inadvertent substitution of the proper technical factors. In many instances radiologists, without training in the proper x-ray technical factors or in what a good mammogram looks like, and without appreciation of the indications and limitations of the procedure, have been coerced or cajoled into the procedure by their enthusiastic surgical colleagues. The technologist, also lacking in training, fails to understand the necessity of

observation of the precise radiographic technical factors that do not follow the present trend of high kilovoltage, fast films and intensifying screens, and rapid processing.

Interpretative error is not the source of very great difficulty, as all mammographers attach the same significance to each change on the mammogram, hence, we all make the same diagnoses, as well as the same mistakes, for the same exact reasons.

With the use of screen-film receptors, interpretative ability has been lessened to a degree by the lack of recognition of very fine structures, by the introduction of screen-film mottle, and by the reduced latitude of the receptors, making the use of the bright light less helpful.

The comparative diagnostic accuracy of technically good mammography depends almost entirely on two things: the age of the patient and the stage of the disease. The latitude of the technique compensates to a great extent for the wide variability of densities and sizes of breasts. Even with this markedly improved technical quality of mammography, small breasts with a minimum of fat pose problems. Here, calcifications or secondary signs of carcinoma must be present to prevent a false negative diagnosis.

FALSE POSITIVE DIAGNOSES

Numerically, the false positive, a benign process interpreted as carcinoma, is the greatest source of error (Figs. 34–1 to 34–3). Such lesions are usually infected cysts, abscesses, fibrosis, fat necrosis, extra-abdominal desmoids, chronic inflammatory processes, or sclerosing adenosis and indurative

614

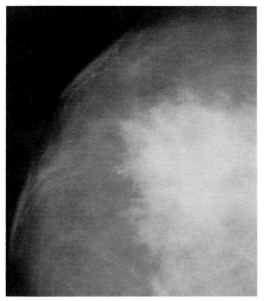

Figure 34–1. Mammographic error of interpretation. This infected cyst produced an irregular 2 × 2.5 cm mass, adjacent skin changes of flattening and thickening, and increased vascularity. Clinically the mass was 4 × 5 cm, and the breast presented with skin changes associated with carcinoma. The patient, a 52-year-old woman, had noted a painful lump in her breast for seven or eight days.

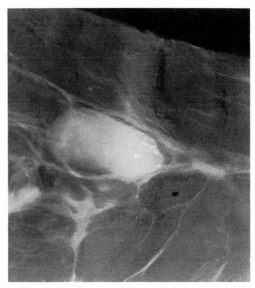

Figure 34–2. Calcified fibroadenoma interpreted as cancer on the mammogram. A 62-year-old woman, four years previously having had a right mastectomy for carcinoma, presented with a hard mass in the left axilla; clinically metastasis. Mammography: 1 × 1.5 cm lobulated circumscribed carcinoma containing fine stippled calcification. Pathology (whole-organ specimen): metastasis to left axilla from right breast; left breast, fibroadenoma (shown).

processes or mastopathies. This 10 per cent error is of little concern to the surgeon, as it does not represent lack of treatment of cancer; also, he is accustomed to submitting three to ten breasts to biopsy in order to demonstrate one cancer.

FALSE NEGATIVE DIAGNOSES

The false negative—carcinoma labeled benign—is the greatest source of concern to the clinician and radiologist. Such errors are usually the result of:

Figure 34–3. Fibroadenoma with marked increase in vascularity. A 58-year-old woman with a breast lump; no family history. Mammography: lobulated, homogeneous 1.8 × 2.2 cm mass, surrounding rim of fat, no calcification, with marked increase in vascularity. Pathology: fibroadenoma. No malignancy in five years of follow-up.

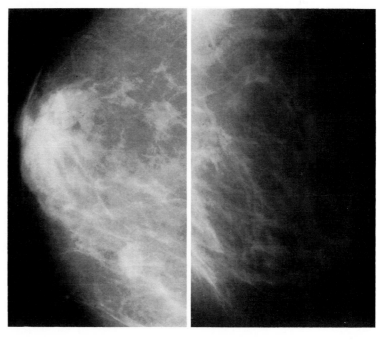

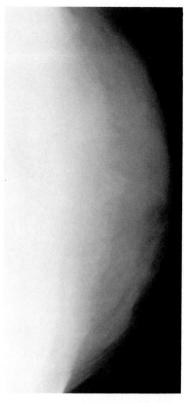

Figure 34–4. Mammographic error of interpretation. There was a 1.5 × 2 cm invasive ductal carcinoma in this breast of a 49-year-old woman who had observed a lump for five weeks. In such a dense breast calcification, encroachment on the subcutaneous adipose tissue or secondary changes would alert the radiologist. No such changes were evident; the carcinoma was overlooked.

1. A lesion that is too small to produce a recognizable density or that is the same density as the surrounding tissues (Figs. 34–4 and 34–5).

2. A carcinoma that is discounted as part of a benign process (Figs. 34–6 to 34–9).

3. A carcinoma that is partially or completely obscured by a benign process (Fig. 34–10).

4. A carcinoma, usually in the extreme periphery of the breast medially or just below the clavicle, that is not projected onto the mammogram (Fig. 34–11).

It then is immediately apparent that with the acceptable mammograms the degree of fatty infiltration of the breast is the most crucial factor in accuracy of diagnosis. The most reliable single index, although exceptions do occur, in predicting the overall accuracy of mammography, is the age of the patient. The first part of our mammography report is an indication of the relative amounts of fat and fibroglandular tissue in the breast, telling the clinician what the degree of reliability of the procedure is in this particular patient.

The uninitiated radiologist has been led in many instances to suspect that almost any fleck of calcification seen in the breast is associated with carcinoma. This is not so, and it is hoped that sufficient examples of calcification in both benign and malignant diseases have been presented to clarify this point. At times, errors will certainly occur in

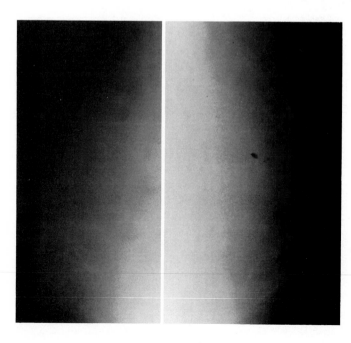

Figure 34–5. Carcinoma missed in young dense breast. A 35-year-old woman with persistent pain in LIQ of the right breast; no family history; gravida 2, para 2; no nursing. Clinically: normal breasts. Mammography: almost homogeneously dense breasts; technically good mammograms could not be obtained. The difference in density was thought to be technical. One year later she noted a lump in the area of pain, but there was no clinical dominant nodule; no mammograms. Five months later a 2 cm mass was palpable with overlying skin flattening. Pathology: duct carcinoma with scirrhous element. Modified radical mastectomy; 0 of 16 axillary lymph nodes positive. Seven years later there was no evidence of disease.

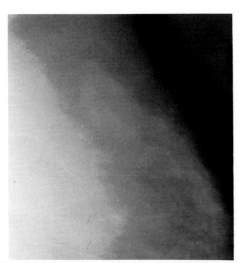

Figure 34–6. Mammographic error of intrepretation. Clinically suspicious 2 cm nodule is seen in the breast of a 43-year-old woman who had a breast lump for four weeks. The mass proved to be a circumscribed carcinoma. This obvious dominant nodule is partially obscured by background fibrocystic disease. Prominent ducts are present; the lesion was diagnosed as probably benign. This may well represent an error of commission.

interpretation of the significance of certain calcifications (Fig. 34–12).

INTERPRETATIVE ERRORS

In every diagnostic medical procedure, errors are encountered. This is true of mammography. On one end of the scale is the unequivocally normal breast, and on the other end is the precise histologic diagnosis of a breast lesion. The intervening gray area existing in the diagnosis of a breast lesion by radiography represents the error in mammography (Figs. 34–13 to 34–15). This area is relatively small, compared with the accuracy of radiographic diagnosis in other procedures, but this is the area of concentration. It is here that improvement in results may be expected.

BENIGN VS MALIGNANT PROCESSES

The list of benign lesions presenting a malignant pattern on mammography is long. In each instance the radiologist must err in a false positive manner so that a carcinoma will not be allowed to progress. This was adamantly pointed out in consideration of clustered calcifications not associated with a mass. The odds against predicting which area of fat necrosis is noncancerous is 100 to 1 (Figs. 34–16 and 34–17); similar odds exist with inflammatory processes and particularly abscesses (Fig. 34–18). A hematoma, such as in Figure 34–19, must be considered malignant, especially with very strong sonographic indications. Mirror-image lesions in both breasts that arouse suspicion must be treated

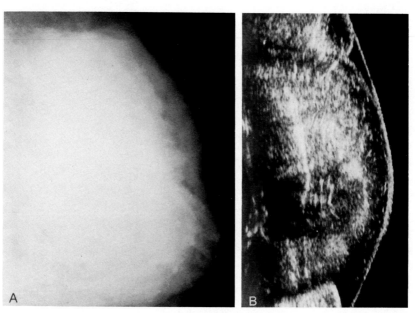

Figure 34–7. Sonography helps confirm diagnosis. A 54-year-old woman with a suspicious mass in the breast. *A,* Mammography: 4 × 5 cm poorly defined mass, upper central breast, containing punctate calcifications. *B,* Sonography: demarcated irregular hypoechoic mass with nonhomogeneous internal echoes; attenuation. Pathology: moderately differentiated duct carcinoma with marked lymphatic invasion. Modified radical mastectomy; metastases to an intramuscular lymph node and to 2 of 13 axillary lymph nodes.

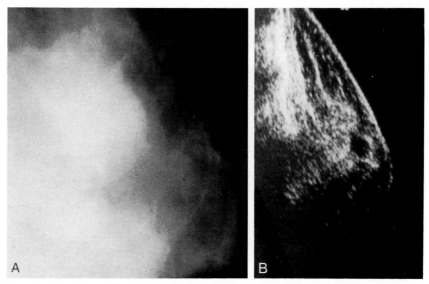

Figure 34–8. Sonography confused diagnosis. A 50-year-old woman seen for checkup following a left mastectomy six years before. *A*, Mammography: 9 × 12 mm moderately invasive carcinoma medially below the level of the nipple against nodular fibrocystic disease. *B*, Sonography: cysts demonstrated in three frames. The irregular density with a few internal echoes without increased through-transmission almost passed as a cyst instead of the carcinoma. Pathology: duct carcinoma, minimal fibrosis. Modified radical mastectomy; all 19 axillary lymph nodes free of tumor. The patient was alive and well two years later.

equally. One should not biopsy the worse of the two, and, if it is benign, ignore the other lesion.

One of the growing challenges to the clinician, radiologist, and pathologist is consideration of the "premalignant" breast (Fig. 34–20).

OBSERVATIONS

In the elderly the dominant nodule, regardless of its smooth borders and at times

a fat line, should be regarded with extreme suspicion.

Additional mammographic criteria are needed for dominant nodules with smooth borders for all age groups. Of 315 consecutive

Text continued on page 623

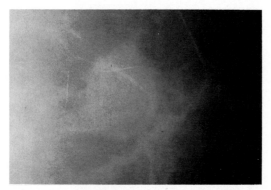

Figure 34–9. Mass of carcinoma that was more benign in appearance. A 47-year-old woman with a clinically suspicious mass; mother had breast cancer. Mammography: 1.5 × 1.7 cm homogeneous circumscribed mass; no secondary changes but without a rim of surrounding fat. Pathology: duct carcinoma; all nodes negative; modified radical mastectomy. The patient was free of disease 11 years later.

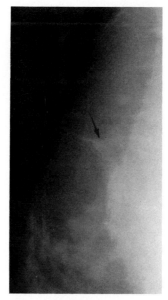

Figure 34–10. Mammographic error of interpretation. This 62-year-old woman had a 1 cm intraductal carcinoma with focal invasion. She had noted a lump for seven weeks that clinically was a 2 × 2.5 cm dominant nodule, probably benign. On the mammograms a 1 cm nodule (arrow) was identified; it was partially obscured by fibrocystic disease and was interpreted as benign.

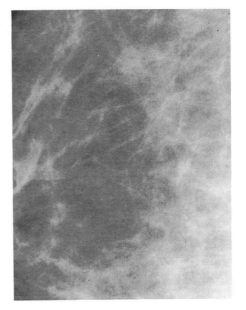

Figure 34–11. Far lateral carcinoma. A 54-year-old woman with a breast lump for two weeks; clinically carcinoma. Mammography: 1.2 cm highly invasive carcinoma seen only on severely rotated cranio-caudad view. Pathology: duct carcinoma with fibrosis. Modified radical mastectomy; 1 of 20 axillary lymph nodes with metastasis. The patient was alive and well nine years later.

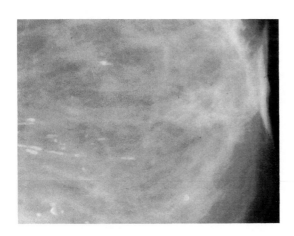

Figure 34–12. Borderline calcification. Just beneath the areola there is a 1 cm area of faint stippled calcification in the breast of a 67-year-old woman with retracted nipple; clinically, it is a benign process. There is obviously present evidence of old secretory disease, subareolar fibrosis, nipple and areolar changes, and, on the original study, increased vascularity. The radiologist is readily led to favor carcinoma; in this case it was subareolar fibrosis.

Figure 34–13. Circumscribed carcinoma in breast. The patient, a 58-year-old woman, had noted a lump in her breast for eight months. Clinically, this was a 4 × 6 cm carcinoma; mammographically, a 4 cm carcinoma. Histopathologic study showed a 4 cm infiltating duct carcinoma with metastasis to multiple axillary lymph nodes.

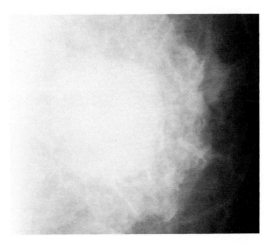

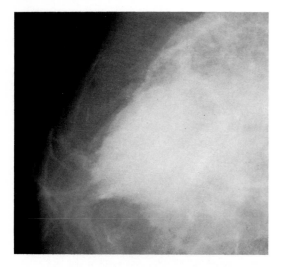

Figure 34–14. Blue-domed cyst. A 3.5 × 4.5 cm blue-domed cyst is shown in a 54-year-old woman who had a lump in her breast for seven weeks. Clinically, this was thought to be a 4 × 5 cm carcinoma; mammographically, a 3.5 × 4.5 cm carcinoma. Ill-defined portions of the periphery, increased vascularity, and straightening and prominence of the ducts tended toward the diagnosis. Cyst was proved by biopsy.

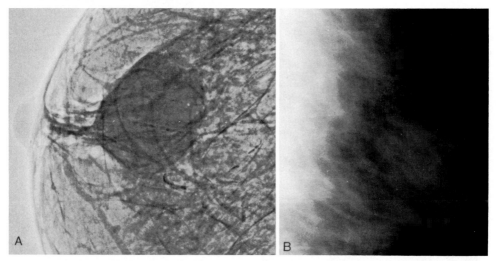

Figure 34–15. Clinically confusing cyst. A 66-year-old woman with a breast lump for five days. *A*, Xeroradiography: Despite the age of the patient, the appearance is that of a cyst. Aspiration was carried out, but some residual thickening remained in the area. Pathology on the fluid was negative for tumor cells. *B*, Mammography was then done; no abnormality except for ductal hyperplasia. No recurrence on follow-up.

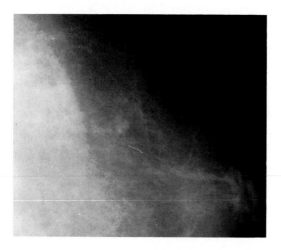

Figure 34–16. Fat necrosis vs carcinoma. A 63-year-old woman seen for baseline study. Mammography: asymmetric density in upper breast, with slight increase in vascularity. Pathology: fat necrosis. After mammograms she was asked about trauma, but nothing specific was revealed.

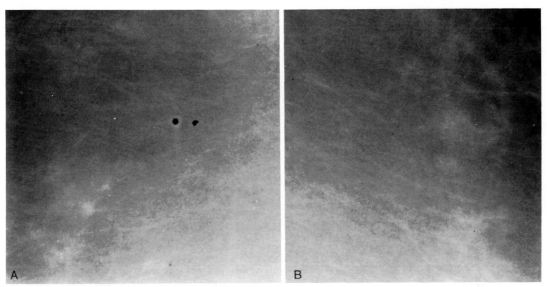

Figure 34–17. Biopsy for fat necrosis; carcinoma found. A 70-year-old woman had a recent aspiration attempt on the right breast. Mammography: 4 × 6 mm density containing several flecks of calcification (*B*); localized area of density containing flecks of calcification (*A*). The areas were localized and bilateral biopsies carried out. Pathology: fat necrosis with a nearby focus of intraductal and duct carcinoma (*B*); fibrocystic disease and sclerosing adenosis (*A*). Right modified radical mastectomy; no residual tumor; all 21 axillary lymph nodes free of tumor. The patient was free of disease three years later.

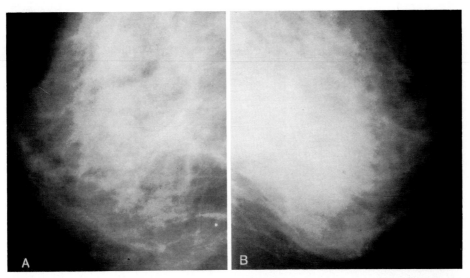

Figure 34–18. A and B, Inflammation vs malignancy. A 45-year-old woman with several masses in the left breast for three weeks. Mammography: approximately 2 × 2.5 cm ill-defined density, left lower breast; increased vascularity; surrounding breast architectural changes; most likely carcinoma. With a lesion of this size, a carcinoma should cause more secondary changes. An inflammatory process cannot be excluded. Pathology: acute mammary duct ectasia associated with chronic inflammation, foreign body giant cells, histiocytic infiltration; ductal hyperplasia. The lesion responded to conservative therapy.

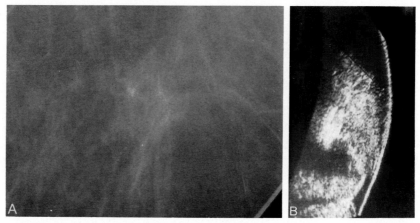

Figure 34–19. Hematoma presenting as carcinoma. A 62-year-old woman with a mass and overlying skin dimpling. *A,* Mammography: 1.5 × 2.2 cm dense, poorly defined mass not present 21 months before; poorly defined carcinoma. *B,* Sonography: irregular, hypoechoic area with marked shadowing; carcinoma. Pathology: organizing hematoma with red cells and fibrosis. No history of trauma elicited.

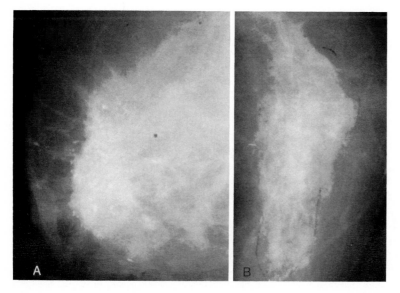

Figure 34–20. What to do for a "premalignant" breast? A 58-year-old woman with a suspicious right breast mass. Mammography: Within a 6 cm comedocarcinoma was a 1.5 × 2.5 cm moderately invasive duct carcinoma; bilateral ductal hyperplasia. Pathology: comedo, duct, mucoid, and papillary forms of carcinoma with areas of productive fibrosis (*A*); florid and sclerosing adenosis, complete range of proliferative activity from hyperplasia to atypia (*B*): a premalignant breast.

breast cancers, 237 produced a nodule on the mammogram. Of the 237, 18 of the masses were smoothly rounded. From the mammograms, five were labeled cancer, four suspicious, and nine benign; clinically there were four cancers, three suspicious lesions, and 11 benign lesions. Ages ranged from 25 to 78 years; eight were under and ten were over age 50 years.

Provisions must be made for indeterminate studies; this is just as necessary for the radiologist as for the pathologist. The radiologist, even with the best technical quality in the ideal subject, cannot be expected to approach the accuracy of the pathologist in the diagnosis of breast lesions. It is only by providing for the recognition of these indeterminate studies, by the radiologist and clinician, that mammography will be fully utilized.

Although the most detailed mammograms will not be obtained of the young adult and lactating breasts (and in many very dense breasts purposely included throughout) and although carcinoma is seen less frequently in these groups, such a high percentage of satisfactory studies is obtained that there should be no hesitation in performing mammography on these patients. This is particularly so when we realize that mammograms, even in this type of breast, may clearly depict signs of carcinoma before they can be appreciated clinically.

The unfortunate and unforgettable errors in mammography have not in a large sense detracted from the procedure. They have brought about the realization that there must be honest and strenuous efforts on the part of the referring physician, surgeon, radiologist, and pathologist to develop precise means of communication with each other. They have promoted appreciation of the contribution of each specialty for better treatment of the breast cancer patient. Furthermore, as each adds his contribution to the diagnostic problem, much of the gray area in the approach of each specialist is erased.

Data on Breast Cancer

35

BACKGROUND

General

Unless otherwise specified, reference to breast data in this volume refers specifically to that obtained on women referred for mammography from the Emory University Clinic. This includes all consecutive patients sent for mammography for a breast problem, as routine follow-up study, as a baseline screening examination, or as part of a clinical work-up. Treatment was carried out by members of the Winship Clinic, the oncologic clinic of Emory University Clinic.

A separate, unique, independent breast-imaging clinic had been established by the author to gather data on mammography, related cancer detection, and diagnostic procedures; particularly to improve detection of breast cancer; and to establish a high-risk breast cancer population. Preliminary discussions had been carried out with the Emory Section of Biostatistics and Computer Center to evaluate the feasibility of such a new approach.

In planning this study in 1962, Emory University was chosen: (1) Emory's Oncologic Clinic had been in existence since 1938; (2) there was strong interest in breast diseases by both surgeons and pathologists; and (3) an unusual population was available, with

98 per cent of the patients being white, 84 per cent Protestant, and nearly 100 per cent at higher socioeconomic levels—a group with interest in preventive medicine and one that provided good follow-up. Most of the patients had been examined by usually two, or possibly three, physicians prior to referral, and most obviously suspicious breast lumps had been removed. A limited number of progressive and innovative oncologic surgeons treated the women. Modified radical mastectomy was the choice of surgical procedures, an unusually high percentage of the cancers at that time being histologically Stage 0 and Stage I. Almost all the breast surgical pathology was under the direction of one pathologist, with only three being primarily involved over the period of this study. Referring physicians were cooperative in providing follow-up on patients not routinely returning to the clinic.

Almost all mammographic recorded reports were by the author, made without knowledge of clinical findings so that the contribution of mammography could be assessed. Mammography technologists were selected for maturity, interest in breast diseases, and dedication to helping the breast cancer patient. All were provided one year to learn about breast diseases, the technique of mammography and breast examination, and how to deal with the frightened women. Intra- and interobservation were evaluated periodically, being carried out with the technologists both in mammographic interpretation and in history taking.

The clinic physicians completed the data forms in their offices. The radiologic technologists compiled the history forms. The radiologist independently recorded radiographic findings; afterward he may have used other available information in reaching a radiologic opinion but without ever changing his coded analysis.

It had been postulated that age and sex were overwhelming epidemiologic factors in breast cancer that might be augmented by other indicators, each being weak when used alone but additive when used in combination or in tandem. But selection of breast cancer indicators posed many problems. Indicators were selected as being aptly associated with breast cancer. They were gathered from papers by leading oncologists of the world and replies to a personal invitation to over 200 oncologists in the United States who were interested in breast cancer. The latter were asked to share new thoughts or personal ideas, even if too underdeveloped for publication. Imperfect as our gleanings from widespread opinions were, we nevertheless became operational, with retrieval of data possible from 1963.

The data accession program was thoroughly planned at Emory University and meticulously set into operation for complete prospective data. Besides the able planning force, two full-time biostatisticians were an integral part of the Mammography Section, where they had their offices, computer terminals, programmers, and research assistants.

Additional assistance was provided for analysis and follow-up information of our patients through the Emory University Clinic Tumor Registry, Emory University Tumor Registry, Emory Hospital and Clinic records, the American Cancer Society, the Atlanta Cancer Surveillance Center (SEER), Georgia Department of Human Resources, Georgia Tumor Registry Association, and the many physicians in the metropolitan Atlanta area.

Lobular carcinoma in situ, metastatic cancer, proven cancer prior to the first visit, or inoperable advanced cancers are not included in our general discussions of breast cancer. Certain cases have been recalled for specific analyses, e.g., Chapter 26 on inflammatory breast carcinoma.

Cyst Aspiration

In the early 1960s, aspiration of cysts of the breast was not a common practice even by oncologic surgeons. As the practice increased more cyst fluid contents were sent for cytologic evaluation. Frequently, suspicious reports appeared on the charts of patients whose cyst's contents had been guaiac-negative and whose mass had completely disappeared. The surgeon was then obligated to obtain an open biopsy breast tissue specimen for histopathologic evaluation. These invariably showed no abnormality so the practices of cytologic studies were abandoned unless the fluid was guaiac-positive. There was no attempt to aspirate multiple cysts, as the possibility of one not being completely aspirated would necessitate a biopsy. Many cysts on mammography were not palpable; many more were apparent on sonography. A number of cysts were aspirated at different times from the same breast, or both breasts—so often that poor records were available. Such inconsistent and unreliable practices led to the abandonment of cyst aspiration in the data base. With no cytologist at Emory University encouraging aspiration tissue biopsies, there was only rare use of this method. It usually was reserved for advanced and inoperable breast lesions to avoid open biopsy.

EMORY UNIVERSITY DATA

Reference Base

During the 20-year period from 1963 to 1982 over 27,000 women were referred from the Emory University Clinic for various numbers of combined clinical and mammographic examinations of the breast (Table 35–1). During that period, 2209 primary operable breast cancers had their primary treatment at Emory University and were studied by the Emory University Pathology Department. The age distribution of the patients was as follows: 26.7 per cent were 35 years or younger; 39.3 per cent were age 36 to 50 years; 24.4 per cent were age 51 to 65 years; and 9.5 per cent were over age 65 years. An almost equal percentage of the women in each age group had breast biopsies, except that older women did have some increase in biopsy rate. Yet, nearly 40 per cent of the biopsies under age 35 years were for fibroadenoma, while 60 per cent of the biopsies in women over age 65 years were for cancer (Table 35–2).

Number of pregnancies, deliveries, periods of nursing, or previous episodes of breast disease indicated no increased risk for breast cancer (Tables 35–3 and 35–4). History of breast cancer in the mother, grandmothers, and aunts had no significant effect. However, one sister with breast cancer doubled the risk and two sisters tripled the risk. The risk of families with numerous breast cancers is not applicable to the general population; these families occur so infrequently.

TABLE 35–1. Patients Studied, Biopsies, and Results (Emory University)

Age (Yrs.)	Patients No.	Patients %	Examinations No.	Examinations %	Biopsies No.	Biopsies %	Benign Biopsies	Malignant Biopsies No.	Malignant Biopsies %
0–20	525	1.9	1021	1.7	206	2.6	206	2	0.1
21–30	4132	15.0	7272	12.4	1096	13.6	1062	55	2.5
31–35	2684	9.8	5685	9.7	619	7.7	593	92	4.2
36–40	3320	12.1	7515	12.8	784	9.7	709	116	5.3
41–45	3838	14.0	8987	15.3	1150	14.3	889	231	10.5
46–50	3608	13.2	8519	14.5	1042	12.9	739	271	12.3
51–55	2638	9.6	6161	10.5	865	10.7	611	310	14.0
56–60	2378	8.7	4770	8.1	745	9.2	339	282	12.8
61–65	1689	6.1	3402	5.8	521	6.5	285	276	12.4
66–70	1337	4.7	2686	4.6	360	4.5	210	182	8.2
71–75	613	2.2	1233	2.1	245	3.0	69	149	6.7
76–80	411	1.5	820	1.4	268	3.3	82	157	7.1
81–90	278	1.0	558	1.0	135	1.7	49	72	3.3
>90	21	0.08	26	0.04	17	0.2	1	14	0.6
Total	27,472	100.0	58,655	100.0	8053	100.0	5844	2209	100.0

TABLE 35–2. Examinations, Biopsies, and Results During 2209 Primary Operable Breast Cancers (Emory University)

Age (Yrs.)	No. Exams	No. Biopsies*	Per Cent Biopsy	No. Cancer	Per Cent Exams Cancer	Per Cent Biopsy Cancer	Per Cent Biopsy Fibroadenoma
≤35	13,978	1921	13.7	60	0.42	3.17	38.77
36–50	25,021	2976	11.9	639	*2.55	21.47	13.84
51–65	14,333	2131	14.9	896	6.25	42.05	3.57
>65	5,323	1025	19.3	614	11.53	59.90	2.46
Total	58,655	8053	13.7	2209	3.77	27.43	15.60

*Excludes cyst aspiration.

TABLE 35–3. Number of Pregnancies of Emory University Patients, With Rates of Biopsy and Pathology

Number of Pregnancies	Per Cent of Total Patients	Per Cent Benign, Pregnancies	Per Cent Fibroadenoma, Pregnancies	Per Cent Cancer, Pregnancies
None	21.4	8.1	4.1	3.5
1	15.6	8.5	1.1	4.0
2	23.9	8.2	1.8	3.8
3	18.9	7.0	1.9	3.5
4	10.3	7.8	2.0	4.5
≥5	9.9	6.7	1.0	3.4

TABLE 35–4. Nursing of Emory University Patients, With Rates of Biopsy and Pathology

Number Months Nursing	Per Cent of Total Patients	Per Cent Benign, Nursing	Per Cent Fibroadenoma, Nursing	Per Cent Cancer, Nursing
None	53.4	8.2	2.7	3.1
1	7.0	9.3	2.1	2.9
2–3	7.9	6.6	2.0	4.2
4–6	8.0	6.8	1.3	2.7
7–10	7.2	7.4	1.0	3.6
11–15	5.5	7.0	2.1	4.2
16–20	3.8	10.0	1.5	6.9
21–30	3.5	7.0	0.4	6.1
31–40	1.7	4.3	0.0	11.1
41–50	0.9	3.3	0.0	19.7
51–60	0.4	11.1	0.0	3.7
61–99	0.7	10.0	2.0	6.0

Women with surgical menopause had only 50 per cent the incidence of breast cancer as those with natural menopause. The 50 per cent of the women who were premenopausal had only 21 per cent of the cancers, while the 43 per cent who were postmenopausal had 74 per cent of the cancers. The women themselves discovered 80 per cent of their breast cancers. Moderate or severe pain occurred in 41 per cent of the women with cancer. Clinical tenderness was noted in 16 per cent of the cancer patients but also was present in 17 per cent of all the breasts.

Sixty-three per cent of cancers occurred in clinically soft breasts, representing 43 per cent of the total population, while 14 per cent of the cancers occurred in x-ray dense breasts, or 34 per cent of the total population. Soft and radiolucent breasts are at the highest risk for cancer, usually representing physiologically older breasts. X-ray ductal hyperplasia had the same risk as atrophic (fatty) breasts (Table 35–5). Bloody nipple discharge from a single duct occurred in 1.3 per cent

of the women but was associated with cancer in only 0.01 per cent of the patients. Clinical multiple nodules were present in less than 2 per cent of the cancers. Cancers were well defined (38 per cent) and firm (14.2 per cent) (Table 35–6). Fibroadenomata were also firm. A hard mass was cancer nearly 50 per cent of the time. Soft masses were produced by 13.8 of the cancers and cystic masses 3.1 per cent of the time. Breast size was poorly related to the incidence of breast cancer (Table 35–7).

In 18 per cent of the cancers there was only a thickening, a nonspecific finding; this was present in 44 per cent of the breasts without cancer. On x-ray, 14 per cent of the cancers had only an increased density, a finding noted in only 2.5 per cent of the patients but a significant finding when reported by the radiologist Altered architecture was even more specific by x-ray, as it was reported in only 0.9 per cent of the breasts but represented 11 per cent of the cancers.

Clinically 86 per cent of the breasts harboring a cancer had some finding, yet only 73 per cent strongly enough for staging by oncologic surgeons steeped in the tradition of staging cancers. Since thickening, when present, clinically involved the UOQ 87 per cent of the time and over 50 per cent of the cancers were in the UOQ (Table 35–8), it is difficult to separate the two.

Ninety-one per cent of the cancers were coded malignant by the radiologist (Table 35–9), exclusive of delayed diagnoses, with 66 per cent being unequivocally coded. This compared with 47 per cent coded as definite cancer by clinical examination. The detection of the 139 cancers in women under the age of 35 years is evaluated with difficulty. This

TABLE 35–5. Radiographic Parenchymal Patterns in Association With 27,472 Patients With 2209 Primary Operable Breast Cancers (Emory University)

Parenchymal Pattern	Per Cent of Patients	Per Cent of Cancers
Fatty	16.1	30.2
Glandular	42.8	22.5
Homogeneously dense	7.1	4.2
Coarsely nodular	20.3	14.5
Ductal hyperplasia		
Fatty	3.8	12.5
Dense	6.8	9.9
Finely nodular	3.1	6.2
Total	100.0	100.0

TABLE 35–6. Clinical Masses Occurring in 23.9 Per Cent of Emory University Patients, With Type, Frequency, and Pathology

Type Mass	Total Masses (%)	Benign With Each Mass Type (%)	Fibroadenoma With Each Mass Type (%)	Cancer With Each Mass Type (%)
Soft	7.8	22.3	3.8	13.8
Firm	67.7	22.7	11.2	14.2
Cystic	17.7	9.8	2.4	3.1
Hard	6.8	10.5	7.0	49.1

TABLE 35–7. Breast Size, Biopsies, and Primary Operable Cancers in 27,472 Emory University Patients

Breast Size	Total Breasts (%)	Benign Biopsied This Size (%)	Fibroadenoma This Size (%)	Cancer This Size (%)
Very small	1.0	7.7	3.1	3.1
Small	18.1	10.1	2.1	3.9
Medium	63.3	7.6	3.9	2.5
Large	17.9	7.6	4.4	1.8
Very large	1.7	10.6	1.8	1.8

TABLE 35–8. Location and Follow-Up on 2209 Primary Operable Breast Carcinomas (Emory University)

Location in Breast	Number	Per Cent of Total	Follow-Up in Years				
			<5	5–9	10–14	15–19	≥20
UOQ	1095	49.6	706	253	109	22	5
UIQ	315	14.3	195	85	30	5	0
LOQ	245	11.1	158	52	25	10	0
Central	241	10.9	165	48	23	3	2
LIQ	154	7.0	100	31	15	6	2
Diffuse	127	5.7	100	24	2	1	0
Axillary tail	26	1.2	21	3	1	1	0
Inframammary crease	6	0.3	6	0	0	0	0
Total	2209	100.0	1451	496	205	48	9

TABLE 35–9. Method of Detection and Age at Detection of Breast Cancer During First Examination*

Age (Yrs.)	X-Ray +, PE −	X-Ray +, PE +	X-Ray −, PE +	X-Ray −, PE −
0–30	5	32	8	12
31–34	9	30	19	24
35–39	22	64	12	8
40–44	43	101	25	36
45–49	55	149	32	25
50–54	81	190	23	21
55–59	82	191	6	14
60–69	119	327	31	21
≥70	69	291	21	11
Total	485	1375	177	172
Per Cent	22.0	62.2	8.0	7.8

*On subsequent examinations 172 cancers were detected (Emory University).

PE = physical examination.

is dealt with more objectively in Chapter 30. In those 103 women with proven cancer shortly after the initial mammogram, 27, or 26 per cent, of the cancers were not definite by x-ray. They were frequently coded as a benign dominant nodule, not a cancer code. In approximately one third of these, the cancer per se or secondary signs, if present, were obscured by the dense fibroglandular tissue. Fourteen, or 13.5 per cent, of the cancers were discovered solely by mammography without physical findings. Many of these lesions, and particularly those in other young women referred for mammography, may have been followed clinically, or even had an attempted aspiration, prior to the request for mammography. All these facets simply emphasize the problems of detection of breast cancer in the young woman.

The code system used by both the surgeon and the radiologist was:

0. Normal
1. Benign, no mass
2. Mass, benign
3. Mass, probably benign
4. Mass, probably malignant
5. Malignant
6. Secondary signs of cancer

For the radiologist, 0 to 2 were no cancer, and 3 to 6 were cancer. For the surgeon, 0 to 1 were no cancer, and 3 to 6 were cancer. The surgeon was allowed six weeks to evaluate a mass, benign (#2): If no biopsy, then it was no cancer; if biopsy was indicated, it could be reclassified.

Of 1844 primary operable breast cancers, 79.3 per cent were free of axillary lymph node metastasis or had metastasis to three or fewer low axillary lymph nodes. In the treatment of 2209 cancers a number did not have axillary lymph node evaluation, since the lesions were in situ or were small, less aggressive tumors. However, 381, or 17.2 per cent, of the cancers had metastasis to more than three low axillary lymph nodes or had a higher level involvement (Table 35–10). We estimate from these data that approximately 82.5 per cent of the primary operable breast cancers at Emory University were histologically Stage 0 or Stage I lesions.

The histologic types of cancers occurring in the 2209 primary operable cancers are shown in Table 35–11. The multiple histologic cancer types in the same breast represent a minimal estimate of the actual occurrence, as whole-organ studies were not done. However, following our whole-organ study from 1965 through 1969 the pathologists became more acutely aware of the possibility of multiple types of cancer in the same breast and made additional efforts to demonstrate them on routine studies. In situ carcinomas were listed only if they were the only histologic type present or if they occurred with some type other than that of their histologic infiltrative component. Multiple tumors in the same breast interfere with clear-cut evaluation of prognosis associated with each individual histologic type of tumor.

Of the total patients, 5.6 per cent reported contusion, while 8.7 per cent with cancer had noted contusion. Twenty per cent of the total

TABLE 35–10. Age at Cancer Detection and Presence of Axillary Lymph Node Metastasis From 2209 Primary Operable Breast Cancers With Sufficient Operative Tissue for Satisfactory Study (Emory University)

Age (Yrs.)	Positive Axillary Lymph Nodes					
	None	≤3, Low	≥3, Low	Low, Mid	All Levels	Total
0–29	24	6	0	3	6	39
30–34	32	10	0	14	10	66
35–39	57	18	1	10	7	93
40–44	120	27	2	22	7	178
45–49	157	33	3	22	21	236
50–54	159	37	4	21	31	252
55–59	155	43	7	28	27	260
60–69	286	55	7	39	31	418
70	215	29	5	25	28	302
Total	1205	258	29	184	168	1844*

*365 axillae not examined pathologically, e.g., in situ, lumpectomy, biopsy only.

TABLE 35–11. Primary Operable Breast Cancers Occurring Singly or With One or Two Other Histologic Types

Type Cancer	Total	Single	Double	Triple
ID comedo	32	32	0	0
ID solid duct	156	97	58	1
ID papillary	48	48	0	0
LCIS	133	55	73	51
Comedocarcinoma	234	213	21	0
Duct	861	794	62	5
Lobular	112	68	42	2
Scirrhous	430	380	49	1
Tubular	16	15	1	0
Papillary	145	127	18	0
Med/no lymph stroma	27	16	1	0
Metaplastic	4	4	0	0
Apocrine	9	9	0	0
Med/lymph stroma	68	48	17	3
Intracystic papillary	19	5	13	1
Mucinous	66	18	44	4
Carcinoid	2	2	0	0
Anaplastic	3	3	0	0
Paget's/mass	17	15	2	0
Paget's/no mass	25	24	1	0
Sarcoma	8	6	1	1
Lymphoma	4	4	0	0
Other	8	5	3	0
Total	2427	1998	406	23
Cases	—	1998	203	8
Total cases 2209				

patients had used the contraceptive pill, while 5.7 per cent with cancer had used the pill. Delays of less than seven days occurred with 23 per cent of the women with cancer, 7 to 30 days' delay by 34.7 per cent, one to two months' delay by 32.4 per cent, and more than 12 months' delay by 9.9 per cent. There was no clinical lesion associated with 26.3 per cent of the cancers, and 24.8 per cent of the cancer patients had no mass lesion by x-ray.

In 1977 we made available all our Emory University data to any interested colleagues in the United States and many places in the world. These efforts of data gathering had been partially funded by the Cancer Control Program, USPHS, a tax-supported federal agency. The data were presented in three volumes—two volumes listing raw data and one volume consisting of several hundred contingency tables used by us to consolidate these data.

Supplementary Data

Concurrent with the patients referred from Emory University Clinic and the Winship Clinic there have been women referred for mammography from a large number of phy-sicians in the metropolitan Atlanta area. These women were evaluated, treated, and/ or followed for their problems in numerous facilities and situations outside Emory University. Although not in our reference data base, they have been sources of clinical trials and training materials and may at times be used as illustrative teaching cases. Follow-up information usually results from correspondence with their primary care physicians. During many years these women constituted more than 50 per cent of the clinical practice in the breast imaging center.

Originally, local radiologists were trained to do most of the mammography. Despite this policy our patient load approached 50 women per day at one point. Women referred from outside Emory University Clinic during the study period were estimated to number 108,000.

A lesser number of women have been referred from the Grady Memorial Hospital, located in downtown Atlanta, which serves as the main teaching hospital for Emory University. These patients, often indigent and of lower socioeconomic levels, provide more advanced breast lesions for teaching purposes but not for data analysis.

A number of cohorts for comparison with

TABLE 35–12. Diagnosis Reported and Coded on 3818 Consecutive Mammograms, M.D. Anderson Hospital, May 1956–May 1962

| Type of Lesion | Total | Coded | | | Clinically Negative* |
		Benign	Negative	Malignant	
Biopsy					
Malignant	728	11	10	707	85
Benign	482	438	0	44	0
No lesion	7	0	7	0	0
No biopsy					
Benign	1437	1437	0	0	—
No lesion	1164	0	1664	0	1664

*Breast normal to palpation.

our younger women in the reference base were gleaned from primarily outside referrals for mammography. It is true that reliance on cooperating physicians had to be made for diagnosis and care. These physicians over the years have been exceedingly cooperative.

From 1973 through 1985 the Breast Imaging Center and the Pathology Department of Emory University participated in the ACS/NCI BCDDP screening program as outlined in Chapter 37. These women provide cases for that chapter but are not an integral part of our reference base. They too are treated primarily throughout the metropolitan Atlanta area.

COMPLEMENTARY DATA

M.D. Anderson Hospital and Tumor Institute

From May 1956 through May 1962, 2352 new patients were admitted to the breast clinic at the University of Texas M.D. Anderson Hospital and Tumor Institute, with a total of 1787 malignant and 565 benign biopsied lesions. During this period 3821 mammograms were performed on women with 728 malignant and 489 benign breast lesions coming to biopsy. No study was excluded for technical reasons. Three patients without

TABLE 35–13. Benign Breast Lesions in 3818 Consecutive Mammograms at M.D. Anderson Hospital With X-Ray Diagnosis and Those Confused With Cancer

Type Lesion	Pathologic Diagnosis	Total	Benign X-Ray Diagnosis	Coded as Malignant
Benign lesions with biopsy	Fibrocystic disease	267	261	6
	Fibroadenoma	86	82	4
	Abscess	45	32	13
	Sclerosing adenosis	21	14	7
	Dilated ducts	6	6	0
	Intraductal papillomata	10	8	2
	Benign fibrosis	10	4	6
	Sebaceous cyst	2	2	0
	Cystosarcoma phylloides	7	7	0
	Scleroderma morphea	2	1	1
	Ectopic breast	1	1	0
	Gynecomastia	9	9	0
	Granulomatous tissue	1	0	1
	Fatty infiltration	1	1	0
	Lipoma	5	5	0
	Fat necrosis	2	1	1
	Apocrine gland hyperplasia	1	0	1
	Granular cell myoblastoma	1	1	0
	Lobular hyperplasia	1	0	1
	Neurofibroma	1	1	0
	Hematoma	1	1	0
	Tuberculosis	2	1	1
	Fibrocystic disease (no biopsy)	1437	1437	0
	Total	1919	1875	44

adequate follow-up were excluded. A breast containing clinically obvious cancer or seen after a diagnosis of cancer was established by biopsy was not studied; the opposite breast was examined under such circumstances.

For objectivity in evaluating the procedure, the radiographic diagnosis was made without benefit of the clinical findings. The diagnosis was designated by a specific code symbol at the time of the initial interpretation so that in review no confusion would arise as to the original conclusion. No provision was made for indeterminate studies.

The pathologists' most recent opinion of the breast biopsy tissue, the mastectomy specimen, or the post-mortem findings was used as the diagnosis in each case. In the absence of biopsy, those lesions diagnosed benign were considered verified by typical radiographic and clinical findings, which remained constant on follow-up. The follow-up period ranged from one month to more than six years.

Table 35–12 tabulates the diagnosis of the 3818 consecutive mammographic studies. In a cancer institution where this series of mammograms was carried out, one should expect a high incidence of malignant disease and an older patient group, in whom mammography is more easily accomplished. Many of the lesions were advanced, as this was the first clinical application of mammography. In many cases x-ray of the obvious cancerous breast was omitted not only because the diagnosis was obvious but also to prevent soiling the film holder with blood or pus oozing from the lesions. Some of these earlier cases were used to illustrate the more severe forms of secondary changes of cancer in discussion of malignant diseases of the breast.

These data emphasize the enormous impact that mammography had on diagnosis and subsequent care of the breast patient. Unfortunately, this was a local phenomenon in an isolated institution, which for the most part excited incredulity in other institutions without such a firsthand experience. The finding of 85 carcinomas, unsuspected clinically and still nonpalpable upon localization by x-ray, was the impetus for wide-ranging thoughts about mass screening and replacement of mutilating surgery with conservation of some breast tissue.

Many of the benign lesions encountered (Table 35–13) still have acquired no further specific radiographic identifying characteristics than those seen on these original studies. The same differential diagnoses with cancer radiographically also persist.

36

Probability of Breast Cancer

BACKGROUND

Establishing the probability of a woman having or likely to develop breast cancer has become important now that it is possible to detect and localize that lesion by mammography a number of years before any clinical evidence is discernible. Placement in a high-

risk breast cancer group can alert that woman to practice BSE, see her family physician, and have periodic mammography. This can be done without unduly alarming that woman.

Light Microscopy

The greatest single probability of the presence of breast cancer is established by diagnosis by light microscopy on permanently fixed and properly stained tissue material. Enhancement by electron microscopy or other supplementary procedures is so seldom used in clinical practice that there is little impact from additional studies. The percentage of precise proper diagnoses as assessed by an individual pathologist is based on his most recent experience and the estimate of his present competence. Malignant tumors from a source outside the breast, lesions such as cystosarcoma phylloides or intracystic papillary tumors that do not have absolute criteria for malignancy, and borderline lesions, especially early intraductal ones, detract from the accuracy of diagnosis. With all necessary tissues (deeper cuts, wider sampling), as many stains as desired, and as much time as needed for study, most pathologists contend a 98 per cent, or higher, accuracy in diagnosis. Other pathologists may think 95 per cent accuracy is the top attainable figure.

Frozen Section

The next greatest probability of breast cancer is associated with a positive frozen-section diagnosis. Here the pathologist expects a lesser degree in accuracy of prediction as to whether a lesion is malignant, with no expectation of pinpointing the source of the malignant cells. An accuracy of 95 per cent may be possible when attempted with breast cancer, but in many instances the diagnosis

633

must be deferred to permanent preparations. A 90 per cent accuracy may be a more workable estimate. In our breast lesions requiring localization, biopsy, and specimen radiography, errors were so frequent and so often impossible to correct owing to loss or mutilation of tissue that our policy is to study only permanently fixed mounts. Diagnosis of breast cancer by cytologic means is practiced sporadically and espoused by select proponents with varying experience; hence, the probability of breast cancer based on this diagnostic approach is difficult to establish.

Mammography

The probability of breast cancer based on mammography is highly variable. A typical spiculated mass with fine stippled calcifications is practically pathognomonic, whereas a cluster of three or four calcifications may be biopsied on the basis of mammography, with an infrequent diagnosis of cancer. Judgment of the accuracy of mammography may be based on a one-time episode (50 per cent of the cancers of the Breast Cancer Detection Demonstration Project (BCDDP) were not detected on the first examination) or follow-up examination, with the last examination being considered in the diagnostic scheme. The quality of the examination based on the type of radiographic receptor, the age of the woman, and the density of the breast as well as the interpretation of vague x-ray reports in review all influence the accuracy of the procedure. Well-trained radiologists practicing good-quality mammography all make the same diagnoses and the same mistakes for the same reasons. These individual radiologists predict the presence of 90 per cent of the prevalent cancers convincingly. With other imaging modalities there are reduced probabilities of breast cancer. From Table 36–1 it can be seen that the relative risk of a positive x-ray examination is 18.7 times that of a normal examination.

Physical Examination

Physical examination is highly variable in predicting the probability of breast cancer. On average, the cancer found on physical examination usually has a poorer prognosis. This, of course, is related to the inability to detect those cancers seen on mammography prior to signs and symptoms. In the BCDDP a positive physical examination resulted in a 52 per cent probability of cancer.

CLINICAL EXAMINATION

Clinical examination of the breast has been the time-honored approach to establish the presence of breast diseases. The decision to biopsy was based on physical findings that increased the probability of breast cancer. Once the decision was made to biopsy the breast, the surgeon's direction for the care of the patient was dependent solely upon the results of the consultation with the pathologist. Until the establishment of clinical mammography in 1956, the probability of detection of a breast cancer with a ten-year salvage was one chance in four, and that by the leading breast centers of the world. Overt signs had to be present and were usually advanced unless there was investigation of some low-risk change, such as nipple discharge or vague clinical complaint.

Emory University

Some abnormality was detected in the first clinical examination of 70.2 per cent of primary operable breast cancers demonstrated at Emory University. Those findings sufficient to be considered suspicious were the ones that usually warranted biopsy. No definite conclusion could be reached as to whether the finding was related to the cancer or to some other area of that breast. This pickup could be considered maximum for

TABLE 36–1. Clinical Examination and Mammography on a Series of 8385 Consecutive Emory University Patients: Epidemiologic, Clinical, Radiographic, and Pathologic Data on 2662 Biopsies and 628 Cancers

	X-Ray – PE –	X-Ray + PE –	X Ray – PE +	X Ray + PE +	Total
No pathology	13,658	166	262	56	14,142
Benign biopsy	1,452	142	354	86	2,034
Cancer	21 (3%)	125 (20%)	50 (8%)	432 (68%)	628

PE = physical examination. Breasts tabulated individually.
+ = Cancer diagnosis; – = no cancer diagnosis.

this group of patients, many with Stage 0 or Stage I tumors. Table 36–1 shows that the relative risk of a positive physical examination is 6.2 times that of a normal examination.

Breast Cancer Detection and Demonstration Project (BCDDP)

Clinical examination was less useful in predicting the probability of breast cancer in a woman's breast in the BCDDP. Only 56 per cent of the cancers were suspected on clinical examination or demonstrated positive findings in one breast. During the first several years of that study the recording forms did not indicate that the clinical findings and cancer were in the same breast. However, 6 per cent of cancers that were missed by x-ray were detected by physical examination.

Observations

Clinical examination alone does not provide the optimal method for establishing sufficiently increased probability of breast cancer for application to the general population. Physical examination, without question, is an absolutely necessary part of the examination of the breast for disease. A noncontributory mammogram should never be used to deter a breast biopsy with a positive clinical finding. Screening for breast cancer has been practiced with physical examination alone and to a lesser extent, in the Health Insurance Program of New York (HIP) study, in which more emphasis was placed on good physical examination than on quality mammography.

EPIDEMIOLOGIC DATA

Single epidemiologic factors are related to a low probability of breast cancer in an individual woman. Yet the epidemiologists have continued their search for that single risk marker for breast cancer without success. Combined epidemiologic factors, or these factors combined with clinical characteristics, fail to select women at risk for breast cancer. Increasing age and female sex (100 female breast cancers per 1 male cancer) have remained the only constant applicable risk markers for breast cancer. Even these strong factors do not provide a hint to the selection of that one female baby girl of 11 born who will develop breast cancer.

Emory University

Our prospective epidemiologic, clinical radiographic, and, when available, pathologic data over nearly 20 years have not provided significant applicable risk markers for breast cancer. Pregnancies, deliveries, nursing, color, race, religion, status of menstruation, hormone exposure, previous breast biopsy for benign disease, and family history add little to the probability of breast cancer except under unusual circumstances. One exception is that 8.5 per cent of naturally postmenopausal women had breast cancer as opposed to 4 per cent of those with surgical menopause, a greater than twofold increase. A mother with breast cancer added no risk to a daughter, but one sister with breast cancer nearly doubled the risk, while two sisters almost tripled the risk. However, the history of two sisters with breast cancer occurred in only 1.4 per cent of the women, hardly applicable to the general population. The risk when the mother and one sister had cancer was highly significant, but this occurred extremely rarely.

Reported

The medical literature is replete with epidemiologic risk factors for breast cancer. In some, as reported by Anderson, on whole families of all females with breast cancer there is an extremely high, almost 100 per cent, probability of breast cancer. Yet these females are extremely few in number. In a general population of women the probability of breast cancer may be increased only by factors of 1.1 to 1.3 times, as suggested by Kelsey (1979): fibrocystic disease, 1.1 times; sister with breast cancer, 1.2 times; and so forth.

ANCILLARY FACTORS

Increased vascularity by infrared photography promised to become a risk marker for breast cancer. In our hands the superficial veins could easily be portrayed by photography, but the test was nonspecific in establishing risk for breast diseases. The experience with vein diameter ratios was similar. Telethermography, then contact thermography, was highly acclaimed as a preselector for mammography and high risk for breast cancer. In practice, thermography proved no more specific than increased vascularity. In the BCDDP its value was deemed so noncontributory that it was discontinued.

RADIOGRAPHIC PARENCHYMAL PATTERNS

Very early in our studies of the breast with high-quality mammography, the hyperplastic process of ductal epithelial hyperplasia was recognized as a frequent companion to breast cancer (see Chapter 16). In 1962 this led us to incorporate in our efforts to collect data on breast cancer 72 possible radiographic descriptive terms of ductal and parenchymal patterns of the breast. No additional pattern suggestive of an increased breast cancer risk was found except in the physiologically older pattern of the breast.

A number of years later Wolfe (1976) adopted one of our descriptive terms of "prominent ducts" for an x-ray pattern of increasing density of breast tissues. For his risk factor to be operative it must be preceded by a normal mammogram and physical examination. Such criteria would remove the probability of an overt cancer developing in a fatty breast. With these criteria we could demonstrate a small increase in developing cancers in dense breasts, but not 37 times as he reported in his two and one-half year study. Our much longer and thorough study showed that after 36 months the incidence of breast cancer reverted to the expected normal incidence. Furthermore, the cancers developing in the dense breast were far advanced compared with those detected in the less dense breasts. Carlile et al. (1985) reported on a four-year study involving four BCDDP on breast parenchymal patterns, all reviewed by Wolfe, and concluded that the increased incidence of breast cancer in dense breasts was due to the masking effect reported by Egan and McSweeney (1979); that no clinical application of breast parenchymal patterns was useful (Wolfe had not recognized ductal hyperplasia); and that after a normal mammogram of fatty breasts, the woman could be better assured that there was little risk of breast cancer.

REGIONAL DISCRIMINANT ANALYSIS

Background

Numerous efforts by oncologists, epidemiologists, biostatisticians, biologists, genet-

icists, radiologists, and pathologists to identify markers for breast cancer risk have been nonproductive. Factors such as cancer in all the close female family members or a mother who had bilateral breast cancer at an early age may be highly predictive but apply to such a small fraction of a per cent of women that they are not useful in large populations. Other factors, such as a mother with breast cancer, may have only a 1.1 times risk that carries a low level of confidence in segregating the women at risk.

Modalities complementary to physical examination, such as thermography, infrared photography, transillumination, ultrasound, and mammography, may aid in demonstration of an occult breast cancer without predictive element of risk.

Since mammography is far superior to all prebiopsy modalities and since it is the standard, it has been widely accepted as a valuable procedure in evaluation of breast abnormalities and as a screening procedure. There is a real problem of cost, personnel, and time in screening large segments of the population with mammography. Identification of those women at increased risk, concentrating mammographic screening efforts on them while reducing its use in women at low risk, would produce a vast reduction in both the theoretical problem of radiation and the real problem of logistics.

Well over $100 million was required for five screenings of 280,000 women in the NCI/ACS BCDDP. Many women never finished all screenings. This number of women represented only approximately 0.6 per cent of the women in the United States over age 40 years. To screen similarly the more than 45 million women in the United States over age 40 years would require $16.1 billion.

Differences in women who have breast cancer or who have signs that are later associated with breast cancer, and differences in serial mammograms before the recognition of clinical cancer, provide a basis for predicting the relative risk of breast cancer.

Systems of statistical techniques, including recently developed stronger and more refined regional discriminant analysis, can assess the relative risk of breast cancer through interaction of various potential risk factors from historical, clinical, and radiologic indicators. This assessment is used on women (1) to determine who has early breast cancer requiring immediate intervention to prevent its becoming life-threatening and (2) to identify those at risk of developing breast cancer.

Patients at higher risk who are referred routinely for clinical and x-ray evaluation of breast problems would receive more frequent concentrated studies, suspicious lesions would receive treatment without delay, and breast biopsies would be more productive. Patients at lower risk, on the other hand, would be spared costs, radiation, and breast cancer concern.

The ultimate aim would be a computerized system for widespread application to provide the clinician with a highly objective and totally consistent assessment of breast cancer for each of his patients.

Thus, it seems logical to utilize the available Emory University experience (Table 36–1), which had established the ability to gather, collate, edit, and analyze data on breast cancer patients since 1963. Various mathematical methods have been investigated to use large numbers of items of data in combination to define profiles for cancer and noncancer patients. Linear discriminant analysis proved to be the most feasible and effective means for defining these profiles, and the extension and refinement of that process has further improved the delineation of the women at risk.

Method

Although the linear discriminant function produced the best results of all available analytic systems, it could not yield comparable results when applied to independent validation samples of cancerous and noncancerous breasts. Additional diminution in the separation of the groups occurred when this instrument was applied to the prediction of future breast cancer. For these reasons, and because the assumptions underlying the linear discriminant analysis model were poorly met by the data employed in the analysis, a more robust system of discriminant analysis was sought.

The process of identifying patients at high risk of subsequent breast cancer was envisioned as an extrapolation of the diagnostic process over time. An adequate assessment of risk of future breast cancer incorporates a continuous, or at least an incremental, time parameter so that risk within any future time interval can be estimated. It is not adequate to specify that a patient has an 80 per cent probability of breast cancer over her lifetime when she, in fact, has a 70 per cent chance of having current breast cancer. For this reason, the discriminant procedure used to de-

lineate relative risk had to be capable of predicting current or imminent breast cancer and of incorporating rather static variables, such as family history of breast cancer, that were indicative of general underlying levels of risk of breast cancer.

The linear discriminant function had the capability of utilizing a number of variables in concert to assess relative risk, but the contribution of each observed risk factor was independent of the particular observed levels of other risk factors for the same patient. There were no interaction effects. The effect of a family history of breast cancer on the composite risk level was the same when overt signs of breast cancer were present and when they were absent. The level of family history of breast cancer did not alter greatly the composite relative risk of breast cancer in the presence of overt signs of the disease, so it did not greatly alter the assessed risk in the absence of overt signs when the linear discriminant function was used. To circumvent this problem, either overt signs of breast cancer must be removed from the analysis, which eliminates information concerning current or imminent breast cancer; or a procedure must be used that evaluates each risk factor differently depending on the level of all other risk factors. Because of the need to evaluate risk of current or imminent breast cancer and because of the difficulty in determining which risk factors pertain only to current breast cancer, the second approach was undertaken.

In 1976, Mosteller, of the Emory University Section of Mammography, developed a completely new type of discriminant analysis called regional discriminant analysis, which he applied to both calibration and validation cancer and noncancer samples and which operates as follow:

The linear discriminant function is estimated from the data, and estimates of the discriminant score are obtained for each breast.* For each breast the contribution of each risk factor is assessed to determine which is most indicative of cancer. The contributions of the remaining risk factors are then adjusted by regression for the particular level of the first variable in the hierarchy; the variable among them that is most indicative of cancer is taken as the second variable in the hierarchy for that particular breast. The process continues until no further variables

---

*Previously described in Ph.D. dissertation, Mosteller, 1976.

TABLE 36–2. Reordering of Several Risk Factors to Illustrate the Value of Discriminant Analysis on 540 Cancer and 641 No-Cancer Women*

	Raw Frequency		After Discriminant Analysis	
	Times Occur	Cancer to No-Cancer	Times Occur	Cancer to No-Cancer
Increased density by x-ray	80 CA	15:1	347	69:1
	6 NO CA		5	
Post menopause, natural	275	25:1	215	107:1
	113		2	
Axillary nodes, clinical	112	28:1	112	28:1
	4		4	

*Obvious changes, such as clinically positive axillary nodes, provide no improvement in the score.

are considered to be indicative of cancer (determined by an arbitrary criterion). The process then stops, resulting in an ordered hierarchy of at least 1 and up to 65 risk factors for each breast—the total risk factors in the scheme.

At the completion of this process for each breast in the analysis sample (540 cancerous and 641 noncancerous breasts), the complete cross classification was partitioned according to the occurrence of each risk factor at each order of the hierarchy. This partitioning constituted a cross classification by risk regions that could then be analyzed by linear discrim-

inant analysis in analogy with the hierarchic regression analysis discussed previously (Table 36–2).

Results

A validation sample of entirely different patients, consisting of 73 cases of cancer and 462 of noncancer, was similarly analyzed. The validation varied only very slightly from the calibration results.

The following summarizes our findings:

Mathematical procedures, some unique to this study, were applied to 114 suggested

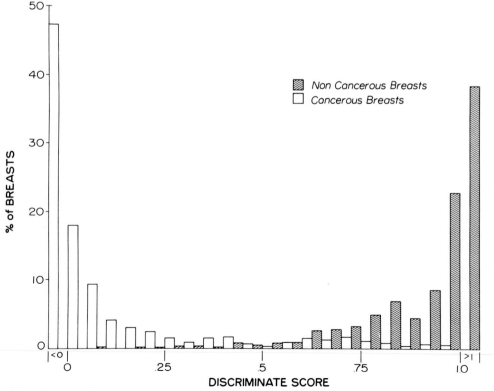

Figure 36–1. Separation of cancer and no-cancer patients by discriminant scores. There is minimal overlapping centrally to cause confusion in assigning risk.

TABLE 36–3. Relative Effectiveness of Selection of Patients for Biopsy for Breast Cancer by Clinical Evaluation by Discriminant Analysis in 16,176 Initial Breast Examinations Containing 624 Proven Cancers and 2028 Benign Lesions at That Examination, With a Projected Total of 734 Cancers

	Per Cent Noncancer Biopsied	Predicted Cancers at Risk		Cancer/Benign Ratio
		No.	Per Cent	
Clinically	12.5	552	71	1:4
Discriminant analysis	11.9	674	92	1:2.8
	10.2	603	82	1:2.7
	5.6	513	70	1:1.8

"Clinically" includes all available data; the same used for RDA.

risk factors, with as many as ten subsets, from history, physical examination, and x-ray examination on 30,904 breast studies on 7252 patients referred from the Emory University Clinic since 1963. One fifth of the cancers were related to symptoms; 82 per cent of the cancers were free of axillary lymph node metastasis. There was no sign or symptom that predicted preclinical cancer. Interaction of numerous indicators subjected to strong statistical procedures could contribute to establishing risk of even early breast cancer. The results of hierarchic discriminant analyses demonstrated the feasibility of using simultaneously large numbers of risk factors in a systematic way to pinpoint patients with mammary cancer (Fig. 36–1). Based on the usual clinical and x-ray assessment of the women, 12.5 per cent of the noncancer patients required biopsy to demonstrate 70 per cent of the cancers, with a cancer to benign rate of 1:4. Using the same data with discriminant analyses, 5.6 per cent of the patients would require biopsy, at the rate of 1 cancer to 1.8 benign lesions; 92 per cent of the cancer patients could be placed in 11.9 per cent of the population. A computerized system has been developed for widespread application to provide the clinician with a highly objective and totally consistent assessment of risk for breast cancer in each of his patients (Tables 36–3 to 36–5).

Observation

Of 540 cancers diagnosed by the pathologist, 132 had been interrupted at the in situ or minimally invasive stage without a mass. The statistical scheme, based on profiles similar to those cancers associated with mass, predicted that 524 cancers should have developed a mass (Fig. 36–2). It seems improbable that the scheme erred this widely, as it did predict the 408 cancers having a mass to have one and an additional 116, of the 132 without mass, to have a mass. The number of basic profiles indicating a mass in the data base of the calibration sample probably was limited and not all-inclusive. This seems reasonable, as of the 1181 patients in the calibration sample, 1170 did have different profiles. Another possibility, assuming that to be life-threatening any cancer must proceed through the mass stage, is that some of those

TABLE 36–4. Regional Discriminant Analysis (RDA) Risk Factor as Expressed in Numerical Value with the Corresponding Numbers of 540 Cancer and 641 Noncancer Patients Within Each Range of This Value

RDA Risk Factors*	Cancers per 100 Women (per cent) With Risk Factors	Noncancers per 100 Women (per cent) With Risk Factors	Cancer/Noncancer Occurrence
0.00–0.149	100	0	338:0
0.15–0.299	98	2	92:2
0.30–0.399	98	2	40:1
0.40–0.499	63	37	19:11
0.50–0.599	38	63	15:25
0.60–0.699	31	69	19:42
0.70–0.799	17	83	11:55
0.80–0.899	5	95	6:109
0.90–0.999	0	100	0:227
1.00	0	100	0:169

*0.00 is cancer and 1.00 is noncancer.

TABLE 36–5. One Hundred Eighty-Six Women Who Developed Primary Breast Cancer Following Normal Clinical And Mammography Examination, With Initial and Subsequent RDA Scores

Number of Women	Initial Score	Subsequent Scores
46	Low	Low
39	Low	Lower
58	Medium to high	Sudden drop
15	Medium	Dropped more than 2 scores
13	High	Dropped more than 3 to 5 scores
15	Medium to high	Medium to high

pathologically similar cancers are nonlethal. With expansion of the number of profiles in the data base, there should emerge subsets of profiles for various histologic types of cancers as suggested in Figure 36–3—those producing axillary metastasis and noninvasive cancers that become invasive, remain noninvasive, or even regress. This observation suggests a tremendously far-reaching impact on knowledge of breast cancer and its treatment.

The 21 cancers with initial no-cancer examinations in Table 36–1 were proved by biopsy within six months of these examinations. In our best attempt to estimate the prevalence of breast cancers based on these data, the 3 per cent was judged four times too large in this dense cancer population, so one quarter of the 3 per cent, or 0.75 per cent, was used to project a total of 734 prevalent cancers (14,142 × 0.75%, or 106 additional cancers, for a total of 734 prevalent cancers being present).

IN VIVO OPTICAL SPECTROSCOPY (INVOS)*

Background

Analytical optical spectroscopy involves the identification of chemical composition of substances by the use of light. Information is gathered by detecting how a given substance affects specific light waves. Each molecular structure can be simplistically considered to be a collection of atomic masses connected by forces that in many ways act as springs. If light strikes such a molecule with a frequency that causes these atomic masses and springs to vibrate, the light energy will be absorbed, and light of that frequency or wavelength cannot be transmitted through many such molecules. These discrete frequencies of absorption, which increase in number with molecular complexity, form a "signature" of absorbing optical frequencies characteristic of each molecular structure. For simple molecular structures, chemical identification through such signatures of absorption is relatively straightforward. For collections of complex molecules, such as those found in biologic systems, understanding which of them causes the absorption pattern may be very difficult. In such cases, empirical means are used to relate the optical results to specific biologic behavior and characteristics.

For over 50 years optical spectroscopy has been employed by laboratories to measure the chemical composition of specific inert

---

*Somanetics Corporation, Troy, MI.

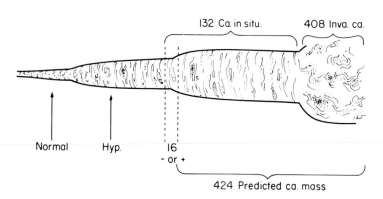

Figure 36–2. Schematic portrayal of progression from normal ductal epithelium to breast cancer. The scheme predicted a mass of cancer in 524 cases. Only the 16 borderline cases were in doubt; progression to frank cancer and reversion to a nonlethal process are suggested possibilities.

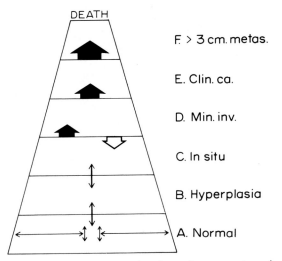

DEATH

F. > 3 cm. metas.

E. Clin. ca.

D. Min. inv.

C. In situ

B. Hyperplasia

A. Normal

Figure 36–3. A suggested pathway for progression of breast cancer to a lethal stage. Vacillations at *A* and *B* are probable as well as from *B* to *C* and *C* to *D*. However, the pathway from *D* to *C* is possible but perhaps less frequent than the more likely one from *C* to *B*.

substances. Numerous applications of infrared spectroscopy have been reviewed by Parker (1971). The uses have been primarily in the study of specific, usually purified, compounds. Differences have been noted in the spectra of oxyhemoglobin and reduced hemoglobin. Infrared absorption spectra for normal and cancerous tissues have been related to substances such as RNA and DNA. Cartwright (1930), May and Grenell (1985), Curcio and Petty (1951), and Cooke and Kuntz (1974) reported on overall infrared transmission and absorption in body tissues. Specific types of tissues and disease processes were not considered. These studies did not include continuous investigation over a wide range of wavelengths to establish organ patterns. No pattern study of broad areas of wavebands had been reported.

Our work in 1980 with wavelengths of light 630 to 680 nanometers showed that poorly oxygenated blood markedly attenuated this beam, whereas well-oxygenated blood had little effect on it. This led to a study in vitro as well as in vivo of the disorganized circulation about a breast cancer, where there was a decided attenuation of the beam as it traversed areas of hypoxic blood. A study of 200 breast masses revealed a characteristic pattern with breast cancer, but benign masses were poorly coordinated. Based on this reproducible pattern of cancer we were encouraged to expand this preliminary work.

More recently, spectroscopy has been shown to be effective in agriculture, in which it is used to determine the difference in the chemical properties of plants and meat as a quality control measure (Conway et al., 1984). The technology has also been used to perform in vitro tests on human blood and tissues (Siggaard-Andersen et al., 1972). Conway also used spectroscopy to determine the fat percentiles in humans and animals. In vivo spectroscopy has been used in extensive experimentation on humans and animals with directly monitored fetal arterial Po_2 as a measurement of hemoglobin oxygenation (Seeds et al., 1984). Another more recent example is the measurement of brain oxygen during anesthesia (Friesen, 1985), using the spectral absorption of metabolic enzymes such as cytochromes. The use of in vivo optical spectroscopy is rapidly opening up new arenas in medical research and diagnostic techniques.

Possible applications of the technology include identification of more complex blood gases and cancer pathology. A potentially beneficial application of in vivo spectroscopy is the detection of possible cancers of the human breast. In this procedure, light of extremely specific and harmless wavelengths is projected into predetermined breast locations. By measuring the absorption of the light by various breast tissues it is possible to determine the likelihood of cancer.

The breasts are well suited to the use of this technique for several reasons: They are partially separated from the other body organs; they are relatively translucent in the employed spectrum; and they are two highly symmetric organs for purposes of comparing data. The result is a sensitive nonimaging demonstration of the modification of the biophysiology of breast tissues, with highly reproducible patterns that depend on biochemistry of the lesions. It is quite distinct from simple mapping of shadows or imaging associated with transillumination involving macroscopic physical properties, as practiced by Cutler (1931) and Carlsen (1982).

Our aim with the use of in vivo optical spectroscopy (INVOS) was a physician-independent unit to select women with a higher risk for breast cancer to ensure referral to more definitive diagnostic procedures, such as mammography.

Clinical Investigation

Since there had been no application of optical spectroscopy to study the structures of the breast or its disease processes, it was necessary for us to pursue the most basic laboratory investigations. We avoided any possible exposure to harmful ultraviolet or infrared light by eliminating by filters all wavelengths less than 500 nm or greater than 1500 nm.

Methods

Spectral curves over a wide range of wavelengths were measured for fat, water, and hemoglobin, then the effects of varying the percentages of fat and water and varying the concentration and oxygenation of hemoglobin in human blood were evaluated. Samples of dissected fatty tissues, fibrous tissues, and combinations of the two from human breast specimens were measured in vitro using specially designed chambers (Egan et al., 1987).

For furthering the design and implementation of the unit, four scans (Somagram) were done on each breast of 400 women having routine mammography. Next, 750 women provided clinical adaptation of the instrument and established Somagram patterns. Three women of childbearing age were followed weekly with Somagrams through three complete menstrual cycles.

Reproducibility of studies on the same unit was monitored by periodic scanning of phantoms and by repeating studies on the same women. Comparison between units was similarly monitored with phantoms and by scans of the same women on different units.

Differences in spectroscopic properties of the two breasts, displayed by attenuation and scatter, that related to hemoglobin, fibrous tissue, fat, water, and other constituents provided parameters for dichotomy of women into cancer and no-cancer groups. Criteria for separation into relative risk (probability of cancer) groups related to how these constituents changed with age of the patient. Certain such criteria were used in an algorithm for computer evaluation of Somagrams. These computer interpretations removed all subjectivity and observer bias. The algorithm produced a numerical in vivo optical spectroscopy (INVOS) value with a range of 32 to 325, the higher score indicating a greater probability of cancer.

A prototype machine was constructed (Fig. 36–4), consisting of a light source, selected light filters, a fiberoptic cable and probe for projecting the light into the breast tissue, and a computer. The optics portion consists of a halogen lamp and a series of narrow-band

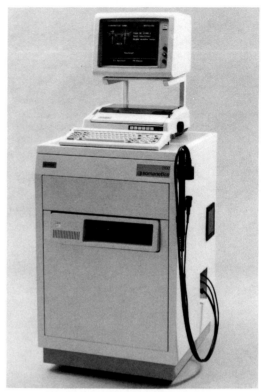

Figure 36–4. The complete unit is compact and readily movable. The CRT displays instruction to the operator and an immediate result of the scans plus relative risk number, INVOS value. The printer then delivers a permanent record.

optical filters to cover the specific wavelength range between 0.5 and 1.5 μ. This micron range represents the window between high water absorption in the infrared region to high hemoglobin absorption in the visible region.

A fiberoptic probe is sequentially placed at four specific locations on each breast (Fig. 36–5). A receiver fiberoptic cable on the opposite side of the breast picks up the transmitted light, which is converted to an electrical signal, amplified, digitized, processed on the computer, and finally displayed on the cathode ray tube (CRT). These specific locations allow for an ample sampling of breast tissue with transmitted light. In addition to the transmitted light, internal back-scattered light is measured with a fiberoptic probe placed in close proximity to the incident light beam. This back-scattered light probe was found necessary to eliminate the effects of skin pigmentation between subjects of different races, and at the same time eliminate the effect of incident light variations. Calculations were made to take signal infor-

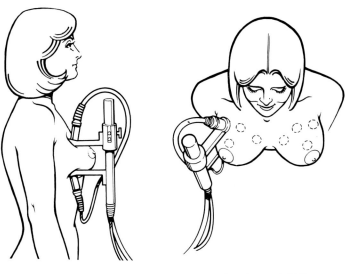

Figure 36–5. Four sites of light probe on each breast. In each site the light traverses the upper as well as the lower portions of the breast.

Lateral View   Craniocaudal View

mation characteristic only of the internal breast tissue.

The examination procedure was standardized so that the technique would be repeatable, independent of operator or patient interface. The probe is positioned on each patient in a prescribed sequential pattern, with the operator relocating the probe as prompted by the computer display. The angle of the probe was designed to ensure maximal and yet gentle contact with the skin, while projecting the necessary volume of light, without leakage (Fig. 36–6).

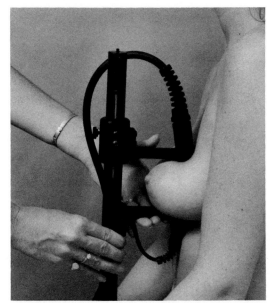

Figure 36–6. Probe in contact with the breast, with firm gentle pressure eliminating ambient light.

The examination can be conducted in any examination room, as long as the room can be darkened to control ambient light, which interferes with the machine's sensitive optic receivers. It is possible to accomplish an examination of both breasts in five minutes or less by using the established standardized approach.

The direct result of the examination is a calculation of the absorption characteristics of the tissue at specific wavelengths. Although analysis of the raw data can be very complicated, a simple graphic representation of the absorption coefficients can be instructive. Therefore, the computer is used to create graphs of the absorption coefficients for each of the light test locations (Fig. 36–7).

Eight hundred studies were carried out to establish risk criteria and 732 studies for validation of the criteria. Equal numbers of 1739 women were from each of the two institutions. A total of 166 breast biopsies were performed, with 89 no-cancer and 77 cancer diagnoses by histology. These women provided a number of subsets, including: clinical no-risk, x-ray no-risk, clinical risk and/or x-ray risk, ductal hyperplasia, and clustered calcifications not associated with a mass.

INVOS data were compared with both x-ray and pathologic diagnoses.

Results

By using this type of optically determined composition information, one can determine a ''physiologic age'' of the patient's breast as contrasted to its chronologic age. Since the

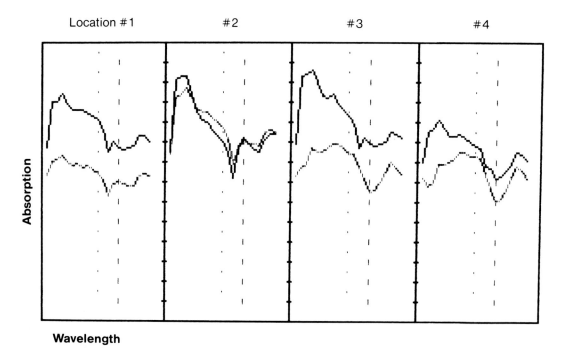

Figure 36–7. Tracings for the four positions of each breast: lateral, central anteriorly, central posteriorly, and medial. Right breast information is the heavy line, and left breast information is the lighter line. Hemoglobin window is at the left of the tracing; the light dashed line is the fat window and the heavy dashed line (vertical) is the water window. INVOS is not shown.

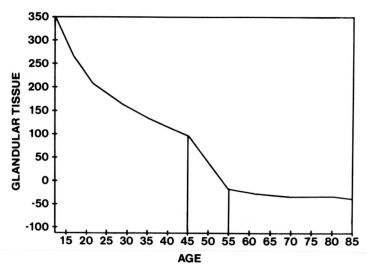

Figure 36–8. Glandular tissue as measured by in vivo optical spectroscopy as function of age. A more rapid fatty infiltration occurs during menopausal years.

human breast, beyond maturity, gradually loses its glandular tissue and gains fatty tissue, the height of the water absorption peak in relation to the fatty, absorption peak is a definite measure of this process (Fig. 36–8). The measurement clearly shows the rapid drop in glandular tissue during menopause. The physiologic age of the breast is well known to be associated with risk for breast cancer.

The equipment software derives much of its sensitivity from a comparison of the calibration population (normal and known biopsy-confirmed pathology) with the breast tissue of the women being examined (Figs. 36–9 and 36–10).

The level of detailed information collected during the examination precludes simple analysis. A sophisticated computer analysis is critical in determining the extremely subtle differences between a woman's breasts, or between a given breast and the normal. The prototype machine analyzes the critical data as well as other patient information (age, weight, height) immediately and stores it for future reference and comparison.

An arbitrary INVOS value of 125 or greater selected 87 per cent of the cancers while including only 26 per cent of the no-cancer cases (Table 36–6; Figs. 36–11 and 36–12). Sensitivity and specificity of the INVOS studies were similar for the two institutions as well as for the women over or under age 50 years (Table 36–7).

Menstrual status had no significant effect on the INVOS values.

The procedure was readily acceptable to all participating women.

Clinical Application

Primary

The least controversial statistic of breast cancer is that the size and histologic stage of the tumor relates inversely to the length of survival of the woman. Mammography has been accepted as the most effective method to detect small breast cancers and to provide the best opportunity for cure or long-term survival. But cost, radiation, and lack of appeal for clinical application in asymptomatic women remain objections to routine mammography. Since 30 per cent of our cancers in women referred to mammography and 60 per cent of cancers in the American Cancer Society–National Cancer Institute Breast Cancer Detection and Demonstration Project

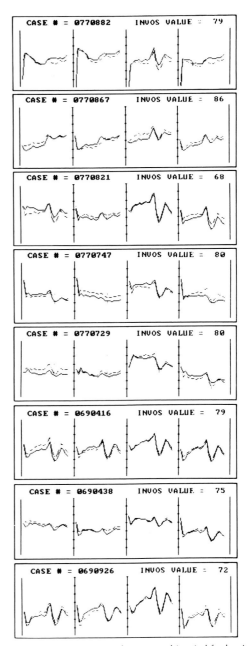

Figure 36–9. Somagrams for women biopsied for benign breast diseases. Tracings are symmetric and similar and have normal fat/water ratios and low INVOS values.

were clinically unsuspected (Baker, 1982), and since there is no applicable epidemiologic risk factor for breast cancer, there is just no reliable way for selection of women for mammography.

A more precise method of selection of that one women in 11 having or destined to have breast cancer would obviate these deterrents to routine mammography. No single, simple risk marker for breast cancer is known. The

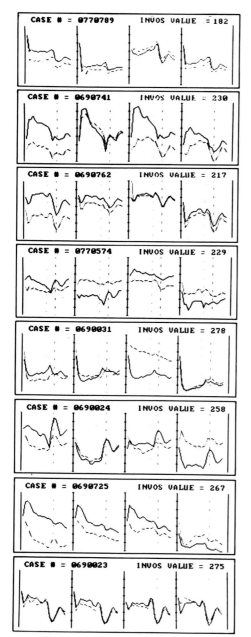

Figure 36–10. Somagrams of women with biopsy-proven primary breast carcinomas. The tracings are often markedly asymmetric, unlike those of normal women, and have high INVOS values.

Once an increased risk is established, the smaller number of women could easily be persuaded to accept mammography.

The application of this strategy is unlimited. Placement of the device in areas readily accessible to women will persuade many who otherwise would not have a breast examination to accept this nonthreatening procedure. Many companies (e.g., Bell Telephone) employing numbers of women of cancer age for years have sought practical screening for breast cancer. Obstetricians and gynecologists are already being urged by their national organization as well as by some women to promote mammography. Somagrams obtained in their offices under the direction of a radiologist are preferable to the x-rays of mammography units operated by nonradiologists, who either make their own interpretations or send the studies to a radiologist who must accept the quality of the examinations. Any woman desiring mammography will not be denied, while an additional 25 per cent of the women, representing a total population, will have mammography. The radiologist will then do that many more mammograms, with a high percentage of early breast cancers being identified.

Secondary

High-Risk Subsets. Seven intraductal (noninfiltrating) carcinomas had an average age INVOS score of 169, with a range of 79 to 267; only one score was below the 125 value. These breasts were biopsied for clustered calcifications not associated with a mass. Twenty-eight similar clusters of calcifications that proved benign had an INVOS score of 89, with a range of 52 to 122. Seven duct carcinomas, primarily in dense nodular breasts radiographically and not clear-cut on x-ray as cancer, had average scores of 200.4,

need then becomes clearly apparent for the development and application of a prescreening tool to select women for mammography.

These data, the relatively inexpensive INVOS unit, its ease of production, it being operator (physician)–independent, its computer-evaluated results, its simplicity in appeal, and the lack of ionizing radiation satisfy criteria for premammography screening.

TABLE 36–6. Separation into High and Low Risk for Breast Cancer in 1739 Women Based on INVOS Values Above and Below 125

	Cancer	No Cancer	Total
INVOS +	67	432	499
INVOS −	10	1230	1240
Total	77	1662	1739

Sensitivity:	87.0%
Specificity:	74.0%
Positive predictive value:	13.4%
Negative predictive value:	99.2%
Relative risk of cancer with positive INVOS:	16.5 times

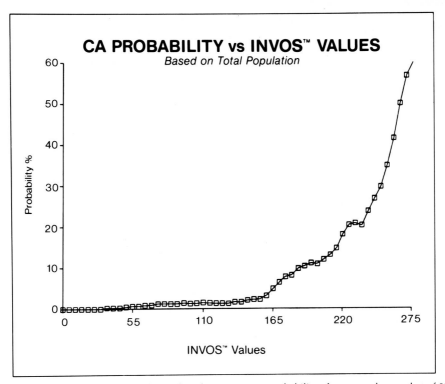

Figure 36–11. An INVOS value of 130 indicates less than 2 per cent probability of cancer, whereas that of 270 indicates well over 50 per cent chance of cancer.

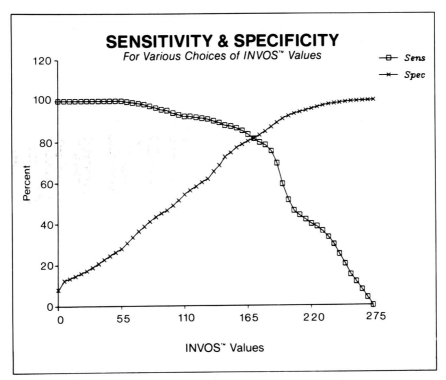

Figure 36–12. Selection of an INVOS value for cancer/no cancer is arbitrary. If greater sensitivity is the goal, lesser specificity must be accepted; e.g., with a 98 per cent sensitivity, specificity may be only 40 per cent.

TABLE 36–7. INVOS Values at Two Institutions for Two Age Groups (1739 Cases)

	Sensitivity (%)	Specificity (%)
Institution A	87.1	76.0
Institution B	86.8	71.8
Combined	87.0	74.0
<50 years of age	84.1	75.5
≥50 years of age	88.3	72.7

with a range of 136 to 278 (Fig. 36–13). This constitutes a group of women at very high risk and most difficult to diagnose accurately by mammography. But with a high INVOS the severe accompanying fibrocystic disease is better evaluated and the women biopsied or followed with more confidence. The calcifications also represent a very early form of carcinoma. The sensitivity of the INVOS was just as high with these early cancers as it was with advanced highly infiltrative lesions.

Another subset of breasts most difficult to evaluate with mammography are flagged with high INVOS numbers at times. The INVOS not only selects these women for mammography but also tends to aid in their study (Fig. 36–14).

Complement to Mammography. The radiologist will be more careful in interpretation of the mammograms and in disposition of a woman with a high INVOS value. More subtle mammographic changes will be biopsied, but more in situ cancers will be found (just as with the introduction of mammography).

The high negative predictive value should be reassuring to the woman falling into the low-risk category. Projected from this highly dense cancer population it should be even more reassuring in the less dense cancer rate in a screening setting.

The sensitivity of the noninfiltrating smaller carcinomas was just as high as that of all the cancers. Since the radiologic and INVOS false negative cases are not the same, INVOS has a potential for increasing the risk-predictive level of mammography.

Economics. Economics greatly favors the radiologist and the patient as each breast-imaging center becomes more active and productive, resulting in better performances for the women. Third-party payers can no longer consider a mammogram for a high INVOS value as screening.

The simplicity of the procedure may appeal to the woman, and the examination may be established in the same way as the Pap smear for cervical cancer.

Liability. Borderline cases will not be dismissed, as the woman will be impressed with the importance of returning for follow-up studies, reducing the dangers of litigation.

Mammograms on the dense breasts will be interpreted with more confidence. The "forgotten" woman under age 35 years will have the opportunity for investigation of her breast cancer rather than being told that it's a "milk duct" or being given antibiotics for months. In younger women the specificity rate may be lowered so that fewer women will require mammography but at the cost of a lowered sensitivity rate.

Since there were instances in which a high INVOS value in a breast that was noncancerous clinically and by x-ray prefaced the histologic diagnosis of cancer, it may be prudent to follow closely other women under similar circumstances (Fig. 36–15). Neither the women nor their physicians object to this more careful program.

Observations

Noninvasive in vivo optical spectroscopy (INVOS) consistently delineates important compositional and physiologic properties of breast tissues as a premammography marker for cancer and a high-assurance no-risk predictor. This new nonimaging approach depends on the biochemistry of tissues rather than on the macroscopic physical properties involved with most breast-imaging modalities. Having established the procedure as inexpensive, physician-independent, simple, requiring only a few minutes, and appealing to women, one can readily adapt it clinically as a premammography screening procedure. Continued studies of over 5000 women in the United States and 3000 women in the Willemin Clinic in Paris have maintained, or surpassed, the sensitivity and specificity rates.

The procedure is designed to increase the use of mammography. If a woman is to have a mammogram, somagraphy can be of only secondary value. Somography is that much-needed means of bringing women to breast x-ray—those women who would not ordinarily receive mammography.

Once a risk is established, the woman calmly accepts it simply as an increased risk compared with that of the general population, not cancer per se, so that she can

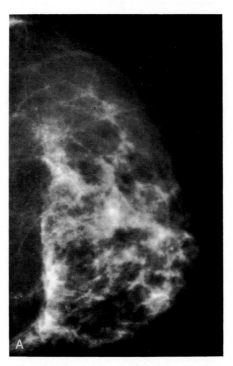

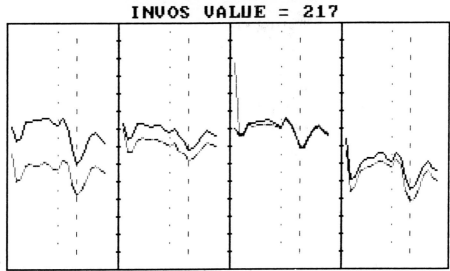

Figure 36–13. Calcification of intraductal carcinoma. A 55-year-old woman seen for routine annual checkup. Clinically: normal breasts. *A,* Mammography: Below nipple level near left chest wall is a cluster of calcifications, not associated with a mass, that have increased in number since the last examination one year before. Localization, biopsy, and specimen radiography is required. *B,* INVOS value: 217. Pathology: intraductal carcinoma of the right breast. Modified radical mastectomy; all 21 axillary lymph nodes free of tumor.

cooperate with her BSE, physician's examinations, and mammograms. A positive IN-VOS does indicate a 16.5 times increased relative risk of breast cancer.

A low INVOS score indicates a 98 per cent negative predictive value. However, the woman can still have her usual care and mammography as desired. No false sense of security should result.

INVOS in many ways is similar to magnetic resonance studies. It strongly supports the hypothesis that breast cancer is a diffuse disease of the intramammary epithelial cells.

In evaluating these data the Emory University Biometry Department attempted to remove all subjectivity and observer bias. In the algorithm for computer analysis, only the raw optical spectroscopic data and the patient

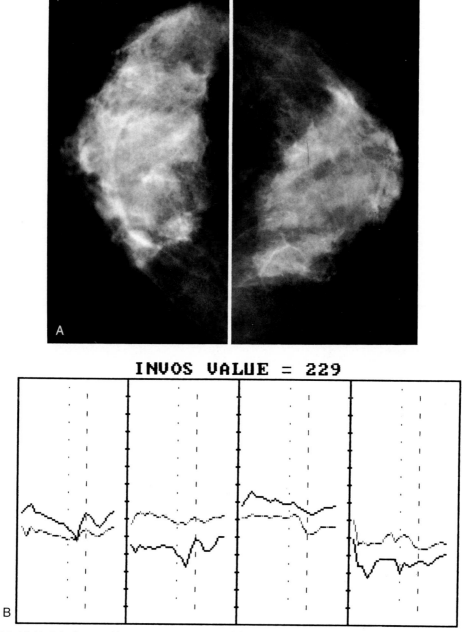

Figure 36–14. Nodular breast with carcinoma. A 49-year-old woman seen for a baseline mammogram; there had been five previous breast biopsies. Clinically: nodular breasts, one area in left, dominant. Aspiration attempted, no fluid. *A*, Mammography: dense, coarsely nodular breasts. *B*, INVOS value: 229. Pathology: intraductal carcinoma, left, with only minimal invasion. Biopsy performed on clinical basis, and noncontributory aspiration attempt.

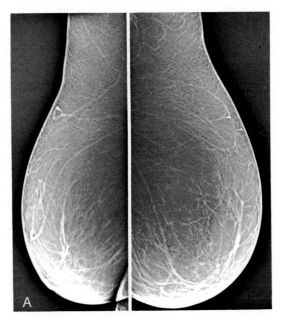

INVOS VALUE = 221

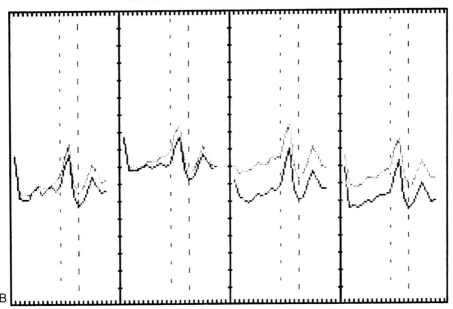

Figure 36–15. Painful breasts. A 76-year-old woman with pain in clinically normal breasts. *A,* Mammography: fatty involution, few small and benign axillary and intramammary lymph nodes. No dominant nodules or secondary signs of carcinoma. *B,* INVOS value: 221.

TABLE 36–8. INVOS Positive (Numbers in Parentheses) of 77 Cancers That Were Palpable, Nonpalpable, X-ray Positive, or X-ray Negative

	Palpable		Nonpalpable		
	X-ray +	X-ray −	X-ray +	X-ray −	**Total**
Institution B	29(26)	3(2)	14(12)	1(0)*	47(41)
Institution A	24(22)	3(2)	3(2)	0	30(26)
Total	53(48)	6(4)	17(14)		77(67)

*Unsuspected in prophylactic mastectomy following mastectomy on opposite breast for carcinoma.

age were utilized. The INVOS value (probability of cancer) was firmly established in all cases prior to biopsy and without benefit of any clinical or radiographic information.

From Table 36–8 it is apparent that women selected to be at risk included those with false negative results by mammography, boosting cancer detection in this series to 96 per cent. This suggests merely a complementary role for spectroscopy but emphasizes effecting closer scrutiny of the mammograms, more credence to vague changes by x-ray, or less likelihood of dismissing a high-risk patient completely.

REFERENCES

Baker LH (1982): Breast Cancer Detection Demonstration Project: five year summary report. CA 32:194.

Carlile T, Kopecky KJ, Thompson DJ, et al (1985): Breast cancer prediction and the Wolfe classification of mammograms. JAMA 254:1050.

Carlsen E (1982): Transillumination light scanning. Diagn Imaging, April:28.

Cartwright CH (1930): Infrared transmission of the flesh. JOSA 20:81.

Conway JM, Norris KH, Bodwell CE (1984): A new approach for the estimation of body composition: infrared interactance. Am J Clin Nutr 40:1123.

Cooke R, Kuntz IO (1974): The properties of water in biological systems. Annu Rev Biophys Bioeng 3:95.

Curcio JA, Petty CC (1951): The near absorption of water. JOSA 41:302.

Cutler M (1931): Transillumination of the breast. Ann Surg 93:223.

Egan RL, McSweeney MB (1979): Mammographic parenchymal patterns and the risk of breast cancer. Radiology 133:65.

Egan RL, Dolan PA, Stoddart HF (1987): In vivo measurement of breast composition using optical spectroscopy. Contemp Surg 30:53.

Friesen RH (1985): Pulse oximetry during pulmonary artery surgery. Anesth Analg 64:376.

Kelsey JL (1979): A review of the epidemiology of human breast cancer. Epidemiol Rev 1:74.

May L, Grenell RG (1935): Infrared spectral studies of tissues. Ann NY Acad Sci 171–189.

Parker FS (1971): Applications of Infrared Spectroscopy in Biochemistry, Biology and Medicine. New York, Plenum Press.

Seeds JW, Cefalo RC, Proctor HH, et al (1984): The relationship of intracranial infrared light absorbance to fetal oxygenation. Am J Obstet Gynecol 149:679.

Siggaard-Andersen O, Nargaard-Pedersen B, Rem J (1972): Hemoglobin pigments. Spectrophotometric determination of oxy-, carboxy-, met-, and sulfhemoglobin in capillary blood. Clin Chim Acta 42:85.

Wolfe JN (1976): Risk of breast cancer development determined by mammographic parenchymal patterns. Cancer 37:2486.

Screening for Breast Cancer

37

BACKGROUND

Screening for breast cancer with mammography is a complex undertaking. There is no counterpart in radiology. I have been opposed to a subspecialty of mammography but could condone one for breast screening. Mammographic screening goes beyond the nonchalance of routinely scanning chest films or bone studies, the mechanics of gastrointestinal fluoroscopy, or the technician role in interventional radiography. It is not the lucrative type of study that permits an early P.M. golf appointment. Instead, it constantly challenges boldness to devise and incorporate new approaches; it demands in-depth mastery of radiographic technology, both innovative and efficient; and it requires the ultimate in the art of medicine in establishing women's cooperation, physicians' confidence, and community approval.

After the demonstration of clinical mammography in the mid-1950s, there swelled a chorus of demand to screen all women for breast cancer. There were endless queries by companies with large numbers of female employees, such as Bell Telephone, about how this technique could be initiated. Several radiologists while being trained, and some who returned to pursue the idea, began formulating plans for individual screening programs. Lack of experience, unavailable x-ray units for rapid examinations, undetermined proper subsets of age groups, and many looming problems were not deterrents. Sensing that this helter-skelter approach would contaminate a screening population, knowing that the cervical Pap smear "had been around for 40 years and never evaluated," and hoping to establish regional centers of expertise, we planned a reproducibility study of mammography prior to any screening programs. Already the director of epidemiology of the National Cancer Institute (NCI) had planned a program using mammography to screen the wives of servicemen on the East Coast and was planning and tooling up another such program for Norway.

Reproducibility Study of Mammography

The questions posed by the reproducibility study of mammography were these: (1) Could the Egan technique be learned by other radiologists and the team approach established at their institutions? (2) Could these radiologists produce acceptable diagnostic results?

Prototype for New Technique Evaluation

The systematic implementation of a study to evaluate mammography for clinical use establishes a protocol for appraisal of other imaging techniques for other areas of the body. Prescribed and successive phases were necessary to evaluate the clinical application of mammography. The first phase, or potential, of the procedure had been empirically well documented over a four-year period, hence the term "reproducibility study of mammography."

PHASE I—FEASIBILITY

On Site At M.D. Anderson Hospital (MDAH). This phase included development of the procedure and establishment of criteria for interpretation, application for clinical use, and safety for the woman.

Some 20 radiographic techniques, with many variations, were formulated and investigated under a range of 12 kvp to 22 mev, using radical mastectomy specimens and frozen 5 mm slices of whole breasts. From these, departure to a high-milliamperage, low-kilovoltage technique was devised that could be used on existing x-ray units with only minor variations. Acceptance by patients resulted in a technique with which the women could cooperate insofar as they were comfortable. Its safety was established through extensive physical measurements by the Physics Department: back-scatter and scatter (collimation); air dose and inverse square law; skin dose; half-value layers in aluminum, fat, and fibroglandular tissue; depth dose using sliced frozen slabs of breast; scatter to eye, gonads, and blood-forming bone; anode material; magnification x-ray equipment; and estimation of relative biologic effects.

The procedure was found to be relatively inexpensive (comparable to a cervical spine series). Exquisite radiographic detail provided a high degree of differentiation between benign and malignant processes as well as clinically unsuspected carcinomas. A 97 per cent diagnostic accuracy in advanced cancer at a tumor institution had been established. There was also a potential adaptation to screening of the general population, as 53 cases of carcinoma were clinically unsuspected and detected solely by mammography—the first such report (Egan, 1962). Results of our four years' use of mammography had been carefully monitored by the Epidemiology Department of MDAH. Also, biostatisticians from the United States Public Health Service (USPHS) reviewed these data and verified the clinical application of the procedure. Five world-renowned radiologists visited to learn firsthand of the technique and reported back to the USPHS, "no prior studies remotely comparable."

Off Site. A large number of radiologists and their technologists had received a one-week training course one-on-one on site. They returned to a variety of clinical institutions under conditions found in local communities, instituted a mammography program, indoctrinated their teams in breast cancer, and were diagnosing a high percentage of breast cancer and finding more than 10 per cent of clinically unsuspected cancers.

PHASE II—PLANNING

Some level of feasibility, applicability, acceptability, and potential must be inherent in a procedure before its evaluation is considered. At this phase, planning is paramount and must encompass individuals in every area of instituting, promoting, and evaluating the undertaking. The aims must be simple and attainable and have a finite point that is measurable.

In undertaking this study, a division of responsibility between the Director of the National Cancer Institute, the Director of the M.D. Anderson Hospital, and the Chief of the Cancer Control Program was established. MDAH would supply training of the radiologists by the Principal Investigator, conduct workshops of participants, review mammograms and tissue sections, and supply all technical services as the clinical center of the study. The Cancer Control Program would collect reports of cases, provide statistical evaluation, assist institutions to organize for the study, and supervise compliance with the protocol. The NCI would be responsible for providing statistical consultations and assisting with analysis of the data.

It was agreed that the institutions in which

the study would be carried out would be divided into two groups: ten distributed throughout Texas and the others geographically distributed throughout the United States. These institutions were selected by a committee composed of representatives of the three participating agencies.

Criteria were established as follows for carrying out the study: (1) The population was to be limited to women who were to undergo biopsy of the breast; (2) mammographic studies were to be performed by the Egan technique; (3) mammograms were to be interpreted by the radiologist without clinical information; (4) all breast biopsies were to be included in this study (not selected cases); and (5) each of the study forms was to be set directly to the Cancer Control Program as completed, for collation and analysis.

PHASE III—INDOCTRINATION OF PARTICIPANTS

Radiologists. Training of the radiologists from the participating institutions was accomplished during a five-day visit to MDAH, when the Principal Investigator offered instruction in his technique and in interpretation of mammograms. They were then introduced to case material consisting of 3000 examinations. Special attention was given to those mammograms that demonstrated characteristics of malignant lesions. The radiologists participated actively in obtaining and interpreting mammograms. They were also introduced to the team approach, in which surgeons and pathologists as well as radiologists are involved in the use of mammography.

Four sets of 24 complete mammograms containing normal, benign, and malignant breast lesions were circulated to the 24 participating radiologists, with each filling out diagnostic reporting forms and forwarding them to the data control office. The sets were then rearranged, recirculated, and reinterpreted.

Teams. Each institution was visited, prior to accumulation of study cases, to ensure that each department involved—radiology, surgery, and pathology—understood the requirements of the protocol and the need for cooperation among the departments and to answer questions that may have arisen. Annual seminars, the basis for the Annual Mammography Seminars, were conducted to keep the participants informed and to exchange ideas.

PHASE IV—ACCUMULATION OF DATA

Reports were made independently on six separate forms: A, Clinical Impression; B, Radiological Examination; C, Surgical Examination (operative report); D, Pathology Report; E, M.D. Anderson Radiology Examination; F, M.D. Anderson Pathology Report. The forms were mailed to the Public Health Service as each was completed.

PHASE V—QUALITY CONTROL

All mammograms were reviewed by the Principal Investigator for judgment of quality of the examinations and diagnosis. All histophathologic material of slides and blocks were reviewed by H. Stephen Gallager, M.D., Associate Pathologist at M.D. Anderson Hospital. All results were forwarded to the data control at the Public Health Service.

Results

Of 1580 breasts biopsied and mammographed, 475 were diagnosed with malignant neoplasms, 1081 with benign lesions, and 24 with no disease. Radiologists were able to diagnose correctly 376 of 475 malignant lesions for a true positive rate of 79 per cent. Of the 1105 breasts classified pathologically as nonmalignant, the radiologists correctly diagnosed 999, or 90 per cent. The false positive rate was 10 per cent.

The findings of the reproducibility study indicate that the technique of mammography developed by Egan can be learned by other radiologists, that films of acceptable quality can be produced, and that the interpretation provides information that is useful in the clinical management of breast diseases.

This study was set up to test mammography as a diagnostic tool. This was considered an absolute step prior to any plans to embark on screening the general population for breast cancer. This study is also a landmark in establishing mammography, as commented upon by Luther Terry, then Secretary of the Department of Health: "Mammography shows promise of being an important diagnostic aid in control of cancer of the breast."

CHALLENGE OF SCREENING

To Medicine

Screening mass populations for disease is a form of preventive medicine, e.g., for hypertension to prevent strokes or for diabetes to prevent blindness. The definite practical and conceptual differences between therapeutic and preventive medicine must be recognized. Vigorous thrusts result in outstanding developments in therapeutic medicine. Needs are clear. Costs and efforts are not issues. In contrast, any progress in preventive medicine is happenstance. A by-product of a larger effort must be retained if it proves to be an ingredient to blend preventive and therapeutic medicine.

In the process of perfecting pneumonectomy, the thoracic surgeon became aware of the causative agent of lung cancer. The use of intrathoracic surgery progressed by leaps and bounds, but no amount of public education ended cigarette smoking. Public education with valid health information must be accompanied by an individual's desire to prevent serious threats to his health.

At present there is no prevention of breast cancer. Our aims must be to prevent the serious sequelae of disease, mobidity, and mortality. This can be done through detection while the patient is symptomless, allowing earlier therapeutic intervention—a true blend of preventive and therapeutic medicine. This is possible through screening of the general population of women with physical examination and mammography. But for mammography to be productive, women must use it. These well women are imbued with a fear of breast cancer, yet our educational approach is lacking. These women must be convinced that mammography is their study and that they alone can induce the medical profession to make it possible for every woman to have her screening mammogram. Each woman should no longer think of herself as a mere person but as a patient with a high risk for symptoms, with discomfort about her breasts, in need of an examination and advice, and willing to pay for it in time and money.

To the Radiologist

The prospect of mass screening of the eligible population thrusts upon the radiologist specific questions and concerns: (1) the differences between symptomatic and asymptomatic women; (2) acceptable costs; (3) women's fears of radiation and the discovery of a cancer; (4) primary physician reaction and participation; (5) referral vs non-referral patients; (6) walk-in patients; (7) acceptable biopsy rates; (8) effect on mortality rates; (9) physical examination; and (10) liability.

In a recent American College of Radiology ad hoc group representative of the leading proponents of mammographic screening, it was readily apparent that the problems of screening could not be reduced, in any area, to a simple clinical application. No consensus was even approached during the less than orderly consideration of the limited subjects of symptomatic patients, cost of screening, biopsy rate, and physical examination. Nothing new could be detected in the problems or the approach to these problems. The motivation to screen for breast cancer and to establish breast-imaging centers will need sharp enhancement with more progressive thinking in order to succeed.

Symptomatic vs Asymptomatic Women

The contribution of mammography to the detection of early breast cancer is directly dependent on its use regardless of the reason for performing the examination. Mammographically screening a woman with a cyst to detect a clinically unsuspected cancer is no diffrent from finding a similar cancer in the breast of a symptom-free woman who has the procedure as part of a routine physical examination. Equal percentages of cancers were found by biopsy in our referral mammography patients whether they had symptoms or signs such as mass, discharge, pain, or fullness or whether they were asymptomatic. In fact, all such mammograms could have been screening procedures, with the symptoms being merely the driving force to have mammography.

From the Emory Oncologic Breast Clinic, of the aproximately 1000 new patients referred annually for mammography, 350 had a breast biopsy, of which 100 yielded primary operable cancers. This was a cancer rate nearly ten times that of the BCDDP women, who in turn had a cancer rate of three to four times that of the general population. With almost all women at some time having breast symptoms, with clinical signs usually associated with advanced cancer, and with symptomatic and asymptomatic women having an equal chance of early breast cancer, certainly for screening purposes an attempted distinction only adds confusion. Once radiologists realize this, third-party insurers will no longer categorize women for payment purposes.

Cost Factors

Another thorn that radiologists insist on introducing is diagnostic vs screening mammography. With the simple recognition that mammography is diagnosing nothing and that all mammography is a screening procedure of sorts, this dilemma can be resolved. The sole purpose of mammography is to determine the necessity for further evaluation: high risk for periodic follow-up, needle aspiration, or biopsy. In the presence of clinical findings, the question is investigation of these findings. The clinician assumes much of the responsibility; in this situation the radiologist may be more concerned about changes elsewhere in that breast or in the other breast. He wants good-quality examination of the clinical area, but this is not as essential as the better quality required to search both breasts. As for the clinically normal breast, the radiologist stands alone and must rely entirely upon his x-ray examination. Here he assumes all the responsibility and must have the best examination without the compromise of poorer quality, lower cost, fewer views, or less professional technology. These are the situations in which we insist upon exquisite radiographic quality for evaluation of changes or comparison of breast asymmetries and on coned-down views of xeroradiographic vague changes or calcifications.

In no way may quality be compromised for cost. Costs may be lowered by reduction of professional fees, volunteer help (nonprofessional), efficient use of x-ray units and personnel by proper scheduling and handling a large volume of women, low-cost space for operation (even consideration of a mobile unit), and batch processing and interpretation.

Basically, because mine was a one-man operation involving travel 50 per cent of the time, my referring physicians were geared for certain delays in reports, as they were always rendered in complete batches. The physician could comfortably review any "emergency" study or discuss it with the technologist and avoid any embarrasing surprises. When I was not traveling, a final report was on the physician's desk by noon the next day. Since mammography is not a lucrative part of general radiology income, cutting costs without losing quality may present problems. Yet it seems inconceivable that one radiologist can survive with a $65 routine mammographic charge, whereas in another city the rate is $250 per examination.

Women's Fears

Women's reluctance to undergo mammography may overtly be due to cost, or even to fear of radiation as publicized, but a more powerful force may be operative: the fear of finding some breast abnormality—*cancer*! A graduate nurse at Emory University measured the flow of epinephrine in women who passed through our mammography section and found that this procedure is a highly charged one—particularly at the moments when the x-ray tube is swung into position and when the technologist is observed checking the mammograms. This fear can be alleviated to a degree by women friends meeting to go together to their respective appointments. One of the best ways to overcome the fear of mammography is to begin screening at an earlier age (baseline age 30 to 35 years) so that women are likely to experience several normal studies before they reach the age of increased risk. In other situations, cancerophobia is a driving force to participate in screening.

Apparently, to women the psychologic aspect of breast cancer screening is very important. The premammography attitude—being alerted at an earlier date to a death sentence by a diagnosis of breast cancer—still lingers. Women today retain the indelible image of a family member or friend slowly succumbing to breast cancer. Some have confided to me their thoughts of suicide as a response to the probable diagnosis of breast cancer. This course of self-destruction is manifested by procrastination in seeking that final diagnosis. Once the diagnosis is confirmed and treatment is completed, the self-destructive mood is absolutely banished.

In screening for breast cancer, compassion and understanding are paramount. A setting that is divorced as much as possible from medical activities is beneficial. Away from the hectic routines of the radiology department and away from the hospital, the ambulatory well woman will be more at ease in the bright, cheerful surroundings that can be provided in a separate breast-imaging center. These women do not want to be made to feel that they are merely another x-ray number amid terminal patients. The single theme of a breast-imaging center is devoid of distractions while it enhances the woman's education as well as her care.

Primary Physician Participation

One of the greatest deterrents to widespread use of mammography has been reluctance on the part of the primary care physician. Initially the contention was that (1) there was nothing of importance in the breast that could not be felt, and (2) a great disservice was done by the false sense of security engendered by the noncancer mammogram. The use of mammography was gradually expanded by the surgeons who recognized its value in their practice, by the occasional internist who did not completely trust the surgeon, and by the gynecologists who, although inexperienced in breast surgery, were charged with responsibility for their patients' breast examinations.

Many of the primary care physicians felt awkward sending a woman for an expensive checkup as part of an examination for which he had already charged a fee. Since these physicians willingly participated in the care of the women who for one reason or another had already obtained a mammogram, this could well represent a potent factor in regulating referral for mammography. Also, some obstetricians and gynecologists felt that they had been singled out to refer their patients for mammography based on recommendations of their national society. In our own Emory University gynecology department, mammography referrals wax and wane according to the recentness of detection of the last clinically unsuspected breast cancer.

Many family physicians suggest mammography only for those women whom they consider to be at high risk for individual reasons, and not because they are interested in any phase of surveying for early breast cancer, particularly in older women. Most primary care physicians see only one or possibly two breast cancers per year and become discouraged in that at least 100 women, on the average, must be referred for mammography in order for a single cancer to be detected. The real disaster for screening is the failure of that physician to insist upon annual examinations, gradually swelling the number of women having mammography. Also, the comparative mammogram is the single best means of calling attention to subtle changes that signal an assuredly curable cancer. Only 0.2 per cent of the women had

an interval cancer with annual screening in the BCDDP, a most reassuring fact to the radiologist.

Early in the BCDDP, the primary care physician was unsure of his role in the community screening project. He was being alerted to the presence of suspicious findings in the breasts of his women patients through an unfamiliar modality used at a distant institution. Some of the women were not really his patients. However, educational programs proceeded rapidly and smoothly via the news media, by telephone calls and reports from the screening center, and by the women directly. These same physicians quickly became eager and cooperative participants in evaluating women's breast problems and sharing follow-up data. At least 29 institutions throughout the United States demonstrated these screening techniques and have produced widespread reports of their activities and results. Today few communities should be without well-informed primary care physicians. In many communities these physicians are playing active roles in organizing and supporting breast-imaging centers to screen their women patients.

Referral vs Nonreferral Women: Walk-in Patients

Once the woman is referred for mammography there are few problems in the routine of a well-established breast-screening center. The first self-supporting breast cancer imaging center was organized in Atlanta in the early 1970s by a group of radiologists and surgeons. At that time the local medical society judicial committee questioned the involved radiologists on a number of occasions, threatening punitive action if any patient was received without bona fide physician referral. In the past 16 to 18 years there has been some softening of this philosophy in Atlanta, but the problem merits consideration by the radiologist, particularly if certain communities and states have contrary practices or laws.

The walk-in patient could be examined and furnished with a list of primary physicians, from which she could select one. This physician would pursue any findings from the screening and establish a patient-physician relationship. A negative screen result could be handled as desired; follow-up positive screening results could also be his responsibility. The screening center itself could keep records of follow-up, mailing periodic reminders to delinquent patients with copies to their physicians.

Prior to the opening of the screening center with its attendant publicity, the medical community should be informed through local medical journals, announcements at meetings, and even mailings to individual physicians. The public announcements will attract some walk-in patients. Provisions for handling these patients must be in place from the opening day of the screening centers.

Biopsy Rates

The breast-imaging center will only indirectly control the biopsy rate for cancer. That rate will be greatly influenced by the individual primary care physician and his surgeon, reflecting their clinical findings and practices. The nonpalpable 0.5 cm infiltrative mass may be readily palpable when the surgeon is directed to the specific site in the breast. However, the borderline calcification not associated with a mass, asymmetric density, or area of architectural distortion will require close cooperation between radiologist and surgeon, since localization and biopsy radiography must be the routine approach. Biopsy of lesions can be based only on radiographic findings. In our practice, with meticulous radiography one of three of the borderline calcifications has proved to be cancer; however, several workers using xeroradiography of the breast report a biopsy rate of 1 in 10 to 1 in 12 as cancer. Our less specific changes, particularly altered architecture, have had an even higher biopsy ratio of cancer to benign lesions.

As a general rule, the surgeon is not overly concerned with mammographic false positive lesions. His concern, and the bane of the mammographer, is the false negative mammogram—the undiagnosed cancer. The important concern is not the cancer/benign ratio rate but the establishment of good rapport with the surgeons and the pathologists. This is the easiest of all, as each strives vigorously to treat curable cancer.

Effect on Mortality Rates

It is safe to assume that not all intraductal carcinomas are particularly lethal, but the evidence is overwhelming that most, if not treated, will be lethal. On the other hand, all intraductal carcinomas demonstrated by light microscopy will not be cured by mastectomy. Some may have metastasized, or unsuspected lesions in the opposite breast may produce metastasis. Probably one fourth of histologic Stage I carcinomas are actually Stage II or III at the time of treatment.

Generally, a better prognosis with breast cancer is related to fewer axillary lymph node metastases and to a smaller sized tumor. At Emory University a greatly improved survival with breast cancer was associated with absence of axillary lymph node metastasis: 70 per cent ten-year salvage without metastasis and 29 per cent ten-year salvage with metastasis. "Mammographic cancers," nonpalpable and often small in size, have ten-year and even 20-year survival of 95 to 98 per cent.

These data should be sufficient encouragement for a breast-imaging center to screen vigorously for breast cancer, currently our only hope to combat this macabre disease.

Physical Examination

Breast-screening centers attract a high percentage of younger women, since these women are more apt to practice preventive medicine. Physicial examination is more difficult in the firmer, more glandular breasts of young women than in the fatty, atrophic breast of older women. A high number of cancers found during mammographic screening are not suspected by clinical examination (over one half in the BCDDP).

Yet physical examination must be a part of a screening program. Seven per cent of the cancers in the BCDDP were picked up on physical examination. In the screening of referred women, the physical examination can be the responsibility of the referring physician. Some radiologists prefer to examine all their patients, which produces no problems. The problem of physical examination arises when the woman has not been referred or when there is no assurance that she has had a physical examination. Nurses, technologists, and paramedical personnel can be trained to do a creditable job. In some states this is not permitted, however, and provision must be made for a physician to do the physical examination. Unless there is a nearby examiner, a full-time physician may be required, often at prohibitive cost.

Liabilities

Radiologists may be called upon for a legal opinion as to whether a certain diagnostic procedure should have been done or if a proper radiologic examination had been conducted and interpreted. Most of the original depositions I have been involved with concerned these questions: Should a mammogram have been performed? If so, would it have aided in reaching the proper diagnosis at an earlier stage, and if so, would it have changed the patient's prognosis? Most of these cases included younger women who had been observed or treated symptomatically while their cancer spread overtly to an incurable stage. Fortified by unsurpassed experience in mammography, intelligent discussions of the cases led to acceptable out-of-court decisions and settlements. Straightforward, unambiguous, timely comments backed by well-established data were helpful to both plaintiffs and defendants. This form of judicial activity does not relate directly to screening for breast cancer.

However, every mammographic examination and its interpretation, with subsequent recommendations or lack of recommendations, involves every breast screening center. The responsible radiologist first must have full knowledge of the state-of-the-art mammography. This includes the shortcomings and relative benefits of his approach and technique and how it compares generally with acceptable radiographic quality of x-ray examinations of the breast. For example, he must be aware of the increased radiation from xeroradiography and its inherent problems in imaging, of the necessity for severe compression during screen-film mammography, and of the sacrifice of radiographic detail to reduce radiation to the breast by faster film emulsions. He must be knowledgeable about the use of supplemental mammographic views and aware of its necessity. In essence, he must be prepared to substantiate what he did and why in exploiting the x-ray procedure for reaching a diagnosis.

Once the well-conducted and exhaustive x-ray examination has been obtained, the radiologist is responsible for assembling maximal information from the procedure, followed by meticulously categorizing that information for its best utilization in care of the patient. This requires a thorough knowledge of the radiographic appearance of the normal breast, normal variants, and changes associated with disease processes both benign and malignant. Information may be gleaned for the immediate care of the patient or for suggesting future care, e.g., increased risk of breast cancer.

All pertinent data, their interpretation, and resultant recommendations must be concisely transferred in a written report to the primary care physician. The screening procedure for breast cancer is still a medical consultation and must be treated as such. It is of utmost importance that the consultation report be clear in specifying the findings; be unambiguous in the probability of the diagnosis whether normal, benign, or malignant; and be straightforward, based on facts and past experience, in recommending the proper clinical application.

In many screening centers, procedures such as various types of thermography or sonography may be available. There are strong arguments favoring the availability of all diagnostic approaches, including needle aspiration and biopsy, in breast-screening centers. However, it is strongly urged that because these are supplementary procedures to mammography, they should not be routinely done to augment fees. Only after well-conducted mammography has been exhausted, and under proven specific indications, are other studies added singly or possibly in tandem, e.g., sonography to determine if all masses against a background of fibrocystic disease are cystic.

The radiologist must be aware that there are practitioners with as much as 30 years' experience in mammography. This does not imply that all of them have conducted controlled mammographic practices, gathered data on their patients prospectively, and had the opportunity for thorough analysis of these data that qualifies them as experts. It does suggest, however, that the less experienced mammographer who is responsible for his screening program become thoroughly familiar with mammographic medical literature. He then can supplement his own experience with well-validated data from others' experience and be in a position at all times to defend his practice. Throughout this volume, problems with poor images, nonspecific changes or poorly delineated pathology, and simply nondiagnostic changes have been illustrated. Some radiologists confidently claim easy differentiation of borderline calcifications not associated with a mass into benign or malignant character. Odds are good that this is possible in some cases, but overall odds are great that such a practice is inviting certain litigation. Defense of a Stage II lesion that develops under observation of these flecks of calcification, as opposed to a nearly 100 per cent cure for a Stage 0 lesion, is difficult on the witness stand. Placing confidence in the risk factors claimed for parenchymal patterns causing wholesale amputations of young women's normal breasts is highly risky when Carlile et al. (1985) concluded after an extensive four-year study, "We strongly believe that mammographic patterns should not be used in decisions for prophylactic mastectomy, clinical management or screening intervals." These examples stress the need for awareness of controversial claims so that they can be cleanly avoided.

RADIATION RISK

Bailar (1976), reflecting on the radiation risk of mammography, voiced the possibility that routine mammography caused more cancer deaths than it prevented. This led to a National Cancer Institute report by Breslow et al. (1977) on radiation risk to the breast.

These investigators reported an excess number of breast cancers found in three populations previously exposed to radiation: (1) Japanese women ten years and older who had survived atomic bomb blasts in Hiroshima and Nagasaki; (2) women who had had extensive fluoroscopy examinations to monitor pneumothorax treatments for tuberculosis; and (3) women who had been treated by radiation therapy for postpartum mastitis. In all instances the women received either whole-body or half-torso large doses of very high-energy radiation, approaching the level of radiation therapy. During fluoroscopies some of the women received as much as 4000 rads to the breast, with many of them developing erythematous skin reactions. Radiation was estimated retrospectively in all but the mastitis cases.

A linear dose-response hypothesis was used to determine that the risk of mammography was approximately 3.5 to 7.5 new cases of breast cancer per 1 million women aged 35 or older at risk per year per rad to both breasts, from the tenth year after exposure throughout the remainder of life. A single mammographic examination with an average dose of less than 1 rad should increase the risk of developing breast cancer by much less than 1 per cent of the natural risk (from 7.0 to 7.07 per cent) at age 35, and by progressively smaller percentages with increasing age.

These data, the basis of the foregoing claims, have been severely criticized. Also,

conclusions using these data to determine the risk of mammography would be questioned for two reasons: (1) Linear hypothesis for radiation effects presumed that the effects at very high levels of radiation exposure could be extrapolated downward to 0; and (2) all possible benefits of mammography were based on a breast cancer screening program by Health Insurance Plan (HIP) of New York City.

The linear extrapolation hypothesis was used despite the warning issued in Bulletin 43, released in 1975 by the National Council of Radiation Protection and Measurements. This followed the NAS-BEIR Report of 1972, which warned against using linear extrapolation from high- to low-dose radiation because "there is such a high possibility of overestimating the actual risk as to be of only marginal value, if any, for purposes of realistic risk-benefit evaluation."

Of just as much importance, the clinical study used was an outdated one—the HIP study begun in the early 1960s. We had planned simply to determine if screening by physical examination and mammography for breast cancer would reduce the mortality from that disease. Not one attempt was even suggested as an evaluation of mammography (see HIP Study).

Numerous reports followed, all hypothetical, with most downplaying the role of the very low dose of radiation during mammography with lessened effects after age 30 years. Jayaraman et al. (1986) considered age at the start of screening, frequency of screening, dose per examination, and cumulative lifetime dose. They concluded that with an assumed radiation dose of 0.5 rad per examination, a phased program of biennial screening beginning at age 30, annual screening beginning at age 40, and semiannual screening after age 55 appears to be appropriate.

Based on less exacting science, the American Cancer Society considered the risk of a mammogram to a woman equivalent to smoking one fourth of a cigarette or to a 60-year-old woman just breathing for 20 minutes. Based on our physicists' meticulous measurements during mammography in our breast center, we reached the following conclusion: To double the risk of breast cancer by mammography, at 20 minutes per examination, the woman would have to be x-rayed for 50 days and nights. (Noah's flood lasted only 40 days and nights.)

SCREENING PROGRAMS FOR BREAST CANCER

HIP Study

Background

Efforts to use mammography in screening for breast cancer appeared after our first publication on the application of clinical mammography (Egan, 1960) and grew more vigorously after the report of 53 clinically unsuspected cancers (Egan, 1962). One such proposal was to screen female personnel and dependents of the United States Public Health Service (USPHS) on the East Coast and compare these women's cancers with a similar group of women in the United States Army or Navy. Another proposal was for screening of women in Norway. The Director of NCI presided at a meeting to discuss this latter proposal, already prepared in final form for distribution by membrs of the Epidemiology Section of NCI.

My premonition was that the time was not quite ripe for such an undertaking because better training of radiologists and better education of the involved physicians was needed. Too rapid an exposure might be good for the designers of the proposal, but an ill-advised exercise could send mammography back into oblivion without the semblance of a clinical trial. My cohorts, interested in preventing mammography from being scuttled, battled for the whole day for the Reproducibility Study, which was already into its early phases. Fortunately, the chairman was persuaded to await the outcome of the Reproducibility Study before funding any screening programs. Yet even at this early date the full impact of the proponents of screening American women for breast cancer was felt from the heat of the seething cauldron.

The inevitable happened. A New York–Washington, D.C. coalition pressed for the HIP of New York City Screening Study in preparation for envisioned good results of the Reproducibility Study. Even as chance instigator of the HIP study, I did not encourage it but felt obliged to help plan, monitor quality, and review progress even though I pressed for a companion study to avoid possible irretrievable damage to mammography. The project radiologist's philosophy differed sharply from mine (the highest quality mammography for the smallest cancer), his being "Get as many women in as possible and process them; the finding of one cancer will be better than none."

The quality of the mammograms was poor with very limited hope for improvement, as only 23 of the total of 35 medical groups had agreed to participate. Furthermore, skin dose averaged 8 R per exposure and was as high as 12 R, as measured by a competent physicist, Dr. Carl Braestrop. This compared with 2 R to the skin as measured by Drs. Warren Sinclair, Robert Shalek, and Dale Trout with our technique. Since the only mission of the project was to see if early diagnosis meant increased salvage, I agreed to continue on the project, shaky as it was. To halt this study already funded and set in motion amid difficulties would threaten total cessation of screening mammography. The quality of the 15 per cent of the mammograms (10 per cent routine and 5 per cent questionable pathology) reviewed by me was barely tolerable.

Protocol

The Health Insurance Plan of Greater New York City had a series of 35 participating medical groups that supplied their members with prepaid physician health care. Each group was geographically separated, and each carried out its own medical practice.

Central headquarters housed the biostatistical group, the project surgeon, and the project radiologist. I traveled to New York City on numerous occasions to give lectures and demonstrations on mammography and its interpretation. My chief technologist traveled by subway to each of the participating centers several times to institute acceptable mammography. The local radiologists selected and used their equipment as they desired.

A total of 64,000 women were assigned to the project, with 32,000 being randomly selected to have four annual screenings by physical examination and mammography. The other 32,000 continued their routine medical care.

Results

At five years there was a 30 per cent decrease in mortality due to breast cancer in the screened group compared with the controls. Only after 18 years was there an undisputed substantial similar decrease in mortality in those women under age 50 years. This latter was corroborated by Tabár (1987).

Comments

The HIP Study has been a milestone in mammography and has made a tremendous contribution to the study of breast cancer: a truly clinical trial demonstrating that mass screening for breast cancer with physical examination and mammography can markedly reduce the mortality from breast cancer. That was the only purpose for which it was designed. It was not designed to, and cannot be used to, evaluate mammography; skin doses of 8 to 12 rads per exposure does not indicate state-of-the-art mammography.

BCDDP

Background

By 1971 mammography had become established in many institutions throughout the United States as an indispensable complement to detection and diagnosis of breast diseases. The local chapters of the American Cancer Society had been active in support of screening for breast cancer at the Guttmann Clinic, under the direction of Strax, following the optimistic early outcome of the HIP study (Strax et al. 1967). American Cancer Society Breast Cancer Detection Projects were planned for four cities; they were to be of two years' duration to demonstrate to the public and to medical communities the feasibility of breast screening with physical examination and mammography. The communities then could carry on the projects if desired. The goals and protocol were clearly identified and designed. Emory University was site-visited on July 31, 1972 and was the first center approved to begin operation on November 1, 1972 to screen 5000 women for each of two years.

However, much confusion resulted from the termination of this project and its replacement by one cosponsored by the National Cancer Institute. Again, Emory University (with Georgia Baptist Hospital in Atlanta) was the first institution to be approved. The aims and methods of the study became highly complicated for a rocky start "sometime" in 1973.

On July 1, 1973 the Atlantic American Cancer Society/National Cancer Institute Breast Cancer Detection Demonstration Project (BCDDP) began its breast cancer screening program with the author as principal investigator. The overall program has been amply summarized by Baker (1982). Each of 27 communities was to screen 10,000 volunteer, asymptomatic women over age 35 years for five annual physical examinations and mammograms. At Emory University 2043 women, and at Georgia Baptist Medical Center (GBMC) 8058 women, were enrolled. Each woman was to supply the name of her own physician, to whom the screening report could be mailed or with whom the results could be discussed. Treatment was planned and carried out by various surgeons using numerous approaches with varying expertise. All women for whom breast biopsies were recommended and two matching cohorts were then followed for an additional five years. A ten-year follow-up is presented.

The quota of 10,000 patients was filled for only the first screening of all subjects. There was a slow but steady decrease in number for the first three screenings, averaging 9392 per screening. Then the 1975–1976 radiation scare took greater tolls, as certain screenees were restricted by the NCI. All women have been followed. Equal numbers of cancers were detected during the first and second screenings, dropping sharply after that. Almost all the interval cancers (11 of 16) occurred during the first year of screening. These facts reflect the "on-the-job training" during the first year to establish proper x-ray examination.

Georgia Baptist Medical Center Results

The Georgia Baptist Medical Center is located in metropolitan Atlanta. Although great efforts were made to remove symptomatic patients from the study, it is postulated that signs or symptoms of breast disease are found more frequently in the clientele of an urban medical center than of one on a university campus. It is possible, especially initially, that the personnel were less experienced, as they were trained by the Emory University staff prior to the institution of the screening program. Oncologic surgeons as well as experienced pathologists were present in both arms of the project.

There was a definite tendency for breast carcinoma (all cancers in both projects were carcinomas) to be more lethal in women under age 50 years (Tables 37–1 to 37–5). But even in the worst situation (under age 50 years and the carcinoma greater than 1 cm in diameter), the results of screening are excellent—83.3 per cent ten-year salvage rate (Table 37–2). These same women contributed to the poor prognosis indicated by the clini-

TABLE 37–1. Georgia Baptist Medical Center: Ten-Year Survival Under and Over Age 50 Years

Age (yrs.)	Number	Dead	Alive	Percentage
<50	44	7	37	84
≥50	76	4	72	94.7
Total	120	11	109	90.8

TABLE 37–3. Georgia Baptist Medical Center: Ten-Year Survival With Cancer 1 cm or Less in Diameter

Age (yrs.)	Number	Dead	Alive	Percentage
<50	27	3	24	88.9
≥50	55	2	53	96.4
Total	82	5	77	93.9

cally palpable lesion (Table 37–4). Screening mammography in the younger woman still accounts for better prognosis than when breast carcinomas are palpable (Tables 37–4 and 37–5).

In the total BCDDP results (Baker, 1982) 41.6 per cent of the carcinomas detected by mammography compared with 52 per cent at Georgia Baptist, and 56 per cent were palpable compared with 408 per cent at Georgia Baptist. This indicates earlier detection of carcinoma at Georgia Baptist.

Emory University Results

The 2043 women screened at Emory University were presumably asymptomatic. Yet, it was later discovered that one woman who had a palpable cancer was aware of the presence of that lump. Another woman, under age 50 years, who was being denied screening as she did not fit the criteria revised by NCI, returned for mammography for a growing breast mass that was obviously clinically carcinoma. Three other cancer patients during routine screening physical examinations had some abnormality of the breast that could not be determined to be related to a malignancy. In the first half of the study, clinical abnormalities were not localized to one breast or the other owing to inadequacy of the recording forms. During the first year there were three interval carcinomas, and only half the total carcinomas were detected, presumably owing to use of xeroradiography and inexperience of the radiologist. After that, closer scrutiny of the xerographs by the technologists and coned-down views on non-screen film resolved most problems. Any

area of asymmetry, trabecular distortion, or grouping of calcifications required improved study over that possible by xeroradiography. The calcifications were usually coarse ones, so conned views were used to see if they were associated with fine diagnostic ones; on this was based the decision to biopsy or not to biopsy. Only one interval carcinoma occurred with this practice, and only eight carcinomas were detected during the last three screens.

Our studies were not the only ones lacking in radiographic quality. Near the end of the first year of the project, when I was a member of a committee to judge radiographic quality at all the centers, it was found that all studies were totally unacceptable. This included both film and xeroradiography. As the quality suffered, so did the radiation to the breast become excessive. By then our physics centers were coming into activity and helped to remedy these problems. Oddly, the real reason for this review was the concern over the quality of thermography, blamed for the lack of specificity in flagging carcinomatous breasts. However, the quality of the thermography turned out to be excellent, to the amazement of the most severe critics.

Nine carcinomas were noninvasive, two microscopically focally invasive, and 14 invasive. Only two lesions were greater than 1 cm in diameter; both were approximately 1.5 cm in size and were the two that were definitely palpable. Each of these had one low axillary lymph node with metastasis, and a third invasive carcinoma also had one low positive axillary lymph node. There was a total of 110 breast biopsies, a ratio of 4.4 benign to 1 malignant lesion.

TABLE 37–2. Georgia Baptist Medical Center: Ten-Year Survival With Cancer Greater Than 1 cm in Diameter

Age (yrs.)	Number	Dead	Alive	Percentage
<50	17	3	14	82.4
≥50	21	3	18	85.7
Total	38	6	32	84.2

TABLE 37–4. Georgia Baptist Medical Center: Ten-Year Survival With Clinically Palpable Cancer

Age (yrs.)	Number	Dead	Alive	Percentage
<50	18	3	15	83.3
≥50	31	4	27	87.1
Total	49	7	42	85.7

TABLE 37–5. Georgia Baptist Medical Center: Ten-Year Survival With X-ray Detected Cancer

Age (yrs.)	Number	Dead	Alive	Percentage
<50	17	2	15	88.2
≥50	45	0	45	100.0
Total	62	2	60	96.8

TABLE 37–7. Emory University: Ten-Year Survival With Cancer Greater Than 1 cm in Diameter

Age (yrs.)	Number	Dead	Alive	Percentage
<50	1	0	1	100.0
≥50	1	0	1	100.0
Total	2	0	2	100.0

Treatment consisted of six radical mastectomies, 13 modified radical mastectomies, and six total mastectomies. In the early 1970s, radical mastectomy was still being used in the Atlanta area for small breast lesions, although it had been mainly discontinued at Emory University.

None of the Emory University cancer patients died from breast cancer during the years of active screening or during the five-year follow-up period. Six of the cancer patients did die, but no death was related to breast cancer, and in no instance was there evidence of persistent or metastatic disease. All were subject to ten-year follow-up. With no cancer-related deaths, the Emory University data would be better than those of the Georgia Baptist Medical Center (Tables 37–6 to 37–10).

Within the five-year period, nine former subjects developed breast cancer. The extent of disease was remarkably different from that detected during the screening years and usually was directly proportional to the elapsed time since the last mammogram. For example, one physician kept up her yearly screening mammogram, with detection of an intraductal comedocarconoma four years after completion of the regular screening program. In contrast, another woman presented with a breast mass four years after her last mammogram (the fifth in the screening program) that proved to be a scirrhous duct carcinoma. It was 4.5 cm in size, and 10 of 16 axillary lymp nodes at all levels had metastasis (Table 37–11).

Combined Results

The combined total of 145 cancers in the Atlanta BCDDP (Tables 37–12 to 37–16) is a rate of 14.5 per 1000 cancers in this volunteer population as opposed to a prevalence rate of 1 or 2 per 1000 women in the general population, depending on the age group. Since 37 per cent of the cancers occurred in women under age 50 years, the rate becomes even more impressive.

One of the most important data is that one third of the cancers were found in women under age 50 years, yet one third of the total cancers less than 1 cm in diameter were in this age group. This strongly attests to the value of mammographic screening in younger women, the very ones the NCI barred from the program after the radiation scare. Too, a curable breast cancer detected at age 40 years offers the potential for many more productive years of life than a similar one detected in an 88-year-old woman.

It is true that at present we do less well with mammography in younger women than in older women, but the difference is not that great. With more care in performing examinations in younger women, by raising the level of concern over breast cancer, and through communicating our desire to help these forgotten women, screening will provide rich rewards. In 1956, when I introduced clinical mammography, my wildest hopes did not encompass 95 per cent ten-year cure rates for breast cancer (Table 37–14).

Overall, despite sudden changes in the program, many obstacles, and harsh publicity the BCDDP continued and succeeded. Besides finding early breast cancer and saving lives, this project has demonstrated to physicians and to the public the value of breast cancer screening, has increased public awareness of the disease, has shown that a large-scale screening program is feasible, and

TABLE 37–6. Emory University: Ten-Year Survival Under and Over Age 50 Years

Age (yrs.)	Number	Dead	Alive	Percentage
<50	9	0	9	100.0
≥50	16	0	16	100.0
Total	25	0	25	100.0

TABLE 37–8. Emory University: Ten-Year Survival With Cancer 1 cm or Less in Diameter

Age (yrs.)	Number	Dead	Alive	Percentage
<50	8	0	8	100.0
≥50	15	0	15	100.0
Total	23	0	23	100.0

TABLE 37–9. Emory University: Ten-Year Survival With Clinically Palpable Cancer

Age (yrs.)	Number	Dead	Alive	Pecentage
<50	2	0	2	100.0
≥50	3	0	3	100.0
Total	5	0	5	100.0

TABLE 37–10. Emory University: Ten-Year Survival With X-Ray Detected Cancer

Age (yrs.)	Number	Dead	Alive	Percentage
<50	7	0	7	100.0
≥50	13	0	13	100.0
Total	20	0	20	100.0

has gone far to educate the physician and the public about early breast cancer and the necessity for early diagnosis and proper follow-up.

The many dedicated and tenacious people who made this endeavor such a great success will long be remembered.

European Experience

A number of European centers have evaluated mass screening for breast cancer with mammography.

Nijmegen, the Netherlands

Following a grant to the University of Utrecht, a screening program using xeroradiography of the breast in women aged 50 to 64 years was started in 1974. Mass screening of a larger target population of women over age 35 years was officially started in January 1975. A total of 30,000 women were invited to a biennial examination and analyzed by a case-control design. The study included 62 breast cancer deaths matched with 310 controls. The breast cancer mortality in the screened group was 0.53 times as low as in the unscreened group (Verbeek, 1984).

Sweden

Breast cancer screening by single-view mammography was started in Gavleborg County, Sweden, in 1974; 74,000 women aged 40 years or older in a total population of 300,000 were invited to participate. Screening intervals varied from two to five years. There was no significant difference in observed and expected incidence of cancer, but there was a substantial reduction in the expected late-stage cancer cases with screening, and a reduction of 35 per cent mortality with screening (Lundgren, 1984).

Beginning in 1977, in Kopparberg and Ostergotland Countries, Sweden, 161,000 women over age 39 years were randomized into 94,000 subjects in a study population and 67,000 in a control group for mass screening for breast cancer, using a single oblique mammographic view. Attendance was 92.5 per cent. The prevalence of breast cancer in the study group was 7 per 1000 compared with 2.2 per 1000 in control group. Stage 0 or Stage I lesions made up 34 per cent of the control group cases, while these stages made up 55.8 per cent of the total study population (Tabar et al., 1985).

Also in 1977 in Malmö, Sweden, a breast cancer screening program was begun with 21,000 study and 21,000 control subjects aged 45 to 65 years. Oblique and craniocaudad views were used. In the control group 52 per cent of the women had Stages II to IV lesions, whereas only 20 per cent of the screened subjects were in corresponding stages (Andersen, 1984).

TABLE 37–11. Emory University: Features of Nine Carcinomas Diagnosed Following BCDDP

Histologic Type	Patient Age (yrs.)	Tumor Size	Palpable	X-Ray Detected	Axillary Nodes	Treatment	Survival (yrs.)	Disease Present
ID, duct	70	2.1 cm	−	+	−	Mod. rad.	2	−
Duct	49	0	−	+	−	" "	3	−
Duct	74	6 mm	+	+	−	" "	1	−
Duct, scirrhous	56	7 × 9 mm	+	+	−	" "	6	−
Duct	50	3.5 cm	−	+	−	" "	1	−
Duct	49	1.8 cm	+	+	−	" "	3	−
Duct	43	1.5 cm	+	+	1/17	" "	5	−
ID, comedo	60	0	−	+	−	" "	5	−
Duct, scirrhous, tubular	49	4.5	+	+	10/16	" "	1	−

TABLE 37–12. Combined Results, Emory University and Georgia Baptist Medical Center: Ten-Year Survival Under and Over Age 50 Years

Age (yrs.)	Number	Dead	Alive	Percentage
<50	53	7	46	86.8
≥50	92	4	88	95.7
Total	145	11	134	92.4

TABLE 37–14. Combined Results, Emory University and Georgia Baptist Medical Center: Ten-Year Survival With Cancer 1 cm or Less in Diameter

Age (yrs.)	Number	Dead	Alive	Percentage
<50	35	3	32	91.4
≥50	70	2	68	97.1
Total	105	5	100	95.2

Canadian Experience

A total of 23,101 women underwent mammography in a randomized screening trial at five centers in Canada. Of the 206 cancers that were confirmed, 174 were detected at first screening, with an average follow-up of 3.2 years for all women. Overall, the five screening centers achieved a sensitivity of 69 per cent, a specificity of 94 per cent, and a negative predictive value of 99.75 per cent.

BREAST-IMAGING CENTERS

The concept of a center strictly limited to the detection and diagnosis of breast diseases is not new. The author was the first to embark on such a program in 1964 at Emory University. The specific objectives were to teach, evaluate, and accumulate data on mammography and related procedures. This unit was completely separated physically and administratively from all other radiographic activities but still remained within the Department of Radiology. Approximately one quarter of the effort was related to patient care, one quarter to teaching, one quarter to data accession, and the remainder to research into all aspects of diagnostic imaging of the breast. Financial support was through grants and fees for service.

When I served as consulting advisor in the early 1970s, a private breast clinic was established in a large medical office building to offer all available breast diagnostic modali-

ties. These include instruction in breast self-examination, physical examination, thermography, mammography, and xeroradiography. This clinic flourished and was in great demand until the radiation scare in 1976, when it closed.

Private breast clinics, both associated with institutions and privately endowed, have been opened in various parts of the United States and other countries. Ideally, all imaging modalities should be available at each center, complementing mammography and physical examination when optimally combined. These include thermography, ultrasound, transillumination, and a screen-film mammography unit equipped for compression of the breast, grid, and magnification. Some radiologists may prefer xeroradiography. All equipment should be evaluated periodically for safety, accuracy, and effectiveness. Radiation should be at the lowest possible level, no more than 1 rad midbreast for a two-view study.

Each center must provide expertise in technology and a radiologist with demonstrated experience and competence in mammography. Provision must be made for physical examination of the breast and teaching of BSE. Ongoing correlation of center recommendations with histopathology must provide estimates of competence.

Each breast-imaging center should make a constant effort to keep cost realistic in order to assure continued patient volume. Charges should reflect the service and the least number of procedures necessary for a proper

TABLE 37–13. Combined Results, Emory University and Georgia Baptist Medical Center: Ten-Year Survival With Cancer Greater Than 1 cm in Diameter

Age (yrs.)	Number	Dead	Alive	Percentage
<50	18	3	15	83.3
≥50	22	3	19	86.4
Total	40	6	34	85.0

TABLE 37–15. Combined Results, Emory University and Georgia Baptist Medical Center: Ten-Year Survival With Clinically Palpable Cancer

Age (yrs.)	Number	Dead	Alive	Percentage
<50	23	3	17	85.0
≥50	34	4	30	88.2
Total	57	7	47	87.0

TABLE 37–16. Combined Results, Emory University and Georgia Baptist Medical Center: Ten-Year Survival With X-Ray Detected Cancer

Age (yrs.)	Number	Dead	Alive	Percentage
<50	24	2	22	91.7
≥50	58	0	58	100.0
Total	82	2	80	97.6

evaluation. Where possible, outside funding should be sought from the community to decrease patient fees even more.

The radiologist can only be a member of the team that diagnoses and treats the patient. The woman must be referred to or provided with a primary care physician. Most breast-imaging centers will be active in screening, and this provisions for walk-in patients are mandatory.

Close rapport and cooperation should be established with third-party carriers to defray costs of examinations, where possible. A prompt and detailed written report of findings should be provided by the radiologist for purposes of both patient care and insurance claims.

The American Cancer Society has provided wide exposure to screening with mammography in the detection of early breast cancer through its scientific validation of the value of screening mammography in the BCDDP. This has been accepted by the medical profession to the extent that many communities will now subsidize breast-imaging centers. This interest of the American Cancer Society will continue and will be an asset to any fledgling breast-imaging center.

The course via breast-imaging centers has now been charted. Challenges to save countless lives remain: optimal imaging, accurate interpretation, competent personnel, adequate facilities, wide availability, and reasonable cost.

OBSERVATIONS

From its inception in May 1956, this author has considered mammography a breast screening procedure: Aid in assessing the questionable breast nodule is of less importance than screening the other three quadrants of the clinically abnormal breast as well as the opposite breast for serious disease. If the mass in question is malignant and is to be biopsied, the pathologist then can aid the surgeon. Breast cancer is most often detected as a result of investigation of cysts, as they provide the opportunity to study the breast by x-ray. Pain is perhaps the second most common complaint leading to mammographic discovery of breast cancer. Complaints of pain or lumps are bona fide reasons for referral for mammography. Only 0.1 per cent of our "symptomatic" patients mentioned cancerophobia in the hope of getting an x-ray examination of the breast. Yet in the BCDDP, 10 per cent of the women used that as an impossible-to-quantify symptom in order to be admitted to the program—a 100-fold increase. For various such reasons, meaningful separation of women into subsets of symptomatic categories is not possible or warranted.

Throw-away medical literature stresses such differences. There are even suggestions that the "screening" mammography should be done at half price and use half the film and effort of "diagnostic" mammography. Lack of experience fosters that concept, so dramatically demonstrated in the first year of the BCDDP, when half the prevalent cancers went undetected. The savings effected by substitution of inferior receptors for convenience, cutting back 1 mrad in radiation and halving the price of mammography represents a Phyrrhic victory and results in loss in the woman's life. Unfortunately, each cancer missed by mammography promotes pressure against screening by this method.

For over 30 years we have searched for a replacement for mammography, and particularly for a premammography risk marker, to reduce the cost of the procedure and the required number of examinations. Until the widespread adoption of optical spectroscopy of the breast as that risk marker, it remains necessary to produce good-quality mammograms on all women regardless of the cost. Currently the cost of a missed cancer to the woman, her family, and the community exceeds $75,000. Mammographic screening is economically sound even though $15,000 to $25,000 may be required to detect a curable cancer, depending upon the particular age group. There is no question that to the more than 50 million women in the United States who are eligible, screening mammography is a bargain.

This seemed particularly a bargain to the women in the Emory University BCDDP who continued their screening, to have their carcinomas detected at a reasonably curable stage. Unfortunately, the two women who started the program before age 50 and took the advice of NCI guidelines and dropped out developed a carcinoma that was advanced at the time of detection.

PHYSICIANS

Over 95 per cent of the women in the United States have come to trust their obstetricians and gynecologists, first for delivery of their babies, then for correction of their gynecologic problems, and then, in time trusting all their ailments to them. The gynecologists, particularly those seeing more cancer-age women, should be a first line in directing women to have their breasts screened and evaluated. But they, as a group, are just not overly interested in women's breast problems. Already harassed with litigation arising from obstetric and gynecologic problems, they are now being lined up for lawsuits related to breast disorders. Sharing that responsibility with a colleague by breast screening is the ideal and logical safeguard for them and a boon to their women patients. Breast societies formed by gynecologists have not flourished. More pressures for such societies are needed.

The success of breast screening centers ultimately rests on cooperation and utilization by women in the breast cancer age group. Without them, failure is inevitable. For mammography to be productive, women must use it. It is necessary that we direct their thinking. For example, the physician may use the following approach: Concentrate on rewards for the detection of early breast cancer. Emphasize the psychosexual rewards of avoiding mutilation and preserving femininity. Downplay adverse images. Capitalize on women's inherent fear of breast cancer to increase receptivity to screening procedures if this fear can be gently maneuvered as an impetus to seek help. Prior to the diagnosis of breast cancer this fear is centered on loss of a breast, whereas after a cancer diagnosis is established there is a shift toward fear of loss of life. National and international women leaders who have experienced breast cancer could publicly motivate women not to wait as long as they did for detection procedures, or to take advantage of detection procedures as they did with their early curable cancers. Start screening early in life, at least by age 30 or preferably younger, to establish a series of normal examinations. Expectation of future normal examinations will alleviate fears.

These women must be convinced that mammography is their study and that they alone can create the milieu for every woman to have screening mammography.

REFERENCES

Andersen I (1984): Breast cancer screening in Malmö. *In* Brunner S, Langfeldt B, Andersen PE (eds): Early Detection of Breast Cancer. Berlin, Springer-Verlag, p 114.

Bailar J (1976): Mammography, a contrary view. Ann Intern Med *84*:77.

Baines CJ, Miller AB, Wall C, McFarlane DV, Simor IS, et al (1986): Sensitivity and specificity of first screen mammography in the Canadian National Breast Screening Study: A preliminary report from five centers. Radiology *160*(2):295.

Baker LH (1982): Breast Cancer Detection Demonstration Project. Five-year summary report. CA *32*:194.

Breslow I, Thomas LB, Upton AC (1977): Final report: the NCI Ad-Hoc Working Group on the risk associated with mammography in mass screening for detection of breast cancer. J Nat Cancer Inst *59*:467.

Carlile T, Kopecky KJ, Thompson DJ, et al (1985): Breast cancer prediction and the Wolfe classification of mammograms. JAMA *254*:1050.

Clark RL, Copeland MM, Egan RL, et al (1965): Reproducibility of the technique of mammography (Egan) for cancer of the breast. Am J Surg *100*:127.

Egan RL (1962): Fifty-three cases of carcinoma of the breast, occult until mammography. AJR *58*:1095.

Jayaraman S, Lanzl LH, Agarwal SK, Chung-Bin A (1986): Analysis of radiation risk versus benefit in mammography. Appl Radiol Mar/Apr:45.

Letton AH, Mason EM(1986): Routine breast screening. Survival after 10.5 years' follow-up. Ann Surg *203*(5) 470.

Lundgren B (1984): Breast cancer screening: Expected and observed incidence and stage of female breast cancer in Gavelborg County, Sweden, and implications for mortality. *In* Brunner S, Langfeldt B, Andersen PE (eds): Berlin, Springer-Verlag, p 101.

Strax P, Venet L, Shapiro S, Gross S (1967): Mammography and clinical examination in mass screening for cancer of the breast. Cancer *20*:2184.

Tabár L (September 1987): Personal Communication.

Tabár L, Gad A, Holmberg LH, et al (1985): Reduction in mortality from breast cancer after mass screening with mammography. Randomized trial from the Breast Cancer Screening Working Groups of the Swedish National Board of Health and Welfare. Lancet *1*:829.

Verbeek AL, Hendriks JH, Holland R, Mravunac M, Sturmans F, Day NE (1984): Reduction of breast cancer mortality through mass screening with modern mammography. Lancet 1: 1222.

Index

A page number in italics indicates a figure; the letter t following a page number indicates a table.

671

674   INDEX